The
Language
of
Medicine

Davi-Ellen Chabner, B.A., M.A.T.

The Language of Medicine

A Write-In Text
Explaining
Medical Terms

FIFTH

EDITION

W.B. SAUNDERS COMPANY
A Division of Harcourt Brace & Company

Philadelphia   London   Toronto   Montreal   Sydney   Tokyo

W.B. SAUNDERS COMPANY
A Division of Harcourt Brace & Company

The Curtis Center
Independence Square West
Philadelphia, Pennsylvania 19106

Library of Congress Cataloging-in-Publication Data

Chabner, Davi-Ellen.
   The language of medicine : a write-in text explaining medical
terms / Davi-Ellen Chabner. — 5th ed.

       p.   cm.

   Includes index.

   ISBN 0–7216–6026–6

   1. Medicine—Terminology.   I. Title.
   [DNLM: 1. Nomenclature.   2. Nomenclature—examination questions. W 15 C427L 1996]
   R123.C43 1996
   610′.14—dc20

   DNLM/DLC   95–5451

The Language of Medicine: A Write-In Text Explaining Medical Terms, Fifth Edition   ISBN 0–7216–6026–6

Printed in the United States of America

Last digit is the print number: 9   8   7   6   5   4   3

To Catherine F. Scott
mentor, colleague, and friend
who envisioned this book before I did
and
In memory of my father,
Bernard H. Rosenzweig, 1914–1994,
whose confidence and belief in me
continues to nurture and support my spirit

Preface to the Fifth Edition

The Language of Medicine is now 20 years old! Having successfully made its way through infancy, latency, and teen-age years into young adulthood, here is an interesting, practical, logical, and effective system for learning medical terminology. In the spring of 1975, Elizabeth J. Taylor, editor at W.B. Saunders Company, and I met for lunch in Washington, D.C. We organized and planned the publication of a medical terminology text based on materials developed for my students at Montgomery College and at the National Institutes of Health. Little did I realize that 20 years later I would be refining, revising, and improving on that original idea!

This new, fifth edition of *The Language of Medicine* reflects my continued interest and fascination with teaching medical terminology and, more importantly, the valuable comments of both students and teachers who find it helpful. In particular, I am grateful for the suggestions received from long-time users of *The Language of Medicine*. I have made every attempt to incorporate their comments and suggested changes in the text.

The intrinsic, basic features of the *The Language of Medicine* have remained the same. They are:

- Simple, nontechnical explanation of medical terms with descriptions of anatomy, physiology, and pathology (no previous knowledge of biology is presumed or needed).
- A workbook format with spaces to write in meanings of terms, respond to exercises, label diagrams, and complete review sheets.
- Organization by body systems with additional chapters on oncology, radiology, nuclear medicine, and radiotherapy, pharmacology, and psychiatry.
- Explanations of clinical procedures, laboratory tests, and abbreviations related to each body system and to other specialized areas of medicine.
- Phonetic Pronunciation of Terms lists that include and review new words introduced in each chapter.
- Practical Applications sections that are short examples of medical language in actual written context: case reports, operative and diagnostic lists, autopsy records, and laboratory and x-ray reports.
- Comprehensive glossaries and appendices that will be a useful reference on the job after completion of your medical terminology studies.

In addition to these basic features, the fifth edition has new aspects. It contains improved and additional diagrams, charts, and tables, designed with particular attention to using different shades of color to enhance understanding of terminology and concepts. In page formatting, diagrams are placed close to explanations so that labeling is easier. Additional lined spaces are provided on the Pronunciation of Terms lists so that meanings can be written alongside each term.

Since *The Language of Medicine* emphasizes explanation of terminology rather than mere memorization of terms, each chapter was carefully read and questions and explanations rewritten to meet criteria of simplicity and understandability. Noncurrent and nonsense terms were weeded out and newer and more practical terms included.

All exercise questions were reviewed; some (spelling exercises) are now omitted, and others (new short vignette questions describing and illustrating disease conditions) are added. New exercise questions with surgical terminology are included as well. In many chapters, there are additional multiple-choice questions with practical applications paragraphs.

A new appendix gives normal values for hematologic tests and implications for high and low values. This is designed as a reference for work situations and for study in the text.

As with previous editions, audiotapes to accompany the text are available from the publisher. These tapes include all the terms on the Pronunciation of Terms list in each chapter. Each term is pronounced and used in a sentence to illustrate its meaning.

The most noticeable change in this edition is the inclusion of two software disks at the back of the book. These contain questions (multiple-choice, short-answer, diagram and word matching, paragraph matching) to test understanding of terminology in each chapter.

Undeniably, the study of medical language requires commitment and hard work, but the benefits are many. You are learning a language that will enable you to interact more effectively in the medical workplace and as an allied health professional. This book aims at bringing the language alive by making the study interesting, logical, and easy to follow.

Thank you for choosing this text. Please continue to communicate your comments and suggestions to me so that future editions and students may benefit. Work hard, but have fun with *The Language of Medicine*.

Davi-Ellen Chabner

To the Teacher

The instructor's manual that accompanies this new edition is greatly expanded and contains the following features:

- Information about using the text and the instructor's manual, proposals for courses, and classroom methods.
- Description of audiotape, software, and testbank materials.
- A paper on teaching medical terminology by Ellen Drake, C.M.T.
- The following quizzes and materials for each chapter, designed to be easy to photocopy and use with students:
  Multiple-Choice Quiz
  Exercise Quiz (based on the exercises at the end of each chapter)
  Spelling Quiz
  Audiotape Quiz
  Diagram Quiz (in systems chapters)
  Crossword Puzzle
  Practical Applications (with multiple-choice questions to use in class)
  Answers to the quizzes and puzzle
  Answers to the Combining Forms and Terminology sections
- Analysis of a medical paper (for optional use in class or for independent study).
- More examples of Practical Applications covering a wide range of medical fields.
- A new section, "Teacher to Teacher," which is the result of a survey sent to users of *The Language of Medicine,* asking them to share their teaching experiences. I have included these responses, with names and affiliations of teachers. Hopefully, this will disseminate new ideas and stimulate communication among instructors of medical terminology.
- A list of common usage terms and medical terminology bloopers and jokes.
- Reference material (dictionaries, texts, and magazines), and Resources (such as sources for patient education materials).

A computerized testbank of questions for generating quizzes and examinations as well as color transparencies for classroom use are also part of *The Language of Medicine* learning system. Please contact the publisher or sales representative for these products.

I am grateful to you for choosing *The Language of Medicine* and for helping it grow through the years. Please continue to write to me and tell me about your experiences using the text and its ancillaries.

DAVI-ELLEN CHABNER

Acknowledgments

This edition and its ancillary features (instructor's manual, audiotapes, software disks, computerized testbank, color transparencies) owes a lion's share of gratitude to Scott W. Weaver, W.B. Saunders editor extraordinaire! Providing intelligent guidance and keeping the project on track at a time when my life was in constant flux, Scott was an energetic, responsive, patient, and reliable partner in this endeavor.

In preparation for this edition, many long-term users of *The Language of Medicine* were asked to review the book. I am grateful to the following instructors, who offered suggestions and shared so much of their talents. Thank you to Renee Braun, Phyllis Broughton, Ellen Drake, Carol Fitzpatrick, Stephen Gavalchik, Patricia Giles, Gail Ingram, Margie Konik, Vickie Lantz, Ranaye Marsh, Rebecca Newsome, Kimberly Rubesne, Connie Schoon, Barbara Singer, Barb Struck, and Susan Webb. I am particularly appreciative to Susan Webb for sending and sharing her course materials and expressing her enthusiasm for *The Language of Medicine.*

During the last 2 years I was fortunate to speak at the Sue Covel Educator's Conferences sponsored by the American Association of Medical Transcriptionists. There I learned about new teaching methods and had an opportunity to share experiences with many interesting, imaginative, creative, and dedicated instructors of medical terminology. Thanks to all the many teachers who took the time to write to me throughout the years and especially recently to Peggy Fuller, Sondra Sue Hein, Frances Prokop, Flo Willoughby, and Chester Halterman.

Kathleen Moore, once again, skillfully compiled and typed the instructor's manual—a daunting job, considering its expanded size. I am grateful to Margaret Biblis, allied health editor, and to Glenn Edelmayer, of the art department, at W.B. Saunders Company, for their many contributions to this edition and to Dolphin Productions for their work on the computer software.

My daughter, Elizabeth S. Chabner, M.D., took time from her busy schedule as intern and resident to read each chapter critically and write the clinically oriented vignettes for each chapter. I am grateful, as well, to Daniel Simon, M.D., for his timely and helpful suggestions for the cardiovascular chapter and to Patrice Gallelli, P.T., for her comments on the musculoskeletal chapter.

Finally, I owe a lifetime of gratitude to Bruce A. Chabner, M.D., who not only patiently answers all my medically oriented questions but listens to and solves most of my nonmedical problems as well.

Table of Contents

9   *Male Reproductive System* 276

10   *Nervous System* 300

11   *Cardiovascular System* 344

16   *Skin*   559

17   *Sense Organs: The Eye and the Ear*   591

18   *Endocrine System*   637

19   *Cancer Medicine (Oncology)*   680

Basic Word Structure

This Chapter is divided into the following sections

In this Chapter you will

- Become familiar with basic objectives to keep in mind as you study the medical language;
- Divide medical words into their component parts;
- Find the meaning of basic combining forms, prefixes, and suffixes of the medical language; and
- Use these combining forms, prefixes, and suffixes to build medical words.

I. Objectives in Studying the Medical Language

There are three objectives to keep in mind as you study medical terminology.

1. **Analyze words by dividing them into component parts.** Your goal is to learn the *tools* of word analysis that will make the understanding of complex terminology easier. Do not simply memorize terms; think about dividing terms into component parts. This text will show you how to separate both complicated and simple terms into understandable word elements. Medical terms are very much like individual jigsaw puzzles. They are constructed of small pieces that make each word unique, but the pieces can be used in different combinations in other words as well. As you become familiar with word parts and learn what each means, you will be able to recognize those word parts in totally new combinations in other terms.

Figure 1–1

Urinary system. (From Chabner DE: Medical Terminology: A Short Course. Philadelphia, WB Saunders, 1990.)

2. **Relate the medical terms to the structure and function of the human body.** Memorization of terms, although essential to retention of the language, should not become the primary objective of your study. A major focus of this text is to *explain* terms in the context of how the body works in health and disease. Medical terms explained in their proper context will also be easier to remember. Thus, the term **hepatitis,** meaning inflammation **(-itis)** of the liver **(hepat),** is better understood when you know where the liver is and how it functions. No previous knowledge of biology, anatomy, or physiology is needed for this study. Explanations in the text are straightforward and basic.

3. **Be aware of spelling and pronunciation problems.** Some medical terms are pronounced alike but are spelled differently, which accounts for their different meanings. For example, **ilium** and **ileum** have identical pronunciations, but the first term, **ilium,** means a part of the pelvis (hip bone), whereas the second term, **ileum,** means a part of the small intestine. Even when terms are spelled correctly, terms can be misunderstood because of incorrect pronunciation. For example, the **urethra** (ū-RĒ-thrăh) is the tube leading from the urinary bladder to the outside of the body, whereas a **ureter** (ŪR-ĕ-tĕr) is one of two tubes each leading from a single kidney and inserting into the urinary bladder. Figure 1–1 illustrates the difference between the urethra and the ureters.

II. Word Analysis

Studying medical terminology is very similar to learning a new language. The words at first sound strange and complicated, although they may stand for commonly known English terms. The terms **otalgia,** meaning ear ache, and **ophthalmologist,** meaning eye doctor, are examples.

Your first job in learning the language is to understand how to divide words into their component parts. The medical language is logical in that most terms, whether complex or simple, can be broken down into basic parts and then understood. For example, consider the following term:

HEMATOLOGY

The **root** is the *foundation of the word.* All medical terms have one or more roots. The root **hemat** means **blood.**

The **suffix** is the *word ending.* All medical terms have a suffix. The suffix **-logy** means **study of.**

The **combining vowel** (usually o) *links the root to the suffix or the root to another root.* A combining vowel has no meaning of its own; it only joins one word part to another.

It is useful to read the meaning of medical terms *starting from the suffix back to the beginning of the term.* Thus, the term **hematology** means **study of blood.**

Here is another familiar medical term:

ELECTROCARDIOGRAM

The root **electr** means **electricity.**
The root **cardi** means **heart.**
The suffix **-gram** means **record.**
The entire word means **record of the electricity in the heart.**

Notice that there are two combining vowels in this term. They link the two roots (**electr** and **cardi**) as well as the root (**cardi**) and suffix (**-gram**).

Try another term:

GASTRITIS

The root **gastr** means **stomach.**
The suffix **-itis** means **inflammation.**

The entire word, reading from the end of the term (suffix) to the beginning, means **inflammation of the stomach.**

Note that the combining vowel, o, is missing in this term. This is because the suffix, **-itis,** begins with a vowel. The combining vowel is dropped before a suffix that begins with a vowel. It is retained, however, between two roots, even if the second root begins with a vowel. Consider the following term:

GASTROENTEROLOGY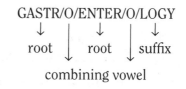

The root **gastr** means **stomach.**
The root **enter** means **intestines.**
The suffix **-logy** means **study of.**
The entire term means **study of the stomach and intestines.**

Notice that the combining vowel is used between **gastr** and **enter,** even though the second root, **enter,** begins with a vowel. When a term contains two or more roots related to parts of the body, often anatomical position determines which root goes before the other. For example, the stomach receives food first, before the small intestine, thus, **gastroenteritis,** not enterogastritis.

In summary, remember three general rules:
1. Read the meaning of medical terms from the suffix back to the beginning of the term and across.
2. Drop the combining vowel (usually o) before a suffix beginning with a vowel: **gastritis** *not* **gastroitis.**
3. Keep the combining vowel between two roots: **gastroenterology** *not* **gastrenterology.**

In addition to the root, suffix, and combining vowel, there are two other word parts commonly found in medical terms. These are the **combining form** and **prefix.** The combining form is simply the root plus the combining vowel. For example, you are already familiar with the following combining forms and their meanings:

HEMAT/O   means   **blood**

root + combining vowel = COMBINING FORM

GASTR/O   means   **stomach**

root + combining vowel = COMBINING FORM

CARDI/O   means   **heart**

root + combining vowel = COMBINING FORM

Combining forms can be used with many different suffixes, so it is useful to know the meaning of a combining form to decipher the meaning of a term.

The **prefix** is a small part that is attached to the *beginning of a term*. Not all medical terms contain prefixes, but the prefix can have an important influence on meaning. Consider the following examples:

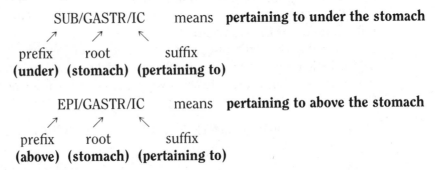

SUB/GASTR/IC   means   **pertaining to under the stomach**

prefix   root   suffix
(under) (stomach) (pertaining to)

EPI/GASTR/IC   means   **pertaining to above the stomach**

prefix   root   suffix
(above) (stomach) (pertaining to)

In summary, the important elements of medical terms are:
1. **Root:** foundation of the term
2. **Suffix:** word ending
3. **Prefix:** word beginning
4. **Combining vowel:** vowel (usually o) that links the root to the suffix or the root to another root
5. **Combining form:** combination of the root and the combining vowel

---

III. Combining Forms, Suffixes, and Prefixes

In previous examples you have been introduced to the combining forms **gastr/o** (stomach), **hemat/o** (blood), and **cardi/o** (heart). The following list contains new combining forms, suffixes, and prefixes with examples of medical words using those word parts. Your job is to write the *meaning* of the medical term in the space provided. As you do this, you may wish to divide the term into its component parts by using slashes (for example: **aden/oma**).

If you have a question about the correct pronunciation of a term, consult the Pronunciation of Terms section at the end of the chapter. The audiotapes that accompany this text contain these terms and their meanings, so you may find it helpful as a study aid. Although most medical terms can be divided into component parts and understood, others will defy simple explanation. Additional information is provided in the text when those terms are introduced, and you may wish to consult a medical dictionary as well.

To test your understanding of word parts and terminology in this chapter, complete the exercises on pages 12 to 19 and check your answers on pages 19 to 21. Then, as a final review, give the meanings for the combining forms, suffixes, and prefixes on the Review Sheet, pages 26 and 27.

Write the meaning of the medical terms that follow in the spaces provided. The notes in italics below the term will help you define it. Simple definitions are best. The first one has been filled in as an example.

Combining Forms

Combining Form	Meaning	Terminology	Meaning
aden/o	gland	adenoma _tumor of a gland_	
		The suffix -oma means tumor or mass.	
		adenitis _____	
		The suffix -itis means inflammation.	
arthr/o	joint	arthritis _____	
bi/o	life	biology _____	
		biopsy _____	
		The suffix -opsy means process of viewing. Living tissue is removed from the body and viewed under a microscope.	
carcin/o	cancerous, cancer	carcinoma _____	
		A carcinoma is a cancerous tumor. Carcinomas grow from epithelial (surface or skin) cells that cover the outside of the body and line organs, cavities, and tubes within the body.	
cardi/o	heart	cardiology _____	
cephal/o	head	cephalic _____	
		(sĕ-FAL-ĭk) The suffix -ic means pertaining to.	

cerebr/o	cerebrum (largest part of the brain)	cerebral _____

The suffix -al means pertaining to. A cerebrovascular accident (CVA) occurs when damage to blood vessels (vascul/o means blood vessels) in the cerebrum causes injury to nerve cells of the brain. This condition is also called a stroke.

cis/o	to cut	incision _____

The prefix in- means into and the suffix -ion means process.

excision _____

The prefix ex- means out.

crin/o	secrete (to form and give off)	endocrine glands _____

The prefix endo- means within; endocrine glands (for example: thyroid, pituitary, and adrenal glands) secrete hormones directly within (into) the bloodstream. Other glands, called exocrine glands, secrete chemicals (saliva, sweat, tears) through tubes (ducts) to the outside of the body.

cyst/o	urinary bladder; a sac or a cyst (sac containing fluid)	cystoscopy _____

(sĭs-TŎS-kō-pē) The suffix -scopy means process of visual examination.

cyt/o	cell	cytology _____

derm/o **dermat/o**	skin	dermatitis _____

hypodermic _____

The prefix hypo- means under, below.

electr/o	electricity	electrocardiogram _____

The suffix -gram means record. Also called an ECG or EKG.

encephal/o	brain	electroencephalogram _____

Also called an EEG.

enter/o	intestines (usually the small intestine)	enteritis _____

The small intestine is narrower and longer than the large intestine (colon).

erythr/o	red	erythrocyte _____

The suffix -cyte means cell. Erythrocytes carry oxygen in the blood.

gastr/o	stomach	gastrectomy _____

The suffix -ectomy means excision or removal.

gastrotomy _____

The suffix -tomy means incision or cutting into.

gnos/o	knowledge	diagnosis _____

The prefix dia- means complete. The suffix -sis means state of. A diagnosis is made after sufficient information has been obtained about the patient's condition.

prognosis _____

The prefix pro- means before. Literally, knowledge before, a prognosis is a prediction about the outcome of an illness, but it is always given after the diagnosis has been determined.

gynec/o	woman, female	gynecology _____
hemat/o	blood	hematology _____
hem/o		hematoma _____

In this term, -oma means a mass or collection of blood, rather than a growth of cells (tumor). A hematoma occurs when blood is lost from blood vessels and collects as clotted blood in a cavity or organ or under the skin.

hepat/o	liver	hepatitis _____
iatr/o	treatment	iatrogenic _____

The suffix -genic means pertaining to producing, produced by, or produced in. Iatrogenic conditions are unexpected side effects that result from treatment by a physician.

leuk/o	white	leukocyte _____

This blood cell helps the body fight disease.

nephr/o	kidney	nephritis _____
		nephrology _____
neur/o	nerve	neurology _____
onc/o	tumor	oncology _____
		oncologist _____

The suffix -ist means one who specializes in a field of medicine.

ophthalm/o	eye	ophthalmoscope _____

(ŏf-THĂL-mō-skōp) The suffix -scope means an instrument for visual examination.

oste/o	bone	osteitis _____
		osteoarthritis _____

This condition is actually a degeneration of bones and joints that occurs as the body ages. It is often accompanied by inflammation.

path/o	disease	pathology _____
		pathologist _____

A pathologist examines biopsy samples microscopically and examines a dead body to determine the cause of death.

ped/o	child	pediatric _____

An orthopedist (orth/o means straight) was originally a doctor who straightened children's bones and corrected deformities. Nowadays, an orthopedist specializes in disorders of bones and muscles of people of all ages.

psych/o	mind	psychology _____
		psychiatrist _____

radi/o	x-rays	radiology _____

ren/o	kidney	renal _____

Ren/o (Latin) and nephr/o (Greek) both mean kidney. Ren/o is used with -al to describe the kidney, whereas nephr/o is used with other suffixes to describe abnormal conditions and operative procedures.

rhin/o	nose	rhinitis _____

sarc/o	flesh	sarcoma _____

This is a cancerous (malignant) tumor. A sarcoma grows from cells of "fleshy" connective tissue such as muscle, bone, and fat, whereas a carcinoma (another type of cancerous tumor) grows from epithelial cells that line the outside of the body or the inside of organs in the body.

sect/o	to cut	resection _____

The prefix re- means back. A resection is a cutting back in the sense of cutting out or removal (excision). A gastric resection is a gastrectomy, or excision of the stomach.

thromb/o	clot, clotting	thrombocyte _____

These cells help clot blood and are also known as platelets. A thrombus is the actual clot that forms, and thrombosis (-osis means condition) is the condition of clot formation.

ur/o	urinary tract, urine	<u>ur</u>ology _____

A urologist is a surgeon who operates on the organs of the urinary tract and the organs of the male reproductive system.

Suffixes			
Suffix	Meaning	Terminology	Meaning
-ac	pertaining to	cardi<u>ac</u> _____	
-al	pertaining to	neur<u>al</u> _____	
-algia	pain	arthr<u>algia</u> _____	
		neur<u>algia</u> _____	
-cyte	cell	leuko<u>cyte</u> _____	
		erythro<u>cyte</u> _____	
		thrombo<u>cyte</u> _____	
-ectomy	excision, removal	nephr<u>ectomy</u> _____	
-emia	blood condition	leuk<u>emia</u> _____	

Literally, this term means a blood condition of white (blood cells). Actually, it is a large increase in the number of cancerous, abnormal white blood cells.

-genic	pertaining to producing, produced by, or produced in	carcino<u>genic</u> _____

Cigarette smoke is carcinogenic.

patho<u>genic</u> _____

A virus or a bacterium is a pathogenic organism.

iatro<u>genic</u> _____

In this term, -genic means produced by.

-gram	record	electroencephalo<u>gram</u> _____
-ic, -ical	pertaining to	gast<u>ric</u> _____
		neurolog<u>ical</u> _____
-ion	process	excis<u>ion</u> _____
-ist	specialist	gynecolog<u>ist</u> _____

-itis	inflammation	cyst<u>itis</u> _____
-logy	study of	endocrin<u>ology</u> _____
-oma	tumor, mass, swelling	hepat<u>oma</u> _____
-opsy	process of viewing	bi<u>opsy</u> _____
-osis	condition, usually abnormal (slight increase in numbers when used with blood cells)	nephr<u>osis</u> _____
		leukocy<u>tosis</u> _____

This condition, a slight increase in normal white blood cells, occurs as white blood cells multiply to fight an infection.

-pathy	disease condition	entero<u>pathy</u> _____

(ĕn-tĕ-RŎP-ă-thē)

adeno<u>pathy</u> _____

(ă-dĕ-NŎP-ă-thē)

-scope	instrument to visually examine	endo<u>scope</u> _____

Endo- means within. A cystoscope is an endoscope.

-scopy	process of visually examining	endo<u>scopy</u> _____

(ĕn-DŎS-kō-pē)

-sis	state of	progno<u>sis</u> _____
-tomy	process of cutting, incision	osteo<u>tomy</u> _____

(ŏs-tē-ŎT-tō-mē)

-y	process, condition	gastroenterolog<u>y</u> _____

Prefixes			
Prefix	Meaning	Terminology	Meaning
a-, an-	no, not, without	<u>an</u>emia _____	

Anemia means a decreased number of erythrocytes or an abnormality of the hemoglobin (a chemical) within the red blood cell. The result is decreased delivery of oxygen to cells of the body. Anemic patients looked so pale that they were thought to be "without blood."

auto-	self	autopsy _____

Actually, an autopsy is the examination of a dead body (with one's own eyes) to determine the cause of death and nature of disease.

dia-	through, complete	diagnosis _____
endo-	within	endocrinologist _____
epi-	above, upon	epigastric _____
		epidermis _____

The outermost layer of skin, lying above the middle layer of skin (called the dermis).

ex-	out	excision _____
exo-	out	exocrine glands _____
hyper-	excessive, above, more than normal	hyperglycemia _____

glyc/o means sugar.

hypo-	deficient, below, less than normal	hypogastric _____

When hypo- is used with a part of the body, it means below.

hypoglycemia _____

In this term, hypo- means deficient.

in-	into, in	incision _____
peri-	surrounding, around	pericardium _____

The suffix -um means a structure. The pericardium is a membrane surrounding the heart.

pro-	before	prognosis _____
re-	back, backward, again	resection _____

An operation in which an organ is "cut back" or removed.

retro-	behind	retrocardiac _____
sub-	below, under	subhepatic _____
trans-	across, through	transhepatic _____

IV. Exercises

The exercises that follow are designed to help you learn the terms that are presented in the chapter. Writing terms over and over again is a good way to remember this new language. Answers are presented in Section V so that they are easy to refer to as you work. *Check your answers carefully* to gain additional information from the correct answers. Each exercise is designed not as a test, but rather as an opportunity for you to learn the material.

A. Complete the following sentences.

1. Word beginnings are called _____ .

2. Word endings are called _____ .

3. The foundation of a word is known as the _____ .

4. A letter linking a suffix and a root, or linking two roots, in a term is called the

    _____ .

5. The combination of a root and a combining vowel is known as the _____ .

B. Give the meanings for the following combining forms.

1. cardi/o _____

2. aden/o _____

3. bi/o _____

4. cerebr/o _____

5. cephal/o _____

6. arthr/o _____

7. carcin/o _____

8. cyst/o _____

9. cyt/o _____

10. derm/o or dermat/o _____

11. encephal/o _____

12. electr/o _____

C. Give the meanings for the following suffixes.

1. -oma _____

2. -al _____

3. -itis _____

4. -logy _____

5. -scopy _____

6. -ic _____

7. -gram _____

8. -opsy _____

D. Using slashes, divide the following terms into parts and give the meaning of the entire term.

1. cerebral _____

2. biopsy _____

3. adenitis _____

4. cephalic _____

5. carcinoma _____

6. cystoscopy _____

7. electrocardiogram _____

8. cardiology _____

9. electroencephalogram _____

10. dermatitis _____

11. arthroscopy _____

12. cytology _____

E. Give the meanings for the following combining forms.

1. erythr/o _____

2. enter/o _____

3. gastr/o _____

4. gnos/o _____

5. hemat/o _____

6. cis/o _____

7. nephr/o _____

8. leuk/o _____

9. iatr/o _____

10. hepat/o _____

11. neur/o _____

12. gynec/o _____

F. Complete the medical term from its meaning given below.

1. white blood cell: _____ cyte

2. inflammation of the stomach: gastr _____

3. pertaining to produced by treatment: _____ genic

4. study of kidneys: _____ logy

5. red blood cell: _____ cyte

6. mass of blood: _____ oma

7. view of living tissue: bi _____

8. pain of nerves: neur _____

9. process of viewing the eye: _____ scopy

10. inflammation of the small intestine: _____ itis

G. *Match the English term in column I with its combining form in column II.*

Column I
English Term

Column II
Combining Form

1. kidney _____reno_____   psych/o
                                  ophthalm/o
2. disease _____patho_____   oste/o
                                  path/o
3. eye _____opthalmo_____   ren/o
                                  rhin/o
4. to cut _____seot_____   radi/o
                                  onc/o
5. nose _____rhino_____   sarc/o
                                  thromb/o
6. flesh _____sarc_____   ur/o
                                  sect/o
7. mind _____psych_____

8. urinary tract _____uro_____

9. bone _____oste_____

10. x-rays _____radi'_____

11. clotting _____thrombo_____

12. tumor _____sare onc_____

H. *Underline the suffix in each term and give the meaning of the entire term.*

1. ophthalmoscopy _____

2. ophthalmoscope _____

3. oncology _____

4. osteitis _____

5. psychosis _____

6. thrombocyte _____

7. renal _____

8. nephrectomy _____

9. osteotomy _____

10. resection _____

11. carcinogenic _____

12. sarcoma _____

I. Match the suffix in column I with its meaning in column II. Write the meaning in the space provided.

Column I
Suffix

Column II
Meaning

1. -algia _____pain_____

2. -ion _____

3. -emia ____blood condition____

4. -gram _____record_____

5. -scope ___view_____

6. -osis ____abnormal_____

7. -ectomy ___remove_____

8. -genic ___produced by_____

9. -pathy ___disease_____

10. -tomy ___incision_____

11. -itis ____inflammation_____

12. -cyte _____cell_____

abnormal condition
record
pertaining to produced by or produced in
instrument to visually examine
pain
blood condition
removal, excision, resection
process
inflammation
cell
disease condition
incision, process of cutting into

J. Select from the following terms to complete the sentences below.

leukocytosis	leukemia	endocrine glands
arthralgia	hematoma	exocrine glands
enteropathy	carcinogenic	iatrogenic
cystitis	neuralgia	hepatoma

1. Cigarette smoke is an example of a (an) _____ *carcinogenic* substance.

2. When there is an abnormal condition of slight increase in white blood cells due to infection in the body,

   the condition is called _____ *leukocytosis* _____.

3. A tumor of the liver is a (an) _____ *hepatoma* _____.

4. The medical term for pain from joints is _____ *arthralgia* _____.

5. Organs that secrete chemicals (hormones) directly into the blood are called _____ *endocrine*

   _____ *glands* _____.
   Examples are the thyroid gland (in the neck), the pituitary gland (at the base of the brain), and the
   adrenal glands (on top of the kidneys).

6. Organs that secrete chemicals out of the body through tubes (ducts) are called _____ *exocrine*

   _____ *glands* _____ . Examples are sweat, tear, and salivary glands.

7. The medical term for pain from nerves is _____ *neuralgia* _____.

8. Ms. Walsh went to her doctor with complaints of pain when urinating. The doctor's diagnosis of her

   condition was inflammation of the urinary bladder, also known as _____ *cystitis* _____.

9. A collection (mass) of blood (under the skin) is a (an) _____ *hematoma* _____.

10. Mr. Bell's white blood cell count is 10 times higher than normal. Examination of his blood shows

    cancerous white blood cells. His diagnosis is _____ *leukemia* _____.

11. After receiving treatment for her urinary tract infection, Ms. Ball developed a severe rash and fever from

    the medication prescribed by the doctor. Her condition is said to be _____ *iatrogenic* _____.

12. After coming back from his trip and eating strange foods, Mr. Cameron had a disease (condition) of his

    intestines, called _____ _____.

K. Give the meanings for the following prefixes.

1. dia- _____   3. auto- _____

2. pro- _____   4. a-, an- _____

5. hyper- _____   10. trans- _____

6. hypo- _____   11. peri- _____

7. epi- _____   12. ex- _____

8. endo- _____   13. sub- _____

9. retro- _____   14. re- _____

L. Underline the prefix in the following terms and give the meaning of the entire term.

1. diagnosis _____

2. prognosis _____

3. subhepatic _____

4. pericardium _____

5. hyperglycemia _____

6. hypodermic _____

7. epigastric _____

8. resection _____

9. hypoglycemia _____

10. anemia _____

M. Complete the following terms (describing areas of medicine) from their meanings given below.

1. study of urinary tract: _____ logy

2. study of women and women's diseases: _____ logy

3. study of blood: _____ logy

4. study of tumors: _____ logy

5. study of the kidneys: _____ logy

6. study of nerves: _____ logy

7. treatment of children: _____ iatrics

8. study of x-rays: _____ logy

9. study of the eyes: _____ logy

10. study of the stomach and intestines: _____ logy

11. study of glands that secrete hormones: _____ logy

12. treatment of the mind: _____ iatry

13. study of disease: _____ logy

14. study of the heart: _____ logy

N. Give the meaning for the underlined word part and then define the term.

1. <u>cere</u>brovascular accident _____

2. <u>en</u>cephalitis _____

3. <u>cysto</u>scope _____

4. an<u>emia</u> _____

5. <u>trans</u>hepatic _____

6. <u>iatro</u>genic _____

7. <u>hypo</u>gastric _____

8. <u>endo</u>crine glands _____

9. osteo<u>tomy</u> _____

10. neur<u>ectomy</u> _____

O. Select from the following terms to complete the sentences below.

anemia	nephrologist	neuropathy
biopsy	psychiatrist	psychologist
oncologist	urologist	oncogenic
pathogenic	thrombocyte	leukemia
prognosis	thrombosis	diagnosis
osteoarthritis		

1. Seventy-two-year-old Ms. Crick suffers from a degenerative joint disease that is caused by wearing away of tissue around her joints. This condition, which literally means inflammation of bones and joints, is

   called _____osteoarthritis_____.

2. The _____biopsy_____ sample was removed during surgery and sent to a pathologist to be examined under the microscope for a proper diagnosis.

3. A (an) _____nephrologist_____ performed surgery to remove Mr. Simon's cancerous kidney.

4. Ms. Rose has suffered from hyperglycemia for many years. This condition is also known as diabetes and can lead to long-term complications such as disease of nerves called ___neuropathy___.

5. A virus or a bacterium produces disease and is therefore a (an) _____ organism.

6. Mr. Jordan has a disease caused by abnormal hemoglobin in his erythrocytes. The erythrocytes change shape, collapsing to form sickle-shaped cells that can become clots and stop the flow of blood. He has a condition called sickle-cell ___anemia___.

7. A (an) ___oncologist___ is a doctor who treats carcinomas and sarcomas.

8. A cell that helps blood to clot is called a platelet or ___thrombocyte___.

9. Dr. Susan Parker told Mr. Jones that his condition would improve with treatment. Her ___prognosis___ was for total recovery in 6 months.

10. A (an) ___psychiatrist___ is a medical doctor who treats mentally ill patients and can prescribe medications for them.

P. *Select the correct term to complete each sentence.*

1. Mrs. Brody had a cough and fever. Her doctor instructed her to go to the (pathology, radiology, hematology) department for a chest x-ray.

2. Mrs. Leaf had problems holding her urine. She made an appointment with a (gastroenterologist, neurologist, urologist).

3. The doctor told the patient she had lost much blood during delivery of her child. She therefore had (anemia, leukocytosis, adenitis).

4. Mr. Preston was having chest pain during his morning walks. He made an appointment to see a (nephrologist, neurologist, cardiologist).

5. After the skiing accident, Dr. Curtin suggested (cystoscopy, biopsy, arthroscopy) to visually examine my swollen, painful knee.

V. Answers to Exercises

A

1. prefixes
2. suffixes
3. root
4. combining vowel
5. combining form

B

1. heart
2. gland
3. life
4. cerebrum, largest part of the brain
5. head
6. joint
7. cancer, cancerous
8. urinary bladder
9. cell
10. skin
11. brain
12. electricity

C

1. tumor, mass
2. pertaining to
3. inflammation
4. process of study
5. process of visual examination
6. pertaining to
7. record
8. process of viewing

D

1. cerebr/al—pertaining to the cerebrum or largest part of the brain
2. bi/opsy—process of viewing life (removal of living tissue and viewing it under the microscope)
3. aden/itis—inflammation of a gland
4. cephal/ic—pertaining to the head
5. carcin/oma—tumor that is cancerous (cancerous tumor)
6. cyst/o/scopy—process of visually examining the urinary bladder
7. electr/o/cardi/o/gram—record of the electricity in the heart
8. cardi/o/logy—process of study of the heart
9. electr/o/encephal/o/gram—record of the electricity in the brain
10. dermat/itis—inflammation of the skin
11. arthr/o/scopy—process of visual examination of a joint
12. cyt/o/logy—process of study of cells

E

1. red
2. intestines (usually small intestine)
3. stomach
4. knowledge
5. blood
6. to cut
7. kidney
8. white
9. treatment
10. liver
11. nerve
12. woman, female

F

1. leukocyte
2. gastritis
3. iatrogenic
4. nephrology
5. erythrocyte
6. hematoma
7. biopsy
8. neuralgia
9. ophthalmoscopy
10. enteritis

G

1. ren/o
2. path/o
3. ophthalm/o
4. sect/o
5. rhin/o
6. sarc/o
7. psych/o
8. ur/o
9. oste/o
10. radi/o
11. thromb/o
12. onc/o

H

1. ophthalmoscopy —process of visual examination of the eye
2. ophthalmoscope —instrument to visually examine the eye
3. oncology —study of tumors
4. osteitis —inflammation of bone
5. psychosis —abnormal condition of the mind
6. thrombocyte —clotting cell (platelet)
7. renal —pertaining to the kidney
8. nephrectomy —removal (excision) of the kidney
9. osteotomy —incision of (to cut into) a bone
10. resection —process of cutting back (in the sense of "out" or removal)
11. carcinogenic —pertaining to producing cancer
12. sarcoma —tumor of flesh (cancerous tumor of flesh tissue, such as bone, fat, and muscle)

I

1. pain
2. process
3. blood condition
4. record
5. instrument to visually examine
6. abnormal condition
7. removal, excision, resection
8. pertaining to producing or produced by
9. disease condition
10. incision, process of cutting into
11. inflammation
12. cell

J

1. carcinogenic
2. leukocytosis
3. hepatoma
4. arthralgia
5. endocrine glands
6. exocrine glands
7. neuralgia
8. cystitis
9. hematoma
10. leukemia
11. iatrogenic
12. enteropathy

K

1. complete, through
2. before
3. self
4. no, not, without
5. excessive, above, more than normal
6. deficient, below, less than normal
7. above, upon
8. within
9. behind
10. across, through
11. surrounding
12. out
13. below, under
14. back

L

1. diagnosis—complete knowledge; a decision about the nature of the patient's condition after the appropriate tests are done
2. prognosis—before knowledge; a prediction about the outcome of treatment, and given after the diagnosis
3. subhepatic—pertaining to below the liver. A combining vowel is not needed between the prefix and the root.
4. pericardium—the membrane surrounding the heart
5. hyperglycemia—condition of excessive sugar in the blood
6. hypodermic—pertaining to under the skin
7. epigastric—pertaining to above the stomach
8. resection—process of cutting back (in the sense of cutting out)
9. hypoglycemia—condition of deficient (low) sugar in the blood
10. anemia—blood condition of low numbers of erythrocytes or deficient hemoglobin in the red blood cells

M

1. urology
2. gynecology
3. hematology
4. oncology
5. nephrology
6. neurology
7. pediatrics (combining vowel *o* has been dropped between ped and iatr)
8. radiology
9. ophthalmology
10. gastroenterology
11. endocrinology
12. psychiatry
13. pathology
14. cardiology

N

1. cerebrum (largest part of the brain). A cerebrovascular accident is damage to the blood vessels of the cerebrum leading to death of brain cells; also called a stroke.
2. brain. Encephalitis is inflammation of the brain.
3. urinary bladder. A cystoscope is an instrument to visually examine the urinary bladder. The cystoscope is placed through the urethra into the bladder.
4. blood condition. Anemia is a low number of red blood cells or abnormal hemoglobin in red blood cells.
5. across, through. Transhepatic means pertaining to across or through the liver.
6. treatment. Iatrogenic means pertaining to an adverse side effect produced by treatment.
7. under, below, deficient. Hypogastric means pertaining to below the stomach.
8. within. Endocrine glands secrete hormones within the body. Examples of these are the pituitary, thyroid, and adrenal glands.
9. incision. Osteotomy is incision of bone.
10. excision. Neurectomy is the removal of a nerve.

O

1. osteoarthritis
2. biopsy
3. urologist (a nephrologist is a medical doctor who treats kidney disorders but does not operate on patients)
4. neuropathy
5. pathogenic
6. anemia
7. oncologist
8. thrombocyte
9. prognosis
10. psychiatrist (a psychologist can treat mentally ill patients but is not a medical doctor and cannot prescribe medications)

P

1. radiology
2. urologist
3. anemia
4. cardiologist
5. arthroscopy

VI. Pronunciation of Terms

The markings ¯ and ˘ above the vowels (a, e, i, o, and u) indicate the proper sounds of the vowels. When ¯ is above a vowel its sound is long, that is, exactly like its name; for example:

ā as in āpe
ē as in ēven
ī as in īce
ō as in ōpen
ū as in ūnit

The ˘ marking indicates a short vowel sound, as in the following examples:

ă as in ăpple
ĕ as in ĕvery
ĭ as in ĭnterest
ŏ as in ŏlive
ŭ as in ŭnder

To test your understanding of the terminology in this chapter, write the meaning of each term in the space provided. In addition, you may wish to cover the terms and write them by looking at your definitions. Make sure your spelling is correct. The page number after each term indicates where it is defined or used in the text so you can easily check your responses.

Term	Pronunciation	Meaning
adenitis (5)	ăd-ĕ-NĪ-tĭs	_____
adenoma (5)	ăd-ĕ-NŌ-mă	_____
adenopathy (10)	ăd-ĕ-NŎP-ă-thē	_____

anemia (10)	ă-NĒ-mē-ă	_____
arthralgia (9)	ăr-THRĂL-jă	_____
arthritis (5)	ăr-THRĪ-tĭs	_____
autopsy (11)	ĂW-tŏp-sē	_____
biology (5)	bī-ŎL-ō-jē	_____
biopsy (5)	BĪ-ŏp-sē	_____
carcinogenic (9)	kăr-sĭ-nō-JĔN-ĭk	_____
carcinoma (5)	kăr-sĭ-NŌ-mă	_____
cardiac (9)	KĂR-dē-ăk	_____
cardiology (5)	kăr-dē-ŎL-ō-jē	_____
cephalic (5)	sĕ-FĂL-ĭk	_____
cerebral (6)	sĕ-RĒ-brăl or SĔR-ĕ-brăl	_____
cystitis (10)	sĭs-TĪ-tĭs	_____
cystoscopy (6)	sĭs-TŎS-kō-pē	_____
cytology (6)	sī-TŎL-ō-jē	_____
dermatitis (6)	dĕr-mă-TĪ-tĭs	_____
dermatology (6)	dĕr-mă-TŎL-ō-jē	_____
diagnosis (7)	dī-ăg-NŌ-sĭs	_____
electrocardiogram (6)	ē-lĕk-trō-KĂR-dē-ō-grăm	_____
electroencephalogram (6)	ē-lĕk-trō-ĕn-SĔF-ă-lō-grăm	_____
endocrine glands (6)	ĔN-dō-krĭn glăndz	_____
endocrinologist (11)	ĕn-dō-krĭ-NŎL-ō-jĭst	_____
endocrinology (10)	ĕn-dō-krĭ-NŎL-ō-jē	_____
endoscope (10)	ĔN-dō-skōp	_____
endoscopy (10)	ĕn-DŎS-kō-pē	_____
enteritis (6)	ĕn-tĕ-RĪ-tĭs	_____
enteropathy (10)	ĕn-tĕ-RŎP-ă-thē	_____
epidermis (11)	ĕp-ĭ-DĔR-mĭs	_____

epigastric (11)	ĕp-ĭ-GĂS-trĭk	_____
erythrocyte (6)	ĕ-RĬTH-rō-sīt	_____
excision (6)	ĕk-SĬZH-ŭn	_____
exocrine glands (6)	ĔK-sō-krĭn glăndz	_____
gastrectomy (6)	găs-TRĔK-tō-mē	_____
gastric (9)	GĂS-trĭk	_____
gastroenterology (10)	găs-trō-ĕn-tĕr-ŎL-ō-jē	_____
gastrotomy (7)	găs-TRŎT-ō-mē	_____
gynecology (7)	gī-nĕ-KŎL-ō-jē or jĭn-ĕ-KŎL-ō-jē	_____
gynecologist (9)	gī-nĕ-KŎL-ō-jĭst or jĭn-ĕ-KŎL-ō-jĭst	_____
hematology (7)	hē-mă-TŎL-ō-jē	_____
hematoma (7)	hē-mă-TŌ-mă	_____
hepatitis (7)	hĕp-ă-TĪ-tĭs	_____
hepatoma (10)	hĕp-ă-TŌ-mă	_____
hyperglycemia (11)	hī-pĕr-glī-SĒ-mē-ă	_____
hypodermic (6)	hī-pō-DĔR-mĭk	_____
hypogastric (11)	hī-pō-GĂS-trĭk	_____
hypoglycemia (11)	hī-pō-glī-SĒ-mē-ă	_____
iatrogenic (7)	ī-ăt-rō-JĔN-ĭk	_____
incision (6)	ĭn-SĬZH-ŭn	_____
leukemia (9)	lōō-KĒ-mē-ă	_____
leukocyte (7)	LŪ-kō-sīt	_____
leukocytosis (10)	lū-kō-sī-TŌ-sĭs	_____
nephrectomy (9)	nĕ-FRĔK-tō-mē	_____
nephritis (7)	nĕ-FRĪ-tĭs	_____
nephrology (7)	nĕ-FRŎL-ō-jē	_____
nephrosis (10)	nĕ-FRŌ-sĭs	_____

nephrotomy (7)	nĕ-FRŎT-ō-mē	_____
neural (9)	NŪ-răl	_____
neuralgia (9)	nū-RĂL-jă	_____
neurological (9)	nū-rō-LŎJ-ĭk-ăl	_____
neurology (7)	nū-RŎL-ō-jē	_____
oncologist (7)	ŏn-KŎL-ō-jĭst	_____
oncology (7)	ŏn-KŎL-ō-jē	_____
ophthalmologist (2)	ŏf-thăl-MŎL-ō-jĭst	_____
ophthalmoscope (7)	ŏf-THĂL-mō-skōp	_____
osteitis (8)	ŏs-tē-Ī-tĭs	_____
osteoarthritis (8)	ŏs-tē-ō-ăr-THRĪ-tĭs	_____
osteotomy (10)	ŏs-tē-ŎT-ō-mē	_____
pathogenic (9)	păth-ō-JĔN-ĭk	_____
pathologist (8)	pă-THŎL-ō-jĭst	_____
pathology (8)	pă-THŎL-ō-jē	_____
pediatric (8)	pē-dē-ĂT-rĭk	_____
pericardium (11)	pĕr-ĭ-KĂR-dē-ŭm	_____
prognosis (7)	prŏg-NŌ-sĭs	_____
psychiatrist (8)	sī-KĪ-ă-trĭst	_____
psychiatry (18)	sī-KĪ-ă-trē	_____
psychology (8)	sī-KŎL-ō-jē	_____
radiology (8)	rā-dē-ŎL-ō-jē	_____
renal (8)	RĒ-năl	_____
resection (8)	rē-SĔK-shŭn	_____
retrocardiac (11)	rĕt-rō-KĂR-dē-ăc	_____
rhinitis (8)	rī-NĪ-tĭs	_____
sarcoma (8)	săr-KŌ-mă	_____

subhepatic (11)   sŭb-hĕ-PĂT-ĭk   _____

thrombocyte (8)   THRŎM-bō-sīt   _____

transhepatic (11)   trănz-hĕ-PĂT-ĭk   _____

urology (8)   ū-RŎL-ō-jē   _____

VII. Review Sheet

This review sheet and the others following each chapter are complete lists of the word elements contained in that chapter. The review sheets are designed to pull together the terminology and to reinforce your learning by giving you the opportunity to write the meanings of each word part in the space provided and test yourself. Check your answers with the information in the chapter or in the Glossary (Medical Terms—English) at the end of the book.

Combining Forms

Combining Form	Meaning	Combining Form	Meaning
aden/o	_____	gnos/o	_____
arthr/o	_____	gynec/o	_____
bi/o	_____	hem/o	_____
carcin/o	_____	hemat/o	_____
cardi/o	_____	hepat/o	_____
cephal/o	_____	iatr/o	_____
cerebr/o	_____	leuk/o	_____
cis/o	_____	log/o	_____
crin/o	_____	nephr/o	_____
cyst/o	_____	neur/o	_____
cyt/o	_____	onc/o	_____
derm/o	_____	ophthalm/o	_____
dermat/o	_____	oste/o	_____
electr/o	_____	path/o	_____
encephal/o	_____	ped/o	_____
enter/o	_____	psych/o	_____
erythr/o	_____	radi/o	_____
gastr/o	_____	ren/o	_____
glyc/o	_____	rhin/o	_____

sarc/o _____   thromb/o _____

sect/o _____   ur/o _____

Suffixes

Suffix	Meaning	Suffix	Meaning
-ac		-itis	
-al		-logy	
-algia		-oma	
-cyte		-opsy	
-ectomy		-osis	
-emia		-pathy	
-genic		-scope	
-gram		-scopy	
-ic, -ical		-sis	
-ion		-tomy	
-ist		-y	

Prefixes

Prefix	Meaning	Prefix	Meaning
a-, an-		hypo-	
auto-		in-	
dia-		peri-	
endo-		pro-	
epi-		re-	
ex-		retro-	
exo-		sub-	
hyper-		trans-	

2

Terms Pertaining to the Body As a Whole

In this Chapter you will
- Define terms that apply to the structural organization of the body;
- Identify the body cavities and recognize the organs contained within those cavities;
- Locate and identify the anatomical and clinical divisions of the abdomen;
- Locate and name the anatomical divisions of the back;
- Become acquainted with terms that describe positions, directions, and planes of the body; and
- Find the meanings for new word elements and use them to understand new medical terms.

I. Structural Organization of the Body

Cells

The cell is the fundamental unit of every living thing (animal or plant). Cells are everywhere in the human body—every tissue, every organ is made up of these individual units.

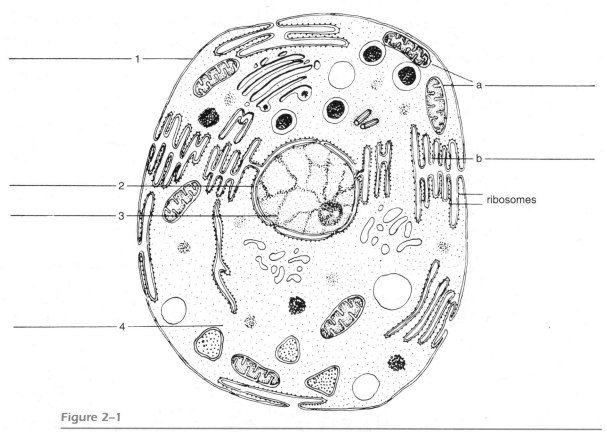

Figure 2–1

Major parts of a cell. Ribosomes *(RĪ-bō-sōmz)* are small granules that help the cell make proteins.

Similarity in Cells. All cells are similar in that they contain a gelatinous substance composed of water, protein, sugar, acids, fats, and various minerals. Several parts of a cell are described below and pictured in Figure 2–1 as they might look when photographed with an electron microscope. Label the structures on Figure 2–1.

(1) **Cell membrane.** This structure not only surrounds and protects the cell, but also determines what passes into and out of the cell.

(2) **Nucleus.** The nucleus is the controlling structure of the cell. It directs the reproduction of the cell and determines the structure and function of the cell.

(3) **Chromosomes.** These are rod-like structures within the nucleus. All human body cells (except for the sex cells, the egg and sperm) contain 23 pairs of chromosomes. The sperm and egg cells have only 23 chromosomes each. After the egg and sperm cells unite to form the embryo, each cell of the embryo then has 46 chromosomes (23 pairs) (Fig. 2–2).

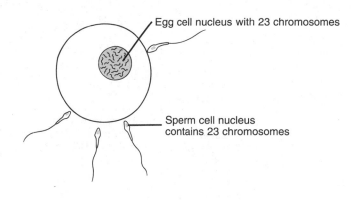

Egg cell nucleus with 23 chromosomes

Sperm cell nucleus contains 23 chromosomes

Figure 2–2

Egg and sperm cells, each containing 23 chromosomes.

Chromosomes contain regions called **genes.** There are several thousand genes, in an orderly sequence, on each chromosome. Each gene is composed of a chemical called **DNA** (deoxyribonucleic acid). DNA regulates the activities of the cell by its sequence (arrangement into genes) on each chromosome. The DNA sequence is like a series of recipes in code. When the code is carried out of the nucleus to the rest of the cell, it directs the activities of the cell, such as cellular reproduction and the manufacture of proteins.

Chromosomes within the nucleus can be analyzed to look at their size, arrangement, and number by doing a **karyotype.** Karyotyping of chromosomes is useful in determining whether chromosomes are normal in number and structure. For example, obstetricians often recommend an amniocentesis (puncture of the sac around the fetus for removal of fluid and cells) of pregnant women to look at the karyotype of the baby. Figure 2–3 shows a karyotype or chromosome "map" of a normal male. The chromosomes have been treated with chemicals so that bands (light and dark areas) can be seen.

If a baby is born with an abnormal number of chromosomes, serious problems can result. In the Down syndrome (previously called mongolism because the patient's facial characteristics resembled those of the mongolian race), the karyotype shows 47 chromosomes instead of the normal number, which is 46. There are three number 21 chromosomes instead of two (either the egg or sperm cell contributes an extra chromosome). Thus, Down

Figure 2–3

Karyotype of a normal male showing 23 pairs of chromosomes. The 23rd pair is the XY pair. In a normal female karyotype, the 23rd pair is XX. (From Behrman RE, Vaughan VC III [eds]: Nelson Textbook of Pediatrics, 13th ed. Philadelphia, WB Saunders, 1987, p 28.)

Figure 2–4

(A) Photograph of a 3½-year-old girl showing typical facial appearance associated with Down syndrome. *(B)* The typical short, broad hand of this child shows characteristic transverse palmar or simian crease *(arrow)*. About one-half of patients with Down syndrome have palms with a single crease, and about 1 per cent of normal persons have this unusual palm pattern. (*A* and *B*, From Bartalos M, Baramki TA: Medical Cytogenetics. Baltimore, Williams & Wilkins, 1967.)

syndrome is also called trisomy-21 syndrome. Its incidence is about once in every 750 live births. The baby is born with physical malformations such as a small, flattened skull; a short, flat-bridged nose; wide-set, slanted eyes; and short, broad hands and feet with a wide gap between the first and the second toes. Reproductive organs are often underdeveloped, congenital heart defects are not uncommon, and some degree of mental retardation is evident (Fig. 2–4).

Continue labeling Figure 2–2.

(4) **Cytoplasm.** Cytoplasm (cyt/o = cell, -plasm = formation) is all the material outside the nucleus and enclosed by the cell membrane. It carries on the work of the cell (in a muscle cell, it does the contracting; in a nerve cell, it transmits impulses). The cytoplasm contains:

(a) **Mitochondria**—small, sausage-shaped bodies that, like miniature power plants, produce energy by burning food in the presence of oxygen. This chemical process is called **catabolism** (cata = down, bol = to cast, -ism = process). During catabolism, complex foods (sugar and fat) are broken down into simpler substances, and energy is released to do the work of the cell.

(b) **Endoplasmic reticulum**—a network (reticulum) of canals within the cell. These canals (containing small structures called ribosomes) are like a cellular tunnel system in which proteins are manufactured for use in the cell. This process of building up complex materials, such as proteins, from simpler parts is called **anabolism** (ana = up, bol = to cast, -ism = process). During anabolism, small pieces of protein are fitted together like links in a chain to make larger proteins.

The two processes, anabolism and catabolism, are known as **metabolism** (meta = change, bol = to cast, -ism = process). Metabolism includes both catabolism and anabolism and is the total of the chemical processes occurring in a cell. If a person has a fast metabolism, then foods, such as sugar and fat, are used up (burned) very quickly and energy is released. If metabolism is slow, foods are burned slowly and fat accumulates in cells.

STUDY SECTION 1

Practice spelling each term and know its meaning.

anabolism	Process of building up complex materials (proteins) from simple materials.
catabolism	Process of breaking down complex materials (foods) to form simpler substances and release energy.
cell membrane	Structure surrounding and protecting the cell. It determines what enters and leaves the cell.
chromosomes	Rod-shaped structures in the nucleus that contain regions of DNA called genes. There are 23 pairs (46) of chromosomes in every cell except for the egg and sperm cells, which contain only 23 each.
cytoplasm	All the material that is outside the nucleus and yet contained within the cell membrane.
DNA	Chemical found within each chromosome. Arranged like a sequence of recipes in code, it directs the activities of the cell.
endoplasmic reticulum	Structure (canals) within the cytoplasm. Site in which large proteins are made from smaller protein pieces.
genes	Regions of DNA within each chromosome.
karyotype	Picture of chromosomes in the nucleus of a cell. The chromosomes are arranged in a numerical order.
metabolism	The total of the chemical processes in a cell. This includes both catabolism and anabolism.
mitochondria	Structures in the cytoplasm in which foods are burned to release energy.
nucleus	Control center of the cell. It contains chromosomes and directs the activities of the cell.

Figure 2–5

Types of cells. Label muscle cell, nerve cell, epithelial cell, and fat cell.

Differences in Cells. Cells are different, or specialized, throughout the body to carry out their individual functions. For instance, a **muscle cell** is long and slender and contains fibers that aid it in contracting and relaxing; an **epithelial,** or skin, **cell** may be square and flat to provide protection; a **nerve cell** may be quite long and have various fibrous extensions that aid in its job of carrying impulses; a **fat cell** contains large, empty spaces for fat storage. These are only a few of the many types of cells in the body. Different types of cells are pictured in Figure 2–5. Label the nerve cell, epithelial cell, fat cell, and muscle cell.

Tissues

A tissue is a group of similar cells working together to do a specific job. A **histologist** (hist/o = tissue) is a scientist who specializes in the study of tissues. Some types of tissues are:

Epithelial Tissue. Epithelial tissue is located all over the body as lining for internal organs, in exocrine and endocrine glands, and as the outer surface of skin covering the body. The term **epithelial** was originally used to describe the tissue above (epi-) the breast nipple (thel/o). Now, it describes tissue that lines the outside of the body and the inner surface of internal organs.

Muscle Tissue. Voluntary muscle is found in arms and legs and parts of the body where movement is voluntary, whereas involuntary muscle is found in the heart and digestive system, as well as other places where movement is not under conscious control. Cardiac muscle is a specialized type of muscle found only in the heart.

Connective Tissue. Examples are **fat** (adipose tissue), **cartilage** (elastic, fibrous tissue attached to bones), bone, and blood.

Nerve Tissue. Nerve tissue conducts impulses all over the body.

Organs

These are structures composed of several kinds of tissue. For example, an organ like the stomach is composed of muscle tissue, nerve tissue, and glandular epithelial tissue. The medical term for internal organs is **viscera** (singular: **viscus**). Examples of abdominal viscera (organs located in the abdomen) are the liver, stomach, intestines, pancreas, spleen, and gallbladder.

Systems

These are groups of organs working together to perform complex functions. For example, the mouth, esophagus, stomach, and small and large intestines are organs that do the work of the digestive system to digest food and absorb it into the bloodstream.

Ten body systems are listed below with their organs. The organs in boldface are ones that you should learn to spell and identify.

System	Organs
Digestive	mouth, **pharynx** (throat), esophagus, stomach, intestines (small and large), liver, gallbladder, pancreas
Urinary or excretory	kidneys, **ureters** (tubes from the kidneys to the urinary bladder), urinary bladder, **urethra** (tube from the bladder to the outside of the body)
Respiratory	nose, pharynx, **larynx** (voice box), **trachea** (windpipe), bronchial tubes, lungs (where exchange of gases takes place)
Reproductive	female: ovaries, uterine (fallopian) tubes, **uterus** (womb), vagina, mammary glands; male: testes and associated tubes, urethra, penis, prostate gland
Endocrine	**thyroid gland** (in the neck), **pituitary gland** (at the base of the brain), sex glands (ovaries and testes), adrenal glands, pancreas (islets of Langerhans), parathyroid glands, thymus gland
Nervous	brain, spinal cord, nerves, and collections of nerves
Circulatory	heart, blood vessels (arteries, veins, and capillaries), lymphatic vessels and nodes, spleen, thymus gland
Muscular	muscles
Skeletal	bones and joints
Skin and sense organs	skin, hair, nails, sweat glands, and sebaceous (oil) glands; the eye, the ear, the nose, and the tongue

STUDY SECTION 2

Practice spelling each term and know its meaning.

adipose tissue	Collection of fat cells.
cartilage	Flexible connective tissue attached to bones at joints, surrounding the trachea, and forming part of the external ear and nose.
epithelial cell	Skin cell that lines the external body surface and the internal surface of organs.
histologist	Specialist in the study of tissues.
larynx (LĂR-ĭnks)	Voice box; located at the upper part of the trachea.
pharynx (FĂR-ĭnks)	Throat. The pharynx is the common passageway for food (from the mouth going to the esophagus) and air (from the nose to the trachea).
pituitary gland	Endocrine gland at the base of the brain.
thyroid gland	Endocrine gland that surrounds the trachea in the neck.
trachea	Windpipe (tube leading from the throat to the bronchial tubes).
ureter	One of two tubes, each leading from a single kidney to the urinary bladder. Spelling clue: ureter has two e's and there are two of them.
urethra	Tube from the urinary bladder to the outside of the body. Spelling clue: urethra has one e and there is only one urethra.
uterus	The womb. The organ that holds the embryo and fetus as it develops.
viscera	Internal organs.

II. Body Cavities

A body cavity is a space within the body that contains internal organs (viscera). Label Figure 2–6 as you learn the names of the body cavities. Some of the important viscera contained within those cavities are listed as well.

Cavity	Organs
(1) Cranial	Brain, pituitary gland.
(2) Thoracic	Lungs, heart, esophagus, trachea, bronchial tubes, thymus gland, aorta (large artery).

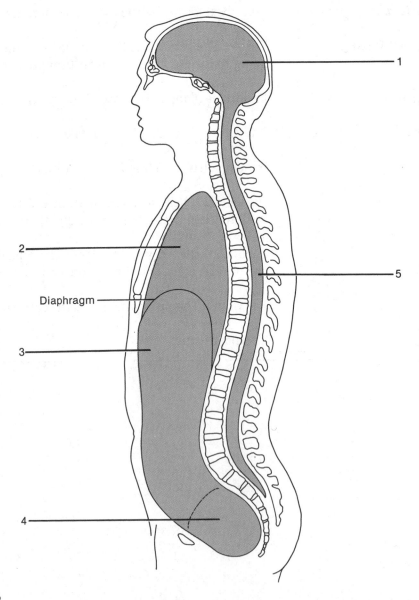

Diaphragm

Figure 2–6

Body cavities. (From Chabner DE: Medical Terminology: A Short Course. Philadelphia, WB Saunders, 1990.)

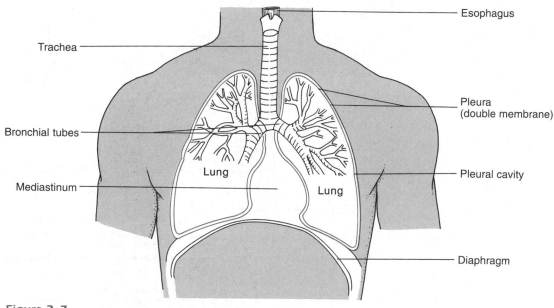

Trachea

Esophagus

Pleura
(double membrane)

Bronchial tubes

Lung

Lung

Mediastinum

Pleural cavity

Diaphragm

Figure 2–7

Divisions of the thoracic cavity. (From Chabner DE: Medical Terminology: A Short Course. Philadelphia, WB Saunders, 1990.)

The thoracic cavity can be divided into two smaller cavities (Fig. 2–7):

a. **Pleural cavity**—space between the membranes that surround each lung. Each pleural cavity is lined with a double-folded membrane called **pleura.** If the pleura becomes inflamed (as in pleuritis or pleurisy), the pleural cavity can fill with fluid.

b. **Mediastinum**—the area between the lungs. It contains the heart, aorta, trachea, esophagus, thymus gland, and bronchial tubes.

(3) Abdominal   Stomach, small and large intestines, spleen, liver, gallbladder, pancreas.

The **peritoneum** is the double-folded membrane surrounding the abdominal cavity (Fig. 2–8). The kidneys are two bean-shaped organs situated at the back (retroperitoneal area) of the abdominal cavity on either side of the backbone (see Fig. 2–10).

(4) Pelvic   Urinary bladder, urethra, ureters; uterus and vagina in the female.

(5) Spinal   Nerves of the spinal cord.

The cranial and spinal cavities are considered **dorsal** body cavities because of their location on the back (posterior) portion of the body. The thoracic, abdominal, and pelvic cavities are considered **ventral** body cavities because they are on the front (anterior) portion of the body.

The thoracic and abdominal cavities are separated by a muscular wall called the **diaphragm.** The abdominal and pelvic cavities are not separated by a muscular wall and together they are frequently called the **abdominopelvic cavity.** Figures 2–9 and 2–10 show the abdominal and thoracic viscera from anterior (ventral) and posterior (dorsal) views.

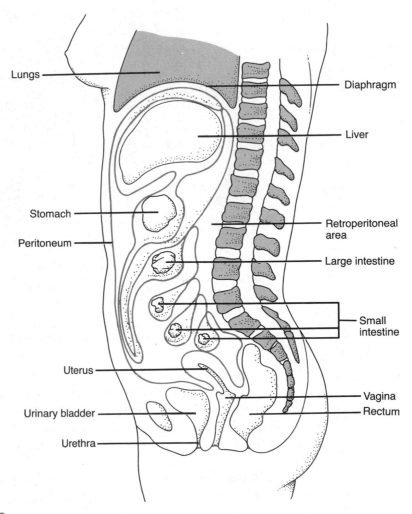

Lungs

Stomach

Peritoneum

Uterus

Urinary bladder

Urethra

Diaphragm

Liver

Retroperitoneal
area

Large intestine

Small
intestine

Vagina

Rectum

Figure 2–8

Side view. The peritoneum surrounds the organs in the abdominal cavity. The retroperitoneal area is behind the peritoneum and contains the kidneys. (From Chabner DE: Medical Terminology: A Short Course. Philadelphia, WB Saunders, 1990.)

STUDY SECTION 3

Practice spelling each term and know its meaning.

abdominal cavity	Space below the chest containing organs such as the liver, stomach, gallbladder, and intestines; also called the **abdomen.**
cranial cavity	Space in the head containing the brain and surrounded by the skull. **Cranial** means **pertaining to the skull.**
diaphragm	Muscle separating the abdominal and thoracic cavities.
dorsal	Pertaining to the back; posterior.
mediastinum	Space between the lungs.
pelvic cavity	Space below the abdomen containing the urinary bladder and reproductive organs. **Pelvic** means **pertaining to the hip bone,** which surrounds the pelvic cavity.
peritoneum	Membrane surrounding the organs in the abdomen.
pleura	A double-layered membrane surrounding each lung.
pleural cavity	Space between the pleural membranes and surrounding each lung.
spinal cavity	Space within the spinal column (backbones) and containing the spinal cord. Also called the **spinal canal.**
thoracic cavity	Space in the chest containing the heart, lungs, bronchial tubes, trachea, esophagus, and other organs.
ventral	Pertaining to the front; anterior.

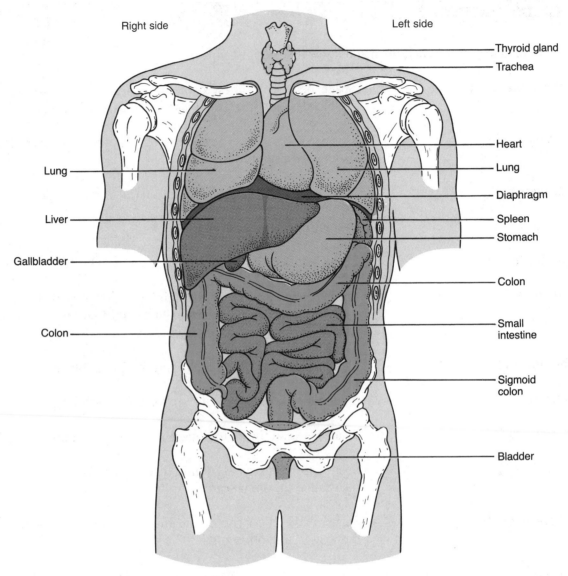

Figure 2–9

Organs of the abdomen and thorax, anterior view.

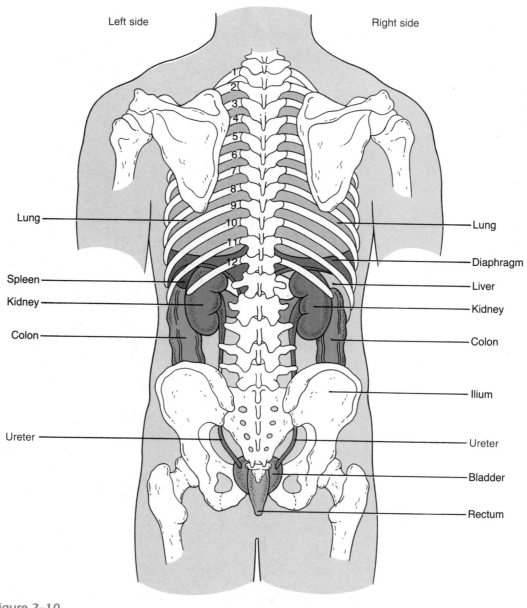

Figure 2–10

Organs of the abdomen and thorax, posterior view.

Figure 2–11

Abdominopelvic regions. These regions can be used clinically to locate internal organs.

III. Abdominopelvic Regions and Quadrants

Regions

Figure 2–11 shows the division of the abdominal and pelvic cavities (abdominopelvic cavity) into nine regions, used by doctors to describe the regions in which internal organs are found. These regions are:

Hypochondriac regions: two upper right and left regions; below the cartilage (chondr/o) of the ribs that extend over the abdomen.

Epigastric region: region above the stomach.

Lumbar regions: two middle right and left regions near the waist.

Umbilical region: region of the navel or umbilicus.

Inguinal regions: two lower right and left regions; near the groin (inguin/o = groin), which is the area where the legs join the trunk of the body. These regions are also known as **iliac** regions because they are near the ilium, which is the upper portion of the hip bone on each side of the body.

Hypogastric region: lower middle region below the umbilical region.

Quadrants

The abdominopelvic area can be divided into four quadrants by drawing two imaginary lines—one horizontally and one vertically through the body. Figure 2–12 shows these quadrants. You add the proper abbreviation on the line under each label on the diagram.

Right upper quadrant, RUQ: contains the liver (right lobe), gallbladder, part of the pancreas, parts of the small and large intestines. & stomach

Left upper quadrant, LUQ: contains the liver (left lobe), stomach, spleen, part of the pancreas, parts of the small and large intestines.

Right lower quadrant, RLQ: contains parts of the small and large intestines, right ovary, right uterine (fallopian) tube, appendix, right ureter.

Left lower quadrant, LLQ: contains parts of the small and large intestines, left ovary, left uterine tube, left ureter.

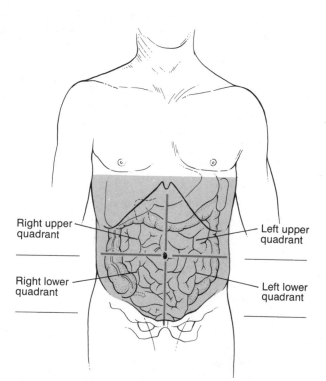

Right upper quadrant

Left upper quadrant

Right lower quadrant

Left lower quadrant

Figure 2–12

Quadrants of the abdomen. (From Swartz MH: Textbook of Physical Diagnosis: History and Examination. Philadelphia, WB Saunders, 1989, p 320.)

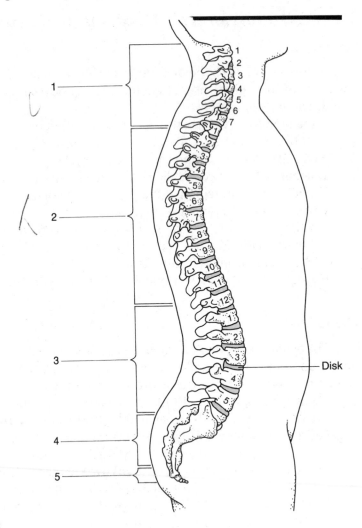

Figure 2–13

Anatomical divisions of the back (spinal column). Disks are shown *in color*. (From Chabner DE: Medical Terminology: A Short Course. Philadelphia, WB Saunders, 1990.)

IV. Divisions of the Back (Spinal Column)

The back is separated into divisions corresponding to regions of the spinal column. The spinal column is composed of a series of bones extending from the neck downward to the tailbone. Each bone is called a **vertebra** (plural: **vertebrae).**

Label the divisions of the back on Figure 2–13 as you study the following:

Division of the Back	Abbreviation	Location
(1) Cervical ✓	C	Neck region. There are 7 cervical vertebrae (C1–C7).
(2) Thoracic ✓	T or D (D = dorsal)	Chest region. There are 12 thoracic vertebrae (T1–T12). Each bone is joined to a rib.
(3) Lumbar ✓	L	Loin (waist) or flank region (between the ribs and the hip bone). There are 5 lumbar vertebrae (L1–L5).
(4) Sacral ✓	S	Five bones (S1–S5) are fused to form one bone, the sacrum.
(5) Coccygeal ✓		The **coccyx** (tailbone) is a small bone composed of 4 fused pieces.

An important distinction should be made between the **spinal column** (back bones or vertebrae) and the **spinal cord** (nerves surrounded by the column). The column is bone tissue, whereas the cord is composed of nerve tissue.

The spaces between the vertebrae (intervertebral spaces) are identified according to the two vertebrae between which they lie; for example, L5–S1 lies between the 5th lumbar and the 1st sacral vertebrae. Within the space and between vertebrae there is a small pad of cartilage called a **disk or disc.** The disk acts as a shock absorber. Occasionally, it moves out of place (ruptures) and puts pressure on a nerve. This is called a **slipped disk,** and it can be very painful.

STUDY SECTION 4

Practice spelling each term and know its meaning.

ABDOMINOPELVIC REGIONS

hypochondriac   Upper right and left regions beneath the ribs.

epigastric   Upper middle region above the stomach.

lumbar	Middle right and left regions near the waist.
umbilical	Central region near the navel.
inguinal	Lower right and left regions near the groin. Also called **iliac regions.**
hypogastric	Lower middle region below the umbilical region.

ABDOMINOPELVIC QUADRANTS

RUQ	Right upper quadrant
LUQ	Left upper quadrant
RLQ	Right lower quadrant
LLQ	Left lower quadrant

DIVISIONS OF THE BACK

cervical	Neck region (C1–C7)
thoracic	Chest region (T1–T12)
lumbar	Loin (waist) region (L1–L5)
sacral	Region of the sacrum (S1–S5)
coccygeal	Region of the coccyx (tailbone)

RELATED TERMS

vertebra	A back bone.
vertebrae	Back bones.
spinal column	Bone tissue surrounding the spinal cavity.
spinal cord	Nervous tissue within the spinal cavity.
disk (disc)	A pad of cartilage between vertebrae.

V. Positional and Directional Terms

The following terms are used to describe the location of organs in relationship to one another throughout the body.

Anterior (ventral)   Front side of the body. *Example:* The abdomen is anterior to the spinal cord. Ventral and anterior are the same position in a human; but in an animal (on four legs), ventral refers to the belly side and anterior to the front near the head.

Posterior (dorsal)   Backbone side of the body. *Example:* The spinal cord is posterior or dorsal to the stomach.

Deep   Away from the surface. *Example:* The stab wound penetrated deep into the abdomen.

Superficial   On the surface. *Example:* Superficial veins can be viewed through the skin.

Proximal   Near the point of attachment to the trunk or near the beginning of a structure. *Examples:* The proximal end of the upper armbone (humerus) joins with the shoulder bone. The proximal end of the stomach is at the esophagus.

Distal   Far from the point of attachment to the trunk or far from the beginning of a structure. *Examples:* At its distal end, the humerus joins with the lower armbones at the elbow. The distal end of the stomach is at the small intestine.

Inferior   Below another structure. *Example:* The large intestine (colon) lies inferior to the stomach and the liver. The term **caudal** (pertaining to the tail) means inferior in humans.

Superior   Above another structure. *Example:* The uterus is located superior to the vagina. The term **cephalic** (pertaining to the head) is also used to mean superior.

Medial   Pertaining to the middle or nearer the medial plane of the body. *Example:* In the anatomical position (see Fig. 2–14), the palms of the hand are faced outward and the fifth finger lies medial to the other fingers.

Lateral   Pertaining to the side. *Example:* The little toes are lateral to the big toes.

Supine   Lying on the back. *Example:* The patient is supine during an examination of the abdomen. The face is **up** in the s**up**ine position.

Prone   Lying on the belly. *Example:* The back bones can be examined with the patient in a prone position. The patient is lying **on** his face in the pr**on**e position.

VI. Planes of the Body

A plane is an imaginary flat surface. Label Figure 2–14 as you study the terms for the planes of the body:

Plane	Location
(1) Frontal (coronal)	Vertical plane that divides the body or structure into anterior and posterior portions. Also called a **coronal** plane. An AP (anterior-posterior) chest x-ray is taken in the frontal plane.
(2) Sagittal (lateral)	Lengthwise vertical plane that divides the body or structure into right and left sides. The **midsagittal** plane divides the body into right and left halves. A **lateral** chest x-ray is taken in the sagittal plane.

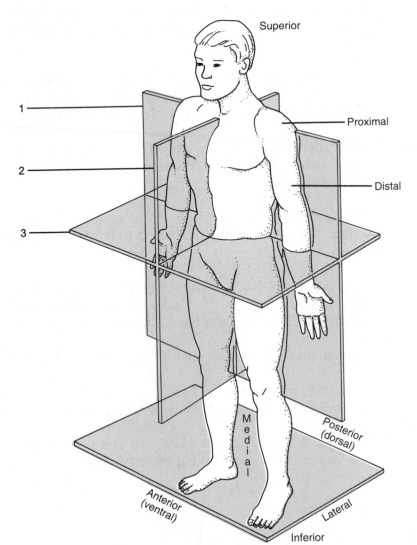

Figure 2–14

Planes of the body. The figure is standing in the anatomical position. In the anatomical position the palms of the hand face outward and the fifth finger lies medial to the other fingers. (From Chabner DE: Medical Terminology: A Short Course. Philadelphia, WB Saunders, 1990.)

(3) Transverse (cross-sectional)   Plane running across the body parallel to the ground (horizontal). It divides the body or structure into upper and lower portions and is also called a **cross-sectional** plane. A CT (computed tomography; also known as computerized axial tomography or CAT) scan is a series of x-ray pictures taken in the transverse plane.

STUDY SECTION 5

Practice spelling each term and know its meaning.

anterior (ventral)	Pertaining to the front (belly side) of the body. (A fish's ventral fin is on its belly side.)
deep	Away from the surface.
distal	Far from the point of attachment to the trunk or far from the beginning of a structure.
frontal (coronal) plane	Vertical plane dividing the body into an anterior and a posterior portion.
inferior (caudal)	Below another structure.
lateral	Pertaining to the side.
medial	Pertaining to the middle or near the medial plane of the body.
posterior (dorsal)	Pertaining to the back of the body. (The dorsal fin of a fish is on its back side.)
prone	Lying on the belly (face down, palm down).
proximal	Near the point of attachment to the trunk or near the beginning of a structure.
sagittal plane	Vertical plane dividing the body into right and left sides. From the Latin sagitta meaning arrow. As an arrow is shot from a bow it enters the body in the sagittal plane, dividing right from left.
superficial	On the surface.
superior (cephalic)	Above another structure.
supine	Lying on the back (face up, palm up).
transverse plane	Horizontal plane dividing the body into upper and lower portions (cross section).

VII. Combining Forms, Prefixes, and Suffixes

Write the meaning of the medical terms that follow in the spaces provided.

Combining Forms			
Combining Form	**Meaning**	**Terminology**	**Meaning**
abdomin/o	abdomen	abdominal _____	
		The abdomen is the region below the chest containing internal organs (liver, intestines, stomach, gallbladder, etc.).	
adip/o	fat	adipose _____	
		The suffix -ose means pertaining to or full of.	
anter/o	front	anterior _____	
		The suffix -ior means pertaining to.	
bol/o	to cast (throw)	anabolism _____	
		The prefix ana- means up. The suffix -ism means process. In this cellular process, proteins are built up (protein synthesis).	
cervic/o	neck (of the body or of the uterus)	cervical _____	
		The cervix is the neck of the uterus. The term cervical can mean pertaining to the neck of the body or the neck (lower part) of the uterus.	
chondr/o	cartilage (type of connective tissue)	chondroma _____	
		This is a benign tumor.	
		chondrosarcoma _____	
		This is a malignant tumor. The term sarc indicates that the malignant tumor is a type of flesh or connective tissue.	
chrom/o	color	chromosomes _____	
		These nuclear structures absorb the color of dyes used to stain the cell. The suffix -somes means bodies. Literally, this term means bodies of color, which is how they first appeared to doctors who saw them under the microscope.	
coccyg/o	coccyx (tailbone)	coccygeal _____	
crani/o	skull	craniotomy _____	
cyt/o	cell	cytoplasm _____	
		The suffix -plasm means formation.	

dist/o	far, distant	distal _____
dors/o	back portion of the body	dorsal _____
hist/o	tissue	histology _____
ili/o	ilium (part of the pelvic bone)	iliac _____
		See Figure 2–10 for a picture of the ilium.
inguin/o	groin	inguinal _____
kary/o	nucleus	karyotype _____
		The suffix -type means classification or picture.
later/o	side	lateral _____
lumb/o	lower back (side and back between the ribs and the pelvis)	lumbosacral _____
medi/o	middle	medial _____
nucle/o	nucleus	nucleic _____
pelv/o	hip, pelvic cavity	pelvic _____
poster/o	back, behind	posterior _____
proxim/o	near	proximal _____
sacr/o	sacrum	sacral _____
sarc/o	flesh	sarcoma _____
spin/o	spine, backbone	spinal _____
thel/o	nipple	epithelial cell _____
		This cell, originally identified as covering nipples, is found covering body surfaces, externally (outside the body) and internally (lining cavities and organs).
thorac/o	chest	thoracic _____
		thoracotomy _____
trache/o	trachea, windpipe	tracheal _____
umbilic/o	navel, umbilicus	umbilical _____

ventr/o	belly side of the body	ventral _____	
vertebr/o	vertebrae, back bones	vertebral _____	
viscer/o	internal organs	visceral _____	

Prefixes			
Prefix	Meaning	Terminology	Meaning
ana-	up	anabolic _____	
cata-	down	catabolism _____	
		The cellular process of breaking down foods to release energy.	
epi-	above	epigastric _____	
hypo-	below	hypochondriac regions _____	
		The Greeks blamed organs (liver and spleen) in the hypochondriac region of the abdomen as the origin of imaginary illnesses. Hence, the term hypochondriac, a person with unusual anxiety about his or her health and with symptoms not attributable to any disease process.	
inter-	between	intervertebral _____	
		A disk (disc) is an intervertebral structure.	
meta-	change	metabolism _____	
		Literally, to cast (bol/o) a change (meta-), meaning the chemical changes (processes) that occur in a cell.	

Suffixes

The following are some new suffixes introduced in this chapter.

Suffix	Meaning	Suffix	Meaning
-eal	pertaining to	**-ior**	pertaining to
-iac	pertaining to	**-ism**	process

-ose	pertaining to, full of		**-somes**	bodies
-plasm	formation		**-type**	picture, classification

VIII. Exercises

Remember to check your answers carefully with those given in Section IX, Answers to Exercises.

A. The following terms are parts of a cell. Match each term with its meaning below.

cell membrane   chromosomes   genes
nucleus   cytoplasm   DNA
mitochondria   endoplasmic reticulum

1. the material of the cell that is outside the nucleus and yet enclosed by the cell membrane

   _____ cytoplasm _____

2. regions of DNA within each chromosome _____ chromosomes _____ gene

3. small, sausage-shaped structures; the place where food is burned to release energy

   _____ mitochondria _____

4. canal-like structure in the cytoplasm; the place where proteins are made ___ E.R. _____

5. the structure that surrounds and protects the cell _____ cell membrane _____

6. the control center of the cell, containing chromosomes _____ neucleus _____

7. a chemical found within each chromosome _____ DNA _____

8. rod-shaped structures in the nucleus that contain regions called genes ___ chromosomes ___

B. Use medical terms or numbers to complete the following sentences.

1. A picture of chromosomes in the nucleus of a cell is called a (an) _____ Kacotype _____

2. The number of chromosomes in a normal male's muscle cell is _____ 23 / 46 _____

3. The number of chromosomes in a female's egg cell is _____ 23 _____

4. The process of building up proteins in a cell is called _____ anabolism _____

5. The process of chemically burning or breaking down foods to release energy in cells is known as

   _____ catabolism _____

6. The total of the chemical processes in a cell is known as _____ *metabolism*

7. A scientist who studies tissues is called a (an) _____ *histology*

8. The medical term for internal organs is _____ *visceral*

C. *Match the part of the body listed with its description below.*

ureter	larynx	urethra
thyroid gland	cartilage	epithelial tissue
pharynx	trachea	adipose tissue
pituitary gland	uterus	pleura

1. the voice box _____ *larynx*

2. membrane surrounding the lungs _____ *pleura*

3. the throat _____ *pharynx*

4. tube from the kidney to the urinary bladder _____ *ureter*

5. collection of fat cells _____ *adipose tissue*

6. an endocrine organ located at the base of the brain _____ *pituitary*

7. windpipe _____ *trachea*

8. flexible connective tissue attached to bones at joints _____ *cartilage*

9. surface cells lining the outside of the body and internal organs _____ *epithelial*

10. an endocrine gland surrounding the windpipe in the neck _____ *thyroid*

11. the womb _____ *uterus*

12. a tube leading from the urinary bladder to the outside of the body _____ *urethra*

D. *Name the five cavities of the body.*

1. the cavity surrounded by the skull _____ *cranium*

2. the cavity in the chest surrounded by the ribs _____ *thoracic*

3. the cavity below the chest containing the stomach, liver, and gallbladder _____ *abdominal*

4. the cavity surrounded by the hip bone _____

5. the cavity surrounded by the bones of the back _____ *spinal*

E. Select from the following definitions to complete the sentences below (1–11).

space surrounding each lung
space between the lungs
muscle separating the abdominal and thoracic cavities
membrane surrounding the abdominal organs
area below the umbilicus (as well as below the stomach)
area above the stomach
area of the navel
areas near the groin
nervous tissue within the spinal cavity
bone tissue surrounding the spinal cavity
a pad of cartilage between each vertebra

1. The hypogastric region is the _____

2. The mediastinum is the _____

3. The spinal cord is _____

4. The diaphragm is a (an) _____

5. An intervertebral disk is _____

6. The pleural cavity is _____

7. The spinal column is _____

8. Inguinal areas are the _____

9. The peritoneum is the _____

10. The umbilical region is the _____

11. The epigastric region is the _____

F. Name the five divisions of the back.

1. region of the neck _____

2. region of the chest _____ thoracic _____

3. region of the waist _____ lumbar _____

4. region of the sacrum _____ sacral _____

5. region of the tailbone _____ ccyx. _____

G. *Give the meanings for the following abbreviations.*

1. LLQ _____

2. L5–S1 _____

3. RUQ _____

4. C3–C4 _____

5. RLQ _____

H. *Give the opposites of the following terms.*

1. deep _____   4. medial _____

2. proximal _____   5. dorsal _____

3. supine _____   6. superior _____

I. *Select from the following medical terms to complete the sentences below.*

vertebra   proximal   frontal
lateral   superior   inferior (caudal)
vertebrae   transverse
distal   sagittal

1. The left lung lies _____ to the heart.

2. The _____ end of the thigh bone joins with the knee cap (patella).

3. The _____ plane is a vertical plane that divides the body into an anterior and a posterior portion.

4. A back bone is called a (an) _____

5. Several back bones are called _____

6. The diaphragm lies _____ to the organs in the thoracic cavity.

7. The _____ plane is a vertical plane that divides the body into right and left portions.

8. The _____ end of the upper armbone is at the shoulder.

9. The _____ plane is a horizontal plane that divides the body into upper and lower portions, like a cross section.

10. The liver lies _____ to the intestines.

J. Give the meanings for the following medical terms.

1. craniotomy _____

2. cervical _____

3. chondroma _____

4. chondrosarcoma _____

5. nucleic _____

6. epigastric _____

7. intervertebral _____

8. pelvic _____

9. posterior _____

10. umbilical _____

K. Give the medical term for the following definitions. Pay attention to spelling!

1. space below the chest containing the liver, stomach, gallbladder, and intestines:

_____

2. flexible connective tissue attached to bones at joints: _____

3. rod-shaped structures in the cell nucleus, containing regions of DNA: _____

4. muscle separating the abdominal and thoracic cavities: _____

5. the voice box: _____

6. vertical plane dividing the body into right and left sides: _____

7. pertaining to the neck: _____

8. tumor (benign) of cartilage: _____

9. control center of the cell; directs the activities of the cell: _____

10. pertaining to the windpipe: _____

L. Complete each term from its meaning given below.

1. pertaining to internal organs: _____ al

2. tumor of flesh tissue (malignant): _____ oma

3. pertaining to the chest: _____ ic

4. picture of the chromosomes in the cell nucleus: _____ type

5. sausage-shaped cellular structures in which catabolism takes place: mito _____

6. space between the lungs: media _____

7. endocrine gland at the base of the brain: _____ ary gland

8. pertaining to skin (surface) cells: epi _____

M. Select the correct term to complete each sentence.

1. Dr. Curnen said the (inguinal, superior, superficial) wound barely scratched the surface.

2. The liver and spleen are on opposite sides of the body. The liver is in the (RUQ, LUQ, LLQ) of the abdominopelvic cavity and the spleen is in the (RUQ, LUQ, RLQ).

3. When a gynecologist examines a patient's pelvis, the patient lies on her back in the (ventral, dorsal, medial) lithotomy position. (Lithotomy = incision to remove a stone—the position also used for removal of ureteral or kidney stones.)

4. Sally's pain was around her navel. The doctor described it as (periumbilical, epigastric, hypogastric).

5. Mrs. Jones was told she was carrying a fetus with trisomy-21. The diagnosis was made by analysis of an abnormal (urine sample, thoracotomy, karyotype).

6. The (spinal, sagittal, abdominal) cavity contains digestive organs.

IX. Answers to Exercises

A

1. cytoplasm	4. endoplasmic reticulum	7. DNA
2. genes	5. cell membrane	8. chromosomes
3. mitochondria	6. nucleus	

B

1. karyotype	4. anabolism	7. histologist
2. 46 (23 pairs)	5. catabolism	8. viscera
3. 23	6. metabolism	

C

1. larynx
2. pleura
3. pharynx
4. ureter
5. adipose tissue
6. pituitary gland
7. trachea
8. cartilage
9. epithelial tissue
10. thyroid gland
11. uterus
12. urethra

D

1. cranial
2. thoracic
3. abdominal
4. pelvic
5. spinal

E

1. area below the umbilicus
2. space between the lungs
3. nervous tissue within the spinal cavity
4. muscle separating the abdominal and thoracic cavities
5. a pad of cartilage between each vertebra
6. space surrounding each lung
7. bone tissue surrounding the spinal cavity
8. areas near the groin
9. membrane surrounding the abdominal organs
10. area of the navel
11. area above the stomach

F

1. cervical
2. thoracic
3. lumbar
4. sacral
5. coccygeal

G

1. left lower quadrant (of the abdominopelvic cavity)
2. between the 5th lumbar vertebra and the 1st sacral vertebra (a common place for a slipped disk)
3. right upper quadrant (of the abdominopelvic cavity)
4. between the 3rd cervical vertebra and the 4th cervical vertebra
5. right lower quadrant (of the abdominopelvic cavity)

H

1. superficial
2. distal
3. prone
4. lateral
5. ventral (anterior)
6. inferior (caudal)

I

1. lateral
2. distal
3. frontal (coronal)
4. vertebra
5. vertebrae
6. inferior (caudal)
7. sagittal
8. proximal
9. transverse
10. superior (cephalic)

J

1. incision of the skull
2. pertaining to the neck (of the body or the cervix of the uterus)
3. tumor of cartilage (benign or noncancerous tumor)
4. flesh tumor of cartilage (cancerous, malignant tumor)
5. pertaining to the nucleus
6. pertaining to above or upon the stomach (upper middle region of the abdominopelvic cavity)
7. pertaining to between the vertebrae
8. pertaining to the hip bone
9. pertaining to the back (dorsal)
10. pertaining to the navel or umbilicus

K

1. abdomen or abdominal cavity
2. cartilage
3. chromosomes
4. diaphragm
5. larynx
6. sagittal—note spelling with two t's.
7. cervical
8. chondroma
9. nucleus
10. tracheal

L

1. visceral
2. sarcoma
3. thoracic
4. karyotype
5. mitochondria—memory tip: catabolism and mitochondria and cat and mouse!
6. mediastinum
7. pituitary gland
8. epithelial

M

1. superficial
2. RUQ; LUQ
3. dorsal
4. periumbilical
5. karyotype
6. abdominal

X. Pronunciation of Terms

To test your understanding of the terminology in this chapter, write the meaning of each term in the space provided. In addition, you may wish to cover the terms and write them by looking at your definitions. Make sure your spelling is correct. The page number after each term indicates where it is defined or used in the text so you can easily check your responses. (If you are not sure what the pronunciation symbols mean, refer to page 21.)

Term	Pronunciation	Meaning
abdomen (39)	ĂB-dō-měn or ăb-DŌ-měn	
abdominal cavity (39)	ăb-DŎM-ĭ-năl KĂ-vĭ-tē	
adipose (35)	ĂD-ĭ-pōs	
anabolism (32)	ă-NĂB-ō-lĭzm	
anterior (49)	an-TĒ-rē-ŏr	
cartilage (35)	KĂR-tĭ-lĭj	
catabolism (32)	kă-TĂB-ō-lĭsm	
cell membrane (32)	sĕl MĔM-brān	
cephalic (49)	sĕ-FĂL-ĭk	
cervical (50)	SĔR-vĭ-kăl	
chondroma (50)	kŏn-DRŌ-mă	
chondrosarcoma (50)	kŏn-drō-săr-KŌ-mă	
chromosome (32)	KRŌ-mō-sōm	
coccygeal (46)	kŏk-sĭ-JĒ-ăl	
coccyx (50)	KŎK-sĭks	
cranial cavity (39)	KRĀ-nē-ăl KĂ-vĭ-tē	
craniotomy (50)	krā-nē-ŎT-ō-mē	
cytoplasm (32)	SĪ-tō-plăzm	
diaphragm (39)	DĪ-ă-frăm	
disk (disc) (46)	dĭsk	
distal (49)	DĬS-tăl	
dorsal (39)	DŎR-săl	
endoplasmic reticulum (32)	ĕn-dō-PLĂZ-mĭk rē-TĬK-ū-lŭm	

epigastric (45)	ĕp-ĭ-GĂS-trĭk	_____
epithelial cell (35)	ĕp-ĭ-THĒ-lē-ăl sĕl	_____
frontal plane (49)	FRŬN-tăl plān	_____
genes (32)	gēnz	_____
histology (51)	hĭs-TŎL-ō-jē	_____
hypochondriac (45)	hī-pō-KŎN-drē-ăk	_____
hypogastric (45)	hĭ-pō-GĂS-trĭk	_____
iliac (51)	ĬL-ē-ăk	_____
inguinal (45)	ĬNG-gwĭ-năl	_____
intervertebral (52)	ĭn-tĕr-VĔR-tĕ-brăl or ĭn-tĕr-vĕr-TĒ-brăl	_____
karyotype (32)	KĂR-ē-ō-tīp	_____
larynx (35)	LĂR-ĭnks	_____
lateral (49)	LĂT-ĕr-al	_____
lumbar (46)	LŬM-băr	_____
lumbosacral (51)	lŭm-bō-SĀ-krăl	_____
medial (49)	MĒ-dē-ăl	_____
mediastinum (39)	mē-dē-ă-STĪ-nŭm	_____
metabolism (32)	mĕ-TĂB-ō-lĭzm	_____
mitochondria (32)	mī-tō-KŎN-drē-ă	_____
nucleic (51)	nū-KLĒ-ĭk	_____
nucleus (32)	NŪ-klē-ŭs	_____
pelvic cavity (39)	PĔL-vĭk KĂ-vĭ-tē	_____
peritoneum (39)	pĕ-rĭ-tō-NĒ-um	_____
pharynx (35)	FĂR-ĭnks	_____
pituitary gland (35)	pĭ-TŪ-ĭ-tăr-ē glănd	_____
pleura (39)	PLOO-ră	_____
pleural cavity (39)	PLOOR-ăl KĂ-vĭ-tē	_____

posterior (49)	pōs-TĒR-ē-ŏr
prone (49)	prōn
proximal (49)	PRŎK-sĭ-măl
sacral (46)	SĀ-krăl
sacrum (45)	SĀ-krŭm
sagittal plane (49)	SĂJ-ĭ-tăl plān
sarcoma (51)	săr-KŌ-mă
spinal cavity (39)	SPĪ-năl KĂ-vĭ-tē
spinal cord (46)	SPĪ-năl kŏrd
spinal column (46)	SPĪ-năl KŎL-ŭm
supine (49)	SŪ-pīn
thoracic cavity (39)	thō-RĂS-ĭk KĂ-vĭ-tē
thoracotomy (51)	thō-ră-KŎT-ō-mē
thyroid gland (35)	THĪ-royd glănd
trachea (35)	TRĀ-kē-ă
tracheal (51)	TRĀ-kē-ăl
transverse plane (49)	trănz-VĔRS plān
umbilical (45)	ŭm-BĬL-ĭ-kăl
ureter (35)	Ū-rĕ-tĕr or ū-RĒ-tĕr
urethra (35)	ū-RĒ-thră
uterus (35)	Ū-tĕ-rŭs
ventral (39)	VĔN-trăl
vertebra (46)	VĔR-tĕ-bră
vertebrae (46)	VĔR-tĕ-brā
vertebral (52)	VĔR-tĕ-brăl or vĕr-TĒ-brăl
viscera (35)	VĬS-ĕr-ă
visceral (52)	VĬS-ĕr-ăl

XI. Review Sheet

Write the meaning of each combining form in the space provided and test yourself. Check your answers with the information in the chapter or in the Glossary (Medical Terms—English) at the end of the book.

Combining Forms

Combining Form	Meaning	Combining Form	Meaning
abdomin/o	_____	lumb/o	_____
adip/o	_____	medi/o	_____
anter/o	_____	nucle/o	_____
bol/o	_____	pelv/o	_____
cervic/o	_____	poster/o	_____
chondr/o	_____	proxim/o	_____
chrom/o	_____	sacr/o	_____
coccyg/o	_____	sarc/o	_____
crani/o	_____	spin/o	_____
cyt/o	_____	thel/o	_____
dist/o	_____	thorac/o	_____
dors/o	_____	trache/o	_____
hist/o	_____	umbilic/o	_____
inguin/o	_____	ventr/o	_____
ili/o	_____	vertebr/o	_____
kary/o	_____	viscer/o	_____
later/o	_____		

Continued on following page

Prefixes

Prefix	Meaning	Prefix	Meaning
ana-	_____	hypo-	_____
cata-	_____	inter-	_____
epi-	_____	meta-	_____

Suffixes

Suffix	Meaning	Suffix	Meaning
-eal	_____	-ose	_____
-ectomy	_____	-plasm	_____
-iac	_____	-somes	_____
-ior	_____	-tomy	_____
-ism	_____	-type	_____
-oma	_____		

Label the regions and quadrants of the abdominopelvic cavity.

Regions

Quadrants

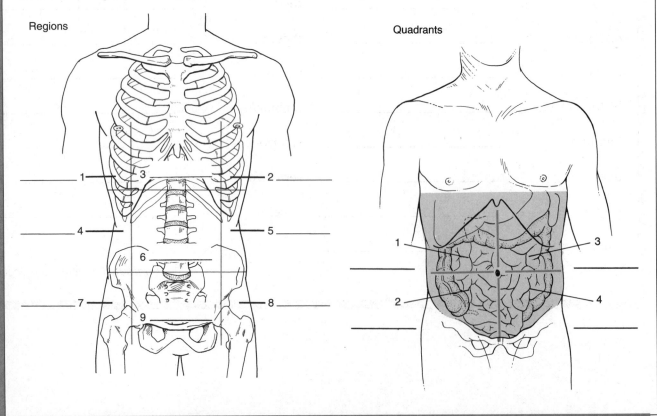

Name the divisions of the spinal column.

neck region (C1–C7) _____

chest region (T1–T12) _____

lower back (loin) region (L1–L5) _____

region of the sacrum (S1–S5) _____

tailbone region _____

Name the planes of the body.

vertical plane that divides the body into anterior and posterior portions

_____

horizontal plane that divides the body into upper and lower portions

_____

vertical plane that divides the body into right and left portions

_____

Name the positional and directional terms.

front of the body _____

back of the body _____

away from the surface _____

on the surface _____

far from the point of attachment to the trunk or far from the beginning of a structure

_____

near the point of attachment to the trunk or near the beginning of a structure

_____

Continued on following page

below another structure _____

above another structure _____

pertaining to the side _____

pertaining to the middle _____

lying on the belly _____

lying on the back _____

Give the meanings of the following terms that pertain to the cell.

chromosomes _____

mitochondria _____

nucleus _____

DNA _____

endoplasmic reticulum _____

cell membrane _____

catabolism _____

anabolism _____

metabolism _____

Give the term that suits the meaning provided.

membrane surrounding the lungs _____

membrane surrounding the abdominal viscera _____

muscular wall separating the thoracic and abdominal cavities _____

space between the lungs, containing the heart, windpipe, aorta _____

a back bone _____

a pad of cartilage between each back bone and the next _____

Suffixes

This Chapter is divided into the following sections

In this Chapter you will

- Define new suffixes and review those presented in previous chapters;
- Gain practice in word analysis by using these suffixes with combining forms to build and understand terms; and
- Name and know the functions of the different types of blood cells in the body.

I. Introduction

This chapter has three purposes. The first is to teach many of the most common suffixes in the medical language. As you work through the entire book, the suffixes mastered in this chapter will appear often. An additional group of basic suffixes is presented in Chapter 6.

The second purpose is to teach new combining forms and use them to make words with suffixes. Your analysis of the terminology in Section III of this chapter will increase your medical language vocabulary.

The third purpose is to expand your understanding of terminology beyond basic word analysis. The appendices in Section IV give additional explanations of many terms listed. In particular, emphasis is placed on learning the names and functions of different types of blood cells. These terms are basic to the vocabulary of a person working in the allied health field.

II. Combining Forms

Read this list and underline those combining forms that are unfamiliar.

Combining Form	Meaning
abdomin/o	abdomen
acr/o	extremities, top, extreme point
acu/o	sharp, severe, sudden
aden/o	gland
agor/a	marketplace
amni/o	amnion (sac surrounding the embryo in the uterus)
angi/o	vessel
arteri/o	artery
arthr/o	joint
axill/o	armpit
blephar/o	eyelid
bronch/o	bronchial tubes (two tubes, one right and one left, that branch from the trachea to enter the lungs)
carcin/o	cancer
chem/o	drug, chemical
chondr/o	cartilage
chron/o	time
col/o	colon (large intestine)
cyst/o	urinary bladder
encephal/o	brain
hydr/o	water, fluid

inguin/o	groin
isch/o	to hold back
lapar/o	abdomen, abdominal wall
laryng/o	larynx (voice box)
lymph/o	lymph

Lymph is clear fluid that bathes tissue spaces and is contained in special lymph vessels and nodes throughout the body.

mamm/o	breast
mast/o	breast
morph/o	shape, form
muc/o	mucus
myel/o	spinal cord, bone marrow

Context of usage indicates which meaning is intended.

my/o	muscle
necr/o	death (of cells or whole body)
nephr/o	kidney
neur/o	nerve
ophthalm/o	eye
oste/o	bone
ot/o	ear
path/o	disease
peritone/o	peritoneum
phag/o	to eat, swallow
plas/o	formation, development
pleur/o	pleura (membranes surrounding lungs and adjacent to chest wall muscles)
pneumon/o	lungs

pulmon/o	lungs
rect/o	rectum
ren/o	kidney
sarc/o	flesh
splen/o	spleen
staphyl/o	clusters
strept/o	twisted chains
thorac/o	chest
thromb/o	clot
tonsill/o	tonsils
trache/o	trachea (windpipe)
ven/o	vein

III. Suffixes and Terminology

Noun Suffixes

The following is a list of the most common noun suffixes. A medical term is given to illustrate the use of the suffix. The basic rule for building a medical word is that the combining vowel, such as **o**, is used to connect the root to the suffix, with the exception that the combining vowel is *not* used before suffixes that begin with a vowel. For example: **gastr/itis**, *not* **gastr/o/itis**.

Numbers above certain terms direct you to an Appendix that follows this list. The Appendix contains additional information that will help you understand the terminology.

Suffix	Meaning	Terminology	Meaning
-algia	pain	arthr<u>algia</u>	joint pain
		ot<u>algia</u>	ear
		neur<u>algia</u>	nerve
		my<u>algia</u>	muscle

-cele	hernia[1]	recto<u>cele</u> _____
		cysto<u>cele</u> _____
-centesis	surgical puncture to remove fluid	thoraco<u>centesis</u> _____
		This term may be shortened to thoracentesis.
		amnio<u>centesis</u>[2] _____
		abdomino<u>centesis</u> _____
		This procedure is also known as a paracentesis.
-coccus (plural: **-cocci**)[3]	berry-shaped bacterium (plural: bacteria)	strepto<u>coccus</u>[4] _____
		staphylo<u>cocci</u> _____
-cyte	cell	erythro<u>cyte</u>[5] _____
		leuko<u>cyte</u> _____
		thrombo<u>cyte</u> _____
-dynia	pain	pleuro<u>dynia</u> _____
		Pain in the chest wall muscles that is aggravated by breathing.
-ectomy	excision, removal, resection	laryng<u>ectomy</u>[6] _____
		mast<u>ectomy</u> _____
-emia	blood condition	an<u>emia</u>[7] _____
		isch<u>emia</u>[8] _____
-genesis	condition of producing, forming	carcino<u>genesis</u> _____
		patho<u>genesis</u> _____
		angio<u>genesis</u> _____

---

[1] See Appendix A.
[2] See Appendix B.
[3] See Appendix C.
[4] See Appendix D.
[5] See Appendix E.
[6] See Appendix F.
[7] See Appendix G.
[8] See Appendix H.

-genic	pertaining to producing, produced by, or in	carcinogenic _____
		osteogenic _____
		An osteogenic sarcoma is a tumor produced by bone tissue.
-gram	record	electroencephalogram _____
		myelogram _____
		Myel/o means spinal cord in this term. This is an x-ray record taken after contrast material is injected into membranes around the spinal cord.
		mammogram _____
-graph	instrument for recording	electroencephalograph _____
-graphy	process of recording	electroencephalography _____
		angiography _____
-itis	inflammation	bronchitis _____
		tonsillitis[9] _____
		blepharitis _____
-logy	study of	ophthalmology _____
		morphology _____
-lysis	breakdown, destruction, separation	hemolysis _____
		Breakdown of red blood cells with release of hemoglobin.
-malacia	softening	osteomalacia _____
		chondromalacia _____
-megaly	enlargement	acromegaly[10] _____
		splenomegaly[11] _____
-oma	tumor, mass, collection of fluid	myoma _____
		This is a benign tumor.

---

[9] See Appendix I.
[10] See Appendix J.
[11] See Appendix K.

myosarc<u>oma</u> _____

This is a malignant tumor. Muscle is a type of flesh (sarc/o) tissue.

multiple myel<u>oma</u> _____

Myel/o means bone marrow in this term. This is a malignant tumor that occurs in bone marrow throughout the body.

hemat<u>oma</u> _____

-opsy	to view	bi<u>opsy</u> _____

necr<u>opsy</u> _____

Autopsy or post mortem examination.

-osis	condition, usually abnormal	necr<u>osis</u> _____

hydronephr<u>osis</u> _____

leukocyt<u>osis</u>[12] _____

lymphocyt<u>osis</u> _____

-pathy	disease condition	cardiomy<u>opathy</u> _____
-penia	deficiency	erythro<u>penia</u> _____

leuko<u>penia</u> _____

thrombocyto<u>penia</u> _____

-phobia	fear	acro<u>phobia</u> _____

Fear of heights.

agora<u>phobia</u> _____

An anxiety disorder marked by fear of venturing out into a crowded place.

-plasia	development, formation, growth	achondro<u>plasia</u>[13] _____
-plasty	surgical repair	angio<u>plasty</u> _____

A narrowed blood vessel is opened using a balloon that is inflated after it is inserted into the blood vessel.

---

[12] See Appendix L.
[13] See Appendix M.

-ptosis[14]	drooping, sagging, prolapse	blepharo<u>ptosis</u> _____
-sclerosis	hardening	arterio<u>sclerosis</u> _____

Atherosclerosis is a form of arteriosclerosis in which the artery becomes clogged with deposits of fat (ather/o means fatty material).

-scope	instrument for visual examination	laparo<u>scope</u> _____
-scopy	process of visual examination	laparo<u>scopy</u>[15] _____
-stasis	stopping, controlling	meta<u>stasis</u> _____

Meta- means beyond. A metastasis is the spreading of a malignant tumor beyond its original site to a secondary organ or location.

hemo<u>stasis</u> _____

Blood flow is stopped naturally by clotting or artificially by compression.

-stomy	opening to form a mouth (stoma)	colo<u>stomy</u> _____
		tracheo<u>stomy</u> _____
-therapy	treatment	hydro<u>therapy</u> _____
		chemo<u>therapy</u> _____
		radio<u>therapy</u> _____
-tomy	incision, to cut into	laparo<u>tomy</u> _____

This is called exploratory surgery.

-trophy	nourishment, development	hyper<u>trophy</u> _____

Cells increase in size, not number. Muscles of weight lifters often hypertrophy.

a<u>trophy</u> _____

Cells decrease in size. Muscles atrophy when they are immobilized in a cast and not in use.

---

[14] See Appendix N.
[15] See Appendix O.

The following are shorter noun suffixes that are usually attached to roots in words.

Suffix	Meaning	Terminology	Meaning
-er	one who	radiograph<u>er</u> _____	
		A technologist who assists in the making of diagnostic x-ray pictures.	
-ia	condition	leukem<u>ia</u> _____	
		pneumon<u>ia</u> _____	
-ist	one who specializes in	nephrolog<u>ist</u> _____	
-ole	little, small	arteri<u>ole</u>[16] _____	
-ule	little, small	ven<u>ule</u> _____	
-um, -ium	structure, tissue, thing	pericard<u>ium</u> _____	
		The pericardium is a membrane around the heart.	
-y	condition, process	nephropath<u>y</u> _____	

Adjective Suffixes

The following are adjective suffixes. There is no simple rule indicating which suffix meaning _pertaining to_ is used with a specific combining form. Your job is to recognize the types of adjectival suffixes in each term.

Suffix	Meaning	Terminology	Meaning
-ac, -iac	pertaining to	cardi<u>ac</u> _____	
-al	pertaining to	periton<u>eal</u> _____	
		inguin<u>al</u> _____	
		pleur<u>al</u> _____	
-ar	pertaining to	tonsill<u>ar</u> _____	

_____

[16]See Appendix P.

-ary	pertaining to	pulm<u>ary</u> _____
		axill<u>ary</u> _____
-eal	pertaining to	laryng<u>eal</u> _____
-ic, -ical	pertaining to	chron<u>ic</u> _____

Acute is the opposite of chronic. It describes a disease that is of rapid onset, severe symptoms, and brief duration.

		patholog<u>ical</u> _____
-oid	resembling	aden<u>oid</u>s[17] _____
		epiderm<u>oid</u> _____

An epidermoid carcinoma is composed of cells that resemble epidermis (outer skin) tissue.

-ose	pertaining to, full of	adip<u>ose</u> _____
-ous	pertaining to	muc<u>ous</u> _____

Mucus (a noun) is the sticky secretion produced by mucous membranes.

-tic	pertaining to	necro<u>tic</u> _____

IV. Appendices

Appendix A: Hernia

A **hernia** is a bulging forth, or protrusion, of an organ or the muscular wall of an organ through the cavity that normally contains it. Some examples of hernias are a hiatal hernia (the stomach protrudes upward into the mediastinum through the esophageal opening in the diaphragm; see Fig. 5–20, page 148) and an inguinal hernia (part of the intestine protrudes downward into the groin region and commonly into the scrotal sac in the male; see Fig. 5–20). A rectocele is a protrusion of the rectum toward the vagina, and a cystocele is a protrusion of the urinary bladder toward the vagina (Fig. 3–1). These hernias often occur in women after many vaginal births. Symptoms appear in older women in the postmenopausal years when estrogen loss weakens tissue supports.

Appendix B: Amniocentesis

The amnion is the sac (membrane) that surrounds the embryo (called the fetus after the 8th week) in the uterus. Fluid accumulates within the sac and can be withdrawn (**amnio-**

---

[17]See Appendix Q.

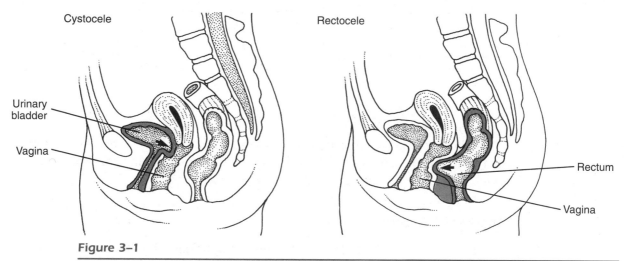

Cystocele

Urinary bladder

Vagina

Rectocele

Rectum

Vagina

Figure 3–1

Cystocele and rectocele. (From Ignatavicius DD, Bayne MV: Medical-Surgical Nursing: A Nursing Process Approach. Philadelphia, WB Saunders, 1991.)

centesis) for analysis after the 13th week of pregnancy. Cells of the fetus are in the fluid and are grown (cultured) for microscopic analysis. A karyotype is made to analyze chromosomes, and the fluid is examined for high levels of certain chemicals that indicate defects in the developing spinal cord and spinal column of the fetus (Fig. 3–2).

Appendix C: Plurals

Words ending in **-us** commonly form their plural by dropping the **-us** and adding **-i.** Thus, nucleus becomes nuclei and coccus becomes cocci (KŎK-sī). A guide to formation of plurals is found in Appendix A at the end of the book.

Appendix D: Streptococcus and Staphylococcus

A **streptococcus** is a berry-shaped bacterium that grows in twisted chains. One group of streptococci are responsible for such conditions as "strep" throat, tonsillitis, rheumatic fever, and certain kidney ailments, whereas another group cause infections in teeth, in the sinuses (cavities) of nose and face, and sometimes in the valves of the heart.

A **staphylococcus** is a bacterium that grows in small clusters, like grapes. Staphylococcal lesions may be external (skin abscesses, boils, styes) or internal (abscesses in bone and kidney). (An abscess is a collection of pus, white blood cells, and protein that is present at

Figure 3–2

Amniocentesis. Under ultrasound (sound wave images) guidance, a needle is inserted through the abdominal and uterine walls into the amniotic cavity. A syringe is attached and amniotic fluid is withdrawn. The doctor uses continuous ultrasound pictures to locate the fetus and other structures within the uterus, and ensure the proper placement of the needle. (From Moore KL, Persaud TVN: Before We Are Born: Essentials of Embryology and Birth Defects, 4th ed. Philadelphia, WB Saunders, 1993, p 89.)

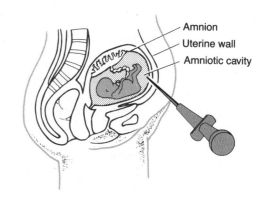

Amnion

Uterine wall

Amniotic cavity

Streptococci

Staphylococci

Figure 3–3

Types of coccal bacteria.

the site of infection.) Figure 3–3 illustrates the pattern of growth of streptococci and staphylococci.

Other bacteria that are coccal in shape include **pneumococci** (pneum/o = lungs), which are the most common cause of bacterial pneumonia in adults, and **gonococci** (gon/o = seed), which invade the reproductive organs and cause gonorrhea.

Appendix E: Blood Cells

Study Figure 3–4 as you read the following to note the differences among the three different types of cells in the blood.

ERYTHROCYTES

(No nucleus;
contains hemoglobin)

On side view

LEUKOCYTES

Granulocytes

Nucleus is
multilobed

(1) eosinophil
granules stain red

(2) basophil
granules stain blue

(3) neutrophil
granules stain purple
(polymorphonuclear
leukocyte)

Agranulocytes

One large
nucleus

(4) lymphocyte

(5) monocyte

THROMBOCYTES

(Platelets)

Figure 3–4

Types of blood cells.

Erythrocytes (red blood cells). These cells are made in the bone marrow (soft tissue in the center of certain bones) and are necessary to carry oxygen from the lungs through the blood to all body cells. The oxygen is then used up by body cells in the process of converting food to energy (catabolism). **Hemoglobin** (globin = protein) is an important protein in erythrocytes that carries the oxygen through the bloodstream.

Leukocytes (white blood cells). There are several types of leukocytes:

Granulocytes (cells with dark-staining granules in their cytoplasm) are formed in bone marrow. There are three types of granulocytes:

1. **Eosinophils** (granules stain red [eosin/o = rosy] with acid stain) are thought to be active and elevated in allergic conditions such as asthma. About 3 per cent of leukocytes are eosinophils.

2. **Basophils** (granules stain blue with basic [bas/o = basic] stain). The function of basophils is not clear, but they play a role in inflammation. Less than 1 per cent of leukocytes are basophils.

3. **Neutrophils** (granules stain blue and red [purple] with neutral stain) are important disease-fighting cells. They are called **phagocytes** (phag/o = eating, swallowing) because they engulf and digest bacteria like tiny Pac men. They are the most numerous disease-fighting "soldiers" and are often called **polymorphonuclear leukocytes** because of their nucleus, which is multilobed (poly = many, morph/o = shape). Almost 60 per cent of leukocytes are neutrophils.

Agranulocytes (cells without dark-staining granules in cytoplasm) are produced by lymph nodes and spleen. There are two types of agranulocytes:

4. **Lymphocytes** (lymph cells) fight disease by producing antibodies and thus destroying foreign cells. They may also attach directly to foreign cells and destroy them. Two types of lymphocytes are T cells and B cells. About 32 per cent of leukocytes are lymphocytes.

5. **Monocytes** (cells with one [mon/o = one] very large nucleus) engulf and destroy cellular debris after neutrophils have attacked foreign cells. Monocytes leave the bloodstream and enter tissues (such as lung and liver) to become **macrophages,** which are large phagocytes. Monocytes make up about 4 per cent of all leukocytes.

Thrombocytes or **Platelets** (clotting cells). These tiny fragments of blood cells are formed in the bone marrow and are necessary for blood clotting.

Appendix F: Pronunciation Clue

Pronunciation clue: The letters **g** and **c** are soft (as in ginger and cent) when followed by an **i** or **e,** and are hard (as in good and can) when followed by an **o** or **a.**

For example: laryngitis (lăr-ĭn-JĪ-tĭs)
laryngotomy (lă-rĭn-GŎT-ō-mē)

Appendix G: Anemia

Anemia literally means no blood. In medical language and usage, anemia refers to a medical condition in which there is a *reduction* in the number of erythrocytes or amount of hemoglobin in the circulating blood. There are many different kinds of anemias, classified on the basis of the many different problems that can arise with red blood cells, their circulation, and content. **Aplastic** (a- = no, plas/o = formation) **anemia** is a severe type in which the bone marrow fails to produce not only erythrocytes but leukocytes and thrombocytes as well.

Appendix H: Ischemia

Ischemia literally means to hold back (isch/o) blood (-emia) from a part of the body. Tissue that becomes **ischemic** loses its normal flow of blood and becomes deprived of oxygen. The ischemia can be caused by mechanical injury to a blood vessel, by blood clots lodging in a vessel, or by the gradual closing off (occlusion) of a vessel owing to collection of fatty material.

Appendix I: Tonsillitis

Tonsils (notice the spelling with one letter l, whereas the combining form has a double letter l) are lymphatic tissue in the throat. They contain white blood cells (lymphocytes) and function to filter and fight bacteria, but they can also become infected and inflamed. Streptococcal infection of the throat can cause **tonsillitis,** which may lead to **tonsillectomy.**

Appendix J: Acromegaly

Acromegaly is an example of an endocrine disorder. The **pituitary gland** attached to the base of the brain produces an excessive amount of growth hormone after the completion of puberty. Hence, a person with acromegaly is of normal height, because the long bones have stopped growth after puberty, but has an abnormally large growth of bones and tissue in the hands, feet, and face. High levels of growth hormone before completion of puberty produce excessive growth of long bones (gigantism) as well as acromegaly.

Appendix K: Splenomegaly

The spleen is an organ in the left upper quadrant of the abdomen (below the diaphragm and to the side of the stomach). It is composed of lymph tissue and blood vessels. Its job is to dispose of dying red blood cells and manufacture white blood cells (lymphocytes) to fight disease. If the spleen must be removed (splenectomy), other organs carry out these functions.

Appendix L: Leukocytosis

When **-osis** is used as a suffix with blood cells, it means an abnormal condition in which there is a slight increase in number of normal circulating blood cells. Thus, in leukocytosis a slight elevation in numbers of *normal* white blood cells occurs in response to the presence of infection in the body. When **-emia** is used as a suffix with blood cells (**-cyte** is usually dropped, as in leukemia), the condition is an *abnormally* high or excessive increase in number of abnormal or cancerous blood cells.

Appendix M: Achondroplasia

Achondroplasia is an inherited disorder in which the bones of the arms and legs fail to grow to normal size owing to a defect in both cartilage and bone. It results in a type of dwarfism characterized by short limbs, a normal-sized head and body, and normal intelligence (Fig. 3–5).

Appendix N: -ptosis

The suffix **-ptosis** is pronounced TŌ-sĭs. The rule is that when two consonants begin a word, the first is silent. If the two consonants are found in the middle of a word, both are

Figure 3–5

A child with achondroplasia. This child also has a curved back and protruding abdomen. (Courtesy of Dr. Harry Medovy, Children's Centre, Winnipeg.)

pronounced. For example blepharoptosis (blĕ-făr-ŏp-TŌ-sĭs). The term **ptosis** is used alone to mean the drooping of or inability to use the upper eyelid.

Appendix O: Laparoscopy

Laparoscopy (also known as peritoneoscopy) is a visual examination of the peritoneal cavity (abdomen) with the use of a laparoscope. The laparoscope is inserted through an incision in the abdomen near the navel, and gas is infused into the peritoneal cavity. This procedure is used to examine the organs in the abdomen for evidence of disease or to perform surgical procedures such as biopsies and tying off of the uterine (fallopian) tubes (Fig. 3–6).

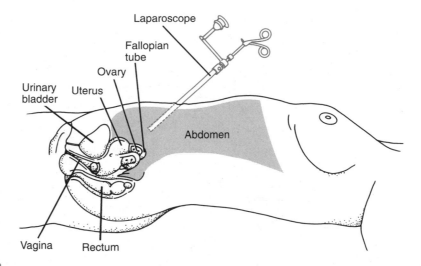

Figure 3–6

Laparoscopy. (From Chabner DE: Medical Terminology: A Short Course. Philadelphia, WB Saunders, 1990.)

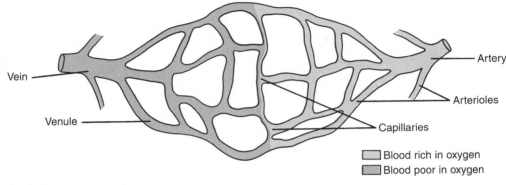

Figure 3–7

Relationship of blood vessels.

Removal of the gallbladder and appendix can also be performed laparoscopically. As a highly accurate diagnostic tool, laparoscopy is used to avoid surgical intervention (laparotomy) and is termed **minimally invasive surgery.**

Appendix P: Arteriole

The relationship between an artery, **arterioles,** capillaries (tiniest of blood vessels), a venule, and a vein is illustrated in Figure 3–7.

Appendix Q: Adenoids

The **adenoids** (the literal meaning is resembling glands, since they are neither endocrine nor exocrine glands) are lymphatic tissue in the part of the throat near the nose and nasal passages. Enlargement of this tissue may cause blockage of the airway from the nose to the throat, and adenoidectomy may be advised. The tonsils are also lymphatic tissue and their location as well as that of the adenoids is indicated in Figure 3–8.

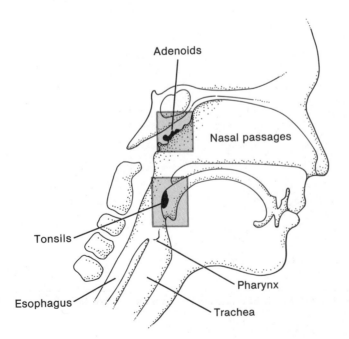

Figure 3–8

Adenoids and tonsils. (From Chabner DE: Medical Terminology: A Short Course. Philadelphia, WB Saunders, 1990.)

V. Exercises

Remember to check your answers carefully with those given in Section VI, Answers to Exercises.

A. Give the meanings for the following suffixes.

1. -cele _____   7. -ectomy _____

2. -emia _____   8. -centesis _____

3. -coccus _____   9. -genesis _____

4. -gram _____   10. -graph _____

5. -cyte _____   11. -itis _____

6. -algia _____   12. -graphy _____

B. Using the following combining forms and your knowledge of suffixes, build the following medical terms.

strept/o	amni/o	laryng/o	carcin/o
staphyl/o	rect/o	isch/o	myel/o
mast/o	cyst/o	ot/o	bronch/o
thorac/o	angi/o	arthr/o	my/o

1. hernia of the urinary bladder _____ cytocele _____

2. pain of muscle _____ myelgeha _____

3. process of producing cancer _____ carcinogensis _____

4. record of the spinal cord _____

5. berry-shaped bacteria in twisted chains _____ streptococcus _____

6. surgical puncture to remove fluid from the chest _____ thoracocentesis _____

7. removal of the breast _____ masectomy _____

8. inflammation of the tubes leading from the windpipe to the lungs _____ bronchitis _____

9. to hold back blood from cells _____ ischemia _____

10. process of recording (x-ray) blood vessels _____

11. record (x-ray) of joints _____

12. berry-shaped bacteria in clusters _____

13. resection of the voice box _____ laryngotomy _____

14. surgical procedure to remove fluid from the sac around the fetus _____ amniocentesis _____

C. Match the following terms that describe blood cells with their meanings below.

eosinophil	monocyte	erythrocyte
thrombocyte	neutrophil	lymphocyte
basophil		

1. a granulocytic white blood cell that destroys foreign cells by engulfing and digesting them; also called

    polymorphonuclear leukocyte _____ neutrophil _____

2. an agranular white blood cell that destroys foreign cells by making antibodies

    _____

3. a clotting cell; also called a platelet _____ thrombocyte _____

4. a leukocyte whose granules turn red with stain and whose numbers are elevated in allergic reactions

    _____ eosinophil _____

5. a red blood cell _____ erythrocyte _____

6. an agranular white blood cell that engulfs and digests cellular debris and contains one large nucleus

    _____ mac monocyte _____

7. a white blood cell containing granules in its cytoplasm and prominent in causing an inflammatory

    reaction _____

D. Give the meanings for the following suffixes.

1. -logy _____   8. -megaly _____

2. -lysis _____   9. -oma _____

3. -pathy _____   10. -opsy _____

4. -penia _____   11. -plasia _____

5. -malacia _____   12. -plasty _____

6. -osis _____   13. -sclerosis _____

7. -phobia _____   14. -stasis _____

E. Using the following combining forms and your knowledge of suffixes, build the following medical terms.

hydr/o	splen/o	cardi/o
blephar/o	hem/o	acr/o
my/o	myel/o	rhin/o
nephr/o	bi/o	arteri/o
chondr/o	morph/o	agor/a
sarc/o		

1. fear of the marketplace (crowds) _____

2. enlargement of the spleen _____

3. study of the shape (of cells) _____

4. softening of cartilage _____

5. abnormal condition of water (fluid) in the kidney _____

6. disease condition of heart muscle _____

7. hardening of arteries _____

8. tumor (benign) of muscle _____

9. flesh tumor (malignant) of muscle _____

10. surgical repair of the nose _____

11. tumor of bone marrow _____

12. fear of heights _____

13. view of living tissue under the microscope _____

14. stoppage of the flow of blood (by mechanical or natural means) _____

15. inflammation of the eyelid _____

F. Match the following terms with their meanings below.

acromegaly	achondroplasia	chemotherapy
laparoscopy	metastasis	hydrotherapy
osteomalacia	laparoscope	hypertrophy
necrosis	colostomy	atrophy

1. treatment using drugs _____ *chemo therapy* _____

2. condition of death (of cells) _____ *necrosis* _____

3. softening of bone _____ *osteo malacia* _____

4. opening of the large intestine to the outside of the body *Colostomy* _____

5. no development; shrinkage of cells _____ *atrophy* _____

6. beyond control; spread of a cancerous tumor to another organ _____

7. instrument to visually examine the abdomen _____ *laparascope* _____

8. enlargement of extremities; an endocrine disorder that causes excess growth hormone to be produced

   from the pituitary gland after puberty _____ *acromegally* _____

9. condition of improper formation of cartilage in the embryo that leads to short bones and dwarf-like

   deformities _____ *a chondro plasia* _____

10. process of viewing the peritoneal (abdominal) cavity _____ *laparoscopy* _____

11. treatment using water _____ *hydrotherapy* _____

12. excessive development of cells (increase in size of individual cells) _____ *hypertrophy* _____

G. Give the meanings for the following suffixes.

1. -ia _____

2. -trophy _____

3. -stasis _____

4. -stomy _____

5. -tomy _____

6. -ole _____

7. -um _____

8. -ule _____

9. -y _____

10. -oid _____

11. -genic _____

12. -ptosis _____

H. Using the following combining forms and suffixes, build the following medical terms.

Combining Forms

pneumon/o	pleur/o
nephr/o	mamm/o
arteri/o	lapar/o
ven/o	radi/o

Suffixes

-gram	-ia	-pathy
-tomy	-ule	-plasty
-scopy	-dynia	-ectomy
-therapy	-ole	

1. incision of the abdomen _____

2. process of visual examination of the abdomen _____

3. a small artery _____

4. condition of the lungs _____

5. treatment using x-rays _____

6. record (x-ray) of the breast _____

7. pain of the chest wall and the membranes surrounding the lungs _____

8. a small vein _____

9. disease condition of the kidney _____

10. surgical repair of the breast _____

I. Underline the suffix in the following terms and give the meaning of the entire term.

1. laryngeal _____

2. inguinal _____

3. chronic _____

4. pulmonary _____

5. adipose _____

6. peritoneal _____

7. axillary _____

8. necrotic _____

9. epidermoid _____

10. mucous _____

J. *Select from the following terms relating to blood and blood vessels to complete the sentences below.*

ischemia	leukemia	hematoma
anemia	multiple myeloma	arterioles
hemostasis	leukocytosis	venules
thrombocytopenia	angioplasty	hemolysis

1. Billy was diagnosed as having excessively high numbers of cancerous white blood cells, a disease known as ___*leukemia*___ . Chemotherapy was prescribed by his doctor, and his prognosis is excellent.

2. Mr. Preston's angiogram showed that he had serious atherosclerosis of one of the arteries supplying blood to his heart. His doctor recommended that ___*angioplasty*___ would be helpful to open up his clogged artery by threading a catheter (tube) through his artery and opening a balloon at the end of the catheter to widen the artery.

3. Mrs. Jackson's blood count showed a greatly reduced number of red blood cells, a condition called ___*thrombocytopenia*___ . The cause of this condition was destruction of her (red) blood cells, known as ___*anemia*___ .

4. Doctors were unable to operate on Joe Hite because his platelet count was so low. His condition is called ___*anemia*___ .

5. Blockage of an artery leading to Mr. Stein's brain led to holding back of blood flow to nerve tissue in his brain. This condition, called ___*ischemia*___ , could lead to necrosis of tissue and a cerebrovascular accident.

6. Small arteries, called ___*arterioles*___ , were broken under Ms. Bein's scalp when she was struck on the head with a rock. She soon developed a mass of blood, called a (an) ___*hematoma*___ , under the skin in that region of her head.

7. Sarah Jones had a staphylococcal infection that caused her white blood cell count to be elevated. This slight elevation of white blood cells is called ___*leukocytosis*___ .

8. The factory for making blood cells is the bone marrow (soft inner tissue within bones). Mr. Brill developed cancerous bone marrow cells in the marrow of his hip, upper arm, and thigh bones, a condition diagnosed as ___*leukocytosis*___ .

9. During surgery, it is important to maintain ___*hemostasis*___ by using clamps to close off blood vessels.

10. Small vessels that carry blood back toward the heart from the capillaries and tissues of the body are

known as _____ *venules* _____ .

K. *Complete the medical term for the following definitions.*

Definition   *Medical Term*

1. The membrane surrounding the heart   peri _____

2. Hardening of arteries   arterio _____

3. Enlargement of the liver   hepato _____

4. New opening of the windpipe to the outside of the body   tracheo _____

5. Inflammation of the tonsils   _____ itis

6. Surgical puncture to remove fluid from the abdomen   abdomino_____

7. Muscle pain   my _____

8. Pertaining to the membranes surrounding the lungs   _____ al

9. Study of the eye   _____ logy

10. Berry-shaped bacteria in clusters   _____ cocci

11. Beyond control (spread of a cancerous tumor)   meta _____

12. Pertaining to the voice box   _____ eal

L. *Select the correct term to complete the following sentences.*

1. Ms. Daley has nine children and presents to her doctor complaining of problems urinating. After examining her, the doctor finds her bladder protruding into her vagina and tells her she has a (rectocele, cystocele, hiatal hernia).

2. Suzy coughed constantly for a week. Her doctor told her that her chest x-ray showed pneumonia. Her sputum (material coughed up from her chest) demonstrated (ischemic, pleuritic, pneumococcal) bacteria.

3. Mr. Manion went to the doctor complaining that he couldn't keep his left upper eyelid from sagging. His doctor told him that he had a neurological problem called Horner's syndrome, characterized by (necrosis, hydronephrosis, ptosis) of his eyelid.

4. After 6 weeks in a cast to set her broken arm, Jill's arm muscles were smaller and weaker. They had (atrophied, hypertrophied, metastasized) and she was advised to have physical therapy to strengthen them.

5. Ms. Brody was diagnosed with breast cancer. The first phase of her treatment included a (nephrectomy, mastectomy, pulmonary resection) to remove her breast and the tumor. Following the surgery her doctors recommended (chemotherapy, radiotherapy, hydrotherapy) using drugs such as methotrexate and 5-fluorouracil.

6. As she grew older, Mrs. Brandwein's facial features became coarser, her hands and tongue became bigger, and doctors told her she had a slowly progressive endocrine condition called (thyromegaly, splenomegaly, acromegaly).

VI. Answers to Exercises

A

1. hernia
2. blood condition
3. berry-shaped bacterium
4. record
5. cell
6. pain
7. removal, excision, resection
8. surgical puncture to remove fluid
9. process of producing, forming
10. instrument to record
11. inflammation
12. process of recording

B

1. cystocele
2. myalgia (myodynia is not used)
3. carcinogenesis
4. myelogram
5. streptococci (bacteria is a plural term)
6. thoracocentesis or thoracentesis
7. mastectomy
8. bronchitis
9. ischemia
10. angiography
11. arthrogram
12. staphylococci
13. laryngectomy
14. amniocentesis

C

1. neutrophil
2. lymphocyte
3. thrombocyte
4. eosinophil
5. erythrocyte
6. monocyte
7. basophil

D

1. process of study
2. breakdown, separation, destruction
3. process of disease
4. deficiency, less than normal
5. softening
6. condition, abnormal condition
7. fear of
8. enlargement
9. tumor, mass
10. process of viewing
11. condition of formation, growth
12. surgical repair
13. hardening, to harden
14. to stop, control

E

1. agoraphobia
2. splenomegaly
3. morphology
4. chondromalacia
5. hydronephrosis
6. cardiomyopathy
7. arteriosclerosis
8. myoma
9. myosarcoma
10. rhinoplasty
11. myeloma (called multiple myeloma)
12. acrophobia
13. biopsy
14. hemostasis
15. blepharitis

F

1. chemotherapy
2. necrosis
3. osteomalacia
4. colostomy
5. atrophy
6. metastasis
7. laparoscope
8. acromegaly
9. achondroplasia
10. laparoscopy
11. hydrotherapy
12. hypertrophy

G

1. condition
2. development, nourishment
3. to stop, control
4. new opening
5. incision, cut into
6. small, little
7. structure
8. small, little
9. condition, process
10. resembling
11. pertaining to producing, produced by or in
12. prolapse, drooping, sagging

H

1. laparotomy
2. laparoscopy
3. arteriole
4. pneumonia (this condition is actually pneumonitis)
5. radiotherapy
6. mammogram
7. pleurodynia
8. venule
9. nephropathy
10. mammoplasty

I

1. laryngeal —pertaining to the voice box
2. inguinal —pertaining to the groin
3. chronic —pertaining to time (over a long period of time)
4. pulmonary —pertaining to the lung

5. adipose —pertaining to (or full of) fat
6. peritoneal —pertaining to the peritoneum (membrane around the abdominal organs)
7. axillary —pertaining to the armpit, under arm

8. necrotic —pertaining to death
9. epidermoid —resembling epidermis (outer layer of skin)
10. mucous —pertaining to mucus

J

1. leukemia
2. angioplasty
3. anemia; hemolysis
4. thrombocytopenia

5. ischemia
6. arterioles; hematoma
7. leukocytosis

8. multiple myeloma
9. hemostasis
10. venules

K

1. pericardium
2. arteriosclerosis
3. hepatomegaly
4. tracheostomy
5. tonsillitis

6. abdominocentesis (this procedure is also known as a paracentesis)
7. myalgia
8. pleural

9. ophthalmology
10. staphylococci
11. metastasis
12. laryngeal

L

1. cystocele
2. pneumococcal
3. ptosis

4. atrophied
5. mastectomy; chemotherapy
6. acromegaly

VII. Pronunciation of Terms

To test your understanding of the terminology in this chapter, write the meaning of each term in the space provided. In addition, you may wish to cover the terms and write them by looking at your definitions. Make sure your spelling is correct. The page number after each term indicates where it is defined or used in the text so you can easily check your responses. (If you are not sure what the pronunciation symbols mean, refer to page 21.)

Term	Pronunciation	Meaning
abdominocentesis (71)	ăb-dŏm-ĭ-nō-sĕn-TĒ-sĭs	_____
achondroplasia (73)	ā-kŏn-drō-PLĀ-zē-ă	_____
acromegaly (72)	ăk-rō-MĔG-ă-lē	_____
acrophobia (73)	ăk-rō-FŌ-bē-ă	_____
acute (76)	ă-KŪT	_____
adenoids (76)	ĂD-ĕ-noydz	_____
adipose (76)	Ă-dĭ-pōs	_____
agoraphobia (73)	ă-gŏr-ă-FŌ-bē-ă	_____
angiogenesis (71)	ăn-jē-ō-JĔN-ĕ-sĭs	_____
amniocentesis (71)	ăm-nē-ō-sĕn-TĒ-sĭs	_____
anemia (71)	ă-NĒ-mē-ă	_____
angiography (72)	ăn-jē-ŎG-ră-fē	_____

angioplasty (73)	ăn-jē-ō-PLĂS-tē	_____
arteriole (75)	ăr-TĒR-ē-ōl	_____
arteriosclerosis (74)	ăr-tē-rē-ō-sklĕ-RŌ-sĭs	_____
arthralgia (70)	ăr-THRĂL-jă	_____
atrophy (74)	ĂT-rō-fē	_____
axillary (76)	ĂK-sĭ-lār-ē	_____
basophil (79)	BĀ-sō-fĭl	_____
biopsy (73)	BĪ-ŏp-sē	_____
blepharitis (72)	blĕ-fă-RĪ-tĭs	_____
blepharoptosis (74)	blĕ-fă-rŏp-TŌ-sĭs	_____
bronchitis (72)	brŏng-KĪ-tĭs	_____
carcinogenesis (71)	kăr-sĭ-nō-JĚN-ĕ-sĭs	_____
cardiomyopathy (73)	kăr-dē-ō-mī-ŎP-ă-thē	_____
chemotherapy (74)	kē-mō-THĚR-ă-pē	_____
chondromalacia (72)	kŏn-drō-mă-LĀ-shă	_____
chronic (76)	KRŎN-ĭk	_____
colostomy (74)	kō-LŎS-tō-mē	_____
cystocele (71)	SĬS-tō-sēl	_____
electroencephalogram (72)	ē-lĕk-trō-ĕn-SĚF-ă-lō-grăm	_____
electroencephalograph (72)	ē-lĕk-trō-ĕn-SĚF-ă-lō-grăf	_____
electroencephalography (72)	ē-lĕk-trō-ĕn-sĕf-ă-LŎG-ră-fē	_____
eosinophil (79)	ē-ō-SĬN-ō-fĭl	_____
epidermoid (76)	ĕp-ĭ-DĔR-moyd	_____
erythrocyte (71)	ĕ-RĬTH-rō-sīt	_____
erythropenia (73)	ĕ-rĭth-rō-PĒ-nē-ă	_____
hematoma (73)	hē-mă-TŌ-mă	_____
hemolysis (72)	hē-MŎL-ĭ-sĭs	_____
hemostasis (74)	hē-mō-STĀ-sĭs	_____

hydronephrosis (73)   hī-drō-nĕ-FRŌ-sĭs   _____

hydrophobia (68)   hī-drō-FŌ-bē-ă   _____

hydrotherapy (74)   hī-drō-THĔR-ă-pē   _____

hypertrophy (74)   hī-PĔR-trō-fē   _____

inguinal (75)   ĬNG-wă-năl   _____

ischemia (71)   ĭs-KĒ-mē-ă   _____

laparoscope (74)   LĂP-ă-rō-skōp   _____

laparoscopy (74)   lă-pă-RŎS-kō-pē   _____

laparotomy (74)   lăp-ă-RŎT-ō-mē   _____

laryngeal (76)   lă-RĬN-jē-ăl or lăr-ĭn-JĒ-ăl   _____

laryngectomy (71)   lăr-ĭn-JĔK-tō-mē   _____

leukemia (75)   lū-KĒ-mē-ă   _____

leukocytosis (73)   lū-kō-sī-TŌ-sĭs   _____

leukopenia (73)   lōō-kō-PĒ-nē-ă   _____

lymphocyte (79)   LĬM-fō-sīt   _____

lymphocytosis (73)   lĭm-fō-sī-TŌ-sĭs   _____

mammogram (72)   MĂM-mō-grăm   _____

mastectomy (71)   măs-TĔK-tō-mē   _____

metastasis (74)   mĕ-TĂS-tă-sĭs   _____

monocyte (79)   MŎN-ō-sīt   _____

morphology (72)   mŏr-FŎL-ō-jē   _____

mucous (76)   MŪ-kŭs   _____

myalgia (70)   mī-ĂL-jă   _____

myelogram (72)   MĪ-ĕ-lō-grăm   _____

myeloma (73)   mī-ĕ-LŌ-mă   _____

myoma (72)   mī-Ō-mă   _____

myosarcoma (73)   mī-ō-săr-KŌ-mă   _____

necrosis (73)   nĕ-KRŌ-sĭs   _____

necrotic (76)	nĕ-KRŎT-ĭk	
nephrologist (75)	nĕ-FRŎL-ō-jĭst	
nephropathy (75)	nĕ-FRŎP-ă-thē	
neuralgia (70)	nū-RĂL-jă	
neutrophil (79)	NŪ-trō-fĭl	
ophthalmology (72)	ŏf-thăl-MŎL-ō-jē	
osteogenic (72)	ŏs-tē-ō-JĔN-ĭk	
osteomalacia (72)	ŏs-tē-ō-mă-LĀ-shă	
otalgia (70)	ō-TĂL-jă	
paracentesis (71)	pă-ră-cĕn-TĒ-sĭs	
pathogenesis (71)	păth-ŏ-JĔN-ĕ-sĭs	
pericardium (75)	pĕr-ē-KĂR-dē-ŭm	
peritoneal (75)	pĕr-ĭ-tō-NĒ-ăl	
platelet (79)	PLĀT-lĕt	
pleurodynia (71)	plŭr-ō-DĬN-ē-ă	
pneumonia (75)	nū-MŌN-yă	
polymorphonuclear leukocyte (79)	pŏl-ē-mŏr-fō-NŪ-klē-ăr LŪ-kō-sīt	
pulmonary (76)	PŬL-mō-nă-rē	
radiotherapy (74)	rā-dē-ō-THĔ-ră-pē	
rectocele (71)	RĔK-tō-sēl	
splenomegaly (72)	splē-nō-MĔG-ă-lē	
staphylococci (71)	stăf-ĭ-lō-KŎK-sī	
streptococcus (71)	strĕp-tō-KŎK-ŭs	
thoracentesis (71)	thō-ră-sĕn-TĒ-sĭs	
thrombocytopenia (73)	thrŏm-bō-sī-tō-PĒ-nē-ă	
tonsillitis (72)	tŏn-sĭ-LĪ-tĭs	
tracheostomy (74)	trā-kē-ŎS-tō-mē	
venule (75)	VĔN-ūl	

VIII. Review Sheet

Write the meanings of each word part in the space provided and test yourself. Check your answers with the information in the chapter or in the glossary (Medical Terms—English) at the end of the book.

Noun Suffixes

Suffix	Meaning	Suffix	Meaning
-algia	_____	-ole	_____
-cele	_____	-oma	_____
-centesis	_____	-opsy	_____
-coccus	_____	-osis	_____
-cyte	_____	-pathy	_____
-dynia	_____	-penia	_____
-ectomy	_____	-phobia	_____
-emia	_____	-plasia	_____
-er	_____	-plasty	_____
-genesis	_____	-ptosis	_____
-genic	_____	-sclerosis	_____
-gram	_____	-scope	_____
-graph	_____	-scopy	_____
-graphy	_____	-stasis	_____
-ia	_____	-stomy	_____
-ist	_____	-therapy	_____
-itis	_____	-tomy	_____
-logy	_____	-trophy	_____
-lysis	_____	-ule	_____
-malacia	_____	-um, -ium	_____
-megaly	_____	-y	_____

Continued on following page

Adjective Suffixes

Suffix	Meaning	Suffix	Meaning
-ac	_____	-oid	_____
-al	_____	-ose	_____
-ary	_____	-ous	_____
-eal	_____	-tic	_____
-ic, -ical	_____		

Combining Forms

Combining Form	Meaning	Combining Form	Meaning
abdomin/o	_____	chem/o	_____
acr/o	_____	chondr/o	_____
aden/o	_____	chron/o	_____
adip/o	_____	col/o	_____
agor/a	_____	cyst/o	_____
amni/o	_____	encephal/o	_____
angi/o	_____	erythr/o	_____
arteri/o	_____	hem/o	_____
arthr/o	_____	hepat/o	_____
axill/o	_____	hydr/o	_____
bi/o	_____	inguin/o	_____
blephar/o	_____	lapar/o	_____
bronch/o	_____	laryng/o	_____
carcin/o	_____	leuk/o	_____
cardi/o	_____	lymph/o	_____

mamm/o	_____	pleur/o	_____
mast/o	_____	pneumon/o	_____
morph/o	_____	pulmon/o	_____
muc/o	_____	radi/o	_____
my/o	_____	rect/o	_____
myel/o	_____	rhin/o	_____
necr/o	_____	sarc/o	_____
nephr/o	_____	splen/o	_____
neur/o	_____	staphyl/o	_____
nucle/o	_____	strept/o	_____
ophthalm/o	_____	thorac/o	_____
oste/o	_____	thromb/o	_____
ot/o	_____	tonsill/o	_____
peritone/o	_____	ven/o	_____
plas/o	_____		

Do you remember the following combining forms from previous chapters?

Combining Form	Meaning	Combining Form	Meaning
anter/o	_____	later/o	_____
cephal/o	_____	onc/o	_____
cervic/o	_____	poster/o	_____
crani/o	_____	ren/o	_____
dist/o	_____	trache/o	_____
dors/o	_____	vertebr/o	_____
gynec/o	_____	viscer/o	_____

4

Prefixes

This Chapter is divided into the following sections

In this Chapter you will

- Define basic prefixes used in the medical language;
- Analyze medical terms that combine prefixes and other word elements; and
- Learn about the Rh condition as an example of an antigen-antibody reaction.

I. Introduction

This chapter on prefixes, like the preceding chapter on suffixes, is designed to give you practice in word analysis and provide a foundation for the study of the terminology of body systems that follows.

The list of combining forms, suffixes, and their meanings in Section II will help you analyze the terminology in the rest of the chapter. The appendices (Section IV) are included to give more complete understanding of the terms and to explain the words with reference to the anatomy, physiology, and diseases of the body.

II. Combining Forms and Suffixes

Combining Forms	
Combining Form	**Meaning**
carp/o	wrist bones
cib/o	meals
cis/o	to cut
cost/o	rib
cutane/o	skin
dactyl/o	fingers, toes
duct/o	to lead, carry
flex/o	to bend
furc/o	forking, branching
gloss/o	tongue
glyc/o	sugar
immun/o	protection
morph/o	shape, form
mort/o	death
nat/i	birth
nect/o	to bind, tie, connect
norm/o	rule, order
ox/o	oxygen
seps/o	infection
somn/o	sleep
son/o	sound

the/o	to put, place
thel/o	nipple
thyr/o	shield; the shape of the thyroid gland resembled (-oid) a shield to those who named it.
top/o	place, position, location
tox/o	poison
trache/o	windpipe, trachea
urethr/o	urethra

Suffixes

Suffix	Meaning
-blast	embryonic, immature
-cyesis	pregnancy
-drome	to run
-fusion	to pour
-gen	producing, forming
-lapse	to slide, fall, sag
-lysis	breakdown, separation, loosening
-meter	to measure
-mission	to send
-or	one who
-partum	birth, labor
-phoria	to bear, carry; feeling (mental state)
-physis	to grow
-plasia	development, formation
-plasm	development, formation

-pnea	breathing	
-ptosis	droop, sag, prolapse	
-rrhea	flow, discharge	
-stasis	to stop, control	
-trophy	nourishment, development	

III. Prefixes and Terminology

Write the meaning of the medical term in the space provided.

Prefix	Meaning	Terminology	Meaning
a-, an-	no, not, without	apnea _____	
		anoxia _____	
ab-	away from	abnormal _____	
		abductor _____	
		A muscle that draws a limb away from the body.	
ad-	toward	adductor _____	
		adrenal glands[1] _____	
ana-	up, apart	anabolism _____	
		analysis _____	
		Psychoanalysis is a psychiatric therapy that explores the mind. Urinalysis (urin/o + [an]alysis) is laboratory examination of urine to aid in diagnosis.	
ante-	before, forward	ante cibum _____	
		a. c. is a notation on prescription orders. It means prior to (before) meals.	
		anteflexion _____	
		ante partum _____	

---

[1] See Appendix A.

anti- against   antisepsis _____

An antiseptic (-sis changes to -tic to form an adjective) substance is used against infections. Anti- is pronounced ăn-tŭh.

antibiotic[2] _____

antigen[3] _____

In this word, anti- stands for antibody.

antibody _____

antitoxin _____

auto- self, own   autoimmune[4] _____

bi- two   bifurcation _____

bilateral _____

brady- slow   bradycardia _____

cata- down   catabolism _____

con- with, together   congenital anomaly[5] _____

connective _____

contra- against, opposite   contraindication _____

Contra- means against in this term.

contralateral[6] _____

Contra- means opposite in this term.

de- down, lack of   dehydration _____

dia- through, complete   diameter _____

diarrhea _____

dialysis[7] _____

dys- bad, painful, difficult, abnormal   dyspnea _____

dysplasia _____

---

[2] See Appendix B.
[3] See Appendix C.
[4] See Appendix D.
[5] See Appendix E.
[6] See Appendix F.
[7] See Appendix G.

ec-, ecto-	out, outside	<u>ec</u>topic pregnancy[8] _____
en-, endo-	in, within	<u>endo</u>tracheal _____
		<u>endo</u>scope _____
		<u>endo</u>cardium _____
epi-	upon, on, above	<u>epi</u>thelium _____
eu-	good, normal	<u>eu</u>thyroid _____

Normal thyroid function.

<u>eu</u>phoria _____

Exaggerated feeling of well-being.

| **ex-** | out, away from | <u>ex</u>ophthalmia _____ |

Protrusion of the eyeball associated with enlargement and overactivity of the thyroid gland.

| **hemi-** | half | <u>hemi</u>glossectomy _____ |
| **hyper-** | excessive, above, | <u>hyper</u>plasia _____ |

Increase in cell numbers.

<u>hyper</u>trophy _____

Increase in size of individual cells.

<u>hyper</u>glycemia _____

hypo-	deficient, under	<u>hypo</u>dermic _____
		<u>hypo</u>glycemia _____
in-	not	<u>in</u>somniac _____
in-	into	<u>in</u>cision _____
infra-	beneath	<u>infra</u>costal _____
inter-	between	<u>inter</u>costal _____
intra-	into, within	<u>intra</u>venous _____
macro-	large	<u>macro</u>cephalic _____

---

[8] See Appendix H.

mal-	bad	malignant _____

From the Latin ignis meaning fire. Benign (ben- = good) tumors are non-cancerous, whereas malignant tumors are cancerous.

malaise _____

From the French malaise meaning a vague feeling of bodily discomfort.

meta-	change, beyond	metamorphosis _____

Meta- means change in this term.

metastasis _____

Meta- means beyond in this term.

metacarpal bones _____

These are five hand bones. They lie beyond the wrist bones, but before the finger bones (phalanges).

micro-	small	microscope _____
neo-	new	neoplasm _____
		neonatal _____
pan-	all	pancytopenia _____

Deficiency of erythrocytes, leukocytes, and thrombocytes.

para-	near, beside, abnormal	parathyroid glands[9] _____
		paralysis _____

Abnormal disruption of the connection between nerve and muscle. Originally from the Greek paralusis meaning to separate, loosen on one side, describing the loss of movement on one side of the body (occurring with stroke patients).

per-	through	percutaneous _____
peri-	surrounding	pericardium _____
		periosteum _____
poly-	many, much	polymorphonuclear _____
		polyneuritis _____
post-	after, behind	post mortem _____
		postnatal _____

[9] See Appendix I.

pre-	before, in front of	precancerous _____
		prenatal _____
pro-	before, forward	prodrome _____

Prodromal symptoms (rash, fever) appear before the actual illness and signal its onset.

prolapse[10] _____

| **pseudo-** | false | pseudocyesis _____ |

Development of signs of pregnancy but without the presence of an embryo.

| **re-** | back, again | relapse _____ |

A disease or its symptoms return after an apparent recovery.

remission _____

Symptoms lessen and the patient feels better.

recombinant DNA[11] _____

retro-	behind, backward	retroperitoneal _____
		retroflexion _____
sub-	under	subcutaneous _____
supra-	above, upper	suprathoracic _____
		suprarenal glands _____
syn-, sym-	together, with	syndactyly _____
		synthesis _____
		syndrome[12] _____

Before the letters b, p, and m, syn becomes sym.

symbiosis[13] _____

symmetry _____

What is asymmetry?

symphysis[14] _____

---

[10] See Appendix J.
[11] See Appendix K.
[12] See Appendix L.
[13] See Appendix M.
[14] See Appendix N.

tachy-	fast	tachypnea _____
trans-	across, through	transfusion _____
		transurethral[15] _____
ultra-	beyond, excess	ultrasonography[16] _____
uni-	one	unilateral _____

IV. Appendices

Appendix A: Adrenal Glands

The **adrenal glands** (also called suprarenal glands) are endocrine glands located above each kidney. They secrete chemicals called hormones that affect the functioning of the body. One of these hormones is called adrenaline (epinephrine). It causes the bronchial tubes to widen, the heart to beat more rapidly, and blood pressure to rise (Fig. 4–1).

Appendix B: Antibiotic

An **antibiotic** is a chemical that destroys or inhibits the growth of microorganisms (small living things) such as bacteria. The first antibiotic, penicillin, was produced from immature plants called molds or fungi.

Appendix C: Antigens and Antibodies; The Rh Condition

An **antigen** is a substance, usually foreign to the body (such as a poison, virus, or bacterium), that stimulates the production of antibodies. **Antibodies** are protein substances made by white blood cells in response to the presence of foreign antigens. For

---

[15] See Appendix O.
[16] See Appendix P.

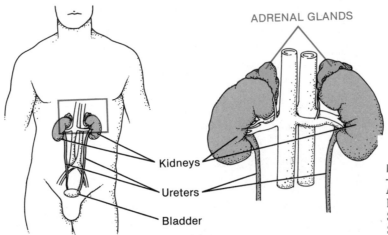

ADRENAL GLANDS

Kidneys
Ureters
Bladder

Figure 4–1

Adrenal glands. (From Chabner DE: Medical Terminology: A Short Course. Philadelphia, WB Saunders, 1990.)

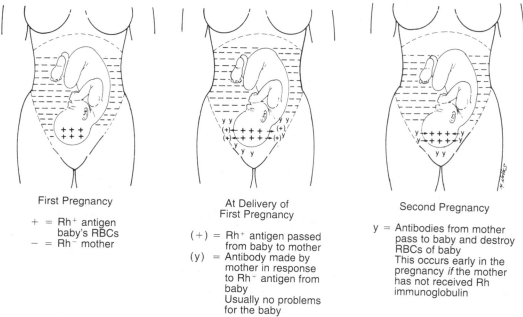

First Pregnancy

\+ = Rh⁺ antigen
baby's RBCs
− = Rh⁻ mother

**At Delivery of
First Pregnancy**

(+) = Rh⁺ antigen passed
from baby to mother
(y) = Antibody made by
mother in response
to Rh⁺ antigen from
baby
Usually no problems
for the baby

Second Pregnancy

y = Antibodies from mother
pass to baby and destroy
RBCs of baby
This occurs early in the
pregnancy *if* the mother
has not received Rh
immunoglobulin

Figure 4–2

Rh condition as an example of an antigen-antibody reaction.

example, the flu virus (antigen) enters the body, causing the production of antibodies in the bloodstream. These antibodies will then attach to and destroy the antigens (viruses) that produced them. The reaction between an antigen and an antibody is called an immune reaction (immun/o means protection).

Another example of an antigen-antibody in the **Rh condition**. A person who is Rh⁺ has a protein coating (antigen) on his or her red blood cells (RBCs). This antigen factor is something that the person is born with and is normal for him or her. A person who is Rh⁻ has normal RBCs as well, but they do not carry the Rh factor antigen.

If an Rh⁻ woman and an Rh⁺ man conceive an embryo, the embryo may be Rh⁻ or Rh⁺. A dangerous condition arises only when the embryo is Rh⁺. During delivery of the first Rh⁺ baby, some of the baby's blood cells containing antigens may escape into the mother's bloodstream. This sensitizes the mother so that she produces a low level of antibodies to the Rh⁺ antigen. Because this occurs at delivery, the first baby is generally not affected and is normal at birth. Sensitization can also occur after a miscarriage or an abortion.

Difficulties arise with the second Rh⁺ pregnancy. If the embryo is Rh⁺ again, during pregnancy the mother's acquired antibodies will enter the infant's bloodstream and attack the infant's RBCs (Rh⁺). The infant's RBCs are destroyed, and the infant attempts to compensate for this loss of cells by making many new immature RBCs (erythroblasts). The infant is born with a condition known as **erythroblastosis fetalis,** or **hemolytic disease of the newborn** (HDN). One of the clinical symptoms of erythroblastosis fetalis is jaundice, or yellow skin pigmentation. The jaundice results from the excessive destruction of RBCs, which causes a substance called **bilirubin** (chemical pigment produced when hemoglobin from dying RBCs is broken down) to accumulate in the blood.

To prevent HDN, Rh immune globulin is given to the mother at 28 weeks of pregnancy and within 72 hours after each Rh⁺ delivery or after every abortion and miscarriage if the father is Rh⁺. The globulin binds to Rh⁺ cells that have escaped into the mother's circulation, and thus prevents the mother from making Rh⁺ antibodies. This ensures that future babies will not develop HDN. Figure 4–2 reviews the antigen-antibody reaction in the Rh condition in diagrammatic fashion.

Appendix D: Autoimmune

Part of the normal immune reaction (protecting the body against foreign invaders) involves making antibodies to fight against viruses and bacteria. However, in an **autoimmune** reaction, the body makes antibodies against its own good cells and tissues, causing inflammation and injury. Examples of autoimmune disorders are rheumatoid arthritis (joints are affected), systemic lupus erythematosus (connective tissues, skin, and internal organs are affected), and Graves disease (hyperthyroidism—the thyroid gland is affected).

Appendix E: Congenital Anomaly

An anomaly is an irregularity in a structure or organ. Examples of **congenital anomalies** (those that an infant is born with) are webbed fingers or toes (syndactyly) and heart defects. Some congenital anomalies are recognized as hereditary (passed to the infant through chromosomes from the father or mother, or both), whereas others are produced by factors during pregnancy (for example, cocaine addiction in the mother produces addiction and brain damage in the infant at birth).

Appendix F: Contralateral

The effect of a stroke (cerebral ischemia or necrosis) on the limbs of the body is **contralateral.** This means that if the brain damage is located on the right side of the brain, the patient will have paralysis on the left side of the body. The muscles on one side of the body are controlled by nerves from the opposite side (contralateral) of the brain. **Ipsilateral (ipsi-** means same) refers to the same side.

Appendix G: Dialysis

Dialysis literally means complete separation. A dialysis machine (artificial kidney) can completely separate out from the blood the harmful waste products of the body that are normally removed by the urine.

Appendix H: Ectopic Pregnancy

In a normal pregnancy, the embryo develops within the uterus. In an **ectopic pregnancy,** the embryo is implanted outside the uterus—most often it is found in the uterine (fallopian) tubes, and sometimes in the ovary or abdominal cavity (Fig. 4–3).

Appendix I: Parathyroid Glands

There are four **parathyroid glands** located on the dorsal side of the thyroid gland. The parathyroids are endocrine glands that produce a hormone and function entirely separately from the thyroid gland. The **parathyroid hormone** increases blood calcium and maintains it at a normal level.

Appendix J: Prolapse

-Lapse means to slide, sag, or fall. If an organ or tissue **prolapses,** it slides forward or downward. Prolapse of the uterus is a common example. If the muscles that hold the uterus in place become weak, the uterus may slide downward toward the vagina (Fig. 4–4).

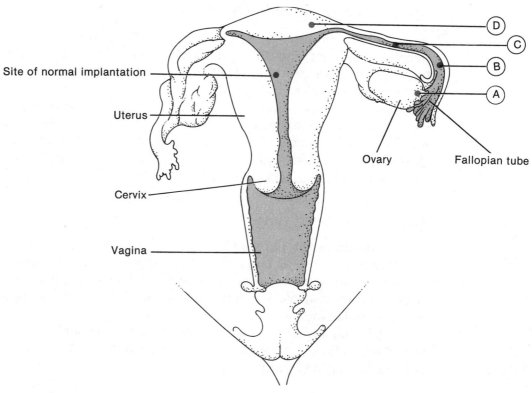

Figure 4–3

Sites of ectopic pregnancies (A, B, C, D). (From Chabner DE: Medical Terminology: A Short Course. Philadelphia, WB Saunders, 1990.)

Ptosis (TŌ-sĭs) is another term that has the same meaning as prolapse. Ptosis of the eyelid occurs when the eyelid muscles are weak and a person has difficulty voluntarily lifting the eyelid to keep the eye open. **Proptosis** (forward prolapse) also is used to refer to the eye and means a bulging or forward protrusion of the eyeball, as in exophthalmia.

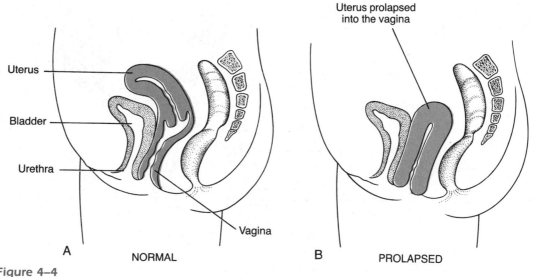

Figure 4–4

Uterine prolapse.

Appendix K: Recombinant DNA

This is the process of taking a gene (region of DNA) from one organism and inserting it (recombining it) into the DNA of another organism. An example is the **recombinant DNA** technique used to manufacture insulin outside the body. The gene that codes for insulin (i.e., contains the recipe for making insulin) is cut out of a human chromosome (using special enzymes) and transferred into a bacterium, such as *Escherichia coli*. The bacterium then contains the gene for making human insulin and, because it divides very rapidly, can produce insulin in large quantities. The insulin is given to diabetic patients who are unable to make their own insulin. Polymerase chain reaction (PCR) is a new method of producing multiple copies of a single gene, and is an important tool for making recombinant DNA.

Appendix L: Syndrome

A **syndrome** is a group of signs or symptoms that commonly occur together and indicate a particular disease or abnormal condition. An example of a syndrome is Reye syndrome, characterized by vomiting, swelling of the brain, increased intracranial pressure, hypoglycemia, and dysfunction of the liver. It can occur in children following a viral infection that has been treated with aspirin.

Fetal alcohol syndrome is a group of symptoms (pre- and postnatal growth deficiency, mental retardation, microcephaly, heart defects) in an infant, caused by the mother's intake of alcohol during pregnancy.

Appendix M: Symbiosis

Symbiosis refers to the living together in close association of two organisms, either for mutual benefit or not. The bacteria that normally live in the digestive tract of humans are an

Figure 4–5

Prostate gland.

Figure 4–6

Ultrasonography. Notice that the 30-week fetus is sucking its thumb. (Courtesy of Stuart Campbell.)

example of symbiosis. **Parasitism** is an example of symbiosis in which one organism benefits and the other does not.

In psychiatry, symbiosis is a relationship between two persons who are emotionally dependent on each other.

Appendix N: Symphysis

A **symphysis** is a type of joint in which the bony surfaces are firmly united by a plate of cartilage. Examples are the pubic symphysis where the pubic bones of the pelvis have grown together and the symphysis of the two halves of the lower jaw bone (mandible) that unite before birth.

Appendix O: Transurethral

A **transurethral** resection of the prostate gland (TURP) is a removal of a portion of the prostate gland by means of an instrument that is passed through **(trans-)** the urethra. The procedure is necessary when the prostatic tissue enlarges (hypertrophies) and interferes with urination. Figure 4–5 shows the location of the prostate gland at the base of the urinary bladder.

Appendix P: Ultrasonography

Ultrasonography is a diagnostic technique using ultrasound waves (inaudible sound waves) to produce an image or photograph of an organ or tissue. The ultrasonic echoes are recorded as they pass through different types of tissue. Figure 4–6 shows an ultrasound image (sonogram) of a fetus.

V. Exercises

Remember to check your answers carefully with those given in Section VI, Answers to Exercises.

A. Give the meanings for the following prefixes.

1. ante- _____

2. ab- _____

3. ana- _____

4. anti- _____

5. a-, an- _____

6. ad- _____

7. auto- _____

8. cata- _____

9. brady- _____

10. contra- _____

11. bi- _____

12. con- _____

B. Match the following terms with their meanings below.

bilateral	adductor	bradycardia
congenital anomaly	antisepsis	apnea
contralateral	analysis	anoxia
ante partum	anteflexion	adrenal

1. bending forward _____

2. a muscle that carries the limb toward the body _____

3. before birth ___ *ante partum* _____

4. slow heartbeat ___ *bradycardia* _____

5. a gland located near (above) each kidney ___ *adrenal* ___

6. not breathing ___ *apnea* _____

7. pertaining to the opposite side ___ *contralateral* ___

8. against infection ___ *antisepsis* _____

9. to separate apart ___ *analysis* _____

10. pertaining to two (both) sides ___ *bilateral* ___

11. condition of no oxygen in tissues ___ *anoxia* ___

12. an irregularity that is present at birth ___ *cong ab* ___

C. *Select from the following terms to complete the sentences below.*

autoimmune   antibody   catabolism
antitoxin   antibiotic   contraindication
antigen   anabolism

1. A chemical substance, such as erythromycin (-mycin = mold), that is made from molds and used against

   bacterial life is a (an) _____ *antibiotic* _____ .

2. The process of burning food (breaking it down) and releasing the energy stored in the food is

   _____ *catabolism* _____ .

3. A reason that a doctor would advise against taking a specific medication would be a (an)

   _____ *contraindication* _____ .

4. A disorder in which the body's own leukocytes make antibodies that damage its own good tissue is a (an)

   _____ *autoimmune* _____ disorder.

5. A foreign agent (virus or bacterium) is known as a (an) _____ *antigen* _____
   because it causes the production of antibodies by white blood cells.

6. A protein made by lymphocytes in response to the presence in the blood of a specific antigen is a (an)

   _____ *antibody* _____ .

7. A type of antibody that acts against poisons that enter the body is a (an) _____ *antitoxin* _____ .

8. The process of building up proteins in cells by putting together small pieces of proteins, called amino

   acids, is called _____ *anabolism* _____ .

D. *Give the meanings for the following prefixes.*

1. ec- _____   9. en- _____

2. dys- _____   10. eu- _____

3. de- _____   11. in- _____

4. dia- _____   12. inter- _____

5. hemi- _____   13. intra- _____

6. hypo- _____   14. infra- _____

7. epi- _____   15. macro- _____

8. hyper- _____

E. Complete the following terms from their meanings given below.

1. normal thyroid function: _____ thyroid

2. painful breathing: _____ pnea

3. pregnancy that is out of place: _____ topic

4. instrument to visually examine within the body: endo _____

5. removal of half of the tongue: _____ glossectomy

6. good feeling (of well-being): _____ phoria

7. pertaining to within the windpipe: endo _____

8. a blood condition of less than normal sugar: _____ glycemia

9. pertaining to (having) a large head: _____ cephalic

10. pertaining to between the ribs: _____ costal

11. pertaining to within a vein: intra _____

12. condition of bad (abnormal) formation (of cells): dys _____

13. condition of excessive formation (numbers of cells): _____ plasia

14. the structure (membrane) that forms the inner lining of the heart: endo _____

15. pertaining to below the ribs: infra _____

16. a blood condition of excessive amount of sugar: hyper _____

F. Match the following terms with their meanings below.

dialysis   incision   metastasis
dehydration   malignant   pancytopenia
diarrhea   metamorphosis   microscope
insomnia   malaise   exophthalmia

1. a vague feeling of bodily discomfort ___malaise___

2. not able to sleep ___insomnia___

3. lack of water ___dehydr___

4. spread of a cancerous tumor to a secondary organ or tissue ___meta___

5. instrument to see small objects ___micro___

6. to cut into an organ or tissue _____ incision _____

7. eyeballs that bulge outward (proptosis) _____ exoph _____

8. condition of change in shape or form _____ meta _____

9. watery discharge (of wastes from the colon) _____ diarrhea _____

10. deficiency of all (blood) cells _____ pancyto _____

11. separation of wastes from the blood by using a machine that does the job of the kidney

_____ dialysis _____

12. harmful, cancerous _____ malignant _____

G. Give the meanings for the following prefixes.

1. mal- _____   11. sub- _____

2. pan- _____   12. supra- _____

3. per- _____   13. re- _____

4. meta- _____   14. retro- _____

5. para- _____   15. tachy- _____

6. peri- _____   16. syn- _____

7. poly- _____   17. uni- _____

8. post- _____   18. trans- _____

9. pro- _____   19. neo- _____

10. pre- _____   20. epi- _____

H. Underline the prefix in the following terms and give the meaning of the entire term.

1. periosteum _____

2. percutaneous _____

3. retroperitoneal _____

4. postnatal _____

5. polyneuritis _____

6. retroflexion _____

7. transurethral _____

8. subcutaneous _____

9. tachypnea _____

10. unilateral _____

11. pseudocyesis _____

I. Match the following terms with their meanings below.

syndrome	parathyroid	relapse	recombinant DNA
prodrome	suprarenal	prolapse	syndactyly
paralysis	remission	neoplasm	ultrasonography

1. disease or its symptoms return _____ *remission* *prolapse* *relapse*

2. loss of movement in muscles _____ *paralysis*

3. a congenital anomaly in which fingers or toes are webbed (formed together)

_____

4. four endocrine glands that are located near (behind) another endocrine gland in the neck

_____ *parathyroid*

5. glands that are located above the kidneys _____ *suprarenal*

6. symptoms that come before the actual illness _____ *prodrome*

7. the technique of transferring genetic material from one organism into another

_____ *rec DNA*

8. sliding, sagging downward or forward _____ *prolapse*

9. new growth or tumor _____ *neoplasm*

10. process of using sound waves to create an image of organs and structures in the body

_____ *ultrasono*

11. group of symptoms that occur together and indicate a particular disorder

_____ *prodrome* *syndrome*

12. Symptoms lessen and a patient feels better _____ *remission*

J. Complete the following terms from their meanings given below.

1. pertaining to new birth: neo _natal_

2. after death: post _Mortum_

3. spread of a cancerous tumor: meta _stasis_

4. branching into two: bi _____

5. increase in development (size of cells): hyper _trophy_

6. pertaining to a chemical that works against bacterial life: _antibiotic_ biotic

7. hand bones (beyond the wrist): _meta_ carpals

8. protein produced by leukocytes to fight foreign organisms: anti _body_

9. group of symptoms that occur together: _syn_ drome

10. surface or skin tissue of the body: _epi_ thelium

K. Select the correct term to complete each sentence.

1. A (synthesis, contralateral, contraindication) to surgery would be a bleeding disorder, such as thrombocytopenia.

2. Medical science was revolutionized by the introduction of (antigens, antibiotics, antibodies) in the 1940s. Now we can treat many infections with only one dose.

3. The elderly gentleman was having (malaise, dialysis, insomnia) despite taking the sleeping medication that his doctor prescribed.

4. During her pregnancy, Ms. Payne described pressure on her (pituitary gland, parathyroid gland, pubic symphysis), making it difficult for her to find a comfortable position.

5. Many people with diabetes accidentally take too much insulin. This results in the lowering of their blood sugar so much that they may be admitted to the Emergency Room (ER) with (hyperplasia, hypoglycemia, hyperglycemia).

VI. Answers to Exercises

A

1. before, forward	5. no, not, without	9. slow
2. away from	6. toward	10. against, opposite
3. up, apart	7. self, own	11. two
4. against	8. down	12. together, with

B

1. anteflexion	5. adrenal	9. analysis
2. adductor	6. apnea	10. bilateral
3. ante partum	7. contralateral	11. anoxia
4. bradycardia	8. antisepsis	12. congenital anomaly

C

1. antibiotic
2. catabolism
3. contraindication
4. autoimmune
5. antigen
6. antibody
7. antitoxin
8. anabolism

D

1. out, outside
2. bad, painful, difficult
3. down, lack of
4. through, complete
5. half
6. deficient, under
7. upon, on, above
8. excessive, above, beyond
9. in, within
10. good, well
11. in, not
12. between
13. within
14. below, inferior
15. large

E

1. euthyroid
2. dyspnea
3. ectopic
4. endoscope
5. hemiglossectomy
6. euphoria
7. endotracheal
8. hypoglycemia
9. macrocephalic
10. intercostal
11. intravenous
12. dysplasia
13. hyperplasia
14. endocardium
15. infracostal
16. hyperglycemia

F

1. malaise
2. insomnia
3. dehydration
4. metastasis
5. microscope
6. incision
7. exophthalmia
8. metamorphosis
9. diarrhea
10. pancytopenia
11. dialysis
12. malignant

G

1. bad
2. all
3. through
4. change, beyond
5. near, beside, abnormal
6. surrounding
7. many, much
8. after, behind
9. before, forward
10. before, in front of
11. under
12. above
13. back, again
14. behind, backward
15. fast
16. together, with
17. one
18. across, through
19. new
20. above, upon, on

H

1. periosteum—membrane (structure) surrounding bone
2. percutaneous—pertaining to through the skin
3. retroperitoneal—pertaining to behind the peritoneum
4. postnatal—pertaining to after birth
5. polyneuritis—inflammation of many nerves
6. retroflexion—bending backward
7. transurethral—pertaining to through the urethra
8. subcutaneous—pertaining to below the skin
9. tachypnea—rapid, fast breathing
10. unilateral—pertaining to one side
11. pseudocyesis—false pregnancy (no pregnancy occurs)

I

1. relapse
2. paralysis
3. syndactyly
4. parathyroid
5. suprarenal (adrenal glands)
6. prodrome
7. recombinant DNA
8. prolapse
9. neoplasm
10. ultrasonography
11. syndrome
12. remission

J

1. neonatal
2. post mortem
3. metastasis
4. bifurcation
5. hypertrophy
6. antibiotic
7. metacarpals
8. antibody
9. syndrome
10. epithelium

K

1. contraindication
2. antibiotics
3. insomnia
4. pubic symphysis
5. hypoglycemia

VII. Pronunciation of Terms

To test your understanding of the terminology in this chapter, write the meaning of each term in the space provided. In addition, you may wish to cover the terms and write them by looking at your definitions. Make sure your spelling is correct. The page number after each term indicates where it is defined or used in the text so you can easily check your responses. (If you are not sure what the pronunciation symbols mean, refer to page 21.)

Term	Pronunciation	Meaning
abductor (101)	ăb-DŬK-tŏr	_____
adductor (101)	ă-DŬK-tŏr	_____
adrenal glands (101)	ă-DRĒ-năl glăndz	_____
analysis (101)	ă-NĂL-ĭ-sĭs	_____
anoxia (101)	ă-NŎK-sē-ă	_____
anteflexion (101)	ăn-tē-FLĔK-shŭn	_____
ante partum (101)	ĂN-tē PĂR-tŭm	_____
antibiotic (102)	ăn-tĭ-bī-ŎT-ĭk	_____
antibody (102)	ĂN-tĭ-bŏd-ē	_____
antigen (102)	ĂN-tĭ-jĕn	_____
antisepsis (102)	ăn-tĭ-SĔP-sĭs	_____
antitoxin (102)	ăn-tĭ-TŎK-sĭn	_____
apnea (101)	ĂP-nē-ă or ăp-NĒ-ă	_____
autoimmune (102)	ăw-tō-ĭ-MŪN	_____
benign (104)	bē-NĪN	_____
bifurcation (102)	bī-fŭr-KĀ-shŭn	_____
bilateral (102)	bī-LĂT-ĕr-ăl	_____
bradycardia (102)	brăd-ē-KĂR-dē-ă	_____
congenital anomaly (102)	kŏn-JĔN-ĭ-tăl ă-NŎM-ă-lē	_____
contraindication (102)	kŏn-tră-ĭn-dĭ-KĀ-shŭn	_____
contralateral (102)	kŏn-tră-LĂT-ĕr-ăl	_____
dehydration (102)	dē-hī-DRĀ-shŭn	_____
dialysis (102)	dī-ĂL-ĭ-sĭs	_____
diarrhea (102)	dī-ă-RĒ-ă	_____
dysplasia (102)	dĭs-PLĀ-zē-ă	_____
dyspnea (102)	DĬSP-nē-ă or dĭsp-NĒ-ă	_____
ectopic pregnancy (103)	ĕk-TŎP-ĭk PRĔG-năn-sē	_____
endocardium (103)	ĕn-dō-KĂR-dē-ŭm	_____

endoscope (103)	ĔN-dō-skōp	_____
endotracheal (103)	ĕn-dō-TRĀ-kē-ăl	_____
epithelium (103)	ĕp-ĭ-THĒ-lē-ŭm	_____
euphoria (103)	ū-FŎR-ē-ă	_____
euthyroid (103)	ū-THĪ-royd	_____
exophthalmia (103)	ĕk-sŏf-THĂL-mē-ă	_____
hemiglossectomy (103)	hĕm-ē-glŏs-SĔK-tō-mē	_____
hyperglycemia (103)	hī-pĕr-glī-SĒ-mē-ă	_____
hyperplasia (103)	hī-pĕr-PLĀ-zē-ă	_____
hypertrophy (103)	hī-PĔR-trō-fē	_____
hypodermic (103)	hī-pō-DĔR-mĭk	_____
hypoglycemia (103)	hī-pō-glī-SĒ-mē-ă	_____
infracostal (103)	ĭn-fră-KŎS-tăl	_____
insomniac (103)	ĭn-SŎM-nē-ăk	_____
intercostal (103)	ĭn-tĕr-KŎS-tăl	_____
intravenous (103)	ĭn-tră-VĒ-nŭs	_____
macrocephalic (103)	măk-rŏ-sĕ-FĂL-ĭk	_____
malaise (104)	măl-ĀZ	_____
malignant (104)	mă-LĬG-nănt	_____
metamorphosis (104)	mĕt-ă-MŎR-fŏ-sĭs	_____
metastasis (104)	mĕ-TĂS-tă-sĭs	_____
microscope (104)	MĪ-krō-skōp	_____
neonatal (104)	nē-ō-NĀ-tăl	_____
neoplasm (104)	NĒ-ō-plăzm	_____
pancytopenia (104)	păn-sī-tō-PĒ-nē-ă	_____
paralysis (104)	pă-RĂL-ĭ-sĭs	_____
parathyroid (104)	păr-ă-THĪ-royd	_____
percutaneous (104)	pĕr-kū-TĀ-nē-ŭs	_____

periosteum (104)	pĕr-ē-ŎS-tē-ŭm
polymorphonuclear (104)	pŏl-ē-mŏr-fō-NŪ-klē-ăr
polyneuritis (104)	pŏl-ē-nū-RĪ-tĭs
post mortem (104)	pōst MŎR-tĕm
postnatal (104)	pōst-NĀ-tăl
precancerous (105)	prē-KĂN-sĕr-ŭs
prodrome (105)	PRŌ-drōm
prolapse (105)	PRŌ-lăps
pseudocyesis (105)	sū-dō-sī-Ē-sĭs
recombinant DNA (105)	rē-KŎM-bĭ-nănt DNA
relapse (105)	RĒ-lăps
remission (105)	rē-MĬ-shŭn
retroflexion (105)	rĕt-rō-FLĔK-shŭn
retroperitoneal (105)	rĕt-rō-pĕr-ĭ-tō-NĒ-ăl
subcutaneous (105)	sŭb-kū-TĀ-nē-ŭs
suprarenal (105)	soo-pră-RĒ-năl
suprathoracic (105)	soo-pră-thō-RĂ-sĭk
symbiosis (105)	sĭm-bē-Ō-sĭs
symmetry (105)	SĬM-mĕ-trē
symphysis (105)	SĬM-fĭ-sĭs
syndactyly (105)	sĭn-DĂK-tĭ-lē
syndrome (105)	SĬN-drōm
synthesis (105)	SĬN-thĕ-sĭs
tachypnea (106)	tă-KĬP-nē-ă or tăk-ĭp-NĒ-ă
transfusion (106)	trăns-FŪ-zhŭn
transurethral (106)	trăns-ū-RĒ-thrăl
ultrasonography (106)	ŭl-tră-sŏn-ŎG-ră-fē
unilateral (106)	ū-nē-LĂT-ĕr-ăl

VIII. Review Sheet

Write out the meanings of each word part in the space provided and test yourself. Check your answers with the information in the chapter or in the Glossary (Medical Terms—English) at the end of the book.

Prefixes

Prefix	Meaning	Prefix	Meaning
a-, an-		hemi-	
ab-		hyper-	
ad-		hypo-	
ana-		in-	
ante-		infra-	
anti-		inter-	
auto-		intra-	
bi-		macro-	
brady-		mal-	
cata-		meta-	
con-		micro-	
contra-		neo-	
de-		pan-	
dia-		para-	
dys-		per-	
ec-, ecto-		peri-	
en-, endo-		poly-	
epi-		post-	
eu-		pre-	
ex-		pro-	

pseudo- _____ syn-, sym- _____

re- _____ tachy- _____

retro- _____ trans- _____

sub- _____ ultra- _____

supra- _____ uni- _____

Combining Forms

Combining Form	Meaning	Combining Form	Meaning
carp/o	_____	nect/o	_____
cib/o	_____	norm/o	_____
cost/o	_____	ophthalm/o	_____
cutane/o	_____	ox/o	_____
dactyl/o	_____	ren/o	_____
duct/o	_____	seps/o	_____
flex/o	_____	somn/o	_____
furc/o	_____	son/o	_____
gloss/o	_____	the/o	_____
glyc/o	_____	thyr/o	_____
immun/o	_____	top/o	_____
later/o	_____	tox/o	_____
morph/o	_____	trache/o	_____
mort/o	_____	urethr/o	_____
nat/i	_____	ven/o	_____
necr/o	_____		

Continued on following page

Suffixes

Combining Form	Meaning	Combining Form	Meaning
-blast	_____	-phoria	_____
-crine	_____	-physis	_____
-cyesis	_____	-plasia	_____
-drome	_____	-plasm	_____
-gen	_____	-pnea	_____
-lapse	_____	-ptosis	_____
-lysis	_____	-rrhea	_____
-mission	_____	-stasis	_____
-partum	_____	-trophy	_____

Prefixes with Similar Meanings

Prefix	Meaning
a- (an-), in-	_____
ante-, pre-, pro-	_____
anti-, contra-	_____
con-, syn- (sym-)	_____
de-, cata-	_____
dia-, per-, trans -	_____
dys-, mal-	_____
ec- (ecto-), ex-	_____
en- (endo-), in-, intra-	_____
epi-, hyper-, supra-	_____
hypo-, infra-, sub-	_____
re-, retro-, post-	_____
ultra-, meta-	_____

Digestive System

This Chapter is divided into the following sections

In this Chapter you will
- Name the organs of the digestive system and describe their locations and functions;
- Describe disease processes and symptoms that affect these organs; and
- Define combining forms for organs and the meaning of related terminology using these word parts.

I. Introduction

The digestive system, also called the **alimentary canal** or **gastrointestinal tract,** begins with the mouth, where food enters the body, and ends with the anus, where solid waste material leaves the body. The primary functions of the organs of the digestive system are threefold.

First, complex food material taken into the mouth must be **digested,** or broken down, mechanically and chemically, as it travels through the gastrointestinal tract (passageway). Digestive **enzymes** speed up chemical reactions and help in the breakdown (digestion) of complex nutrients. Complex proteins are digested to simpler **amino acids;** complicated sugars are reduced to simple sugars, such as **glucose;** and large fat molecules (triglycerides) are broken down to **fatty acids** and glycerol.

Second, the digested food must be **absorbed** into the bloodstream by passing through the walls of the small intestine. In this way, valuable nutrients, such as sugar and amino acids, can travel to all the cells of the body. Cells then catabolize (burn) nutrients in the presence of oxygen to release energy stored within the food. Cells also use amino acid nutrients to anabolize (build) large protein molecules needed for growth and development. Although the walls of the small intestine also absorb fatty acids and glycerol, these nutrients enter lymphatic vessels rather than blood vessels. Digested fats eventually enter the bloodstream as lymph vessels join with blood vessels in the upper chest region.

The third function of the digestive system is the **elimination** of the solid waste materials that cannot be absorbed into the bloodstream. The large intestine concentrates these solid wastes, called **feces,** and the wastes finally pass out of the body through the anus.

II. Anatomy and Physiology

Oral Cavity

The alimentary canal begins with the oral cavity, or mouth. Label Figure 5–1 as you learn the major parts of the oral cavity.

The **cheeks** (1) form the walls of the oval-shaped oral cavity, and the **lips** (2) surround the opening to the cavity.

The **hard palate** (3) forms the anterior portion of the roof of the mouth, and the muscular **soft palate** (4) lies posterior to it. **Rugae** are irregular ridges in the mucous membrane covering the anterior portion of the hard palate. Hanging from the soft palate is a small, soft tissue called the **uvula** (5). The word uvula means little grape. The structure functions to aid in producing sounds and speech.

The **tongue** (6) extends across the floor of the oral cavity, and muscles attach it to the lower jaw bone. It moves food around during **mastication** (chewing) and **deglutition** (swallowing). **Papillae,** small raised areas on the tongue, contain taste buds that are sensitive to the chemical nature of foods and allow discrimination of different tastes as food moves across the tongue.

The **tonsils** (7) are masses of lymphatic tissue located in depressions of the mucous membranes on both sides if the oropharynx (part of the throat near the mouth). They act as filters to protect the body from the invasion of microorganisms and produce lymphocytes, which are white blood cells able to fight disease.

The **gums** (8) are made of fleshy tissue and surround the sockets of the **teeth** (9). Figure 5–2 shows a dental arch with 16 permanent teeth (there are 32 permanent teeth in the entire oral cavity). Label the figure with the following names of teeth:

(1) central incisor	(5) second premolar
(2) lateral incisor	(6) first molar
(3) cuspid or canine	(7) second molar
(4) first premolar	(8) third molar, or wisdom tooth

Dentists use special terms to describe the surfaces of teeth (Fig. 5–2). The **labial** surface (labi/o means lip), for incisor and canine teeth, is nearest the lips. The **buccal** surface (bucc/o means cheek), for premolar and molar teeth, is adjacent to the cheek. These are indicated on the left side of Figure 5–2. Some dentists refer to both the labial and the buccal surfaces as the **facial** surface (faci/o means face). Opposite to the facial surface, all teeth have a **lingual** surface (lingu/o means tongue). The **mesial** surface of a tooth lies nearest to the median line and the **distal** surface, farthest from the medial line. Premolars and molars have an additional

NCS Test Sheet 50

Form No. 98255

Reorder Phone Number
1-800-367-6627

KEY ITEM COUNT

NCS
With Education in Mind™

T F
1. Ⓐ ● Ⓒ Ⓓ Ⓔ
2. Ⓐ Ⓑ Ⓒ Ⓓ ●
3. Ⓐ Ⓑ ● Ⓓ Ⓔ
4. Ⓐ ● Ⓒ Ⓓ Ⓔ
5. Ⓐ Ⓑ Ⓒ Ⓓ ●
6. Ⓐ Ⓑ ● Ⓓ Ⓔ
7. Ⓐ Ⓑ Ⓒ Ⓓ Ⓔ
8. Ⓐ Ⓑ Ⓒ ● Ⓔ
9. Ⓐ ● Ⓒ Ⓓ Ⓔ
10. Ⓐ Ⓑ Ⓒ ● Ⓔ
11. Ⓐ ● Ⓒ Ⓓ Ⓔ
12. Ⓐ ● Ⓒ Ⓓ Ⓔ
13. Ⓐ Ⓑ ● Ⓓ Ⓔ
14. Ⓐ Ⓑ Ⓒ ● Ⓔ
15. Ⓐ Ⓑ ● Ⓓ Ⓔ
16. Ⓐ Ⓑ Ⓒ Ⓓ ●
17. ● Ⓑ Ⓒ Ⓓ Ⓔ
18. Ⓐ Ⓑ Ⓒ Ⓓ ●
19. Ⓐ ● Ⓒ Ⓓ Ⓔ
20. Ⓐ Ⓑ Ⓒ ● Ⓔ
21. Ⓐ Ⓑ ● Ⓓ Ⓔ
22. ● Ⓑ Ⓒ Ⓓ Ⓔ
23. Ⓐ ● Ⓒ Ⓓ Ⓔ
24. Ⓐ Ⓑ ● Ⓓ Ⓔ
25. Ⓐ Ⓑ Ⓒ ● Ⓔ

T F
26. Ⓐ Ⓑ Ⓒ ● Ⓔ
27. Ⓐ Ⓑ Ⓒ Ⓓ ●
28. Ⓐ Ⓑ ● Ⓓ Ⓔ
29. Ⓐ ● Ⓒ Ⓓ Ⓔ
30. ● Ⓑ Ⓒ Ⓓ Ⓔ
31. Ⓐ Ⓑ Ⓒ Ⓓ Ⓔ
32. Ⓐ Ⓑ Ⓒ Ⓓ Ⓔ
33. Ⓐ Ⓑ Ⓒ Ⓓ Ⓔ
34. Ⓐ Ⓑ Ⓒ Ⓓ Ⓔ
35. Ⓐ Ⓑ Ⓒ Ⓓ Ⓔ
36. Ⓐ Ⓑ Ⓒ Ⓓ Ⓔ
37. Ⓐ Ⓑ Ⓒ Ⓓ Ⓔ
38. Ⓐ Ⓑ Ⓒ Ⓓ Ⓔ
39. Ⓐ Ⓑ Ⓒ Ⓓ Ⓔ
40. Ⓐ Ⓑ Ⓒ Ⓓ Ⓔ
41. Ⓐ Ⓑ Ⓒ Ⓓ Ⓔ
42. Ⓐ Ⓑ Ⓒ Ⓓ Ⓔ
43. Ⓐ Ⓑ Ⓒ Ⓓ Ⓔ
44. Ⓐ Ⓑ Ⓒ Ⓓ Ⓔ
45. Ⓐ Ⓑ Ⓒ Ⓓ Ⓔ
46. Ⓐ Ⓑ Ⓒ Ⓓ Ⓔ
47. Ⓐ Ⓑ Ⓒ Ⓓ Ⓔ
48. Ⓐ Ⓑ Ⓒ Ⓓ Ⓔ
49. Ⓐ Ⓑ Ⓒ Ⓓ Ⓔ
50. Ⓐ Ⓑ Ⓒ Ⓓ Ⓔ

STUDENT ID NUMBER

NUMBER CORRECT	29
PERCENT CORRECT	97%
ROSTER NUMBER	
SCORE	
RESCORE	

MARKING INSTRUCTIONS

Use a No. 2 Pencil

Ⓐ ● Ⓒ Ⓓ Ⓔ
Fill oval completely

Ⓐ Ⓑ Ⓒ Ⓓ Ⓔ
Erase cleanly

50 ITEM

NAME   RAJ Kullal
UNIT   Test 11   chapter 13
ROOM   DATE   April 10/98

NCS Test Sheet 50

Form No. 98255

Reorder Phone Number
1-800-367-6627

1

KEY ITEM COUNT

NCS
With Education in Mind™

T F
1. (A)(B)(C)(D)●
2. (A)●(C)(D)(E)
3. (A)(B)(C)●(E)
4. (A)●(C)(D)(E)
5. (A)(B)●(D)(E)
6. (A)●(C)(D)(E)
7. (A)(B)(C)●(E)
8. (A)(B)(C)●(E)
9. (A)(B)(C)(D)●
10. (A)(B)(C)●(E)
11. ●(B)(C)(D)(E)
12. (A)(B)(C)●(E)
13. (A)(B)(C)●(E)
14. ●(B)(C)(D)(E)
15. (A)●(C)(D)(E)
16. ●(B)(C)(D)(E)
17. (A)●(C)(D)(E)
18. (A)(B)(C)●(E)
19. (A)(B)(C)●(E)
20. (A)(B)●(D)(E)
21. (A)(B)●(D)(E)
22. (A)(B)(C)(D)(E)
23. ●(B)(C)(D)(E)
24. (A)●(C)(D)(E)
25. (A)(B)●(D)(E)

T F
26. (A)(B)●(D)(E)
27. (A)●(C)(D)(E)
28. (A)(B)(C)●(E)
29. (A)(B)(C)●(E)
30. (A)●(C)(D)(E)
31. (A)(B)(C)●(E)
32. (A)●(C)(D)(E)
33. (A)(B)●(D)(E)
34. (A)(B)(C)(D)●
35. ●(B)(C)(D)(E)
36. (A)(B)●(D)(E)
37. ●(B)(C)(D)(E)
38. (A)●(C)(D)(E)
39. (A)(B)●(D)(E)
40. (A)(B)●(D)(E)
41. (A)(B)(C)(D)(E)
42. (A)(B)(C)(D)(E)
43. (A)(B)(C)(D)(E)
44. (A)(B)(C)(D)(E)
45. (A)(B)(C)(D)(E)
46. (A)(B)(C)(D)(E)
47. (A)(B)(C)(D)(E)
48. (A)(B)(C)(D)(E)
49. (A)(B)(C)(D)(E)
50. (A)(B)(C)(D)(E)

STUDENT ID NUMBER

NUMBER CORRECT	38
PERCENT CORRECT	95
ROSTER NUMBER	
SCORE	
RESCORE	

MARKING INSTRUCTIONS

Use a No. 2 Pencil

(A) ● (C)(D)(E)
Fill oval completely

(A)(B)(C)(D)(E)
Erase cleanly

50 ITEM

NAME RAJ KULLAR
UNIT Chapter 12
ROOM DATE April 3/98

Pharynx

(8) _____

(9) _____

(3) _____

(4) _____

(5) _____

(7) _____

(1) _____

(6) _____

(2) _____

Figure 5–1

Oral cavity.

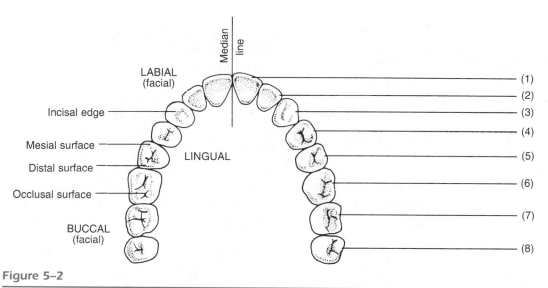

Median line

LABIAL (facial)

Incisal edge

Mesial surface

Distal surface

Occlusal surface

LINGUAL

BUCCAL (facial)

(1) _____

(2) _____

(3) _____

(4) _____

(5) _____

(6) _____

(7) _____

(8) _____

Figure 5–2

Permanent teeth within the dental arch.

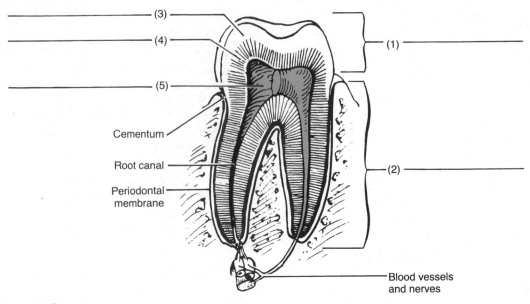

Cementum

Root canal

Periodontal membrane

Blood vessels and nerves

Figure 5–3

Anatomy of a tooth.

occlusal surface (occlusion means to close) that comes in contact with a corresponding tooth in the opposing arch. The incisors and cuspids have a sharp **incisal** edge.

Figure 5–3 shows the inner anatomy of a tooth. Label it as you read the following description:

A tooth consists of a **crown** (1), which shows above the gumline and a **root** (2), which lies within the bony tooth socket. The outermost protective layer of the crown, the **enamel** (3), protects the tooth. Enamel is a dense, hard, white substance—the hardest substance in the body. **Dentin** (4), the main substance of the tooth, lies beneath the enamel and extends throughout the crown. Yellow in color, dentin is composed of bony tissue that is softer than enamel. The **cementum** covers, protects, and supports the dentin in the root. A **periodontal membrane** surrounds the cementum and holds the tooth in place in the tooth socket.

The **pulp** (5) lies underneath the dentin. It is soft and delicate tissue and fills the center of the tooth. Blood vessels, nerve endings, connective tissue, and lymphatic vessels are within the pulp canal (also called the **root canal**). Root canal therapy is often necessary when disease or abscess (pus collection) occurs in the pulp canal. A dentist opens the tooth from above and cleans the canal of infection, nerves, and blood vessels. The canal is then disinfected and filled with material to prevent the entrance of microorganisms and decay.

Three pairs of **salivary glands** (Fig. 5–4) surround the oral cavity. These exocrine glands produce a fluid called **saliva** that contains important digestive **enzymes.** Saliva is released from the **parotid gland** (1), **submandibular gland** (2), and **sublingual gland** (3) on each side of the mouth. Narrow ducts carry the saliva into the oral cavity.

Pharynx

Refer to Figure 5–5. The **pharynx** or **throat** is a muscular tube, about 5 inches long, lined with a mucous membrane. It serves as a common passageway for air traveling from the nose (nasal cavity) to the windpipe (trachea) and food traveling from the oral cavity to the **esophagus.** When swallowing (deglutition) occurs, a flap of tissue, the epiglottis, covers the trachea so that food cannot enter and become lodged there.

Figure 5–6 traces the passage of food from the esophagus through the gastrointestinal tract. Label it as you read the following paragraphs.

Figure 5–4

Salivary glands.

Esophagus

The **esophagus** (1), meaning swallowing (phag/o) inward (eso-), is a 9- to 10-inch muscular tube extending from the pharynx to the stomach. Rhythmic contractions of muscles in the wall of the esophagus propel food toward the stomach. **Peristalsis,** meaning constriction (-stalsis) surrounding (peri-), is this involuntary, progressive, rhythm-like contraction of the esophagus and the other gastrointestinal tubes. The process is like squeezing a marble (the bolus, or semisolid mass of food) through a rubber tube.

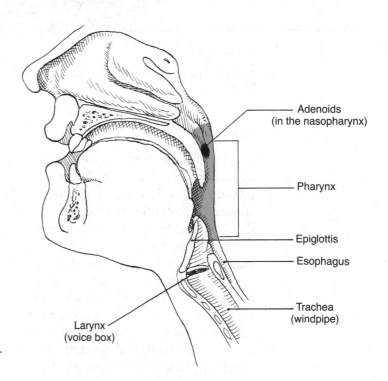

Figure 5–5

The pharynx, a sagittal view.

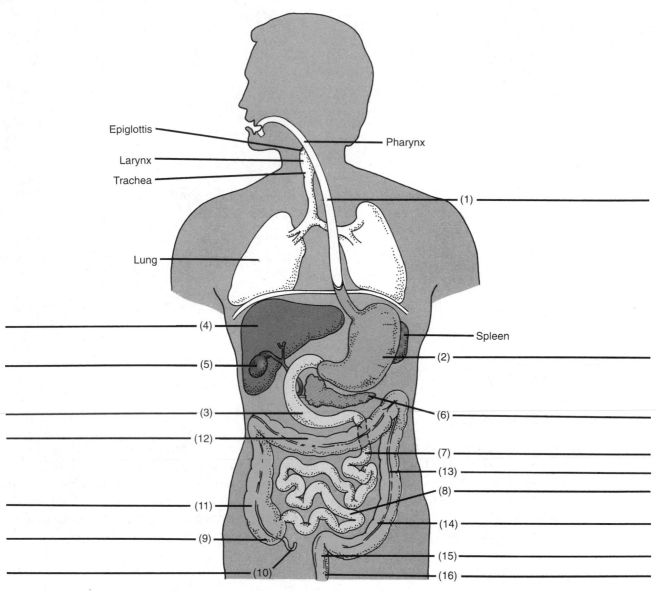

Epiglottis
Pharynx
Larynx
Trachea
(1)
Lung
(4)
Spleen
(5)
(2)
(3)
(6)
(12)
(7)
(13)
(8)
(11)
(14)
(9)
(15)
(10)
(16)

Figure 5–6

The gastrointestinal tract. (From Chabner DE: Medical Terminology: A Short Course. Philadelphia, WB Saunders, 1990.)

Stomach

Food passes from the esophagus into the **stomach** (2). The stomach is composed of an upper portion called the **fundus,** a middle section known as the **body,** and a lower portion, the **pylorus** (Fig. 5–7). Rings of muscles called **sphincters** control the openings into and from the stomach. The **cardiac sphincter** relaxes and contracts to move food from the esophagus into the stomach, whereas the **pyloric sphincter** allows food to leave the stomach when it has been sufficiently digested. Folds in the mucous membrane **(mucosa)** lining the stomach are called **rugae.** The rugae contain digestive glands that produce enzymes and **hydrochloric acid.**

The role of the stomach is to prepare the food chemically and mechanically so that it can be received in the small intestine for further digestion and absorption into the bloodstream. Food does not enter the bloodstream through the walls of the stomach. The stomach controls the passing of foods into the first part of the small intestine so that it proceeds only when it is chemically ready and in small amounts. Food leaves the stomach in 1–4 hours or longer, depending upon the amount and type of food eaten.

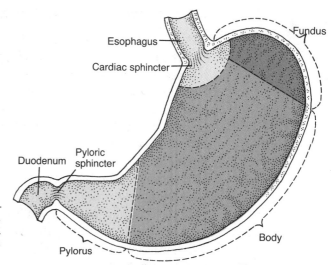

Figure 5–7

Parts of the stomach. (From Ignatavicius DD, Bayne MV: Medical-Surgical Nursing: A Nursing Process Approach. Philadelphia, WB Saunders, 1991, p 1222.)

Small Intestine (Small Bowel)

(Continue labeling Fig. 5–6.)

The **small intestine (small bowel)** extends for 20 feet from the pyloric sphincter to the first part of the large intestine. It has three parts. The **duodenum** (3), only 1 foot in length, receives food from the stomach as well as **bile** from the **liver** (4) and **gallbladder** (5) and pancreatic juice from the **pancreas** (6). Enzymes and bile help to digest food before it passes into the second part of the small intestine, the **jejunum** (7), about 8 feet long. The jejunum connects with the third section, the **ileum** (8), about 11 feet long. The ileum attaches to the first part of the large intestine.

Millions of tiny, microscopic projections called **villi** line the walls of the small intestine. The tiny capillaries (microscopic blood vessels) in the villi absorb the digested nutrients into the bloodstream and lymph vessels. Figure 5–8 shows several different views of villi in the lining of the small intestine.

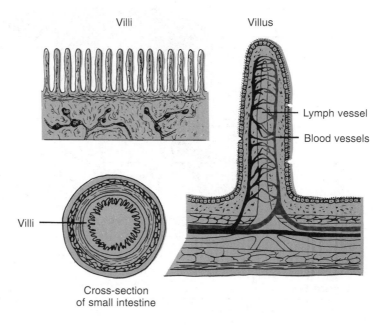

Figure 5–8

Villi in the lining of the small intestine.

Large Intestine (Large Bowel)

(Continue labeling Fig. 5–6.)

The large intestine extends from the end of the ileum to the anus. It is divided into four parts: cecum, colon, sigmoid colon, and rectum. The **cecum** (9) is a pouch on the right side that attaches to the ileum by the ileocecal valve (sphincter). The **appendix** (10) hangs from the cecum. The appendix has no clear function, but it causes problems when inflamed and infected. The **colon** (large intestine), about 5 feet long, has three divisions. The **ascending colon** (11) extends from the cecum to the under surface of the liver, where it turns to the left (hepatic flexure or bend) to become the **transverse colon** (12). The transverse colon passes horizontally to the left toward the spleen, and turns downward (splenic flexure) into the **descending colon** (13). The **sigmoid colon** (14), shaped like an S (sigma), lies at the distal end of the descending colon and leads into the **rectum** (15). The rectum terminates in the lower opening of the gastrointestinal tract, the **anus** (16).

The large intestine receives the fluid waste products of digestion (the material unable to pass into the bloodstream) and stores these wastes until they can be released from the body. Because the large intestine absorbs most of the water within the waste material, the body can expel solid **feces** (stools). Diarrhea, watery stools, can result from lack of absorption of the water through the walls of the large intestine.

Liver, Gallbladder, and Pancreas

Three important additional organs of the digestive system—the liver, gallbladder, and pancreas—play crucial roles in the proper digestion and absorption of nutrients. Label Figure 5–9 as you study the following:

The **liver** (1), located in the right upper quadrant (RUQ) of the abdomen, manufactures a thick, yellowish-brown, sometimes greenish, fluid called **bile.** Bile contains cholesterol (a fatty substance), bile acids, and several bile pigments. One of these pigments, **bilirubin,** is produced from the breakdown of hemoglobin in the liver. The liver combines bilirubin with bile, and then excretes both into the duodenum. They leave the body in feces.

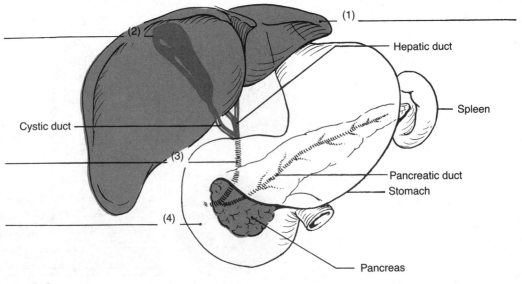

Figure 5–9

Liver, gallbladder, and pancreas.

Figure 5–10

Functions of the pancreas.

The liver continuously releases bile, which then travels down the **hepatic duct** to the **cystic duct.** The cystic duct leads to the **gallbladder** (2), a pear-shaped sac under the liver, which stores and concentrates the bile for later use. After meals, in response to the presence of food in the stomach and duodenum, the gallbladder contracts, forcing the bile out the cystic duct into the **common bile duct** (3), which joins with the **pancreatic duct** just before the entrance to the **duodenum** (4). The duodenum thus receives a mixture of bile and pancreatic juices.

Bile has a detergent-like effect on fats in the duodenum. It breaks apart large fat globules so that enzymes from the pancreas can digest the fats. This is called **emulsification.** Without bile, most of the fat taken into the body would remain undigested.

The liver, besides producing bile, has several other vital and important functions. Some of these are:

1. Keeping the amount of **glucose** (sugar) in the blood at a normal level. The liver removes excess glucose from the bloodstream and stores it as **glycogen** (starch) in liver cells. When the blood sugar level becomes dangerously low the liver can convert stored glycogen back into glucose via a process called glycogenolysis. In addition, the liver can also convert proteins and fats into glucose when the body needs sugar by a process called gluconeogenesis.

2. Manufacture of some blood proteins, particularly those necessary for blood clotting.

3. Destruction of old erythrocytes and release of bilirubin.

4. Removal of poisons (detoxification) from the blood.

The term **hepatic portal system** refers to the blood vessels that bring blood to the liver from the intestines. Digested foods pass into the portal vein directly after being absorbed into the bloodstream from the small intestine, thus giving the liver first chance at using the nutrients.

The **pancreas** is both an exocrine and an endocrine organ. As an exocrine gland, it produces pancreatic juices filled with enzymes (**amylase** and **lipase**) to digest food. These pass into the duodenum through the pancreatic duct.

As an endocrine gland (secreting into the bloodstream), the pancreas secretes **insulin.** This hormone, needed to help release sugar from the blood, acts as a carrier to bring glucose into cells of the body to be used for energy. Figure 5–10 reviews these functions of the pancreas.

Figure 5–11 is a flow chart following the pathway of food throughout the gastrointestinal tract.

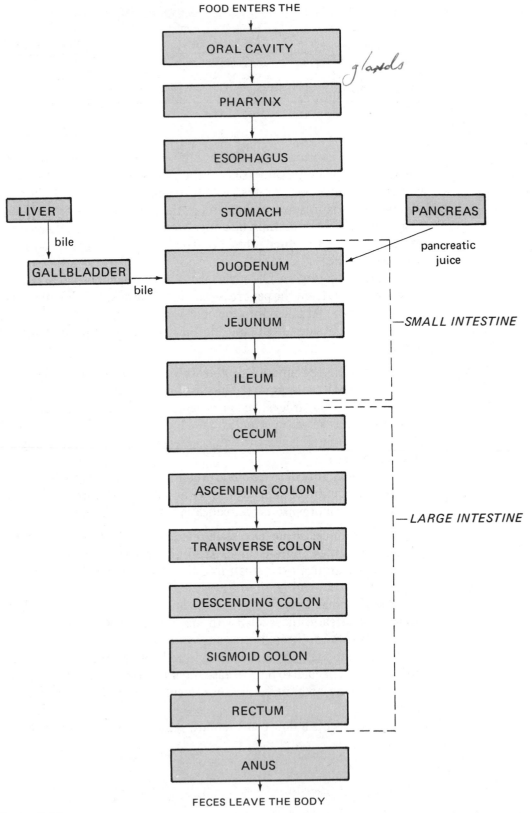

Figure 5–11

Pathway of food through the digestive tract.

III. Vocabulary

This list will help you review many of the new terms introduced in the text. Short definitions will reinforce your understanding of the terms. See Section VIII of this chapter for help in pronouncing the more difficult terms.

absorption	Passage of materials through the walls of the intestine into the bloodstream.
alimentary canal	The digestive tract (canal); aliment means food.
amino acids	Small substances that are the building blocks of proteins and are produced when proteins are digested.
amylase	Enzyme (-ase = enzyme) from the pancreas to digest starch (amyl = starch).
anus	Opening of the digestive tract to the outside of the body.
appendix	Blind pouch hanging from the first part of the colon (cecum). It literally means hanging (pend/o) on (ap-). Usually found in the RLQ.
bile	Digestive juice made in the liver and stored in the gallbladder. It physically breaks up (emulsifies) large fat globules. Bile was originally called gall (Latin *bilis* meaning gall or anger), probably because it has a bitter taste. It is composed of bile pigments, cholesterol, and bile salts.
bilirubin	Pigment released by the liver in bile; produced from the destruction of hemoglobin, a blood protein (-globin).
bowel	Intestine.
canine teeth	Pointed, dog-like (canine) teeth, next to (distal to) the incisors. Also called cuspids or eyeteeth.
cecum	First part of the large intestine.
colon	Large intestine; ascending, transverse, and descending parts.
common bile duct	Carries bile from the liver and gallbladder to the duodenum.
deglutition	Swallowing.
dentin	Major tissue composing teeth, covered by the enamel in the crown and a protective layer of cementum in the root.
digestion	Breakdown of complex foods to simpler forms.
duodenum	First part of the small intestine. Duo = 2, den = 10; the duodenum measures 12 inches in length.
emulsification	Physical process of breaking up large fat globules into smaller globules, thus increasing the surface area that enzymes can use to digest the fat.

enamel	Hard, outermost layer of a tooth.
enzyme	A chemical that speeds up a reaction between substances. Digestive enzymes help in the breakdown of complex foods to simpler foods.
esophagus	Tube connecting the throat to the stomach.
fatty acids	Substances produced when fats are digested.
feces	Solid wastes; stools.
gallbladder	Small sac under the liver; stores bile.
glucose	Simple sugar.
glycogen	Animal starch; glucose is stored in the form of glycogen in liver cells.
hepatic portal system	Capillaries (small blood vessels) that carry blood from the digestive tract to the liver.
hydrochloric acid	Substance produced by the stomach; necessary for digestion of food.
ileum	Third part of the small intestine; from the Greek *eilos* meaning twisted. When the abdomen was viewed at necropsy (autopsy), the intestine appeared twisted and the ileum was often an area of obstruction.
incisor	One of four front teeth in the dental arch.
insulin	Hormone produced by the endocrine cells of the pancreas. It transports sugar into cells from the blood and stimulates glycogen formation by the liver.
jejunum	Second part of the small intestine. The Latin *jejunus* means empty; this part of the intestine was always empty when a body was examined after death.
lipase	Pancreatic enzyme necessary to digest fats.
liver	A large organ located in the RUQ of the abdomen. The liver secretes bile; stores sugar, iron, and vitamins; produces blood proteins; and destroys worn out red blood cells. The normal adult liver weighs about 2½–3 pounds.
mastication	Chewing.
palate	Roof of the mouth. The hard palate is anterior to the soft palate.
pancreas	Organ under the stomach; produces insulin (for transport of sugar into cells) and enzymes (for digestion of foods).
papillae (singular: **papilla**)	Small elevations on the tongue. A papilla is any nipple-like elevation.
parotid gland	Salivary gland near the ear.

peristalsis	Rhythm-like contractions of the tubes of the alimentary tract and other tubular structures.
pharynx	Throat, the common passageway for food from the mouth and air from the nose.
pulp	Soft tissue within a tooth containing nerves and blood vessels.
pyloric sphincter	Ring of muscle at the distal region of the stomach.
rectum	End of the colon.
rugae	Ridges on the hard palate and wall of the stomach.
saliva	Digestive juice produced by salivary glands.
salivary glands	Parotid, sublingual, and submandibular glands.
sigmoid colon	Lower part of the colon; shaped like an **S.**
sphincter	Ring of muscles within a tube. **Ph** sounds like **f.**
stomach	Muscular organ that receives food from the esophagus. Digestion begins in the stomach and continues in the duodenum.
triglycerides	Large fat molecules composed of three molecules of fatty acids with one molecule of glycerol.
uvula	Soft tissue hanging from the soft palate in the mouth.
villi (singular: **villus**)	Tiny microscopic projections in the walls of the small intestine to absorb nutrients into the bloodstream.

IV. Combining Forms, Suffixes, and Terminology

Check Section VIII of this chapter for help with pronunciation of terms. Write the meaning of the medical term in the space provided.

Parts of the Body			
Combining Form	Meaning	Terminology	Meaning
an/o	anus	peri__an__al _____	
append/o	appendix	appendectomy _____	
appendic/o	appendix	appendicitis _____	

See Figure 5–12.

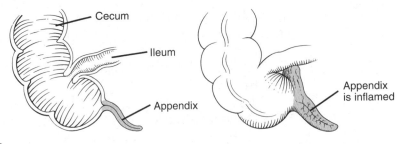

Figure 5–12

(A) Normal appendix and *(B)* appendicitis. (*A* and *B,* From Miller BF, Keane CB: Encyclopedia and Dictionary of Medicine, Nursing, and Allied Health, 5th ed. Philadelphia, WB Saunders, 1992, p 111.)

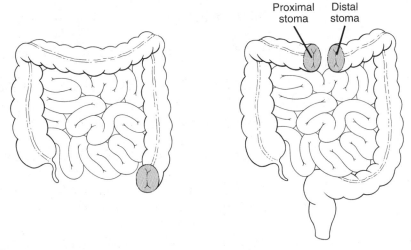

Figure 5–13

Two types of colostomies. *(A)* Sigmoid colostomy is used after resection of the rectum and part of the sigmoid colon. *(B)* Transverse (double-barreled) colostomy is used in emergencies such as intestinal obstruction or perforation (a hole or break in the wall). There are two stomas. The proximal stoma, closest to the small intestine, drains feces. The distal stoma drains mucus.

Figure 5–14

Mesentery and three types of anastomoses.

bucc/o	cheek	buccal mucosa _____

The mucosa is composed of epithelial cells.

cec/o	cecum	cecal _____

celi/o	belly, abdomen	celiac _____

Abdomin/o and lapar/o also mean abdomen. When there is more than one combining form with the same meaning there is no rule indicating when one or the other is used. Your job is to recognize each in its proper context.

cheil/o	lip	cheilosis _____

Labi/o also means lip.

cholecyst/o	gallbladder	cholecystectomy _____

choledoch/o	common bile duct	choledochotomy _____

col/o	colon, large intestine	colostomy _____

-stomy, when used with a combining form for an organ, means an opening to the outside of the body (Fig. 5–13).

colon/o	colon	colonic _____
		colonoscopy _____

dent/i	tooth	dentibuccal _____

Odont/o also means tooth.

duoden/o	duodenum	duodenal _____

enter/o	intestines, usually small intestine	enteropathy _____
		enterocolitis _____

When two combining forms for gastrointestinal organs are in a term, the one closest to the mouth appears first.

enterocolostomy _____

-stomy, when used with two or more combining forms for organs, means the surgical creation of an opening between those organs inside the body. This is also called an anastomosis (ana = up, stom = opening, -sis = state of) (Fig. 5–14).

mesentery _____

This membrane is a part of the double fold of peritoneum that stretches around the organs in the abdomen and holds them in place. It is literally in the middle (mes-) of the intestines, attaching the intestines to the muscle wall at the back of the abdomen (see Fig. 5–14.)

parenteral _____

Par (from para-) means apart from in this term. Parenteral nutrition is food (glucose) given intravenously (IV) and not through the intestinal tract. Parenteral injections can be subcutaneous and intramuscular, as well.

esophag/o	esophagus	esophageal _____

Note that the final g is softened (ji) by changing the suffix from al to eal.

faci/o	face	facial _____
gastr/o	stomach	gastralgia _____
gingiv/o	gums	gingivitis _____
gloss/o	tongue	hypoglossal _____

Lingu/o also means tongue.

hepat/o	liver	hepatoma _____
		hepatomegaly _____
ile/o	ileum	ileocecal sphincter _____

Also called the ileocecal valve.

ileitis _____

ileostomy _____

jejun/o	jejunum	gastrojejunostomy _____

An anastomosis.

choledochojejunostomy _____

An anastomosis.

labi/o	lip	labial _____
lapar/o	abdomen	laparoscopy _____

Also called peritoneoscopy.

lingu/o	tongue	sublingual _____
mandibul/o	lower jaw, mandible	submandibular _____
odont/o	tooth	orthodontist _____

Orth/o means straight.

periodontist _____

endodontist _____

Does root canal therapy.

or/o	mouth	oral _____

Stomat/o also means mouth.

palat/o	palate	palatoplasty _____
pancreat/o	pancreas	pancreatitis _____
pharyng/o	throat	pharyngeal _____
peritone/o	peritoneum	peritonitis _____

The e of the root has been dropped in this term.

proct/o	anus and rectum	proctologist _____
pylor/o	pyloric sphincter	pyloroplasty _____
rect/o	rectum	rectocele _____
sialaden/o	salivary gland	sialadenectomy _____
sigmoid/o	sigmoid colon	sigmoidoscopy _____
stomat/o	mouth	stomatitis _____

Substances

Combining Form	Meaning	Terminology	Meaning
amyl/o	starch	amylase _____	

-ase means enzyme.

bil/i	gall, bile	biliary _____	

The biliary tract includes the organs (liver and gallbladder) and ducts (hepatic, cystic, and common bile ducts) that secrete, store, and empty bile into the duodenum.

bilirubin/o	bilirubin (bile pigment)	hyperbilirubinemia _____	
chol/e	gall, bile	cholelithiasis _____	

lith/o means stone or calculus; -iasis means abnormal condition.

gluc/o	sugar	gluconeogenesis _____	

New sugar is made by liver cells from fats and proteins.

glyc/o	sugar

hyperglycemia _____

glycogen/o	glycogen, animal starch

glycogenolysis _____

Liver cells can change glycogen back to glucose when blood sugar is low.

lip/o	fat, lipid

lipoma _____

lith/o	stone

cholecystolithiasis _____

sial/o	saliva, salivary

sialolith _____

steat/o	fat

steatorrhea _____

Fats are improperly digested (malabsorbed) and appear in the feces.

Suffixes			
Suffix	Meaning	Terminology	Meaning
-ase	enzyme	lipase _____	
-chezia	defecation, elimination of wastes	hematochezia _____	

(hem-ă-tō-KĒ-zē-ă). Bright red blood is found in the feces.

-iasis	abnormal condition	choledocholithiasis _____
-prandial	meal	postprandial _____

Post cibum also means after meals (cib/o means meal).

V. Pathology of the Digestive System

This section is divided into terms that describe symptoms (signs of illness) and terms that describe pathological conditions. The sentences following the definitions use medical words that are familiar to you and often describe the **etiology** (eti/o = cause) of the illness and its treatment. If the etiology is neither known nor understood, it is called **idiopathic** (idi/o = unknown).

Symptoms

achlorhydria   Lack of hydrochloric acid in the stomach.

This can be a symptom of chronic gastritis or gastric carcinoma.

Figure 5–15

Ascites. The patient's abdomen is full of fluid. (From Swartz MH: Textbook of Physical Diagnosis: History and Examination. Philadelphia, WB Saunders, 1989, plate XIIA.)

anorexia	Lack of appetite (-orexia = appetite).

Often a sign of malignancy or liver disease. Anorexia nervosa is loss of appetite owing to emotional problems such as anger, anxiety, and fear. It is an eating disorder and is discussed, along with a similar disorder, bulimia nervosa, in Chapter 22.

ascites Abnormal accumulation of fluid in the abdomen.

This condition, previously called dropsy, occurs when fluid seeps out of the bloodstream and collects in the peritoneal cavity. It can be a symptom of neoplasm or inflammatory disorders in the abdomen, venous hypertension (high blood pressure) caused by liver disease (cirrhosis), and heart failure. Figure 5–15 illustrates ascites.

colic Acute abdominal pain caused by spasms of intestinal muscles.

Colic, commonly occurring in the first 3 months of life, is related to excessive swallowing of air (aerophagia), rapid or overfeeding, allergy to milk, or feeding problems.

constipation Difficult, delayed elimination of feces.

Stools are dry and hard when peristalsis is slow. A medication that encourages movement of feces from the colon is called a laxative. A cathartic is a strong laxative.

diarrhea Loose, watery stools.

The acute onset of postprandial diarrhea suggests an acute infection or toxin. Watery or bloody stools are a symptom of inflammation or disease in the gastrointestinal tract.

dysphagia Difficult, painful swallowing.

This is a symptom of motility (movement) problems in the esophagus or a tumor or swelling that blocks the passage of food.

flatus Gas expelled through the anus.

gastroesophageal reflux Solids and fluids return to the mouth from the stomach.

Heartburn is the burning sensation caused by the regurgitation of hydrochloric acid from the stomach into the esophagus. A **hiatal hernia** (bulging of the stomach wall upward toward the esophagus) can cause this symptom.

hematochezia Bright red blood from the rectum.

> Hematochezia can appear associated with colonic tumors, ulcerative colitis, and hemorrhoids.

jaundice Yellow-orange coloration of the skin and other tissues due to high levels of bilirubin in the blood.

> Jaundice (**icterus**) can occur in three major ways: (1) Malfunction of liver cells (hepatocytes) because of liver disease (hepatopathy) prevents the liver from combining bilirubin with bile; (2) obstruction of bile flow (choledocholithiasis) prevents bilirubin and bile from being excreted into the intestine; and (3) excessive destruction of erythrocytes in hemolysis causes excess bilirubin in the blood.

melena Black, dark brown, tarry stools; feces containing blood.

> This symptom reflects bleeding above the first section of the duodenum, as would be the case with a bleeding ulcer.

nausea Unpleasant sensation from the stomach with a tendency to vomit.

> This term comes from a Greek word meaning seasickness. Irritation of nerve endings in the stomach or other parts of the body sends a message to the vomiting reflex center in the brain. If the sensation becomes intense, vomiting results. Vomiting can be a symptom of the perforation (hole through the wall) of an abdominal organ; obstruction of a bile duct, stomach, or intestine; or toxins (poisons).

steatorrhea Fat in the feces.

> Improper absorption (malabsorption) of fat can cause fat to remain in the intestines. Etiology may be enteritis or pancreatitis.

Pathological Conditions

Oral Cavity and Teeth

aphthous stomatitis Inflammation of the mouth with small ulcers.

> This idiopathic condition is also known as **canker** (KĂNK-ĕr) **sores.** Aphth/o means ulcer.

dental caries Tooth decay (caries means decay).

> Dental plaque is the accumulation of foods, proteins from saliva, and necrotic debris on the tooth enamel. Bacteria grow in the plaque and cause the production of acid that dissolves the tooth enamel resulting in a cavity (area of decay). If the bacterial infection reaches the pulp of the tooth (causing pulpitis), root canal therapy may be necessary.

herpetic stomatitis Inflammation of the mouth (gingiva, lips, palate, and tongue) by infection with the herpesvirus. Commonly called **fever blisters** or **cold sores.**

oral leukoplakia White plaques or patches (-plakia means plaque) on the mucosa of the mouth.

> A precancerous condition; major etiological factors are chronic tobacco and alcohol use.

periodontal disease   Inflammation and degeneration of gums, teeth, and surrounding bone; also called **pyorrhea** (py/o means pus).

Chronic inflammation of gums (gingivitis) occurs from accumulation of dental plaque and calculus (hardened plaque). Gingivectomy may be necessary to remove pockets of pus and allow new tissue to form.

Gastrointestinal Tract

achalasia   Failure of the sphincter muscles of the lower esophagus to relax (-chalasia means relaxation) during swallowing.

When failure of proper peristalsis occurs, food cannot pass through the esophagus easily (dysphagia). The cause of achalasia is unknown, but anxiety and tension aggravate the condition. Physicians often recommend a bland diet low in bulk, and dilation (widening) of the cardiac or lower esophageal sphincter (LES) to relieve symptoms (Fig. 5–16).

anal fistula   Abnormal tube-like passageway near the anus, which may communicate with the rectum (Fig. 5–17). An **anal fissure** is a narrow slit in the anal wall.

colonic polyposis   Polyps (small growths) protrude from the mucous membrane of the colon. Figure 5–17 shows two kinds of polyps.

colorectal cancer   Carcinoma of the colon or rectum, or both.

A theory of colonic carcinogenesis has been proposed linking a diet high in beef and fat with the development of bacteria in the colon that increase the level of bile and fatty acids, which act as carcinogens. The prognosis for patients with colorectal carcinoma depends on the stage (extent of spread) of the neoplasm, upon diagnosis, how easily the cancer can be resected, and its responsiveness to radiotherapy and chemotherapy (Fig. 5–18).

Figure 5–16

Balloon dilatation of the lower esophagus for achalasia. (From Ignatavicius DD, Bayne MV: Medical-Surgical Nursing: A Nursing Process Approach. Philadelphia, WB Saunders, 1991, p 1287.)

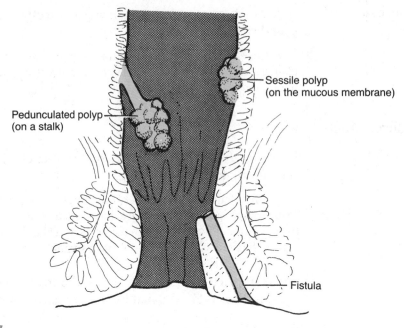

Labels on figure:
- Sessile polyp (on the mucous membrane)
- Pedunculated polyp (on a stalk)
- Fistula

Figure 5–17

Polyps and anal fistula.

Label on figure:
- Carcinoma

Figure 5–18

Carcinoma of the ascending colon. The cancer projects into the lumen (the space within a tube or tubular organ) but has not caused obstruction. (From Kumar V, Cotran RS, Robbins SL: Basic Pathology, 5th ed. Philadelphia, WB Saunders, 1992, p 516.)

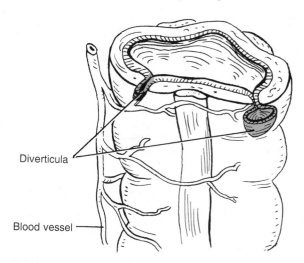

Diverticula

Blood vessel —

Figure 5–19

Diverticula of the large intestine. The mucous lining bulges through the muscular wall to form a diverticulum.

Crohn's disease	Chronic inflammation of the intestinal tract that can affect any part of the digestive tract from the mouth to the anus.
	This chronic relapsing disease causes inflammation with diarrhea, cramping, and fever and commonly affects the last (terminal) part of the ileum. Similar to ulcerative colitis, both are forms of **inflammatory bowel disease** (IBD). Physicians do not know the cause of this disease, and often the disease is treated by medicines or surgical removal of the diseased portion of the intestine, with anastomosis of remaining parts.
diverticula (singular: **diverticulum**)	Abnormal side pockets (outpouchings) in the intestinal wall.
	A common location for diverticulosis is the sigmoid colon. When undigested food or bacteria become trapped in a diverticulum, diverticulitis occurs. Figure 5–19 illustrates diverticula (di = aside, verti = to turn, cul = small).
dysentery	Painful, inflamed intestines.
	Commonly occurring in the colon, the etiology of dysentery is usually ingested food or water containing bacteria (salmonellae or shigellae), amebae (one-celled organisms), or viruses. Colitis, diarrhea, and abdominal cramps occur.
esophageal varices	Swollen, twisted veins around the distal end of the esophagus.
	Liver disease (such as cirrhosis) can cause increased pressure in blood vessels (hepatic portal system), and the pressure can lead to enlarged, twisted esophageal veins with danger of hemorrhage (bleeding).
hemorrhoids	Swollen, twisted, varicose veins in the rectal region.
	Also known as piles, hemorrhoids can be internal (within the wall of the rectum) or external (in the anal area), and they are often caused by chronic constipation and straining, which increases pressure on anal veins.
hernia	Protrusion of an organ or part through the muscle normally containing it.
	A **hiatal hernia** occurs when the upper part of the stomach protrudes through the esophageal opening in the diaphragm. An **inguinal hernia** occurs when a small loop

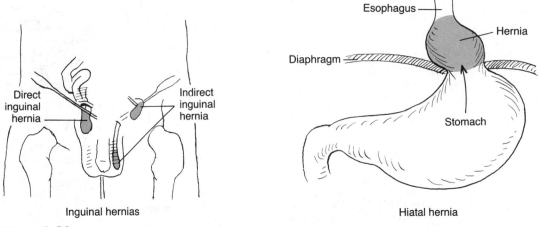

Figure 5–20

Hernias.

of bowel protrudes through a weak place in the lower abdominal muscle wall (groin). Muscle weakness can be inherited or acquired as part of the aging process, pregnancy, obesity, or heavy lifting and coughing (Fig. 5–20).

ileus

Intestinal obstruction.

Etiology may be tumor, failure of peristalsis, or abnormal twisting of the intestine.

intussusception

Telescoping of the intestines.

The condition occurs most commonly in children and usually in the ileocecal region. Treatment involves resection of the intussusception and anastomosis (Fig. 5–21).

irritable bowel syndrome

A group of symptoms (diarrhea and constipation, lower abdominal pain, and bloating) associated with stress and tension. Also called **spastic colon.**

No pathological lesions are found in the intestines. Treatment includes psychotherapy to manage stress and medications (antidiarrheals and bulk-forming

Figure 5–21

Intussusception.

Figure 5–22

Volvulus.

laxatives) to relieve symptoms. A diet high in bran and fiber also helps soften stools and establish regular bowel movements.

ulcer   Open sore or lesion (wound) of skin (epithelial) tissue.

Gastric or duodenal ulcers (both are peptic ulcers) are examples. Duodenal ulcers are now thought to be caused by a bacterium, *Helicobacter pylori.* The combination of bacteria, hyperacidity, and gastric juice (called pepsin) damages epithelial linings. A **perforating ulcer** is one that creates a hole through the entire thickness of an organ. Treatment includes drugs to reduce the production of hydrochloric acid and protect the lining of the stomach and intestine. Research is aimed at finding antibiotics to destroy *H. pylori.*

ulcerative colitis   Chronic inflammation of the colon with the presence of ulcers.

This is an idiopathic, chronic, recurrent diarrheal disease (inflammatory bowel disease). Resection of diseased bowel with colostomy or ileostomy may be necessary as treatment. Unlike Crohn's disease, this inflammatory bowel disease is associated with a higher risk of colon cancer.

volvulus   Twisting of the intestine upon itself.

A surgical emergency, the volvulus must be released immediately (Fig. 5–22).

Liver, Gallbladder, and Pancreas

cirrhosis   Chronic disease of the liver with degeneration of liver cells.

Alcoholism combined with malnutrition is a common etiological factor, but infection and poisons can affect the liver cells as well. Alcohol has a toxic effect on hepatocytes, causing fat cells to accumulate, followed by necrosis and fibrous scarring, and discoloration (cirrh/o refers to the liver's orange-yellow color). As with other liver diseases, jaundice results when the liver cells fail to function and bilirubin is not eliminated from the body.

gallstones   Hard collections of bile form in the gallbladder and bile ducts; also called **chole-lithiasis.**

Calculi (stones) can prevent bile from leaving the gallbladder and bile ducts to enter the duodenum (Fig. 5–23). Conventional treatment has been cholecystectomy or choledo-cholithotomy. More recently, a technique has been developed to remove the gallbladder by laparoscopic technique (laparoscopic cholecystectomy) similar to that used to tie off the fallopian tubes (tubal ligation). In another procedure, an endoscope is passed through

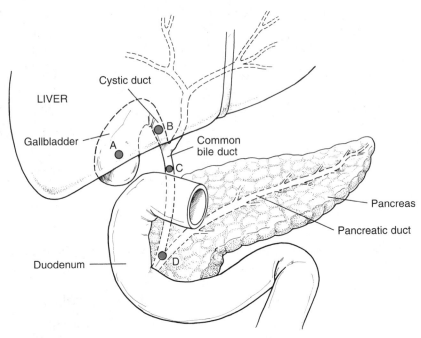

Figure 5–23

Positions in which gallstones can cause symptoms. *(A)* Stone in the gallbladder causing mild or no symptoms. *(B)* Stone obstructing the cystic duct causing pain. *(C)* Stone obstructing the common bile duct causing pain and jaundice. *(D)* Stone at the lower end of the common bile duct and pancreatic duct causing pain, jaundice, and pancreatitis.

the esophagus and stomach to the common bile duct. It snares a stone with a basket-type device and removes the stone orally. In addition, a drug (chenodiol) is now given orally to decrease cholesterol synthesis in the liver and dissolve existing stones.

pancreatitis Inflammation of the pancreas.

Digestive enzymes attack pancreatic tissue, leading to damage to the gland. In most cases the etiology is unknown, but inflammation can develop from alcoholism, gallstones, abdominal trauma, or drugs. Treatment includes drugs to relieve pain, intravenous fluids, careful monitoring of diet, and surgery to remove portions of the gland.

viral hepatitis Inflammation of the liver caused by virus.

There are three major types of viral hepatitis: **Hepatitis A** (caused by type A virus and previously called infectious hepatitis) is a benign, acute, self-limited disorder transmitted by infected water and food (virus is also excreted in feces). **Hepatitis B** (caused by type B virus and called serum hepatitis) is acquired parenterally, through blood (transfusions, hypodermic needles, and dental and surgical instruments) and via body fluids, such as tears, saliva, and semen. A vaccine that provides immunity to hepatitis B is recommended for hospital personnel, dentists, laboratory technicians, and persons requiring frequent transfusions. **Hepatitis C** is transmitted by blood or blood products and close personal contact. In both hepatitis B and hepatitis C, liver enzymes may be elevated, indicating damage to liver tissue. Symptoms include malaise, joint pain, and in severe cases, nausea, anorexia, and jaundice.

VI. Exercises

Remember to check your answers carefully with those given in Section VII, Answers to Exercises.

A. Match the following digestive system structures with their meanings below.

anus   sigmoid colon   ileum
esophagus   pancreas   liver
jejunum   gallbladder   colon
pharynx   cecum   duodenum

1. large intestine ___*cecum* *colon*___

2. small sac under the liver; stores bile ___*gall*___

3. first part of the large intestine ___*duodenum* *cecum*___

4. opening of the digestive tract to the outside of the body ___*anus*___

5. second part of the small intestine ___*jejunum*___

6. tube connecting the throat to the stomach ___*eso*___

7. third part of the small intestine ___*ileum*___

8. large organ located in the RUQ; secretes bile, stores sugar, produces blood proteins

   ___*liver*___

9. throat ___*pharynx*___

10. lower part of the colon ___*sigmoid*___

11. first part of the small intestine ___*duodenum*___

12. organ under the stomach; produces insulin and digestive enzymes ___*pancreas*___

B. Circle the term that correctly fits the definition given. You should be able to define the other terms as well!

1. **tiny, microscopic projections in the walls of the small intestine:**
   papillae   villi   rugae

2. **salivary gland near the ear:**
   submandibular   sublingual   parotid

3. **ring of muscle at the distal end of the stomach:**
   pyloric sphincter   uvula   cardiac sphincter

4. **soft, inner section of a tooth:**
   dentin   enamel   *pulp*

5. **chemical that speeds up reactions and helps digest foods:**
   triglyceride   amino acid   *enzyme*

6. **pigment released with bile:**
   glycogen   *bilirubin*   melena

7. **hormone produced by endocrine cells of the pancreas:**
   insulin   amylase   lipase

8. **rhythm-like movement of the muscles in the walls of the gastrointestinal tract:**
   deglutition   mastication   *peristalsis*

9. **breakdown of large fat globules:**
   absorption   *emulsification*   anabolism

10. **pointed, dog-like tooth medial to premolars:**
    incisor   *canine*   molar

C. Complete the following.

1. labi/o and cheil/o both mean _____

2. gloss/o and lingu/o both mean _____

3. or/o and stomat/o both mean _____

4. dent/i and odont/o both mean _____

5. lapar/o and celi/o both mean _____

6. gluc/o and glyc/o both mean _____

7. lip/o, steat/o, and adip/o all mean _____

8. -iasis and -osis both mean _____

9. chol/e and bil/i both mean _____

10. -ectomy and resection both mean _____

D. Build medical terms.

1. removal of a salivary gland _____

2. pertaining to the throat _____

3. hernia of the rectum _____

4. enlargement of the liver _____

5. surgical repair of the roof of the mouth _____

6. after meals _____

7. visual examination of the anal and rectal region _____

8. study of the cause (of disease) _____

9. incision of the common bile duct _____

10. pertaining to tooth and cheek (the surface of tooth against the cheek) _____

11. disease condition of the small intestine _____

12. new opening between the common bile duct and the jejunum _____

13. pertaining to surrounding the anus _____

14. new opening from the colon to the outside of the body _____

15. pertaining to under the lower jaw _____

16. pertaining to the face _____

E. Match the following doctors or dentists with their specialties.

oral surgeon   endodontist   colorectal surgeon
orthodontist   proctologist   nephrologist
gastroenterologist   periodontist   urologist

1. diagnosis and treatment of disorders of the anus and rectum _proctologist_

2. operates on the organs of the urinary tract _urologist_

3. straightens teeth _ortho_

4. performs root canal therapy _____

5. operates on the mouth and teeth _oral_

6. diagnoses and uses drugs to treat kidney disorders _nephrologist_

7. diagnoses and treats alimentary tract disorders _gastre_

8. treats gum disease _____

9. operates on the intestinal tract _colorectal_

F. Build medical terms to describe the following inflammations.

1. inflammation of the appendix _____

2. inflammation of the large intestine _____

3. inflammation of the tube from the throat to the stomach _____

4. inflammation of the membrane around the abdomen _____

5. inflammation of the gallbladder _____

6. inflammation of the third part of the small intestine _____

7. inflammation of the pancreas _____

8. inflammation of the gums _____

9. inflammation of the liver _____

10. inflammation of the mouth _____

11. inflammation of the salivary gland _____

12. inflammation of the small and large intestine _____

G. Match the following terms with their meanings below.

anastomosis   hyperglycemia   mesentery
mucosa   malabsorption   parenteral
biliary   dysphagia   gluconeogenesis
hepatic portal system hyperbilirubinemia   glycogenolysis

1. high level of blood sugar _____ hyperglycemia _____

2. difficult, painful swallowing _____ dysphagia _____

3. pertaining to administration other than through the intestinal tract _____ parenteral _____

4. a mucous membrane _____ mucosa _____

5. the veins that carry blood to and from the liver _____ hepatic p. sys _____

6. breakdown (conversion) of animal starch to sugar _____ mesentery _____

7. membrane that connects the small intestine to the abdominal wall _____ mucosa _____

8. difficult passage of material into the bloodstream _____ malabsorption _____

9. new surgical connection between two previously unconnected organs _anastomosis_

10. pertaining to bile ducts and organs ___biliary___

11. process of forming new sugar from proteins and fats ___gluconeogenesis___

12. high levels of a bile pigment in the bloodstream ___hyperbili___

H. Give the names of the following gastrointestinal symptoms from their descriptions.

1. bright red blood in stools _____

2. lack of appetite _____

3. discharge of fat in the feces _____

4. black, tarry stools; feces contain blood _____

5. abnormal accumulation of fluid in the abdomen _____

6. lack of hydrochloric acid in the stomach _____

7. acute abdominal pain _____

8. gas expelled through the anus _____

9. an unpleasant sensation from the stomach with a tendency to vomit _____

10. return of solids and fluid to the mouth from the stomach _____

11. loose, watery stools _____

12. difficult, delayed elimination of feces with dry, hard stools _____

I. Give short answers for the following.

1. What is jaundice? _____

2. Give three ways in which a patient can become jaundiced:

   a. _____

   b. _____

   c. _____

3. What does it mean when a disease is described as _idiopathic?_ _____

J. Using the pathological terminology listed below complete the following sentences.

herpetic stomatitis	aphthous stomatitis	achalasia
dental caries	oral leukoplakia	periodontal disease
colorectal cancer	colonic polyposis	anal fistula
Crohn's disease		

1. Ms. Lewis's dysphagia was diagnosed by her doctor as being caused by a failure of the muscles in her lower esophagus to relax during swallowing. Her condition is also known as

   _____ .

2. Mr. Rosen's proctalgia was related to the abnormal tube-like passageway that formed near his anus. His

   doctor performed surgery to close off the _____ *anal fistula* _____ .

3. When bacteria produce acid that eats away at tooth enamel, the result can be tooth decay, otherwise

   known as _____ .

4. Nancy Brand's symptoms of chronic diarrhea, abdominal cramps, and fever led her doctor to suspect that she suffered from an inflammatory bowel disease that affected the distal portion of her ileum. He

   prescribed steroid drugs to heal her condition, also known as _____ *Crohns disease* *colonic polyposis* _____ .

5. The results of President Reagan's colonoscopy revealed the presence of small benign growths protruding from the mucous membrane of his large intestine. His diagnosis was

   _____ *colonic polyposis* _____ .

6. During a routine dental checkup, Dr. Payne discovered white plaques on Jim's buccal mucosa. A chronic smoker and alcoholic, Jim was advised that the lesions were precancerous and should be removed. His

   diagnosis was _____ *oral leukoplakia* _____ .

7. Every time Bob had a stressful time at work he developed a fever blister (cold sore) on his lip, resulting from reactivation of a previous viral infection. His doctor told him his condition was called

   _____ *herpetic stomatitis* _____ .

8. After biopsy of the neoplasm in Mr. Greenberg's ascending colon, and determination that the lesion was

   malignant, Dr. Jones's diagnosis was _____ *colerectal cancer* _____ .
   He advised radical (complete) colectomy followed by colostomy.

9. The small ulcers (canker sores) on Diane's gums and buccal mucosa were both painful and annoying.

   Her dentist told her that the condition was known as _____ *dental car* _____ ,
   and he did not know what caused it.

10. Failure to floss her teeth and remove dental plaque regularly led to Sharon's gingivitis and pyorrhea.

Her dentist called the condition _____
and advised consulting a specialist who could treat her condition.

K. Match the following pathological diagnoses with their definitions.

hepatitis	pancreatitis	cirrhosis
ileus	dysentery	irritable bowel syndrome
diverticula	cholecystolithiasis	hiatal hernia
peptic ulcer	intussusception	volvulus
esophageal varices	ulcerative colitis	hemorrhoids

1. protrusion of the upper part of the stomach through the esophageal opening in the diaphragm

   _____ hiatal hernia _____

2. painful, inflamed intestines caused by bacterial infection _____

3. swollen, twisted veins in the rectal region _____ hemorrhoid _____

4. a sore or lesion of the mucous membrane in the gastric or duodenal region

   _____ peptic ulcer _____

5. intestinal obstruction _____

6. twisting of the intestine upon itself _____

7. swollen, twisted veins around the distal end of the esophagus _____

8. abnormal side-pockets in the intestinal wall _____ diverticula _____

9. chronic inflammation of the large bowel with ulcers _____

10. telescoping of the intestines _____ intussusception _____

11. inflammation of the liver caused by type A, type B, or type C virus ____ hepatitis _____

12. inflammation of the pancreas _____ pancreatitis _____

13. calculi in the sac that stores bile _____

14. chronic liver disease resulting from alcoholism and malnutrition ___ ah cirrhosis ___

15. a group of symptoms (diarrhea and constipation, abdominal pain, bloating) associated with stress and

   tension, but without inflammation of the intestine _____ irritable bowel syndrome ____

L. Complete the following terms from their meanings given below.

1. membrane (peritoneal fold) that holds the intestines together: mes _____

2. removal of the gallbladder: _____ ectomy

3. black, dark brown, tarry stools containing blood: mel _____

4. high levels of pigment in the blood (jaundice): hyper _____

5. pertaining to under the tongue: sub _____

6. twisting of the intestine upon itself: vol _____

7. organ under the stomach that produces insulin and digestive enzymes: pan _____

8. lack of appetite: an _____

9. swollen, twisted veins in the rectal region: _____ oids

10. new connection between two previously unconnected tubes: ana _____

VII. Answers to Exercises

A

1. colon
2. gallbladder
3. cecum
4. anus
5. jejunum
6. esophagus
7. ileum
8. liver
9. pharynx
10. sigmoid colon
11. duodenum
12. pancreas

B

1. Villi. Papillae are nipple-like projections in the tongue where taste buds are located, and rugae are folds in the mucous membrane of the stomach and hard palate.
2. Parotid. The submandibular gland is under the lower jaw, and the sublingual gland is under the tongue.
3. Pyloric sphincter. The uvula is soft tissue hanging from the soft palate, the cardiac sphincter is a ring of muscle between the esophagus and stomach.
4. Pulp. Dentin is the hard part of the tooth directly under the enamel and in the root; and enamel is the hard, outermost part of the tooth composing the crown.
5. Enzyme. A triglyceride is a large fat molecule, and an amino acid is substance produced when proteins are digested.
6. Bilirubin. Glycogen is animal starch that is produced in liver cells from sugar, and melena is dark, tarry stools.
7. Insulin. Amylase and lipase are digestive enzymes produced by the exocrine cells of the pancreas.
8. Peristalsis. Deglutition is swallowing, and mastication is chewing.
9. Emulsification. Absorption is the passage of materials through the walls of the small intestine into the bloodstream, and anabolism is the process of building up proteins in a cell (protein synthesis).
10. Canine. An incisor is one of the four front teeth in the dental arch (not pointed or dog-like), and a molar is one of three large teeth just behind (distal to) the two premolar teeth.

C

1. lip
2. tongue
3. mouth
4. tooth
5. abdomen
6. sugar
7. fat
8. abnormal condition
9. gall, bile
10. removal, excision

D

1. sialadenectomy
2. pharyngeal
3. rectocele
4. hepatomegaly
5. palatoplasty
6. postprandial (post cibum—cib/o means meals)
7. proctoscopy
8. etiology
9. choledochotomy
10. dentibuccal
11. enteropathy
12. choledochojejunostomy
13. perianal
14. colostomy
15. submandibular
16. facial

E

1. proctologist
2. urologist
3. orthodontist
4. endodontists
5. oral surgeon
6. nephrologist
7. gastroenterologist
8. periodontist
9. colorectal surgeon

F

1. appendicitis
2. colitis
3. esophagitis
4. peritonitis (note that the e is dropped)
5. cholecystitis
6. ileitis
7. pancreatitis
8. gingivitis
9. hepatitis
10. stomatitis
11. sialadenitis
12. enterocolitis (when two combining forms for gastrointestinal organs are in a term, use the one that is closest to the mouth first)

G

1. hyperglycemia
2. dysphagia
3. parenteral
4. mucosa
5. hepatic portal system
6. glycogenolysis
7. mesentery
8. malabsorption
9. anastomosis
10. biliary
11. gluconeogenesis
12. hyperbilirubinemia

H

1. hematochezia
2. anorexia
3. steatorrhea
4. melena
5. ascites
6. achlorhydria
7. colic
8. flatus
9. nausea
10. gastroesophageal reflux (regurgitation or heartburn)
11. diarrhea
12. constipation

I

1. yellow-orange coloration of the skin and other tissues (hyperbilirubinemia)
2. a. any liver disease (hepatopathy—such as cirrhosis, hepatoma, or hepatitis), so that bilirubin is not processed into bile and cannot be excreted in feces
b. obstruction of bile flow, so that bile and bilirubin are not excreted and accumulate in the bloodstream
c. excessive hemolysis leading to overproduction of bilirubin and high levels in the bloodstream
3. its cause is not known

J

1. achalasia
2. anal fistula
3. dental caries
4. Crohn's disease
5. colonic polyposis
6. oral leukoplakia
7. herpetic stomatitis
8. colorectal cancer
9. aphthous stomatitis
10. periodontal disease

K

1. hiatal hernia
2. dysentery
3. hemorrhoids
4. peptic ulcer
5. ileus
6. volvulus
7. esophageal varices
8. diverticula (diverticulosis)
9. ulcerative colitis
10. intussusception
11. viral hepatitis
12. pancreatitis
13. cholecystolithiasis (gallstones)
14. cirrhosis
15. irritable bowel syndrome

L

1. mesentery
2. cholecystectomy
3. melena
4. hyperbilirubinemia
5. sublingual
6. volvulus
7. pancreas
8. anorexia
9. hemorrhoids
10. anastomosis

VIII. Pronunciation of Terms

To test your understanding of the terminology in this chapter, write the meaning of each term in the space provided. In addition, you may wish to cover the terms and write them by looking at your definitions. Make sure your spelling is correct. The page number after each term indicates where it is defined or used in the text so you can easily check your responses. If you are not sure what the pronunciation symbols mean, refer to page 21.

Vocabulary and Terminology Sections

Term	Pronunciation	Meaning
absorption (135)	ăb-SŎRP-shŭn	
alimentary canal (135)	ăl-ĕ-MĔN-tăr-ē kă-NĂL	
amino acids (135)	ă-MĒ-nō ĂS-ĭdz	
amylase (135)	ĂM-ĭ-lās	
anus (135)	Ā-nŭs	
appendectomy (137)	ăp-ĕn-DĔK-tō-mē	
appendicitis (137)	ă-pĕn-dĭ-SĪ-tĭs	
appendix (135)	ă-PĔN-dĭks	
bile (135)	BĪL	
biliary (141)	BĬL-ē-ăr-ē	
bilirubin (135)	bĭl-ĭ-ROO-bĭn	
bowel (135)	BŎW-ĕl	
buccal mucosa (139)	BŬK-ăl mū-KŌ-să	
canine teeth (135)	KĀ-nīn tēth	
cecal (139)	SĒ-kăl	
cecum (135)	SĒ-kŭm	
celiac (139)	SĒ-lē-ăk	
cheilosis (139)	kī-LŌ-sĭs	
cholecystectomy (139)	kō-lĕ-sĭs-TĔK-tō-mē	
choledocholithiasis (142)	kō-lĕd-ō-kō-lĭ-THĪ-ă-sĭs	
choledochojejunostomy (140)	kō-lĕd-ō-kō-jĭ-jū-NŎS-tō-mē	

choledochotomy (139)	kō-lĕd-ō-KŎT-ō-mē	_____
cholelithiasis (141)	kō-lē-lĭ-THĪ-ă-sĭs	_____
colon (135)	KŌ-lĕn	_____
colonic (139)	kō-LŎN-ĭk	_____
colonoscopy (139)	kō-lŏn-ŎS-kō-pē	_____
colostomy (139)	kŏ-LŎS-tō-mē	_____
common bile duct (135)	KŎM-ĭn bīl dŭkt	_____
deglutition (135)	dē-gloo-TĬSH-ŭn	_____
dentibuccal (139)	dĕn-tē-BŬK-ăl	_____
dentin (135)	DĔN-tĭn	_____
digestion (135)	dī-JĔST-yŭn	_____
duodenal (139)	dū-ō-DĒ-năl or dū-ŎD-dĕ-năl	_____
duodenum (135)	dū-ō-DĒ-nŭm or dū-ŎD-dĕ-ŭm	_____
emulsification (135)	ē-mŭl-sĭ-fĭ-KĀ-shŭn	_____
enamel (136)	ē-NĂM-ĕl	_____
endodontist (141)	ĕn-dō-DŎN-tĭst	_____
enterocolitis (141)	ĕn-tĕr-ō-kō-LĪ-tĭs	_____
enterocolostomy (139)	ĕn-tĕr-ō-kō-LŎS-tō-mē	_____
enteropathy (139)	ĕn-tĕr-ŎP-ă-thē	_____
enzyme (136)	ĔN-zīm	_____
esophageal (140)	ĕ-sŏf-ă-JĒ-ăl	_____
esophagus (136)	ĕ-SŎF-ă-gŭs	_____
facial (140)	FĀ-shŭl	_____
feces (136)	FĒ-sēz	_____
gallbladder (136)	găl-BLĂ-dĕr	_____
gastralgia (140)	găs-TRĂL-jă	_____
gastrojejunostomy (140)	găs-trō-jĭ-jū-NŎS-tō-mē	_____

gluconeogenesis (142)	gloo-kō-nē-ō-JĚN-ĕ-sĭs	_____
glucose (136)	GLOO-kōs	_____
glycogen (136)	GLĪ-kō-jĕn	_____
glycogenolysis (142)	glī-kō-jĕ-NŎL-ĭ-sĭs	_____
hepatic portal system (136)	hĕ-PĂ-tĭk PŎR-tăl SĬS-tĕm	_____
hepatoma (140)	hĕ-pă-TŌ-mă	_____
hepatomegaly (140)	hĕ-pă-tō-MĔG-ă-lē	_____
hydrochloric acid (136)	hī-drō-KLŎR-ĭk Ă-sĭd	_____
hyperbilirubinemia (141)	hī-pĕr-bĭl-ĭ-roo-bĭ-NĒ-mē-ă	_____
hyperglycemia (142)	hī-pĕr-glī-SĒ-mē-ă	_____
hypoglossal (140)	hī-pō-GLŎ-săl	_____
ileitis (140)	ĭl-ē-Ī-tĭs	_____
ileocecal sphincter (140)	ĭl-ē-ō-SĒ-kăl SFĬNGK-tĕr	_____
ileostomy (140)	ĭl-ē-ŎS-tō-mē	_____
ileum (136)	ĬL-ē-ŭm	_____
incisor (136)	ĭn-SĪ-zŏr	_____
insulin (136)	ĬN-sŭ-lĭn	_____
jejunum (136)	jĕ-JOO-nŭm	_____
labial (140)	LĀ-bē-ăl	_____
laparoscopy (140)	lă-pă-RŎS-kō-pē	_____
lipase (136)	LĪ-pās	_____
liver (136)	LĬ-vĕr	_____
mastication (136)	măs-tĭ-KĀ-shŭn	_____
mesentery (139)	MĔS-ĕn-tĕr-ē	_____
molar teeth (126)	MŌ-lăr-tēth	_____
oral (141)	ŎR-ăl	_____
orthodontist (140)	ŏr-thō-DŎN-tĭst	_____
palate (136)	PĂL-ăt	_____

palatoplasty (141)	PĂL-ă-tō-plăs-tē	_____
pancreas (136)	PĂN-krē-ăs	_____
pancreatitis (141)	păn-krē-ă-TĪ-tĭs	_____
papillae (136)	pă-PĬL-ē	_____
parenteral (140)	pă-RĔN-tĕr-ăl	_____
parotid gland (136)	pă-RŎT-ĭd gland	_____
perianal (137)	pĕ-rē-Ā-năl	_____
periodontist (141)	pĕr-ē-ō-DŎN-tĭst	_____
peristalsis (137)	pĕr-ĭ-STĂL-sĭs	_____
pharyngeal (141)	făr-ăn-JĒ-ăl or fă-RĬN-jē-ăl	_____
pharynx (137)	FĂR-ĭnks	_____
postprandial (142)	pōst-PRĂN-dē-ăl	_____
premolar teeth (126)	prē-MŌ-lăr tēth	_____
proctologist (141)	prŏk-TŎL-ō-jĭst	_____
pulp (137)	pŭlp	_____
pyloric sphincter (137)	pī-LŎR-ĭk SFĬNGK-tĕr	_____
pyloroplasty (141)	pī-LŎR-ō-plăs-tē	_____
rectocele (141)	RĔK-tō-sēl	_____
rectum (137)	RĔK-tŭm	_____
rugae (137)	ROO-gē	_____
saliva (137)	să-LĪ-vă	_____
salivary glands (137)	SĂL-ĭ-vĕr-ē glăndz	_____
sialadenectomy (141)	sī-ăl-ă-dĕ-NĔK-tō-mē	_____
sialolith (142)	sī-ĂL-ō-lĭth	_____
sigmoid colon (137)	SĬG-moyd KŌ-lŏn	_____
sigmoidoscopy (141)	sĭg-moy-DŎS-kō-pē	_____
sphincter (137)	SFĬNGK-tĕr	_____
steatorrhea (142)	stē-ă-tō-RĒ-ă	_____

stomatitis (141)	stō-mă-TĪ-tĭs	
sublingual (140)	sŭb-LĬNG-wăl	
submandibular (140)	sŭb-măn-DĬB-ū-lăr	
triglycerides (137)	trī-GLĬ-sĕ-rīdz	
uvula (137)	Ū-vū-lă	
villi (137)	VĬL-ī	

Pathological Terminology

Term	Pronunciation	Meaning
achalasia (145)	ăk-ăh-LĀ-zē-ă	
achlorhydria (142)	ā-klŏr-HĬD-rē-ă	
anal fistula (145)	Ā-năl FĬS-tū-lă	
anorexia (143)	ăn-ō-RĔK-sē-ă	
aphthous stomatitis (144)	ĂF-thŭs stō-mă-TĪ-tĭs	
ascites (143)	ă-SĪ-tēz	
cholelithiasis (149)	kō-lĕ-lĭ-THĪ-ă-sĭs	
cirrhosis (149)	sĭr-RŌ-sĭs	
colic (143)	KŎL-ĭk	
colonic polyposis (145)	kō-LŎN-ĭk pŏl-ĭ-PŌ-sĭs	
colorectal cancer (145)	kō-lō-RĔK-tăl KĂN-sĕr	
constipation (143)	cŏn-stĭ-PĀ-shŭn	
Crohn's disease (147)	krōnz dĭ-ZĒZ	
dental caries (144)	DĔN-tăl KĂR-ēz	
diarrhea (143)	dī-ăh-RĒ-ă	
diverticula (147)	dī-vĕr-TĬK-ū-lă	
dysentery (147)	DĬS-ĕn-tĕr-ē	
dysphagia (143)	dĭs-PHĀ-jē-ă	

esophageal varices (147)	ē-sŏf-ăh-JĒ-ăl VĂR-ĭ-sēz	
etiology (142)	ē-tē-ŎL-ō-jē	
flatus (143)	FLĀ-tŭs	
gastroesophageal reflux (143)	găs-trō-ē-sŏf-ă-JĒ-ăl RĒ-flŭx	
hematochezia (142)	hēm-ă-tō-KĒ-zē-ă	
hemorrhoids (147)	HĔM-ō-roydz	
herpetic stomatitis (144)	hĕr-PĔT-ĭk stō-măh-TĪ-tĭs	
hiatal hernia (147)	hī-Ā-tăl HĔR-nē-ă	
icterus (144)	ĬK-tĕr-ŭs	
idiopathic (142)	ĭd-ē-ō-PĂTH-ĭk	
ileus (148)	ĬL-ē-ŭs	
inflammatory bowel disease (147)	ĭn-FLĂ-mă-tō-rē BŎW-ĕl dĭ-zēz	
inguinal hernia (147)	ĬNG-wă-năl HĔR-nē-ă	
intussusception (148)	ĭn-tŭs-sŭs-SĔP-shŭn	
irritable bowel syndrome (148)	ĬR-ĭh-tăl-bil BŎW-ĕl SĬN-drōm	
jaundice (144)	JĂWN-dĭs	
melena (144)	MĔL-ĕh-nă or mĕ-LĒ-nă	
nausea (144)	NĂW-zē-ă	
oral leukoplakia (144)	ŎR-ăl lū-kō-PLĀ-kē-ă	
pancreatitis (150)	păn-krē-ă-TĪ-tĭs	
periodontal disease (145)	pĕr-ē-ō-DŎN-tăl dĭ-ZĒZ	
ulcer (149)	ŬL-sĕr	
ulcerative colitis (149)	ŬL-sĕr-ă-tĭv kō-LĪ-tĭs	
viral hepatitis (150)	VĪ-răl hĕp-ă-TĬ-tĭs	
volvulus (149)	VŎL-vū-lŭs	

Additional Suffixes and Digestive System Terminology

This Chapter is divided into the following sections

In this Chapter you will

- Define new suffixes and use them with digestive system combining forms;
- List and explain some laboratory tests, clinical procedures, and abbreviations common to the digestive system.

I. Introduction

This chapter will give you practice in word building, while not introducing a large number of new terms. It is designed to give you a breather after a long and difficult chapter.

Study the new suffixes in Section II first and complete the meanings of the terms in Sections II and III. Checking the meanings of the terms with a dictionary may prove helpful and add additional understanding.

The information included in Section IV (Laboratory Tests, Clinical Procedures, and Abbreviations) should be useful to those of you who work in laboratory or clinical areas and also serve as a helpful reference.

Section V (Practical Applications) is designed to give you examples of medical language in context. Congratulate yourself as you decipher medical sentences, operation reports, case studies, and other material. You may also find this section useful in class as an oral reading exercise.

II. Suffixes

Write the meaning of the medical term in the space provided.

Suffix	Meaning	Terminology	Meaning
-ectasis, -ectasia ✓	stretching, dilation, dilatation	bronchiectasis _____ *Bronchi/o means bronchial tubes.* lymphangiectasia _____	
-emesis	vomiting	hematemesis _____	
-lysis	destruction, breakdown, separation	hemolysis _____ *Red blood cells are destroyed.*	
-pepsia	digestion	dyspepsia _____	
-phagia	eating, swallowing	polyphagia _____ *Appetite is increased.* dysphagia _____	
-plasty	surgical repair	rhinoplasty _____ blepharoplasty _____	
-ptosis	prolapse, fall, sag	proptosis _____ *Pro- means before, forward. This term refers to the forward protrusion of the eye (exophthalmia).*	
-ptysis	spitting	hemoptysis _____ *From the respiratory tract and lungs.*	
-rrhagia, -rrhage	bursting forth of blood	hemorrhage _____ menorrhagia _____ *Men/o means menstrual flow.*	
-rrhaphy	suture	herniorrhaphy _____ *Herni/o means hernia. The hernia is repaired.*	
-rrhea	flow, discharge	menorrhea _____ dysmenorrhea _____	

-spasm	sudden, involuntary contraction of muscles	pylorospasm _____
		cardiospasm _____
		Spasm of the cardiac sphincter at the distal end of the esophagus; achalasia.
-stasis	stopping, controlling	cholestasis _____
		hemostasis _____
-stenosis	tightening, stricture, narrowing	pyloric stenosis _____
		A narrowed lumen (space within a tubular structure).
-tresia ✓	opening	atresia _____
		A structure that should have been open is closed.
		esophageal atresia _____
		A congenital anomaly in which the esophagus does not connect with the stomach. It is commonly accompanied by a tracheo-esophageal fistula.
		biliary atresia _____
		Congenital hypoplasia or nonformation of bile ducts resulting in jaundice.

Many of the suffixes that are listed above are also used alone as separate terms. They are listed below with examples of how the term would be used in a sentence.

ectasia	Mammary duct **ectasia** may cause mastitis.
lysis	The disease caused **lysis** of liver cells.
emesis (emetic)	If a child swallows poison, a drug to induce **emesis** is prescribed. A strong solution of salt or ipecac syrup is an example of an emetic.
ptosis	Mr. Smith's weakened eyelid muscles caused **ptosis** of his lids.
spasm	Eating spicy foods can lead to **spasm** of gastric sphincters.
stasis	Overgrowth of bacteria within the small intestine causes **stasis** of the intestinal contents.
stenosis	Projectile vomiting in an infant during feeding is a symptom of pyloric **stenosis.**

III. Combining Forms and Terminology

Write the meaning of the combining form and then the meaning of the term that includes that combining form in the spaces provided.

Combining Form	Meaning	Terminology	Meaning
bucc/o	_____	buccal _____	
cec/o	_____	cecal volvulus _____	
celi/o	_____	celiac artery _____	
		Carries blood from the aorta to the abdomen.	
cheil/o	_____	cheilosis _____	
chol/e	_____	cholelithiasis _____	
cholangi/o	_____	cholangiectasis _____	
cholecyst/o	_____	cholecystectomy _____	
choledoch/o	_____	choledochal _____	
col/o	_____	colectomy _____	
colon/o	_____	colonoscopy _____	
dent/i	_____	dentalgia _____	
duoden/o	_____	gastroduodenal anastomosis _____	
		_____	
enter/o	_____	gastroenteritis _____	
esophag/o	_____	esophageal atresia _____	
		A congenital anomaly that must be corrected surgically.	
gastr/o	_____	gastrojejunostomy _____	
gingiv/o	_____	gingivectomy _____	
gloss/o	_____	glossopharyngeal _____	
glyc/o	_____	glycolysis _____	

hepat/o _____ hepatomegaly _____

herni/o _____ herniorrhaphy _____

ile/o _____ ileostomy _____

jejun/o _____ cholecystojejunostomy _____

labi/o _____ labioglossopharyngeal _____

lingu/o _____ sublingual _____

lip/o _____ lipase _____

lith/o _____ cholecystolithiasis _____

odont/o _____ periodontal membrane _____

or/o _____ oropharynx _____

The tonsils are in the oropharynx.

palat/o _____ palatoplasty _____

This surgical procedure is performed to correct a congenital anomaly called cleft (split) palate.

pancreat/o _____ pancreatic _____

proct/o _____ proctosigmoidoscopy _____

pylor/o _____ pyloric stenosis _____

rect/o _____ rectosigmoidectomy _____

sialaden/o _____ sialadenectomy _____

splen/o _____ splenic flexure _____

The bend in the transverse colon downward near the spleen.

steat/o _____ steatorrhea _____

stomat/o _____ aphthous stomatitis _____

IV. Laboratory Tests, Clinical Procedures, and Abbreviations

Laboratory Tests

Liver Function Tests

SGOT (serum glutamic oxaloacetic transaminase)
   Also called **AST** (aspartic acid transaminase) or **OT**

These tests reveal the levels of enzymes (transaminases) in the blood serum. Serum is the clear fluid that remains after blood has clotted. Enzyme levels are elevated when there is damage to liver cells because the enzymes leak out of liver cells into the blood. A high SGPT (ALT) level is especially indicative of liver disease.

SGPT (serum glutamic pyruvic transaminase)
   Also called **ALT** (alanine transaminase) or **PT**

alkaline phosphatase

This is another enzyme test done on serum. An increased level of alkaline phosphatase (alk phos) is found in liver disease, cancers, and many other abnormal conditions.

serum bilirubin

High levels of bilirubin in the blood produce a jaundiced condition in the patient. The test is also known as the icterus index.

Figure 6–1

Barium enemas. *(A)* X-ray of a normal colon (note that the splenic flexure is high in the left upper quadrant). *Arrows* indicate residual stool in cecum and ascending colon. *(B)* X-ray of the descending colon showing diverticula *(arrows)*. (A, From Putman CE, Ravin CE: Textbook of Diagnostic Imaging. Philadelphia, WB Saunders, 1988, p 884; B, From Putman CE, Ravin CE: Textbook of Diagnostic Imaging, 2nd ed. Philadelphia, WB Saunders, 1994, p 836.)

Stool Analyses

stool culture

Feces are placed in a growth medium to test for microorganisms that are in large numbers or abnormally present.

stool guaiac or **Hemoccult test**

Test to determine the presence of blood in the feces and an important screening test for colon cancer. Guaiac (GWĪ-ăk) is a chemical from the wood of trees. It is added to a stool sample and reacts with occult blood.

Clinical Procedures

X-Ray Tests

barium enema

Technicians inject barium sulfate, a contrast medium (substance that x-rays cannot penetrate) by enema into the rectum, and x-rays are taken of the rectum and colon. This is also known as a **lower GI series.** Figure 6–1 shows an x-ray of a normal colon and an x-ray of a colon with diverticula.

barium swallow

Barium sulfate is swallowed and x-rays are taken of the esophagus, stomach, and small intestine. This is also known as an **upper GI series.** In a small-bowel follow-through, sequential x-ray pictures of the small intestine are taken as barium passes through. Figure 6–2 shows a barium swallow of a normal esophagus and a barium swallow of an esophagus with diverticulum.

Figure 6–2

Barium swallows. *(A)* Normal esophagus shown by air-contrast esophagogram (gas-containing granules are swallowed with water, followed by barium swallow). *(B)* Air-contrast esophagogram shows a diverticulum *(arrowheads)* arising from the midesophagus. (*A* and *B,* From Putman CE, Ravin CE: Textbook of Diagnostic Imaging, 2nd ed. Philadelphia, WB Saunders, 1994, pp 669, 709.)

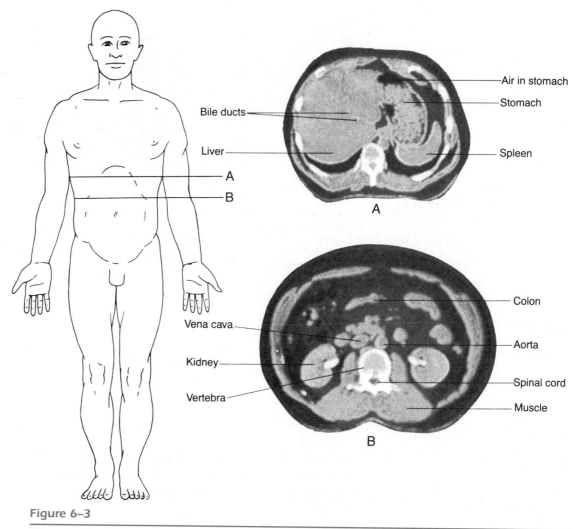

Figure 6–3

CT scans of the abdomen. Lighter color (white) is the most dense tissue (bone) and darker color (black) is the least dense (air). (From Solomon EP, Phillips GA: Understanding Human Anatomy and Physiology. Philadelphia, WB Saunders, 1987, p 21.)

cholangiography	X-ray pictures of the bile vessels. In **percutaneous transhepatic cholangiography,** contrast material is injected via a needle that is inserted through the skin into the liver, and x-rays of bile vessels are taken.
CT (CAT) scan of the abdomen	Computed tomography (computed axial tomography). A series of x-ray pictures are taken and processed by a computer to show a cross-sectional (transverse) image of internal organs. Positioning of the machine gives different cross-sectional pictures of the abdomen (Fig. 6–3). Iodine-based dyes and barium can be used to visualize blood vessels and the gastrointestinal tract. Tomography (tom/o means to cut) means that a *series* of x-rays are taken to see an organ in depth.
endoscopic retrograde cholangiopancreatography (ERCP)	Contrast material (via endoscope) is injected into the pancreatic and bile ducts while x-rays are taken. The endoscope is passed through the mouth, esophagus, and stomach into the duodenum to where the common bile duct and pancreas enter. Retrograde means that the dye is injected in a backward (retro-) direction to the normal flow of substances.

Figure 6–4

(A) Normal liver scan in anterior view. *(B)* Liver scan in anterior view showing multiple metastases from carcinoma of the lung. Multiple "cold" areas (reduced radionuclide uptake) are visible in the liver. (*A* and *B,* From Berk RN: Diagnostic imaging procedures in gastroenterology. *In* Wyngaarden JB, Smith LH Jr [eds]: Cecil Textbook of Medicine, 17th ed. Philadelphia, WB Saunders, 1985, p 653.)

Ultrasound

abdominal ultrasonography   Sound waves are beamed into the abdomen, and a record is made of the echoes as they bounce off the abdominal viscera.

Radioactive

liver scan   Radioactive material is injected intravenously and taken up by the liver cells. An image of the liver (scintiscan) is made using a special scanner that records uptake of radioactive material by the liver cells (Fig. 6–4).

Other Procedures

gastrointestinal endoscopy   A flexible fiberoptic tube is placed through the mouth or anus to visualize parts of the gastrointestinal tract. *Examples:* esophagogastroduodenoscopy, colonoscopy (Fig. 6–5), sigmoidoscopy, proctoscopy. Patients with a family history of gastrointestinal cancer should relate this information to their gastroenterologist so that they receive the appropriate type of endoscopy.

liver biopsy   A needle is inserted percutaneously into the liver, and a sample of liver tissue is removed for microscopic examination. A local anesthetic is injected into the skin overlying the liver so that insertion of the needle is relatively painless. The average sample is less than 1 inch long. This procedure is useful in diagnosis of cirrhosis, chronic hepatitis, and cancerous tumors.

nasogastric intubation   A nasogastric tube (NG tube) is passed through the nose into the stomach and upper region of the small intestine. The procedure is used to remove fluid postoperatively and to obtain gastric or intestinal contents for analysis.

paracentesis (abdominocentesis)   Surgical puncture to remove fluid from the abdomen (peritoneal cavity). This procedure is done to remove fluid from a patient with ascites and for diagnostic purposes.

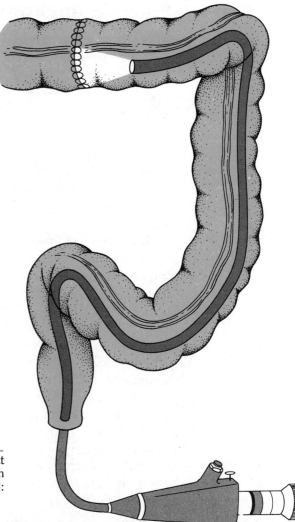

Figure 6–5

Colonoscopy. Note the area of anastomosis that the colonoscope is illuminating. (Redrawn from Routine colonoscopy. Am Fam Physician 35[2]: 264, 1987.)

ABBREVIATIONS

alk phos	alkaline phosphatase
ALT, AST	alanine transaminase, aspartic acid transaminase Enzyme tests of liver function.
BE	barium enema
BRBPR	bright red blood per (through) rectum; hematochezia
BM	bowel movement
CT scan (CAT scan)	computed tomography (computed axial tomography)
EGD	esophagogastroduodenoscopy
ERCP	endoscopic retrograde cholangiopancreatography
GB	gallbladder
GI	gastrointestinal

IBD	inflammatory bowel disease
LFTs	liver function tests; alk phos, bilirubin, AST (SGOT), ALT (SGPT)
NG tube	nasogastric tube
NPO	nothing by mouth (*nulla per os*)
PUD	peptic ulcer disease
SGOT, SGPT	serum glutamic oxaloacetic transaminase, serum glutamic pyruvic transaminase Enzyme tests of liver function.
TPN	total parenteral nutrition This intravenous (IV) solution contains sugar (dextrose), proteins (amino acids), electrolytes (sodium, potassium, chloride), and vitamins.
UGI	upper gastrointestinal

V. Practical Applications

This section contains actual medical reports using terms that you have studied in this and previous chapters. Explanations of more difficult terms are added in brackets.

Colonoscopy Report

The patient is a 73-year-old female who underwent colonoscopy and polypectomy on June 10, 1988. She was thought to have an invasive carcinoma, and on June 12, 1988, she underwent a low anterior resection and coloproctostomy. On August 2, 1989, she was seen in the office for flexible sigmoidoscopy, and a polyp was seen. Colonoscopy was scheduled.

Description of Procedure. The fiberoptic colonoscope was introduced, and I could pass it to about 15 cm, at which point there appeared to be an anastomosis. The colonoscope passed easily through a wide-open anastomosis to 30 cm, at which point a very friable [easily crumbled] polyp, irregular, on a short little stalk, was encountered. This was snared, the coagulating [blood clotting] current was applied, and the pedicle [stalk of the polyp] was severed and recovered and sent to pathology for histological identification. The colonoscope was then reintroduced and passed through the rectum to the sigmoid colon. Again we saw the anastomosis, and proximal to this, we could see the fulgurated [destroyed by high-frequency electric current] base of the removed polyp. No bleeding was encountered, and I continued to advance the colonoscope through the descending colon. We proceeded to advance the colonoscope through the splenic flexure in the transverse colon. In spite of vigorous mechanical bowel preparation and the shortened colon from the previous resection, she had a considerable amount of stool, and it became progressively more difficult to visualize as we approached the hepatic flexure. Finally, at the hepatic flexure, I abandoned further evaluation and began to withdraw the colonoscope. The colonoscope passed through the transverse colon, splenic flexure, descending colon, sigmoid colon, rectum, and anus and was withdrawn. She tolerated the procedure well, but had some nausea. We will await the results of pathology, and in the event that it is not an invasive carcinoma, I would recommend a repeat colonoscopy in 6 months, at which time we will use a 48-hour more vigorous mechanical bowel preparation.

VI. Exercises

Remember to check your answers carefully with those given in Section VII, Answers to Exercises.

A. Give the meanings for the following suffixes.

1. -pepsia _____

2. -ptysis _____

3. -emesis _____

4. -phagia _____

5. -ptosis _____ 11. -ectasis _____

6. -rrhea _____ 12. -stenosis _____

7. -rrhagia _____ 13. -stasis _____

8. -rrhaphy _____ 14. -spasm _____

9. -plasty _____ 15. -ectasia _____

10. -lysis _____

B. Using the suffixes listed in exercise A and the following combining forms, build medical terms.

blephar/o   chol/e   lymphangi/o
hemat/o   men/o   herni/o
hem/o   rhin/o   bronchi/o
pylor/o

1. menstrual flow _____

2. stoppage of bile (flow) _____

3. suture of a hernia _____

4. dilation of lymph vessels _____

5. spitting up of blood (from the respiratory tract) _____

6. vomiting blood (from the digestive tract) _____

7. dilation of tubes leading from the windpipe into the lungs _____

8. surgical repair of eyelids _____

9. stopping blood flow _____

10. surgical repair of the nose _____

11. destruction of blood (red blood cells) _____

12. sudden involuntary contraction of muscles at the distal region of the stomach

_____

13. excessive bleeding (bursting forth of blood) during menstruation _____

14. sudden involuntary contraction of muscles within the bronchial tubes _____

C. Give the meanings for the following terms.

1. dysphagia _____

2. polyphagia _____

3. dyspepsia _____

4. biliary atresia _____

5. proptosis _____

6. cholestasis _____

7. esophageal atresia _____

8. cardiospasm _____

9. emesis _____

10. stenosis _____

D. Match the following surgical procedures with their meanings below.

herniorrhaphy	blepharoplasty	rectosigmoidectomy
cecostomy	gastroduodenal anastomosis	cholecystectomy
sphincterotomy	colectomy	cholecystojejunostomy
gingivectomy	paracentesis	ileostomy

1. removal of the gallbladder _____

2. large bowel resection _____

3. suture of a weakened muscular wall (hernia) _____

4. new opening of the first part of the colon to the outside of the body_____

5. surgical repair of the eyelid _____

6. incision of a ring of muscles _____

7. new surgical connection between the stomach and the first part of the small intestine

   _____

8. opening of the third part of the small intestine to the outside of the body _____

9. removal of gum tissue _____

10. new surgical connection between the gallbladder and the second part of the small intestine

    _____

11. surgical puncture of the abdomen for withdrawal of fluid _____

12. removal of the rectum and sigmoid colon _____

E. Complete the following terms from their meanings.

1. discharge of fat: steat _____

2. painful swallowing: dys _____

3. abnormal condition of gallstones: chole _____

4. pertaining to the cheek: _____ al

5. pain in a tooth: dent _____

6. prolapse of an eyelid: blepharo _____

7. enlargement of the liver: hepato _____

8. pertaining to under the tongue: sub _____

9. removal of the gallbladder: _____ ectomy

10. pertaining to the common bile duct: chole _____

F. Give meanings for the following terms.

1. cecal volvulus _____

2. aphthous stomatitis _____

3. celiac artery _____

4. lipase _____

5. cheilosis _____

6. oropharynx _____

7. glycolysis _____

8. glossopharyngeal _____

9. sialadenectomy _____

10. periodontal membrane _____

G. *Match the name of the laboratory test or clinical procedure with its description.*

CT of the abdomen
liver scan
percutaneous transhepatic
    cholangiography
stool guaiac (Hemoccult)

endoscopic retrograde
    cholangiopancreatography
abdominal ultrasonography
serum bilirubin
barium swallow

stool culture
barium enema
nasogastric intubation
liver biopsy

1. measurement of bile pigment in the blood _____

2. feces are placed in a growth medium for bacterial analysis _____

3. x-ray examination of the lower gastrointestinal tract _____

4. sound waves are used to image abdominal organs _____

5. test to reveal hidden blood in feces _____

6. upper gastrointestinal x-rays _____

7. contrast material is injected through the liver and x-rays are taken of bile vessels

_____

8. tube is inserted through the nose into the stomach _____

9. transverse x-ray pictures of the abdominal organs _____

10. contrast material is injected through an endoscope, and x-ray pictures of the pancreas and bile ducts are

taken _____

11. percutaneous removal of liver tissue followed by microscopic examination

_____

12. radioactive material is injected intravenously, and an image is made of the material as it is taken up by

liver cells _____

H. Match the abbreviation in column I with its meaning in column II. Write the letter of the meaning in the space provided.

Column I

1. TPN _____

2. PUD _____

3. EGD _____

4. IBD _____

5. BE _____

6. SGPT _____

7. LFTs _____

8. NPO _____

Column II

A. liver function tests
B. nothing given by mouth; *nulla per os*
C. includes Crohn's disease and ulcerative colitis—inflammatory bowel disease
D. peptic ulcer disease
E. total parenteral nutrition
F. barium enema
G. esophagogastroduodenoscopy
H. serum glutamic pyruvic transaminase (blood test of liver function)

I. Give the suffix for the following terms.

1. hemorrhage _____

2. flow, discharge _____

3. suture _____

4. dilation _____

5. narrowing, stricture _____

6. vomiting _____

7. spitting _____

8. prolapse _____

9. excision _____

10. digestion _____

11. eating, swallowing _____

12. hardening _____

13. stopping, controlling _____

14. surgical repair _____

15. opening _____

16. surgical puncture _____

17. involuntary contraction _____

18. new opening _____

19. incision _____

20. destruction, breakdown _____

J. Circle the correct term in parentheses to complete each sentence.

1. When Mrs. Smith developed diarrhea and crampy abdominal pain, she consulted a **(urologist, nephrologist, gastroenterologist)** and worried that she might have **(inflammatory bowel disease, esophageal varices, achalasia)**.

2. After taking a careful history and physical, Dr. Blakemore diagnosed Mr. Bean, a long-time drinker, with **(hemorrhoids, pancreatitis, appendicitis).** Mr. Bean had complained of sharp mid-epigastric pain and a change in bowel habits.

3. Many pregnant women cannot lie flat after eating because of a burning sensation in their chest and throat. Doctors call this condition **(volvulus, dysentery, gastroesophageal reflux).**

4. Pediatric surgeons must be wary of **(inguinal hernia, intussusception, oral leukoplakia)** in young infants who have not had a bowel movement in many days and have projectile vomiting.

5. Boris had terrible problems with his teeth. Not only did he need a periodontist for his **(anorexia, ascites, gingivitis),** but also an **(endodontist, oral surgeon, orthodontist)** to straighten his teeth.

VII. Answers to Exercises

A

1. digestion
2. spitting (from the respiratory tract)
3. vomiting
4. eating, swallowing
5. prolapse, falling, sagging
6. flow, discharge
7. bursting forth of blood
8. suture
9. surgical repair
10. destruction, breakdown, separation
11. stretching, dilation, dilatation
12. tightening, narrowed lumen, stricture
13. stopping, controlling
14. sudden, involuntary contraction of muscles
15. dilation, stretching, dilatation

B

1. menorrhea
2. cholestasis
3. herniorrhaphy
4. lymphangiectasis
5. hemoptysis
6. hematemesis
7. bronchiectasis
8. blepharoplasty
9. hemostasis
10. rhinoplasty
11. hemolysis
12. pylorospasm
13. menorrhagia
14. bronchiospasm

C

1. painful swallowing
2. excessive (much) eating
3. difficult digestion
4. biliary ducts are not open (congenital anomaly)
5. forward prolapse (bulging) of the eyes (ex-ophthalmia)
6. stoppage of flow of bile
7. esophagus is not open (closed off) at birth (congenital anomaly)
8. involuntary contraction of muscles at the distal end of the esophagus
9. vomiting
10. tightening, stricture, narrowing

D

1. cholecystectomy
2. colectomy
3. herniorrhaphy
4. cecostomy
5. blepharoplasty
6. sphincterotomy
7. gastroduodenal anastomosis (gastroduodenostomy)—both are acceptable
8. ileostomy
9. gingivectomy
10. cholecystojejunostomy (cholecystojejunal anastomosis)
11. paracentesis (abdominocentesis)
12. rectosigmoidectomy

E

1. steatorrhea
2. dysphagia
3. cholelithiasis
4. buccal
5. dentalgia
6. ptosis
7. hepatomegaly
8. sublingual
9. cholecystectomy
10. choledochal

F

1. twisted intestine in the area of the cecum
2. inflammation of the mouth with small ulcers
3. blood vessel bringing blood to the abdomen
4. enzyme to digest fat
5. abnormal condition of lips
6. the part of the throat near the mouth
7. breakdown of sugar
8. pertaining to the tongue and the throat
9. removal of a salivary gland
10. membrane surrounding a tooth

G

1. serum bilirubin
2. stool culture
3. barium enema
4. abdominal ultrasonography
5. stool guaiac (Hemoccult)
6. barium swallow
7. percutaneous transhepatic cholangiography
8. nasogastric intubation
9. CT scan of the abdomen
10. endoscopic retrograde cholangiopancreatography (ERCP)
11. liver biopsy
12. liver scan

H

1. E	4. C	7. A
2. D	5. F	8. B
3. G	6. H	

I

1. -rrhagia, -rrhage	8. -ptosis	15. -tresia
2. -rrhea	9. -ectomy	16. -centesis
3. -rrhaphy	10. -pepsia	17. -spasm
4. -ectasis, -ectasia	11. -phagia	18. -stomy
5. -stenosis	12. -sclerosis	19. -tomy
6. -emesis	13. -stasis	20. -lysis
7. -ptysis	14. -plasty	

J

1. gastroenterologist; inflammatory bowel disease
2. pancreatitis
3. gastroesophageal reflux
4. intussusception
5. gingivitis; orthodontist

VIII. Pronunciation of Terms

To test your understanding of the terminology in this chapter, write the meaning of each term in the space provided. In addition, you may wish to cover the terms and write them by looking at your definitions. Make sure your spelling is correct. The page number after each term indicates where it is defined or used in the text so you can easily check your responses. (If you are not sure what the pronunciation symbols mean, refer to page 21.)

Term	Pronunciation	Meaning
abdominal ultrasonography (174)	ăb-DŎM-ĭn-ăl ŭl-tră-sō-NŎG-ră-fē	_____
aphthous stomatitis (170)	ĂF-thŭs stō-mă-TĪ-tĭs	_____
atresia (168)	ā-TRĒ-zē-ă	_____
biliary atresia (168)	BĬL-ē-ăr-ē ā-TRĒ-zē-ă	_____
bronchiectasis (167)	brŏng-kē-ĔK-tă-sĭs	_____
buccal (169)	BŬK-ăl	_____
cardiospasm (168)	KĂR-dē-ō-spăzm	_____
cecal volvulus (169)	SĒ-kăl VŎL-vū-lŭs	_____
celiac artery (169)	SĒ-lē-ăk ĂR-tĕr-ē	_____
cheilosis (169)	kī-LŌ-sis	_____
cholangiectasis (169)	kōl-ăn-jē-ĔK-tă-sĭs	_____
cholangiography (173)	kōl-ăn-jē-ŎG-ră-fē	_____
cholangiopancreatography (173)	kŏl-ăn-jē-ō-păn-krē-ă-TŎG-ră-fē	_____
cholecystectomy (169)	kō-lē-sĭs-TĔK-tō-mē	_____

cholecystojejunostomy (170)	kō-lē-sĭs-tō-jĕ-jŭ-NŎS-tō-mē	_____
cholecystolithiasis (170)	kō-lē-sĭs-tō-lĭ-THĪ-ă-sĭs	_____
choledochal (169)	kō-lē-DŎK-ăl	_____
cholelithiasis (169)	kō-lē-lĭ-THĬ-ă-sĭs	_____
cholestasis (168)	kō-lē-STĀ-sĭs	_____
colectomy (169)	kō-LĔK-tō-mē	_____
colonoscopy (169)	kō-lŏn-ŎS-kō-pē	_____
dentalgia (169)	dĕn-TĂL-jă	_____
dysmenorrhea (167)	dĭs-mĕn-ŏr-RĒ-ă	_____
dyspepsia (167)	dĭs-PĔP-sē-ă	_____
dysphagia (167)	dĭs-FĀ-jē-ă	_____
esophageal atresia (168)	ĕ-sŏf-ă-JĒ-ăl ā-TRĒ-zē-ă	_____
gastroduodenal anastomosis (169)	găs-trō-dū-ō-DĒ-năl ă-nă-stō-MŌ-sĭs	_____
gastroenteritis (169)	găs-trō-ĕn-tĕ-RĪ-tĭs	_____
gastrointestinal endoscopy (174)	găs-trō-ĭn-TĔS-tĭn-ăl ĕn-DŎS-kō-pē	_____
gastrojejunostomy (169)	găs-trō-jĕ-jū-NŎS-tō-mē	_____
gingivectomy (169)	gĭn-gĭ-VĔK-tō-mē	_____
glossopharyngeal(169)	glŏs-ō-fă-rĭn-GĒ-al	_____
glycolysis (169)	glī-KŎL-ĭ-sis	_____
hematemesis (167)	hē-mă-TĔM-ĕh-sĭs	_____
hemolysis (167)	hē-MŎL-ĭ-sĭs	_____
hemoptysis (167)	hē-MŎP-tĭ-sĭs	_____
hemorrhage (167)	HĔM-ŏr-ĭj	_____
hemostasis (168)	hē-mō-STĀ-sĭs	_____
hepatomegaly (170)	hĕp-ă-tō-MĔG-ă-lē	_____
herniorrhaphy (170)	hĕr-nē-ŎR-ă-fē	_____

ileostomy (170)	ĭl-ē-ŎS-tō-mē	_____
labioglossopharyngeal (170)	lā-bē-ō-glŏs-ō-fă-RĬN-jē-ăl	_____
lipase (170)	LĪ-pās	_____
lymphangiectasia (167)	lĭm-făn-jē-ĕk-TĀ-zē-ă	_____
menorrhagia (167)	mĕn-ŏr-RĀ-jă	_____
menorrhea (167)	mĕn-ŏr-RĒ-ă	_____
oropharynx (170)	ŏr-ō-FĂR-ĭnks	_____
palatoplasty (170)	PĂL-ă-tō-plăs-tē	_____
pancreatic (170)	păn-krē-ĂH-tĭk	_____
periodontal membrane (170)	pĕr-ē-ō-DŎN-tăl MĔM-brān	_____
polyphagia (167)	pŏl-ē-FĀ-jē-ă	_____
proctosigmoidoscopy (170)	prŏk-tō-sĭg-mŏyd-ŎS-kō-pē	_____
proptosis (167)	prŏp-TŌ-sĭs	_____
pyloric stenosis (168)	pī-LŎR-ĭk stĕ-NŌ-sĭs	_____
pylorospasm (168)	pī-LŎR-ō-spăsm	_____
rectosigmoidectomy (170)	rĕk-tō-sĭg-mŏy-DĔK-tō-mē	_____
rhinoplasty (167)	rī-nō-PLĂS-tē	_____
splenic flexure (170)	SPLĔ-nĭk FLĔK-shŭr	_____

IX. Review Sheet

Write meanings for combining forms and suffixes in the space provided. Check your answers with information in Chapters 5 and 6 or in the Glossary (Medical Terms—English) at the end of the book.

Combining Forms

Combining Form	Meaning	Combining Form	Meaning
amyl/o	_____	dent/i	_____
an/o	_____	duoden/o	_____
append/o	_____	enter/o	_____
appendic/o	_____	esophag/o	_____
bil/i	_____	eti/o	_____
bilirubin/o	_____	gastr/o	_____
bronch/o	_____	gingiv/o	_____
bucc/o	_____	gloss/o	_____
cec/o	_____	gluc/o	_____
celi/o	_____	glyc/o	_____
cervic/o	_____	glycogen/o	_____
cheil/o	_____	hem/o	_____
cholangi/o	_____	hemat/o	_____
chol/e	_____	hepat/o	_____
cholecyst/o	_____	herni/o	_____
choledoch/o	_____	idi/o	_____
cib/o	_____	ile/o	_____
cirrh/o	_____	jejun/o	_____
col/o	_____	labi/o	_____
colon/o	_____	lapar/o	_____

lingu/o	_____	peritone/o	_____
lip/o	_____	pharyng/o	_____
lith/o	_____	proct/o	_____
lymphangi/o	_____	pylor/o	_____
mandibul/o	_____	rect/o	_____
men/o	_____	sialaden/o	_____
necr/o	_____	sigmoid/o	_____
odont/o	_____	splen/o	_____
or/o	_____	steat/o	_____
palat/o	_____	stomat/o	_____
pancreat/o	_____	tonsill/o	_____

Suffixes

Suffix	Meaning	Suffix	Meaning
-ase	_____	-iasis	_____
-centesis	_____	-lysis	_____
-chezia	_____	-megaly	_____
-ectasia	_____	-orexia	_____
-ectasis	_____	-pathy	_____
-ectomy	_____	-pepsia	_____
-emesis	_____	-phagia	_____
-emia	_____	-plasty	_____
-genesis	_____	-prandial	_____
-graphy	_____	-ptosis	_____

Continued on following page

-ptysis	_____	-spasm	_____
-rrhage	_____	-stasis	_____
-rrhagia	_____	-stenosis	_____
-rrhaphy	_____	-stomy	_____
-rrhea	_____	-tomy	_____
-scopy	_____	-tresia	_____

Urinary System

This Chapter is divided into the following sections

In this Chapter you will

- Name the organs of the urinary system and describe their locations and functions;
- Give the meaning of various pathological conditions affecting the system;
- Recognize the use and interpretation of urinalysis as a diagnostic test;
- Detail the meanings of combining forms, prefixes, and suffixes of the system terminology; and
- List and explain some clinical procedures, laboratory tests, and abbreviations that pertain to the urinary system.

I. Introduction

You have just learned how food is brought into the bloodstream by the digestive system. In a future chapter you will learn how oxygen is brought into the bloodstream by the respiratory system. Food and oxygen are combined in the cells of the body to produce energy (catabolism). In the process, however, the substance of the food and oxygen is not destroyed. Instead, the small particles of which the food and oxygen are made are actually rearranged into new combinations. These are waste products. When foods like sugars and fats, which contain particles of carbon, hydrogen, and oxygen, combine with oxygen in cells, the wastes produced are gases called carbon dioxide (carbon and oxygen) and water (hydrogen and oxygen) in the form of vapor. These gases are removed from the body by exhalation through the lungs.

Protein foods are more complicated than sugars and fats. They contain carbon, hydrogen, and oxygen **plus** nitrogen and other elements. The waste that is produced when proteins combine with oxygen is called **nitrogenous waste,** and it is more difficult to excrete (to separate out) from the body than are gases like carbon dioxide and water vapor.

The body cannot efficiently put the nitrogenous waste into a gaseous form and exhale it, so it excretes it in the form of a soluble (dissolved in water) waste substance called **urea.** The major function of the urinary system is to remove urea from the bloodstream so that it does not accumulate in the body and become toxic.

Urea is formed in the liver from ammonia, which in turn is derived from the breakdown of simple proteins (amino acids) in the body cells. The urea is carried in the bloodstream to the kidneys, where it passes with water, salts, and acids out of the bloodstream and into the kidney tubules as **urine.** Urine then travels down the ureters into the bladder and out of the body.

Besides removing urea from the blood, another important function of the kidneys is to maintain the proper balance of water, salts, and acids in the body fluids. Salts, such as sodium and potassium, and some acids are known as **electrolytes** (small molecules that conduct an electrical charge). Electrolytes are necessary for the proper functioning of muscle and nerve cells. The kidney adjusts the amounts of water and electrolytes by secreting some substances into the urine and holding back others in the bloodstream for use in the body.

In addition to forming urine and eliminating it from the body, the kidneys also act as endocrine organs, secreting into the bloodstream substances that act at some distant site in the body. Examples of the kidneys' endocrine function include the secretion of **renin,** a substance important in the control of blood pressure, and **erythropoietin** (erythr/o = red, -poietin = substance that forms), a hormone that regulates the production of red blood cells. The kidneys also secrete an active form of vitamin D, necessary for the absorption of calcium from the intestine. In addition, hormones such as insulin and parathyroid hormone are degraded and extracted from the bloodstream by the kidney.

II. Anatomy of the Major Organs

The organs of the urinary system are (label Figure 7–1 as you read these paragraphs)
(1) Two **kidneys**—bean-shaped organs situated behind the abdominal cavity (retroperitoneal) on either side of the vertebral column in the lumbar region of the spine.

The kidneys are embedded in a cushion of adipose tissue and surrounded by fibrous connective tissue for protection. They are fist-sized and weigh about 4 to 6 ounces each.

The kidneys consist of an outer **cortex** region (cortex means outer portion or bark, as the bark of a tree) and an inner **medulla** region (medulla means marrow or inner portion). The

Large vein to heart

Aorta

Adrenal gland

(1)

Renal artery

Hilum

Renal vein

(1)

Medulla

Cortex

ureters — (2) — (2) — ureters

Trigone — (3)

Prostate gland

urethra (4)

Meatus

Figure 7–1

Organs of the urinary system, in a male.

depression on the medial border of the kidney, through which blood vessels and nerves pass, is called the **hilum.**

(2) Two **ureters**—muscular tubes (16 to 18 inches long) lined with mucous membrane. They convey urine in peristaltic waves from the kidney to the urinary bladder.

(3) **Urinary bladder**—hollow, muscular, distensible sac in the pelvic cavity. It serves as a temporary reservoir for urine. The **trigone** is a triangular space at the base of the bladder where the ureters enter and the urethra leads out.

(4) **Urethra**—membranous tube through which urine is discharged from the urinary bladder. The process of expelling (**voiding**) urine through the urethra is called **micturition.** The external opening of the urethra is called the urethral or urinary **meatus.** The female urethra is about 1½ inches long, lying anterior to the vagina and vaginal meatus. The male urethra is about 8 inches long and entends downward through the prostate gland to the

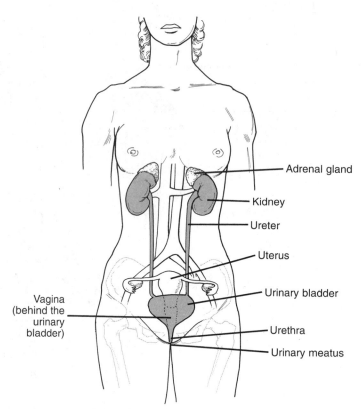

Adrenal gland

Kidney

Ureter

Uterus

Urinary bladder

Urethra

Urinary meatus

Vagina
(behind the
urinary
bladder)

Figure 7–2

Female urinary system.

meatus at the tip of the penis. Figure 7–2 illustrates the female urinary system. Compare it with Figure 7–1, which shows the male urinary system.

III. How the Kidneys Produce Urine

Blood enters each kidney from the aorta by way of the right and left **renal arteries.** After the renal artery enters the kidney (at the hilum), the artery branches into smaller and smaller arteries. The smallest arteries are called **arterioles,** and these are located throughout the cortex of the kidney (Fig. 7–3).

Since the arterioles are small, blood passes through them slowly, but constantly. Blood flow through the kidney is so essential that the kidneys have their own special device for maintaining blood flow. If blood pressure falls in the vessels of the kidney, so that blood flow is diminished, the kidney produces **renin** and discharges it into the blood. Renin leads to the formation of a substance that stimulates the contraction of arterioles so that blood pressure is increased and blood flow in the kidneys is restored to normal.

Each arteriole in the cortex of the kidney leads into a mass of very tiny, coiled and intertwined smaller blood vessels called **capillaries.** The collection of capillaries, shaped in the form of a tiny ball, is called a **glomerulus.** There are about 1 million glomeruli in the cortex region of each kidney (Fig. 7–4).

The kidneys produce urine by a process of **filtration.** As blood passes through the many glomeruli, the walls of each glomerulus (the filter) are thin enough to permit water, salts, sugar, and **urea** (with other nitrogenous wastes such as **creatinine** and **uric acid**) to leave the

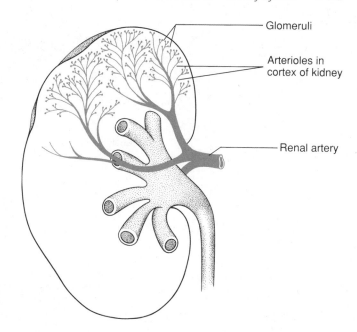

Figure 7–3

Renal artery branching to form smaller arteries, arterioles, and glomeruli.

bloodstream. These materials are collected in a tiny, cup-like structure called a **Bowman's capsule,** which surrounds each glomerulus (Fig. 7–4). The walls of the glomeruli prevent large substances such as proteins and blood cells from filtering into the Bowman's capsule. These substances remain in the blood and normally do not appear in urine.

Attached to each Bowman's capsule is a long, twisted tube called a **renal tubule** (Fig. 7–5). As water, sugar, salts, urea, and other wastes pass through the renal tubule, most of the water, all of the sugar, and some salts return to the bloodstream through tiny capillaries surrounding each tubule. This **reabsorption** assures that the body retains essential substances such as sugar, water, and salts. Only the wastes, some water, and some salts and acids (that are secreted into the tubule from the surrounding capillary bloodstream) remain in the renal tubule. Each renal tubule, now containing urine (95 per cent water, 5 per cent urea, creatinine, salts, and acids) ends in a larger collecting tubule. Thousands of collecting tubules

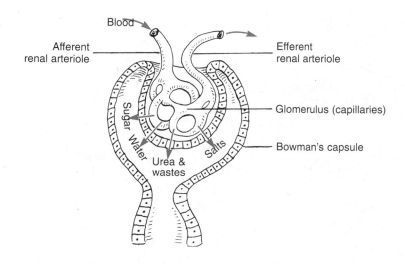

Figure 7–4

Glomerulus and Bowman's capsule. Afferent arteriole carries blood toward *(af-)*. The glomerulus and efferent arteriole carry blood away *(ef)*.

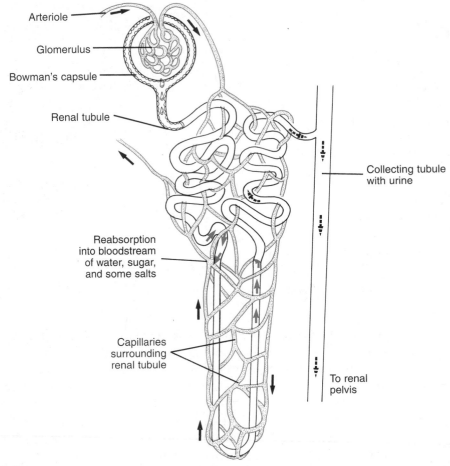

Arteriole

Glomerulus

Bowman's capsule

Renal tubule

Reabsorption
into bloodstream
of water, sugar,
and some salts

Capillaries
surrounding
renal tubule

Collecting tubule
with urine

To renal
pelvis

Figure 7–5

A nephron (the functional unit of the kidney with glomerulus, renal tubule, and surrounding capillaries). *Solid black arrows* indicate flow of blood. *Broken arrows* indicate urine formation and flow. *Solid colored arrows* indicate reabsorption of water, sugar, and salts back into the bloodstream.

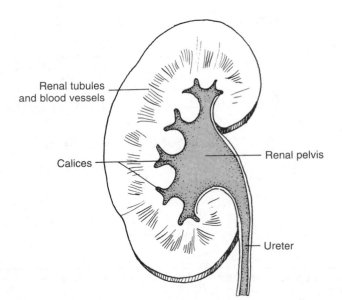

Renal tubules
and blood vessels

Calices

Renal pelvis

Ureter

Figure 7–6

Section of kidney showing renal pelvis, calices, and ureter.

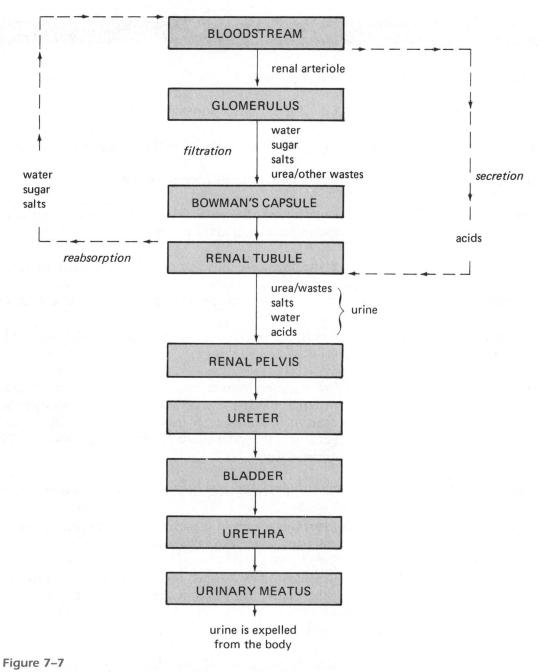

Figure 7–7

Flow diagram of the process of forming and expelling urine.

lead to the **renal pelvis,** a basin-like area in the central area of the kidney. Small, cup-like regions of the renal pelvis are **calices** (singular: **calix** or **calyx**). Figure 7–6 illustrates a section of the kidney showing the renal pelvis and calices.

The renal pelvis narrows into the **ureter,** which carries the urine to the **urinary bladder** where the urine is temporarily stored. The exit area of the bladder to the **urethra** is closed by sphincters that do not permit urine to leave the bladder. As the bladder fills up, pressure is placed on the base of the urethra, which causes the desire to urinate.

Study the flow diagram in Figure 7–7 to trace the process of forming urine and expelling it from the body.

IV. Vocabulary

arteriole	A small artery.
Bowman's capsule	Cup-shaped capsule surrounding each glomerulus.
calix or calyx (plural: **calices**)	Cup-like collecting region of the renal pelvis.
catheter	A tube for injecting or removing fluids.
cortex	Outer region; the renal cortex is the outer region of the kidney (cortical means pertaining to the cortex).
creatinine	Waste product of muscle metabolism; nitrogenous waste excreted in urine.
electrolyte	A chemical that carries an electrical charge in a solution.
erythropoietin	A hormone secreted by the kidney to stimulate the production of red blood cells.
filtration	Process whereby some substances, but not all, pass through a filter or other material. Blood pressure forces materials through the filter. About 180 quarts of fluid are filtered from the blood daily, but the kidney returns 98–99 per cent of the water and salts. Only about 1½ quarts (1500 ml) of urine are excreted daily.
glomerulus (plural: **glomeruli**)	Tiny ball of capillaries (microscopic blood vessels) in cortex of kidney.
hilum	Depression or pit in that part of an organ where blood vessels and nerves enter and leave. Also called a hilus.
kidney	One of two bean-shaped organs located behind the abdominal cavity on either side of the backbone in the lumbar region.
meatus	Opening or canal.
medulla	Inner region; the renal medulla is the inner region of the kidney (medullary means pertaining to the medulla).
micturition	Urination; the act of voiding.
nitrogenous wastes	Substances containing nitrogen and excreted in urine.
reabsorption	The process of accepting again or taking back. Materials necessary to the body are reabsorbed into the blood from the renal tubules as urine is formed.
renal artery	Carries blood to the kidney.
renal pelvis	Central collecting region in the kidney.

renal tubules	Microscopic tubes in the kidney where urine is formed as water, sugar, and salts are reabsorbed (secreted back) into the bloodstream.
renal vein	Carries blood away from the kidney.
renin	A hormone synthesized, stored, and secreted by the kidney; it raises blood pressure by influencing vasoconstriction (narrowing of blood vessels).
trigone ✓	Triangular area in the bladder where the ureters enter and the urethra exits.
urea ✓	Major nitrogenous waste product excreted in urine.
ureter ✓	One of two tubes leading from the kidney to the bladder.
urethra ✓	Tube leading from the bladder to the outside of the body.
uric acid ✓	Nitrogenous waste excreted in the urine.
urinary bladder	Sac that holds urine.
voiding ✓	Expelling urine (micturition).

V. Terminology: Structures, Substances, and Urinary Symptoms

Write the meaning of the medical term in the space provided.

Structures			
Combining Form	Meaning	Terminology	Meaning
cali/o **calic/o**	calix (calyx)	caliectasis _____	
		caliceal _____	
cyst/o	urinary bladder	cystitis _____	
		cystourethrogram _____	
		cystocele _____	
		cystectomy _____	
glomerul/o	glomerulus (collection of capillaries)	glomerular _____	

meat/o   meatus   <u>meat</u>al stenosis _____

                                               <u>meat</u>otomy _____

nephr/o   kidney   par<u>aneph</u>ric _____

                                               <u>neph</u>ropathy _____
(ně-FRŎ-pă-thē)

                                               <u>neph</u>rohypertrophy _____

                                               <u>neph</u>rolithotomy _____

Incision (percutaneous) into the kidney to remove a stone.

                                               <u>neph</u>rosclerosis _____

Arterioles in the kidney are affected.

                                               <u>neph</u>rotomography _____

Tomography is an x-ray process whereby a series of x-ray pictures are taken to show an organ in varying depths. Tom/o means to cut; hence, the x-rays give different views or "cuts" of the organ.

                                               hydro<u>neph</u>rosis _____

Obstruction to urine flow may be caused by renal calculi (Fig. 7–8), stricture (narrowing) of the ureter, or hypertrophy of the prostate gland at the base of the bladder in males.

Figure 7–8

Hydronephrosis caused by a stone (obstruction) in the upper part of a ureter *(left)*, and hydroureter with hydronephrosis caused by a stone in the lower part of the ureter *(right)*. (From Ignatavicius DD, Bayne MV: Medical-Surgical Nursing: A Nursing Process Approach. Philadelphia, WB Saunders, 1991, p 1864.)

pyel/o	renal pelvis	pyelolithotomy _____

Removal of a large calculus that contributes to blockage of urine flow and development of infection.

pyelogram _____

Intravenous (IVP) and retrograde pyelograms are discussed on page 206, Section VIII, under Clinical Procedures.

ren/o	kidney	renal ischemia _____

renal transplantation _____

See page 209, Section VIII, under Clinical Procedures.

renal calculus _____

renal dialysis _____

This includes hemodialysis and peritoneal dialysis. See page 208, Section VIII, under Clinical Procedures.

trigon/o	trigone (region of the bladder)	trigonitis _____

ureter/o	ureter	ureteroplasty _____

ureterolithotomy _____

ureteroileostomy _____

After cystectomy, a segment of the ileum is used in place of the bladder to carry urine from the ureters out of the body. Also called an ileal conduit.

urethr/o	urethra	urethritis _____

urethroplasty _____

urethral stricture _____

A stricture is an abnormal narrowing of an opening or passageway.

vesic/o	urinary bladder	perivesical _____

Do not confuse the term vesical with the term vesicle, which is a small blister on the skin.

vesicoureteral reflux _____

Substances and Symptoms

Combining Form or Suffix	Meaning	Terminology	Meaning
albumin/o	albumin (a protein in the blood)	albuminuria _____	

-uria means urine condition. This symptom can indicate malfunction of the kidney as protein leaks out of damaged glomeruli.

azot/o	nitrogen	azotemia _____	

This is reflected in an elevated BUN (blood urea nitrogen) test.

bacteri/o	bacteria	bacteriuria _____	

Usually a sign of infection.

dips/o	thirst	polydipsia _____	

A sign of diabetes mellitus or diabetes insipidus (see page 205, Section VII, Pathological Terminology).

ket/o **keton/o**	ketone bodies (acids and acetone)	ketosis _____	

Often called ketoacidosis because acids accumulate in the blood and tissues. See page 202, Ketone bodies, in Section VI, Urinalysis.

		ketonuria _____	
lith/o	stone	nephrolithiasis _____	
noct/i	night	nocturia _____	

Noctiphobia is an irrational fear of night or darkness.

olig/o	scanty	oliguria _____	
-poietin	substance that forms	erythropoietin _____	
py/o	pus	pyuria _____	
-tripsy	to crush	lithotripsy _____	

See page 209, Section VIII, under Clinical Procedures.

ur/o	urine (urea)	uremia _____	

This toxic state results when nitrogenous waste products accumulate in the blood (azotemia).

		enuresis _____	

Literally, a condition of being "in urine," and also called bedwetting.

diuresis _____

di- (from dia-) means complete. Caffeine and alcohol can produce diuresis, acting as diuretics to produce a diluted urine.

antidiuretic hormone _____

This substance (a hormone from the pituitary gland, and literally meaning against diuresis) normally acts on the renal tubules to cause water to be reabsorbed into the bloodstream.

urin/o	urine	urinary incontinence _____

Incontinence literally means not (in-) able to hold (tin) together (con-). This is loss of control of the passage of urine from the bladder. Stress incontinence is due to strain on the bladder opening when coughing or sneezing, and urgency incontinence is inability to hold back urination when feeling the urge to void.

urinary retention _____

This symptom results when there is blockage to the outflow of urine from the bladder.

-uria	urination, urine condition	dysuria _____

anuria _____

hematuria _____

glycosuria _____

A symptom of diabetes mellitus.

polyuria _____

A symptom of both diabetes mellitus and diabetes insipidus. See page 205, Section VII, Pathological Terminology.

VI. Urinalysis

Urinalysis is an examination of urine to determine the presence of abnormal elements which may indicate various pathological conditions.

The following are some of the tests made in a urinalysis:

1. **Color**—Normal urine color is yellow (amber) or straw colored. A colorless, pale urine indicates a large amount of water in the urine, whereas a smoky red or brown color of urine is due to the presence of large amounts of blood. Foods, such as beets, and certain drugs can also produce red hues in urine.

2. **pH**—This is a test of the chemical nature of urine. The pH test indicates to what degree a solution (such as urine or blood) is **acid** or **alkaline (basic).** The pH range is from 0

(very acid) to 14 (very alkaline). Normal urine is slightly acid (6.5). However, in infections of the bladder, the urine pH may be alkaline, owing to the actions of bacteria in the urine that break down the urea and release an alkaline substance called ammonia.

3. **Protein**—Small amounts of protein are normally found in the urine but not in sufficient quantity to produce a positive result by ordinary methods of testing. When urinary tests for protein become positive, **albumin** is usually responsible. Albumin is the major protein in blood plasma. If it is detected in urine **(albuminuria),** it may indicate a leak in the glomerular membrane, which allows albumin to enter the renal tubule and pass into the urine.

4. **Glucose**—Sugar is not normally found in the urine. In most cases, when it does appear **(glycosuria),** it indicates **diabetes mellitus.** In diabetes mellitus, there is an excess of sugar in the bloodstream (hyperglycemia), which leads to "spilling over" of sugar into the urine. The renal tubules are unable to reabsorb all the sugar that filters out through the glomerular membrane.

5. **Specific gravity**—The specific gravity of urine reflects the amount of wastes, minerals, and solids in the urine. It is a comparison of the density of urine with that of water. The urine of patients with diabetes mellitus has a higher than normal specific gravity because of the presence of sugar. In kidney diseases such as nephritis, the specific gravity of urine is low because the urine is diluted by large quantities of water that cannot be reabsorbed into the blood.

6. **Ketone bodies**—Ketones (sometimes referred to as **acetones,** which are a type of ketone body) are breakdown products from fat catabolism in cells. Ketones accumulate in large quantities in blood and urine when fat, instead of sugar, is used as fuel for energy in cells. This happens, for example, in diabetes mellitus when cells that are deprived of sugar must use up their available fat for energy. In starvation, when sugar is not available, ketonuria and ketosis (ketones in the blood) occur as fat is abnormally catabolized.

The presence of ketones in the blood is quite dangerous since ketones increase the acidity of the blood **(acidosis).** This can lead to coma (unconsciousness) and death.

7. **Sediment**—Abnormal particles are present in the urine as a sign of a pathological condition. Included are cells (epithelial cells, white blood cells, or red blood cells), bacteria, or crystals.

8. **Pus**—**Pyuria** gives a **turbid** (cloudy) appearance to urine. Large numbers of leukocytes (polymorphonuclears) are present because of infection or inflammation in the kidney or bladder.

9. **Phenylketonuria (PKU)**—Phenylketones are substances that accumulate in the urine of infants born with a special congenital problem. These infants are born lacking an important enzyme. The enzyme (phenylalanine hydroxylase) is necessary in cells to change one amino acid (phenylalanine) to another amino acid (tyrosine). Lack of the enzyme causes phenylalanine to reach high levels in the infant's bloodstream, and this will eventually lead to mental retardation. The PKU test, done just after birth, can detect the phenylketonuria or phenylalanine in the blood. When it is detected, the infant is fed a low-protein diet that excludes phenylalanine so that mental retardation is prevented. This strict diet is necessary until the child is an adult.

10. **Bilirubin**—This pigment substance from hemoglobin breakdown may appear in the urine, darkening it, as an indication of liver or gallbladder disease. The diseased liver has difficulty removing bilirubin from the blood **(hyperbilirubinemia),** which causes excessive bilirubin to appear in the urine **(bilirubinuria).**

VII. Pathological Terminology: Kidney, Bladder, and Associated Conditions

Your expanding knowledge of medical terminology should help you understand the terminology in the following paragraphs.

Kidney

glomerulonephritis

Inflammation of the kidney glomerulus (Bright's disease).

Acute glomerulonephritis may develop as part of a systemic disorder (a condition that affects many organs in the body) or be idiopathic. It can also occur after an acute infection, as in poststreptococcal glomerulonephritis. In this condition, which appears 10–14 days after a streptococcal infection, no bacteria are actually found in the kidney, but inflammation results from an immune (antigen and antibody) reaction in the glomerulus. Most patients recover spontaneously, but in some cases the disease becomes chronic. Chronic glomerulonephritis can result in hypertension (high blood pressure), albuminuria (protein seeps through damaged glomerular walls), renal failure, and uremia. Drugs may be useful to control inflammation, and dialysis or transplant may be necessary if uremia occurs.

interstitial nephritis

Inflammation of the renal interstitium (connective tissue that lies between the renal tubules).

Acute interstitial nephritis is an increasingly frequent disorder that may develop after the administration of drugs. It is characterized by fever, skin rash, eosinophils in the blood and urine, and poor renal function. Recovery may be anticipated when the offending agent is discontinued and may be hastened by use of *corticosteroids* (anti-inflammatory agents).

nephrolithiasis

Kidney stones **(renal calculi).**

Kidney stones are usually composed of uric acid or calcium salts. Although the etiology is often unknown, conditions associated with an increase in the concentration of calcium (parathyroid gland tumors) or high levels of uric acid in the blood **(hyperuricemia—**associated with gouty arthritis) may contribute to the formation of calculi. Stones often lodge in the ureter or bladder as well as in the renal pelvis and may require removal by extracorporeal shock wave **lithotripsy** (see page 209, Section VIII, under Clinical Procedures) or surgery.

nephrotic syndrome

A group of symptoms caused by excessive protein loss in the urine (also called **nephrosis).**

In addition to marked proteinuria, symptoms include **edema** (swelling due to fluid in tissue spaces), hypoalbuminemia, and susceptibility to infections. Nephrotic syndrome may follow glomerulonephritis, exposure to toxins or drugs, and other pathological conditions, such as diabetes mellitus and malignant disease. Drugs may be useful to heal the leaky glomerulus.

Figure 7–9

Polycystic kidneys. The kidneys contain masses of cysts, and the ureters are malformed and abnormally dilated. (From Kumar V, Cotran RS, Robbins SL: Basic Pathology, 5th ed. Philadelphia, WB Saunders, 1992, p 465.)

polycystic kidneys

Multiple fluid-filled sacs (cysts) within and upon the kidney.

This is a hereditary condition that usually remains **asymptomatic** (without symptoms) until adult life. Cysts progressively develop in both kidneys, leading to nephromegaly, hematuria, urinary tract infection, hypertension, and uremia. Figure 7–9 shows polycystic kidney disease in an adult.

pyelonephritis

Inflammation of the renal pelvis.

This common type of kidney disease is caused by bacterial infection. Many small **abscesses** (collections of pus) form in the renal pelvis. Pyuria is found on urinalysis. Treatment consists of antibiotics and surgical correction of any obstruction to urine flow.

renal cell carcinoma

Cancerous tumor of the kidney in adulthood.

This tumor accounts for 2 per cent of all cancers in adults. Its primary symptom is hematuria, and the tumor often metastasizes to the bone and lungs. Survival rate depends on the extent of spread of the tumor. Nephrectomy is the treatment of choice.

renal failure

Failure of the kidney to excrete urine.

The kidney stops excreting nitrogenous waste products and acids derived from diet and body metabolism. Renal failure may be acute or chronic, reversible or progressive, mild or severe. The final phase of chronic renal failure is **end-stage renal disease (ESRD).** If untreated, the condition is fatal. Erythropoietin is used to treat patients with ESRD. It increases red blood cells, with marked improvement in energy level.

renal hypertension	High blood pressure resulting from kidney disease.

Renal hypertension is the most common type of **secondary hypertension** (high blood pressure caused by an abnormal condition, such as glomerulonephritis or renal artery stenosis). If the cause of high blood pressure is not known, it is called **essential hypertension.** Chronic essential hypertension can cause arteriole walls in the kidney to become narrowed and thickened (nephrosclerosis), and this can produce glomerular ischemia, atrophy, and scarring of kidney tissue.

Wilms' tumor	Malignant tumor of the kidney occurring in childhood.

This tumor may be treated with surgery, radiation, and chemotherapy. There is a high percentage of cure if it is treated before metastasis has occurred.

Urinary Bladder

bladder cancer	Malignant tumor of the urinary bladder.

The bladder is the most common site of malignancy of the urinary system. It occurs more frequently in men and in persons over the age of 50, especially industrial workers exposed to dyes and leather. Tobacco is the most damaging nonoccupational carcinogen. Symptoms include gross (visible to the naked eye) or microscopic hematuria and dysuria, and increased urinary frequency. Cystoscopy with biopsy is the most common diagnostic procedure. Staging of the tumor is based on the depth to which the bladder wall (urothelium) has been penetrated and the extent of metastasis. Superficial tumors are removed by electrocauterization (burning). Cystectomy, chemotherapy, and radiation therapy are useful for more invasive disease.

Associated Conditions

diabetes insipidus	Inadequate secretion or resistance of the kidney to the action of antidiuretic hormone (ADH).

Two major symptoms of this condition are polydipsia and polyuria. Lack of ADH prevents water from being reabsorbed into the blood through the renal tubules. Insipidus means tasteless, reflecting that the urine is very dilute and watery, not sweet as in diabetes mellitus. The term **diabetes** is taken from a Greek word meaning siphon. It leads to an inability of the kidneys to hold water in the body, which instead runs through the body as through a siphon (a tube for carrying fluid).

diabetes mellitus	Inadequate secretion or improper utilization of insulin.

Major symptoms of diabetes mellitus are glycosuria, hyperglycemia, polyuria, and polydipsia. Without insulin, sugar is prevented from leaving the bloodstream and cannot be used by body cells for energy. Sugar thus remains in the blood (hyperglycemia) and spills over into the urine (glycosuria) when the kidney cannot reabsorb it through the renal tubules. Mellitus means sweet, reflecting the content of the urine. The term diabetes, when used by itself, usually refers to the more common condition, diabetes mellitus, rather than diabetes insipidus.

VIII. Laboratory Tests, Clinical Procedures, and Abbreviations

Laboratory Tests

blood urea nitrogen (BUN)

This test measures the amount of urea in the blood. Normally the urea level is low since urea is excreted in the urine continuously. When the kidney is diseased or fails, however, urea accumulates in the blood (a condition known as uremia), and this can lead to unconsciousness and death.

creatinine clearance test

This test measures the ability of the kidney to remove creatinine from the blood. A blood sample is drawn and the amount of creatinine concentration is compared with the amount of creatinine excreted in the urine during a 24-hour period. If the kidney is not functioning well in its job of clearing creatinine from the blood, there will be a disproportionate amount of creatinine in the blood compared with the amount in the urine.

Clinical Procedures

X-Rays

CT scans

Transverse x-ray views of the kidney are taken with or without contrast material and are useful in the diagnosis of tumors, cysts, abscesses, and hydronephrosis. Studies may be obtained in renal failure, when contrast material should not be given.

intravenous pyelogram (IVP)

Contrast material is injected within a vein and travels to the kidney where it is filtered into the urine. X-rays are then taken showing the contrast material filling the kidneys, ureters, bladder, and urethra. These x-rays provide a test of renal function as well as show cysts, tumors, infections, hydronephrosis, and calculi. Also called an **excretory urogram.** IVP **tomograms** show a series of images of the kidney and may be required to see details.

kidneys, ureters, and bladder (KUB)

This x-ray record (no contrast material is used) demonstrates the size and location of the kidneys in relation to other organs in the abdominopelvic region.

renal angiography

Contrast material is injected into the bloodstream and x-rays are taken of the blood vessels (vascular system) of the kidney. This procedure is helpful for the diagnosis of kidney tumors and to outline renal vessels in hypertensive patients.

retrograde pyelogram

Contrast material is introduced directly into the bladder and ureters through a cystoscope, and x-rays are taken to determine the presence of stones or obstructions. This technique may be indicated when poor renal function makes it impossible to visualize the kidneys, ureters, and bladder by use of intravenous dye as in an IVP. It may also be used as a substitute for an IVP when a patient is allergic to intravenous contrast material.

voiding cystourethrogram (VCUG)

The bladder is filled with contrast material, as in a retrograde pyelogram, and x-rays are taken of the bladder and urethra as a patient is expelling urine. (Fig. 7–10 shows a VCUG revealing an abnormality of the bladder that causes

Figure 7–10

Voiding cystourethrogram. The urethra is not shown, but note the swollen bladder and left ureter (hydroureter) and hydronephrosis. This condition is due to an abnormality of the bladder causing vesicoureteral reflux of urine on the left. (From James AE Jr, Squire LF: Nuclear Radiology. Philadelphia, WB Saunders, 1973.)

reflux of urine back up toward the kidney. [Normally, urine does not flow back—reflux—into the ureters, the bladder is not dilated, and the urethra is not obstructed.])

Ultrasound

ultrasonography   Kidney size, tumors, hydronephrosis, polycystic kidney, and ureteral and bladder obstruction are some of the many conditions that can be diagnosed using sound waves, but no information about renal function is obtained.

Radioactive

radioisotope studies   A radioactive substance (isotope) is injected into the bloodstream in small amounts and is taken up by the kidneys. Pictures show the size and shape of the kidney **(renal scan)** and its function **(renogram).** These studies can indicate size of blood vessels, diagnose obstruction, and determine the separate function of each kidney.

Magnetic Imaging

magnetic resonance imaging (MRI)   The patient lies surrounded by a cylindrical magnetic resonance machine, and images are made of the pelvic and retroperitoneal regions using magnetic waves. This high-technology machine produces an image of internal organs based upon the movement of small particles called protons. The images can be taken in all three planes of the body—frontal, sagittal, and transverse—and are useful in showing pelvic, retroperitoneal, and vascular anatomy.

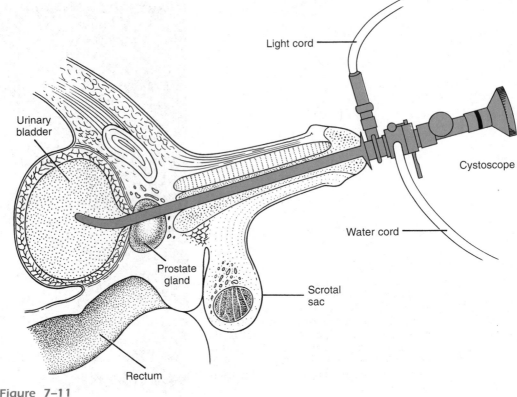

Light cord

Cystoscope

Urinary
bladder

Water cord

Prostate
gland

Scrotal
sac

Rectum

Figure 7–11

Cystoscope.

Other Procedures

cystoscopy

Visual examination of the urinary bladder by means of a cystoscope. A hollow metal tube is introduced into the urinary meatus and passed through the urethra into the bladder. By means of a light source, special lenses, and mirrors, the bladder mucosa is examined for tumors, calculi, or inflammation. By placing a catheter through the cystoscope, urine samples can be withdrawn and contrast material can be injected into the bladder. A cystoscope is shown in Figure 7–11. A **panendoscope** is a cystoscope that gives a wide-angle view of the bladder.

dialysis

Waste materials such as urea are separated from the bloodstream when the kidneys can no longer function. There are two kinds of dialysis:

hemodialysis—using an artificial kidney machine that receives waste-filled blood from the patient's bloodstream, filters it, and returns the dialysed blood to the patient's body.

peritoneal dialysis—using a peritoneal **catheter** (tube), fluid is introduced into the peritoneal (abdominal) cavity. The fluid causes wastes in the capillaries of the peritoneum to pass out of the bloodstream and into the fluid. Fluid (with wastes) is then removed by catheter. Peritoneal dialysis may be performed intermittently (IPD) with the aid of a mechanical apparatus or continuously by the patient without artificial support. The latter technique is known as continuous ambulatory peritoneal dialysis (CAPD) (Fig. 7–12).

extracorporeal shock wave lithotripsy (ESWL)

Shock waves are used to crush urinary tract stones into tiny fragments that can then be passed out with urine. After receiving some type of anesthesia, the patient is immersed in a tank of water and shock waves are generated electrically. Using an x-ray picture screen (fluoroscopy) the physician can position the patient so that the stone will receive the shock waves properly. Figure 7–13 illustrates extracorporeal (outside the body) shock wave lithotripsy.

renal biopsy

Biopsy of the kidney may be performed at the time of surgery (open) or through the skin (percutaneous or closed). When the latter technique is used, the patient lies in the prone position and, following administration of local anesthesia to the overlying skin and muscles of the back, a biopsy needle is inserted with the aid of fluoroscopy (x-rays on a screen) or ultrasonography, and tissue is obtained for microscopic examination by a pathologist.

renal transplantation

A kidney is transplanted into a patient with renal failure from an identical twin (isograft) or other individual (allograft). Best results occur when the donor is closely related to the recipient, and better than 90 per cent of the kidneys survive for 1 year or longer (Fig. 7–14).

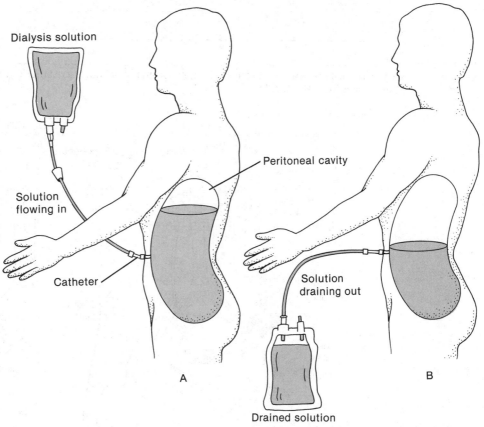

Figure 7–12

Continuous ambulatory peritoneal dialysis (CAPD). *(A)* The dialysis solution (dialysate) flows from a collapsible plastic bag through a catheter into the patient's peritoneal cavity. The empty bag is folded and inserted into undergarments. *(B)* After 4–8 hours, the bag is unfolded, and the fluid is allowed to drain into it by gravity. The full bag is discarded, and a new bag of fresh dialysate is attached. (*A* and *B,* From Chabner DE: Medical Terminology: A Short Course. Philadelphia, WB Saunders, 1990.)

Figure 7–13

Extracorporeal shock wave lithotripsy. (Redrawn from Kandel LB, Harrison LH: New approaches to urinary tract stones. Drug Ther 18:44, 1988.)

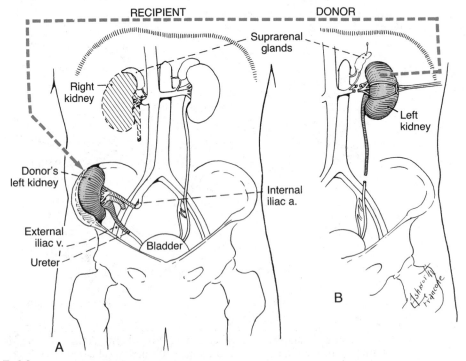

Figure 7–14

(A) Kidney transplanted to right pelvis. (B) Kidney of donor. (A and B, From Jacob SW, Francone CA: Elements of Anatomy and Physiology, 2nd ed. Philadelphia, WB Saunders, 1989, p 274.)

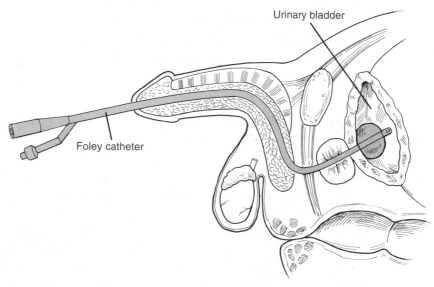

Figure 7–15

Foley catheter in place in the urinary bladder.

urinary catheterization A flexible, tubular instrument is passed through the urethra into the urinary bladder. Catheters are used for drainage of urine, to introduce irrigating solutions into the bladder, or to inflate the bladder. A Foley catheter is an indwelling (left in the bladder) catheter held in place by a balloon inflated with air or liquid (see Fig. 7–15).

ABBREVIATIONS

ADH	Antidiuretic hormone; vasopressin	**HD**	Hemodialysis
ARF	Acute renal failure	**IVP**	Intravenous pyelogram
BUN	Blood urea nitrogen	**K$^+$**	Potassium; an electrolyte
CAPD	Continuous ambulatory peritoneal dialysis	**KUB**	Kidney, ureter, and bladder
Cath	Catheter, catheterization	**Na$^+$**	Sodium; an electrolyte
Cl$^-$	Chloride; an electrolyte excreted by the kidney	**pH**	Symbol for degree of acidity or alkalinity
CRF	Chronic renal failure	**PKU**	Phenylketonuria
cysto	Cystoscopic examination	**UA**	Urinalysis
ESRD	End-stage renal disease	**UTI**	Urinary tract infection
ESWL	Extracorporeal shock wave lithotripsy	**VCUG**	Voiding cystourethrogram
HCO$_3^-$	Bicarbonate; an electrolyte conserved by the kidney		

IX. Practical Applications

This section contains an actual medical report using terms that you have studied in this and previous chapters. Questions are included to test your understanding. Answers are on page 220 under Answers to Exercises.

Urological Case Study

The patient, a 50-year-old woman, presented herself at the clinic complaining of dysuria. This symptom was followed by sudden onset of hematuria and clots. There had been no history of urolithiasis, pyuria, or previous hematuria. Nocturia had been present about 5 years ago. Panendoscopy revealed a carcinoma located about 2 cm from the left ureteral orifice. A partial cystectomy was carried out and the lesion cleared. No ileal conduit was necessary. A metastatic workup was negative. Bilateral pelvic lymphadenectomy revealed no positive nodes.

Questions: Circle the correct answer.

1. Urologic refers to which system of the body?
   (A) digestive
   (B) reproductive
   (C) endocrine
   (D) excretory

2. What was the patient's reason for appearing at the clinic?
   (A) scanty urination
   (B) inability to urinate
   (C) painful urination
   (D) diuresis

3. What acute symptom followed?
   (A) blood in the feces
   (B) blood in the urine
   (C) excessive urea in the blood
   (D) vomiting blood

4. Which of the following was a previous symptom?
   (A) pus in the urine
   (B) blood in the urine
   (C) urinary tract calculi
   (D) excessive urination at night

5. What diagnostic procedure was carried out?
   (A) dialysis
   (B) lithotripsy
   (C) cystoscopy using a wide-angle view of the bladder
   (D) urinalysis

6. The patient's diagnosis was
   (A) malignant tumor of the bladder
   (B) tumor in the proximal ureter
   (C) benign ileal tumor
   (D) malignant tumor with stones

7. Treatment was
   (A) ureteroileostomy
   (B) radical bladder resection
   (C) removal of tumor and subtotal removal of the bladder
   (D) not necessary because of negative lymph nodes

X. Exercises

Remember to check your answers carefully with those given in Section XI, Answers to Exercises.

A. *Using the following terms, trace the path of urine formation from afferent renal arterioles to the point at which urine leaves the body.*

renal pelvis	ureter	Bowman's capsule
glomerulus	urinary meatus	urethra
renal tubule	urinary bladder	

1. _renal tubule_
2. _renal pelvis_
3. _____
4. _____

5. _____
6. _urinary bladder_
7. _urethra_
8. _urinary meatus_

B. *Match the term in column I with the letter of a definition or term of similar meaning in column II.*

Column I

1. voiding _____C_____
2. trigone _____I_____
3. renal cortex _____J_____
4. renal medulla _____G_____
5. urea _____D_____
6. erythropoietin _____A_____
7. renin _____H_____
8. electrolyte _____F_____
9. hilum _____
10. calix (calyx) _____

Column II

A. a hormone secreted by the kidney that stimulates formation of red blood cells
B. notch on the surface of the kidney where blood vessels and nerve enter
C. micturition
D. nitrogenous waste
E. cup-like collecting region of the renal pelvis
F. a small molecule that carries an electric charge in solution
G. inner region of the kidney
H. hormone made by the kidney that causes blood pressure to rise
I. triangular area in the bladder
J. outer section of the kidney

C. Give the meanings for the following medical terms.

1. caliceal _____

2. uric acid _____

3. urinary meatal stenosis _____

4. cystocele _____

5. pyelolithotomy _____

6. trigonitis _____

7. ureteroileostomy _____

8. urethral stricture _____

9. vesicoureteral reflux _____

10. creatinine _____

11. medullary _____

12. cortical _____

D. Select the correct term to complete the sentences below.

1. After diagnosis of renal cell carcinoma (made by renal biopsy), Dr. Davis advised Donna that **(nephrostomy, meatotomy, nephrectomy)** would be necessary.

2. Ever since Bill's condition of gout was diagnosed, he has been warned that uric acid crystals could accumulate in his blood and tissues, leading to **(pyuria, renal calculi, cystocele)**.

3. The voiding cystourethrogram demonstrated blockage of urine flow from Jim's bladder and **(hydronephrosis, renal ischemia, azotemia)**.

4. Narrowed arterioles in the kidney increase blood pressure, and thus **(urinary incontinence, urinary retention, nephrosclerosis)** is often associated with hypertension.

5. Eight-year-old Willy was wetting his bed at night while sleeping. His mother limited Willy's intake of fluids at nighttime to discourage his **(nocturia, oliguria, enuresis)**.

6. David's chronic juvenile diabetes eventually resulted in **(nephropathy, meatal stenosis, urolithiasis)**, which led to renal failure.

7. After Sue's bilateral renal failure, her doctor advised (**nephrotomography, nephrolithotomy, renal transplantation**) to save her life.

8. When Betty's left kidney stopped functioning, her contralateral kidney overdeveloped or (**metastasized, atrophied, hypertrophied**) to meet the increased workload.

E. Give the meanings for the following terms that relate to urinary symptoms.

1. azotemia _____

2. polydipsia _____

3. nocturia _____

4. urinary incontinence _____

5. oliguria _____

6. bacteriuria _____

7. albuminuria _____

8. enuresis _____

9. urinary retention _____

10. dysuria _____

11. polyuria _____

12. glycosuria _____

13. ketosis _____

14. anuria _____

F. Give short answers for the following.

1. What is the difference between hematuria and uremia? _____

2. What is diuresis? _____

3. What is a diuretic? _____

4. What is antidiuretic hormone? _____

G. Match the following terms that pertain to urinalysis with their meanings below.

specific gravity   sediment   proteinuria
bilirubinuria   pyuria   ketonuria
hematuria   glycosuria   phenylketonuria
pH

1. Abnormal particles are present in the urine—cells, bacteria, and crystals.

   _____

2. High levels of a substance appear in urine when a baby is born with a deficiency of an enzyme. The infant can become mentally retarded if she or he is not put on a strict diet that prevents the substance from

   accumulating in the blood and urine. _____

3. Color of the urine is smoky red owing to the presence of blood. _____

4. Urine is turbid (cloudy) owing to the presence of polymorphonuclear leukocytes and pus.

   _____

5. Sugar in the urine; a symptom of diabetes mellitus and a result of hyperglycemia.

   _____

6. This urine test reflects the acidity or alkalinity of the urine. _____

7. High levels of acids and acetones accumulate in the urine as a result of abnormal fat catabolism.

   _____

8. Dark pigment accumulates in urine as a result of liver or gallbladder disease.

   _____

9. This urine test reflects the concentration of the urine. _____

10. Leaky glomeruli can produce this accumulation of albumin in the urine. _____

H. Describe the following abnormal conditions that affect the kidney.

1. renal failure _____

2. polycystic kidney _____

3. interstitial nephritis _____

4. glomerulonephritis _____

5. nephrolithiasis _____

6. renal cell carcinoma _____

7. pyelonephritis _____

8. Wilms' tumor _____

9. nephrotic syndrome _____

10. renal hypertension _____

I. Match the following terms with their meanings below.

edema	stricture	secondary hypertension
abscess	essential hypertension	diabetes insipidus
catheter	diabetes mellitus	

1. high blood pressure that is idiopathic _____

2. swelling, fluid in tissues _____ *edema* _____

3. a narrowed area in a tube _____

4. collection of pus _____

5. inadequate secretion of insulin or improper utilization of insulin leads to this condition

_____

6. high blood pressure caused by kidney disease or another disease _____

7. a tube for withdrawing or giving fluid _____

8. inadequate secretion or resistance of the kidney to the action of antidiuretic hormone

_____

J. Identify the following tests, procedures, or abbreviations.

1. CAPD _____

2. BUN _____

3. cysto _____

4. IVP _____

5. retrograde pyelogram _____

6. KUB _____

7. renal scan _____

8. voiding cystourethrogram _____

9. renal biopsy _____

10. hemodialysis _____

11. UTI _____

12. Na$^+$ _____

13. K$^+$ _____

14. CT scan _____

15. renal angiography _____

16. ESWL _____

K. Match the following surgical procedures with their meanings below.

cystectomy	meatotomy	ureteroileostomy (ileal conduit)
cystostomy	nephrectomy	ureterolithotomy
extracorporeal shock-wave lithotripsy	nephrostomy nephrolithotomy	urethroplasty

1. Excision of a kidney _____

2. Surgical incision into the kidney to remove a stone _____

3. Incision of the urinary meatus for enlargement _____

4. Crushing of stones (with sound waves generated outside the body) _____

5. New opening of the ureters to a segment of ileum (in place of the bladder)

    _____

6. Surgical repair of the urethra _____

7. Creation of an artificial opening into the kidney (via catheter) from the outside of the body

    _____

8. Surgical formation of an opening from the bladder to the outside of the body

    _____

9. Removal of the urinary bladder _____

10. Incision of a ureter to remove a stone _____

XI. Answers to Exercises

A

1. glomerulus
2. Bowman's capsule
3. renal tubule
4. renal pelvis
5. ureter
6. urinary bladder
7. urethra
8. urinary meatus

B

1. C
2. I
3. J
4. G
5. D
6. A
7. H
8. F
9. B
10. E

C

1. pertaining to a calix (collecting cup of renal pelvis)
2. a nitrogenous waste excreted in urine; high levels of uric acid in the blood are associated with gouty arthritis
3. narrowing of the urinary meatus
4. hernia of the urinary bladder
5. incision to remove a stone from the renal pelvis
6. inflammation of the trigone (triangular area in the bladder where the ureters enter and urethra exits)
7. new opening between the ureter and the ileum (an anastomosis); urine then leaves the body through an ileostomy; this surgery is performed when the bladder has been resected
8. narrowing (narrowed portion) of the urethra
9. backflow of urine from the bladder into the ureter
10. a nitrogenous waste produced from muscle metabolism and excreted in the urine
11. pertaining to the inner, middle section (of the kidney)
12. pertaining to the outer section (of the kidney)

D

1. nephrectomy
2. renal calculi
3. hydronephrosis
4. nephrosclerosis
5. enuresis
6. nephropathy
7. renal transplantation
8. hypertrophied

E

1. excess nitrogenous wastes in the bloodstream
2. condition of much thirst
3. excessive urination at night
4. inability to hold urine in the bladder
5. scanty urination
6. bacteria in the urine (sign of infection)
7. protein in the urine
8. bedwetting
9. inability to release urine from the bladder
10. painful urination
11. excessive urination
12. sugar in the urine
13. abnormal condition of ketone bodies (acids and acetones) in the blood and body tissues
14. no urination

F

1. Hematuria is the presence of blood in the urine and uremia is a toxic condition of excess urea (nitrogenous waste) in the bloodstream. Hematuria is a symptomatic condition of the urine (-uria), and uremia is an abnormal condition of the blood (-emia).
2. Diuresis is the excessive production of urine (polyuria).
3. A diuretic is a drug or chemical (caffeine or alcohol) that causes diuresis to occur.
4. Antidiuretic hormone is a hormone produced by the pituitary gland that normally helps the renal tubules to reabsorb water back into the bloodstream. It works against diuresis to help retain water in the blood.

G

1. sediment
2. phenylketonuria (phenylketones in the urine)
3. hematuria (blood in the urine)
4. pyuria (pus in the urine)
5. glycosuria (sugar in the urine)
6. pH
7. ketonuria (ketone bodies in the urine)
8. bilirubinuria (high levels of bilirubin in the urine)
9. specific gravity
10. proteinuria

H

1. kidney does not produce urine
2. multiple fluid-filled sacs form in and on the kidney
3. inflammation of the connective tissue (interstitium) lying between the renal tubules
4. inflammation of the glomerulus of the kidney (may be a complication following a streptococcal infection)
5. condition of kidney stones (renal calculi)
6. malignant tumor of the kidney in adults
7. inflammation of the kidney and renal pelvis (caused by a bacterial infection, such as *Escherichia coli,* that enters the urinary tract from the gastrointestinal tract)
8. malignant tumor of the kidney in children
9. group of symptoms (proteinuria, edema, hypoalbuminemia) that appear when the kidney is damaged by disease; also called nephrosis
10. high blood pressure caused by kidney disease

I

1. essential hypertension
2. edema
3. stricture
4. abscess
5. diabetes mellitus
6. secondary hypertension
7. catheter
8. diabetes insipidus

J

1. continuous ambulatory (walking around) peritoneal dialysis (patient puts fluid in his or her abdomen and wastes from the blood enter the fluid, which is then drained and fresh fluid replaces it)
2. blood urea nitrogen (a blood test showing the amount of nitrogenous waste in the blood)
3. cystoscopy (visual examination of the urinary bladder)
4. intravenous pyelogram (x-ray record of the renal pelvis after injecting dye into a vein)
5. x-ray record of the renal pelvis after injecting dye through the bladder and ureters to the kidney
6. x-ray record of the kidneys, ureters, and bladder (no dye is given)
7. radioactive scan of the kidney after injecting a radioisotope into the veins and visualizing how the kidneys pick it up
8. x-ray record of the bladder and urethra taken while the patient is voiding
9. tissue from the kidney is removed from the body and examined under a microscope
10. removal of nitrogenous wastes from the blood by removing blood and passing it through a filter that separates out the wastes; the blood is then sent back into the body
11. urinary tract infection
12. sodium (an electrolyte)
13. potassium (an electrolyte)
14. x-ray pictures taken in a transverse plane
15. process of recording (x-rays) of blood vessels within the kidney
16. extracorporeal shock wave lithotripsy (kidney and urinary tract stones are crushed by shock waves)

K

1. nephrectomy
2. pyelolithotomy
3. meatotomy
4. extracorporeal shock wave lithotripsy
5. ureteroileostomy
6. urethroplasty
7. nephrostomy
8. cystostomy
9. cystectomy
10. ureterolithotomy

Answers to Practical Applications

1. D
2. C
3. B
4. D
5. C
6. A
7. C

XII. Pronunciation of Terms

To test your understanding of the terminology in this chapter, write the meaning of each term in the space provided. In addition, you may wish to cover the terms and write them by looking at your definitions. Make sure your spelling is correct. The page number after each term indicates where it is defined or used in the text so you can easily check your responses. (If you are not sure what the pronunciation symbols mean, refer to page 21.)

Term	Pronunciation	Meaning
abscess (204)	ĂB-sĕs	_____
albuminuria (200)	ăl-bū-mĭ-NŪ-rē-ă	_____
antidiuretic hormone (201)	ăn-tĭ-dī-ū-RĚ-tĭk HŎR-mōn	_____
azotemia (200)	ă-zō-TĒ-mē-ă	_____
bacteriuria (200)	băk-tē-rē-Ū-rē-ă	_____
caliceal (197)	kā-lĭ-SĒ-ăl	_____
caliectasis (197)	kā-lē-ĔK-tă-sĭs	_____
calix (calyx); calices (196)	KĀ-lĭks; KĀ-lĭ-sēz	_____
catheter (196)	KĂ-thĕ-tĕr	_____

cortex (196)	KŎR-tĕks	_____
cortical (196)	KŎR-tĭ-kăl	_____
creatinine (196)	krē-ĂT-ĭ-nēn	_____
cystectomy (197)	sĭs-TĔK-tō-mē	_____
cystitis (197)	sĭs-TĪ-tĭs	_____
cystocele (197)	SĬS-tō-sēl	_____
cystoscopy (208)	sĭs-TŎS-kō-pē	_____
cystourethrogram (197)	sĭs-tō-ū-RĒ-thrō-grăm	_____
diabetes insipidus (205)	dī-ă-BĒ-tēz ĭn-SĬP-ĭ-dŭs	_____
diabetes mellitus (205)	dī-ă-BĒ-tēz MĔL-ĭ-tŭs	_____
diuresis (201)	dī-ūr-RĒ-sĭs	_____
dysuria (201)	dĭs-Ū-rē-ă	_____
edema (203)	ĕ-DĒ-mă	_____
electrolyte (196)	ē-LĔK-trō-līt	_____
enuresis (200)	ĕn-ū-RĒ-sĭs	_____
erythropoietin (196)	ĕ-rĭth-rō-PŌ-ĭ-tĭn	_____
essential hypertension (205)	ĕ-SĔN-shŭl hī-pĕr-TĒN-shŭn	_____
glomerular (197)	glō-MĔR-ū-lăr	_____
glomerulonephritis (203)	glō-mĕr-ū-lō-nĕ-FRĪ-tĭs	_____
glomerulus; glomeruli (196)	glō-MĔR-ū-lŭs; glō-MĔR-ū-LĪ	_____
glycosuria (201)	glī-kōs-Ū-rē-ă	_____
hematuria (201)	hēm-ă-TŪ-rē-ă	_____
hemodialysis (208)	hē-mō-dī-ĂL-ĭ-sĭs	_____
hilum (196)	HĪ-lŭm	_____
hydronephrosis (198)	hī-drō-nĕ-FRŌ-sĭs	_____
interstitial nephritis (203)	ĭn-tĕr-STĬ-shŭl nĕ-FRĪ-tĭs	_____

intravenous pyelogram (206)	ĭn-tră-VĒ-nŭs PĪ-ĕl-ō-grăm	_____
ketonuria (200)	kē-tōn-Ū-rē-ă	_____
ketosis (200)	kē-TŌ-sĭs	_____
lithotripsy (200)	LĬTH-ō-trĭp-sē	_____
meatal stenosis (198)	mē-Ā-tăl stĕ-NŌ-sĭs	_____
meatotomy (198)	mē-ă-TŎT-ō-mē	_____
meatus (196)	mē-Ā-tŭs	_____
medulla (196)	mĕ-DŪL-ă or mĕ-DŬL-ă	_____
medullary (196)	MĔD-ū-lăr-ē	_____
micturition (196)	mĭk-tū-RĬSH-ŭn	_____
nephrohypertrophy (198)	nĕf-rō-hī-PĔR-trō-fē	_____
nephrolithiasis (203)	nĕf-rō-lĭ-THĪ-ă-sĭs	_____
nephrolithotomy (198)	nĕf-rō-lĭ-THŎT-ō-mē	_____
nephropathy (198)	nĕf-RŎP-ă-thē	_____
nephrosclerosis (198)	nĕf-rō-sklĕ-RŌ-sĭs	_____
nephrotic syndrome (203)	nĕ-FRŎT-ĭk SĬN-drōm	_____
nephrotomography (198)	nĕf-rō-tō-MŎG-ră-fē	_____
nitrogenous waste (196)	nĭ-TRŎJ-ĕ-nŭs wāst	_____
nocturia (200)	nŏk-TŪ-rē-ă	_____
oliguria (200)	ŏl-ī-GŪ-rē-ă	_____
paranephric (198)	pă-ră-NĔF-rĭk	_____
peritoneal dialysis (208)	pĕr-ĭ-tō-NĒ-ăl dī-ĂL-ĭ-sĭs	_____
perivesical (199)	pĕ-rē-VĔS-ĭ-kăl	_____
phenylketonuria (202)	fē-nĭl-kē-tō-NŪ-rē-ă or fĕn-ĭl-kē-tō-NŪ-rē-ă	_____
polycystic kidneys (204)	pŏl-ē-SĬS-tĭk KĬD-nēz	_____
polydipsia (200)	pŏl-ē-DĬP-sē-ă	_____
polyuria (201)	pŏl-ē-ŪR-ē-ă	_____

pyelogram (199)	PĪ-ĕ-lo-grăm	
pyelolithotomy (199)	pī-ĕ-lō-lĭ-THŎT-ō-mē	
pyelonephritis (204)	pī-ĕ-lō-nĕf-RĪ-tĭs	
pyuria (200)	pī-Ū-rē-ă	
renal angiography (206)	RĒ-nal ăn-jē-ŎG-ră-fē	
renal calculi (203)	RĒ-năl KĂL-kū-lī	
renal cell carcinoma (204)	RĒ-năl sĕl kăr-sĭ-NŌ-mă	
renal failure (206)	RĒ-năl FĀL-ŭr	
renal hypertension (205)	RĒ-năl hī-pĕr-TĔN-shŭn	
renal ischemia (199)	RĒ-năl ĭs-KĒ-mē-ă	
renal pelvis (196)	RĒ-năl PĔL-vĭs	
renal transplantation (209)	RĒ-năl trăns-plăn-TĀ-shŭn	
renin (197)	RĒ-nĭn	
retrograde pyelogram (206)	RĔ-trō-grād PĪ-ĕ-lō-grăm	
secondary hypertension (205)	SĔ-kŏn-dă-rē hī-pĕr-TĔN-shŭn	
stricture (199)	STRĬK-shŭr	
trigone (197)	TRĪ-gōn	
trigonitis (199)	trī-gō-NĪ-tĭs	
urea (197)	ū-RĒ-ă	
uremia (200)	ū-RĒ-mē-ă	
ureter (197)	ū-RĒ-tĕr or ŪR-ĕ-tĕr	
ureteroileostomy (199)	ū-rē-tĕr-ō-ĭl-ē-ŎS-tō-mē	
ureterolithotomy (199)	ū-rē-tĕr-ō-lĭ-THŎT-ō-mē	
ureteroplasty (199)	ū-rē-tĕr-ō-PLĂS-tē	
urethra (197)	ū-RĒ-thră	
urethritis (199)	ū-rē-THRĬ-tĭs	
urethroplasty (199)	ū-rē-thrō-PLĂS-tē	

uric acid (197)   Ū-rĭk ĀS-ĭd

urinalysis (201)   ū-rĭn-ĂL-ĭ-sĭs

urinary incontinence (201)   ŬR-ĭ-năr-ē ĭn-KŎN-tĭ-nĕns

urinary retention (201)   ŬR-ī-nĕr-ē rē-TĚN-shŭn

vesicoureteral reflux (199)   vĕs-ĭ-kō-ū-RĒ-tĕr-ăl
                                   RĒ-flŭks

voiding (197)   VOY-dĭng

Wilms' tumor (205)   Wĭlmz TŪ-mŭr

XIII. Review Sheet

Write the meanings for combining forms, suffixes, and prefixes in the space provided. Check your answers with the information in the Chapter or in the Glossary (Medical Terms—English) at the end of the book.

Combining Forms

Combining Form	Meaning	Combining Form	Meaning
albumin/o	_____	meat/o	_____
angi/o	_____	necr/o	_____
arteri/o	_____	nephr/o	_____
azot/o	_____	noct/i	_____
bacteri/o	_____	olig/o	_____
cali/o	_____	py/o	_____
calic/o	_____	pyel/o	_____
cyst/o	_____	ren/o	_____
dips/o	_____	tom/o	_____
glomerul/o	_____	tox/o	_____
glyc/o	_____	trigon/o	_____
glycos/o	_____	ur/o	_____
hydr/o	_____	ureter/o	_____
isch/o	_____	urethr/o	_____
ket/o	_____	urin/o	_____
keton/o	_____	vesic/o	_____
lith/o	_____		

Continued on following page

Suffixes

Suffix	Meaning	Suffix	Meaning
-cele	_____	-rrhea	_____
-ectasis	_____	-sclerosis	_____
-emia	_____	-spasm	_____
-lithiasis	_____	-stenosis	_____
-lithotomy	_____	-stomy	_____
-lysis	_____	-tomy	_____
-megaly	_____	-tripsy	_____
-ole	_____	-trophy	_____
-plasty	_____	-ule	_____
-poietin	_____	-uria	_____
-rrhaphy	_____		

Prefixes

Prefix	Meaning	Prefix	Meaning
a-, an-	_____	en-	_____
anti-	_____	peri-	_____
dia-	_____	poly-	_____
dys-	_____	retro-	_____

Review of Anatomical Terms

Match the number of the urinary system structure in column I with its location or function in column II.

Column I

1. urethra
2. cortex
3. Bowman's capsule
4. calices
5. renal pelvis
6. glomerulus
7. medulla
8. renal tubules
9. urinary bladder
10. ureters

Column II

_____ Tiny structure surrounding each glomerulus; receives filtered materials from blood.

_____ Tubes carrying urine from kidney to urinary bladder.

_____ Tubules leading from Bowman's capsule. Urine is formed there as water, sugar, and salts are reabsorbed into the bloodstream.

_____ Inner (middle) region of the kidney.

_____ Muscular sac that serves as a reservoir for urine.

_____ Cup-like divisions of the renal pelvis that receive urine from the renal tubules.

_____ Tube carrying urine from the bladder to the outside of the body.

_____ Central urine-collecting basin in the kidney that narrows into the ureter.

_____ Collection of capillaries through which materials from the blood are filtered into Bowman's capsule.

_____ Outer region of the kidney.

8

Female Reproductive System

In this Chapter you will
- Name the organs of the female reproductive system, their locations, and combining forms;
- Explain how these organs and their hormones function in the processes of menstruation and pregnancy;
- Identify abnormal conditions of the female reproductive system and of the newborn child; and
- Explain some important laboratory tests, clinical procedures, and abbreviations related to gynecology and obstetrics.

I. Introduction

Sexual reproduction is the union of the nuclei of the female sex cell **(ovum)** and the male sex cell **(sperm)** that results in the creation of a new individual. The ovum and sperm cell are specialized cells differing primarily from normal body cells in one important way. Each sex cell (also called a **gamete**) contains exactly half the number of chromosomes that a normal body cell contains. When the nuclei of ovum and sperm cell unite, the cell produced receives half of its genetic material from its female parent and half from its male parent; thus it contains a full, normal complement of hereditary material.

Gametes are produced in special organs called **gonads** in male and female. The female gonads are the **ovaries,** and the male gonads are the **testes.** An ovum, after leaving the ovary, travels down a duct **(uterine** or **fallopian tube)** leading to the **uterus** (womb). If **coitus** (copulation, sexual intercourse) has occurred, and sperm cells are present in the uterine tube, union of the ovum and sperm may take place. This union is called **fertilization.** The **embryo** (called the **fetus** after the 2nd month) then begins a 40-week (approximately 9-month) period of development **(gestation, pregnancy)** within the uterus.

The female reproductive system consists of organs that produce **ova** and provide a place for the growth of the embryo. In addition, the female reproductive organs supply important hormones that contribute to the development of female secondary sex characteristics (body hair, breast development, structural changes in bones and fat).

Ova mature and are released from the ovary from the onset of **puberty** (beginning of the fertile period when secondary sex characteristics develop) to **menopause** (cessation of fertility and diminishing of hormone production). Women are born with all the eggs that they will possibly release. However, it is not until the onset of puberty that the eggs mature and leave the ovary. If fertilization occurs at any time during the years between puberty and menopause, the fertilized egg may grow and develop within the uterus. Various hormones are secreted from the ovary and from a blood-vessel–filled organ **(placenta)** that grows in the wall of the uterus during pregnancy. If fertilization does not occur, hormone changes result in the shedding of the uterine lining, and bleeding, or **menstruation,** occurs.

The names of the hormones from the ovaries that play important roles in the processes of menstruation and pregnancy, and in the development of secondary sex characteristics, are **estrogen** and **progesterone.** Other hormones that govern the functions of the ovary, breast, and uterus are secreted by the **pituitary gland,** which is located behind the bridge of the nose at the base of the brain.

Gynecology is the study of the female reproductive system (organs, hormones, and diseases); **obstetrics** (obstetrix means midwife) is a specialty concerned with pregnancy and delivery of the fetus; and **neonatology** is the study and treatment of the newborn child.

II. Organs of the Female Reproductive System

Uterus, Ovaries, and Associated Organs

Figures 8–1 and 8–3 should be labeled as you read and study the following paragraphs.

Figure 8–1 is a lateral view of the female reproductive organs and shows their relationship to the other organs in the pelvic cavity. The **ovaries** (1) (only one ovary is shown in this lateral view) are a pair of small almond-shaped organs located in the lower abdomen. The **uterine** or **fallopian tubes** (2) (only one is shown in this view) lead from each ovary to the **uterus** (3), which is a muscular organ situated between the urinary bladder and the rectum. The uterus is normally in a bent forward position and about 3 inches in length in a nonpregnant woman. Midway between the uterus and the rectum is a region in the abdominal cavity known as the **cul-de-sac** (4). This region is often examined for the presence of cancerous growths.

The **vagina** (5) is a tube extending from the uterus to the exterior of the body. **Bartholin's glands** (6) are two small, rounded glands on either side of the vaginal orifice. These glands produce a mucous secretion that lubricates the vagina. The **clitoris** (7) is an organ of sensitive, erectile tissue located anterior to the vaginal orifice and in front of the urethral meatus. The clitoris is similar in structure to the penis in the male.

Figure 8–1

Organs of the female reproductive system, lateral view.

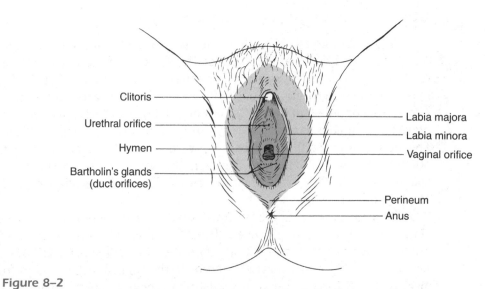

Figure 8–2

External female genitalia (vulva).

Figure 8–3

Female reproductive system, anterior view.

The region between the vaginal orifice and the anus is called the **perineum** (8). This region, at the floor of the pelvic cavity, may be torn in childbirth, resulting in damage to the urinary meatus (if the tear is forward), and the anus (if the tear is backward). To avoid a perineal tear, the obstetrician often cuts the perineum posteriorly before delivery. This incision is called an **episiotomy.** The perineum is then sewn together (repaired) after childbirth.

The external genitalia (organs of reproduction) of the female are collectively called the **vulva.** Figure 8–2 shows the various structures that are part of the vulva. The **labia majora** are the outer lips of the vagina, and the **labia minora** are the smaller, inner lips. The **hymen** is a mucous membrane that normally partially covers the entrance to the vagina. The clitoris and Bartholin's glands are also parts of the vulva.

Figure 8–3 is an anterior view of the female reproductive system. Each **ovary** (1) is held in place on either side of the uterus by **ligaments** (2).

Within each ovary are thousands of small sacs called **graafian follicles** (3). Each graafian follicle contains an **ovum** (4). When an ovum is mature, the graafian follicle ruptures to the surface and the ovum leaves the ovary. The release of the ovum from the ovary is called **ovulation.** The ruptured follicle fills first with blood, and then with a yellow, fat-like material. It is then called the **corpus luteum** (5) (meaning yellow body).

Near each ovary is a duct, about 5½ inches long, called a **uterine** or **fallopian tube** (6). Collectively, the fallopian tubes, ovaries, and supporting ligaments are called the **adnexa** (accessory structures) of the uterus. The egg, after its release from the ovary, is caught up by the finger-like ends of the uterine tube. These ends are called **fimbriae** (7). The tube itself is lined with small hairs that, through their motion, sweep the ovum along. It usually takes the ovum about 5 days to pass through the fallopian tube.

It is within the fallopian tube that fertilization takes place if any sperm cells are present. If coitus takes place near the time of ovulation and no contraception is used, there is a high likelihood that sperm cells will be in the uterine tube when the egg cell is passing through. If coitus has not taken place, the ovum remains unfertilized and, after a day or two, disintegrates.

The fallopian tubes, one on either side, lead into the **uterus** (8), a pear-shaped organ with muscular walls and a mucous membrane lining filled with a rich supply of blood vessels. The

Figure 8–4

The breast.

Know this

rounded upper portion of the uterus is called the **fundus,** and the larger, central section is the **corpus** (body of the organ). The specialized epithelial mucosa of the uterus is called the **endometrium** (9); the middle, muscular layer is the **myometrium** (10); and the outer, membranous tissue layer is the **perimetrium** (11).

The narrow, lower portion of the uterus is called the **cervix** (12) (meaning neck). The cervical opening leads into a 3-inch-long tube called the **vagina** (13), which opens to the outside of the body.

The Breast (Accessory Organ of Reproduction)

Label Figure 8–4 as you read the following description of breast structures.

The breasts are two **mammary** (milk-producing) **glands** located in the upper anterior region of the chest. They are composed of **glandular tissue** (1) that develops in response to hormones from the ovaries during puberty. The breasts also contain **fibrous** and **fatty tissue** (2), special **lactiferous** (milk-carrying) **ducts** (3), and **sinuses** (cavities) (4) that carry milk to the opening or nipple. The breast nipple is called the **mammary papilla** (5), and the dark-pigmented area around the mammary papilla is called the **areola** (6).

During pregnancy, the hormones from the ovaries and the placenta stimulate glandular tissues in the breasts to their full development. After **parturition** (giving birth), hormones from the pituitary gland stimulate the production of milk **(lactation).**

III. Menstruation and Pregnancy

Menstrual Cycle (Fig. 8–5)

The beginning of menstruation at the time of puberty is called **menarche.** Each menstrual cycle is divided into 28 days. These days can be grouped into four time periods, which are useful in describing the events of the cycle. The approximate time periods are:

Days 1–5 (Menstrual Period)

These are the days during which bloody fluid containing disintegrated endometrial cells, glandular secretions, and blood cells is discharged through the vagina.

Days 6–12

After the menstrual period is ended, the lining of the uterus begins to repair itself as the hormone estrogen is released by the maturing graafian follicle in the ovaries. This is also the period of the growth of the ovum in the graafian follicle.

Days 13–14 (Ovulatory Period)

On about the 14th day of the cycle, the graafian follicle ruptures **(ovulation)** and the egg leaves the ovary to travel slowly down the uterine tube.

Days 15–28

The empty graafian follicle fills with a yellow material and becomes known as the **corpus luteum.** The corpus luteum functions as an endocrine organ and secretes two hormones, **estrogen** and **progesterone,** into the bloodstream. These hormones stimulate the building up of the lining of the uterus in anticipation of fertilization of the egg and pregnancy.

If fertilization does *not* occur, the corpus luteum in the ovary stops producing progesterone and estrogen and regresses. At this time, owing to the lowered levels of progesterone and estrogen, some women have symptoms of depression, breast tenderness, and irritability prior to menstruation. These symptoms are known as **premenstrual syndrome (PMS).** About 5 days after the fall in hormones, the uterine endometrium breaks down and the menstrual period begins (days 1–5).

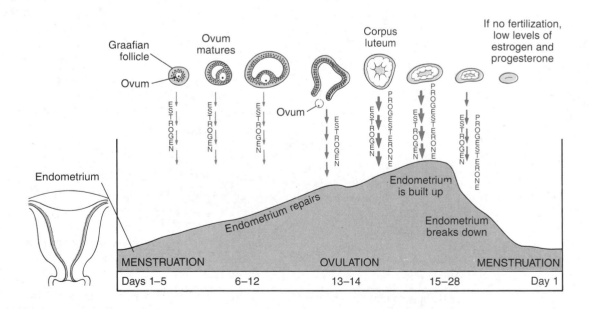

The menstrual cycle.

Pregnancy

If fertilization does occur in the uterine tube, the fertilized egg travels to the uterus and implants in the uterine endometrium. The corpus luteum in the ovary continues to produce progesterone and estrogen, which support the vascular and muscular development of the uterine lining.

The **placenta,** a vascular organ, now forms within the uterine wall. The placenta is derived from maternal endometrium and partly from the **chorion,** the outermost membrane that surrounds the developing embryo. The **amnion** is the innermost of the embryonic membranes, and it holds the fetus suspended in an amniotic cavity surrounded by a fluid called the **amniotic fluid.** The amnion and fluid are sometimes known as the "bag of water." When this breaks, it signals the onset of labor.

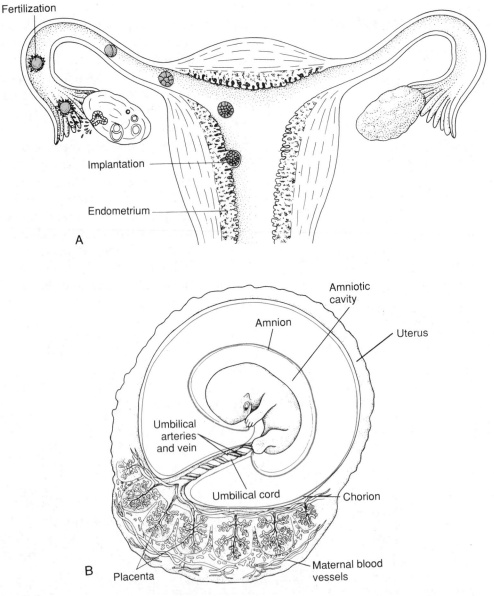

Figure 8–6

(A) Implantation of the embryo. *(B)* Placenta and membranes (chorion and amnion). *(A* and *B,* From Solomon EP, Phillips GA: Understanding Human Anatomy and Physiology. Philadelphia, WB Saunders, 1987, p 348.)

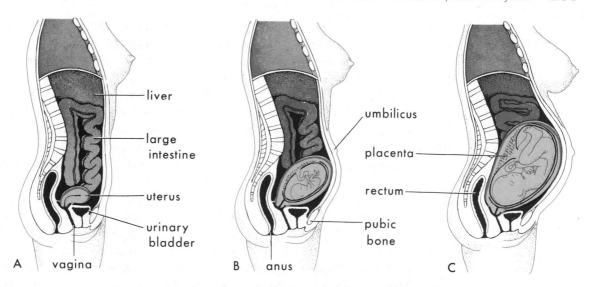

Sagittal sections of a nonpregnant woman *(A)*, a woman 20 weeks pregnant *(B)*, and a woman 30 weeks pregnant *(C)*. (*A–C*, From Moore KL, Persaud TVN: Before We Are Born: Essentials of Embryology and Birth Defects, 4th ed. Philadelphia, WB Saunders, 1993, p 103.)

The maternal blood and fetal blood never mix during pregnancy, but important nutrients, oxygen, and wastes are exchanged as the blood vessels of the baby (coming from the umbilical cord) lie side by side with the mother's blood vessels in the placenta. Figure 8–6 shows the embryo's implantation in the uterus and its relationship to the placenta and enveloping membranes.

The placenta, also known as the **afterbirth** because it separates from the uterus after delivery, produces its own hormone as it develops in the uterus. This placental hormone is called **human chorionic gonadotropin (HCG).** HCG is the hormone tested for in the urine of women who suspect that they are pregnant. HCG stimulates the corpus luteum to continue producing hormones until about the 3rd month of pregnancy, when the placenta itself takes over the endocrine function and releases estrogen and progesterone. Progesterone maintains the development of the placenta. Low levels of progesterone can lead to spontaneous abortion in pregnant women and menstrual irregularities in nonpregnant women.

The uterus normally lies in the pelvis. During pregnancy, the uterus expands as the fetus grows, and it rises out of the pelvic cavity until about 28–30 weeks when it occupies a large part of the abdominopelvic cavity and reaches the epigastric region (Fig. 8–7).

IV. Hormonal Interactions

The events of menstruation and pregnancy are dependent not only upon hormones from the ovary (estrogen and progesterone) but also on hormones from the **pituitary gland.** These pituitary gland hormones are **follicle-stimulating hormone (FSH)** and **luteinizing hormone (LH).** After the onset of menstruation, the pituitary gland begins to secrete FSH and LH, so that their levels rise in the bloodstream. FSH and LH stimulate the maturation of the ovum and ovulation. After ovulation, LH in particular influences the maintenance of the corpus luteum and its production of estrogen and progesterone.

During pregnancy, the high levels of estrogen and progesterone affect the pituitary gland itself by shutting off its production of FSH and LH. This means that while a woman is pregnant, additional eggs do not mature and ovulation cannot occur. This hormonal interaction wherein a high level of hormones (estrogen and progesterone) acts to **shut off** the production of another set of hormones (FSH and LH) is called **negative feedback**. Negative feedback is the principle behind the action of birth control pills. The pills contain varying amounts of estrogen and progesterone. As they are taken, the level of hormones rises in the blood. Negative feedback occurs, and the pituitary does not release FSH or LH. Without FSH or LH, ovulation cannot occur and a woman does not become pregnant. Currently, subdermal implants containing estrogen and progesterone can be effective for up to 5 years.

Other female contraceptive measures include the **IUD (intrauterine device)** and the **diaphragm.** The IUD is a small coil placed inside the uterus by a physician. It prevents implantation of the fertilized egg in the uterine lining. Use of the IUD carries risks including ectopic uterine pregnancy, infection, uterine perforation, and severely increased and painful menstrual flow. The diaphragm is a rubber, cup-shaped device inserted, before coitus, on the outside of the cervix to prevent the entrance of sperm into the uterus.

When the secretion of estrogen from the ovaries lessens and fewer egg cells are produced, **menopause** begins. Menopause is the gradual ending of the menstrual cycle and is a natural process resulting from the normal aging of the ovaries. Other names for menopause are change of life and **climacteric.** Premature menopause occurs before age 35, whereas delayed menopause occurs after age 58. Artificial menopause can occur if the ovaries are removed by surgery or made nonfunctional by radiation therapy.

During menopause, when estrogen levels fall, many women experience hot flashes (the temperature regulation mechanism in the brain is disturbed) and vaginal atrophy (lining of the vagina dries and thins, predisposing it to irritation and discomfort during sexual intercourse). **Estrogen replacement therapy (ERT)**, given orally or as a transdermal patch, is sometimes used to relieve uncomfortable symptoms of menopause, and when combined with progesterone in low doses, it is believed to protect a woman from uterine cancer, the development of porous bones (osteoporosis), and heart disease. ERT has been associated with an increased risk of breast cancer in younger women who take it for longer periods.

V. Vocabulary

This list will help you review many of the new terms introduced in the text. Short definitions will reinforce your understanding of the terms. See Section XII of this chapter for help in pronouncing the more difficult terms.

adnexa	Accessory parts of the uterus; the fallopian tubes and ovaries.
amnion	Innermost membrane around the developing embryo.
areola	Dark-pigmented area around the breast nipple.
Bartholin's glands	Small exocrine glands at the vaginal orifice.
cervix	Lower, neck-like portion of the uterus.
chorion	Outermost layer of the two membranes surrounding the embryo; it is part of the placenta.

clitoris	Organ of sensitive erectile tissue anterior to the urinary meatus.
coitus	Sexual intercourse; copulation. Pronunciation is KŌ-ĭ-tus.
corpus luteum	Empty graafian follicle that secretes estrogen and progesterone after release of the egg cell; literally means yellow (luteum) body (corpus).
cul-de-sac	Region within the pelvis, midway between the rectum and the uterus.
embryo	Stage in development from fertilization of the ovum through the 2nd month of pregnancy.
endometrium	The inner mucous membrane lining the uterus.
estrogen	Hormone produced by the ovaries; responsible for female secondary sex characteristics and buildup of the uterine lining during the menstrual cycle.
fallopian tubes	Ducts through which the egg travels into the ovary; uterine tubes; oviducts.
fertilization	Union of the sperm and ovum (fusion of the two nuclei occurs).
fetus	The embryo from the 3rd month (after 8 weeks) to birth.
fimbriae (plural)	Finger-like ends of the fallopian tubes.
follicle-stimulating hormone (FSH)	Hormone produced by the pituitary gland; stimulates maturation of the ovum.
gamete	Sex cell; sperm or ovum.
genitalia	Reproductive organs; also called genitals.
gestation	Pregnancy.
gonads	Organs in the male and female that produce gametes; ovaries and testes.
graafian follicle	Developing sac enclosing each ovum within the ovary. Only about 400 of these sacs will mature in a woman's lifetime.
human chorionic gonadotropin (HCG)	Hormone produced by the placenta to sustain pregnancy by stimulating (-tropin) the mother's ovaries to produce estrogen and progesterone.
hymen	Mucous membrane partially or completely covering the vaginal orifice.
labia	Lips of the vagina; labia majora are the larger, outermost lips, and labia minora are the smaller, innermost lips.
lactiferous ducts	Tubes that carry milk within the breast.

luteinizing hormone (LH)	Hormone produced by the pituitary gland; promotes ovulation.
menarche	The beginning of the first menstrual period during puberty.
menopause	The gradual ending of menstrual function.
menstruation	The monthly shedding of the uterine lining; menses means month.
myometrium	The muscle layer lining the uterus.
orifice	An opening.
ovaries	Organs in the female lower abdomen that produce ova and hormones; female gonads. The ovaries are almond shaped and about the size of large walnuts.
ovulation	Release of the ovum from the ovary.
ovum (plural: ova)	Egg cell; female gamete.
papilla	A small nipple-shaped projection or elevation. The mammary papilla is the nipple of the breast.
parturition	Act of giving birth.
perimetrium	The membrane surrounding the uterus.
perineum	In females, the area between the anus and the vagina.
placenta	Vascular organ that develops during pregnancy in the uterine wall and serves as a communication between the maternal and the fetal bloodstreams.
progesterone	Hormone produced by the corpus luteum in the ovary and the placenta of pregnant women. Progesterone means hormone (-one) for (pro-) pregnancy (gester).
puberty	Beginning of the fertile period when gametes are produced and secondary sex characteristics appear.
uterine tubes	Fallopian tubes or oviducts.
uterus	Womb; muscular organ in which the embryo develops. The upper portion is the fundus; the middle portion is the corpus; and the lower, neck portion is the cervix. (See Fig. 8–8, page 240.)
vagina	A tube extending from the uterus to the exterior of the body.
vulva	External genitalia of the female; includes the labia, hymen, and clitoris.

VI. Terminology: Combining Forms, Suffixes, and Prefixes

Write the meaning of the medical term in the space provided.

Combining Forms

Combining Form	Meaning	Terminology	Meaning
amni/o	amnion	amniocentesis	
		amniotic fluid	
cervic/o	cervix, neck	endocervicitis	
chori/o **chorion/o**	chorion	choriogenesis	
		chorionic	
colp/o	vagina	colporrhaphy	
		colposcopy	
culd/o	cul-de-sac	culdocentesis	

A needle is placed through the posterior wall of the vagina, and fluid is withdrawn from the cul-de-sac for diagnostic purposes.

| **episi/o** | vulva | episiotomy | |

An incision is made through the skin of the perineum to enlarge the vaginal orifice through which the baby will pass.

| **galact/o** | milk | galactorrhea | |

Abnormal, persistent discharge of milk, commonly seen with pituitary gland tumors.

| **gynec/o** | woman, female | gynecomastia | |

One or both breasts enlarge in a male. It often occurs with puberty or with aging or is drug related.

| **hyster/o** | uterus, womb | hysterectomy | |

Abdominal: removal through the abdominal wall; vaginal: removal through the vagina. A total abdominal hysterectomy (TAH) is removal of the entire uterus (including the cervix) through an abdominal incision (Fig. 8–8).

| **lact/o** | milk | lactogenesis | |
| | | lactation | |

The normal secretion of milk.

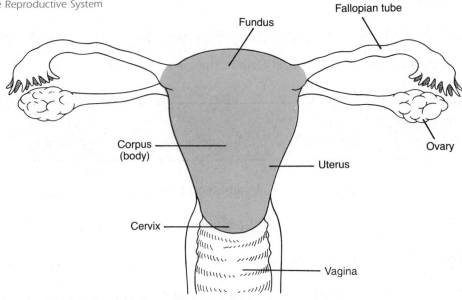

Figure 8–8

Total (complete) hysterectomy. The entire uterus (fundus, corpus, and cervix) is removed, but the ovaries and fallopian tubes remain. (From Chabner DE: Medical Terminology: A Short Course. Philadelphia, WB Saunders, 1990.)

mamm/o	breast	mammary _____
		mammoplasty _____
		Includes reduction and augmentation (enlargement) operations.
mast/o	breast	mastitis _____
		mastectomy _____
		Mastectomy procedures are discussed under carcinoma of the breast (see page 248, Section VII, Pathology).
men/o	menses, menstruation	amenorrhea _____
		Absence of menses for 6 months or for longer than 3 of the patient's normal menstrual cycles.
		dysmenorrhea _____
		oligomenorrhea _____
		Infrequent menstrual periods (interval varies from 36 days to 6 months).
		menorrhagia _____
		Profuse or prolonged menstrual bleeding occurring at regular intervals; fibroids (see page 245 Section VII, Pathology) are a leading cause of menorrhagia.
metr/o **metri/o** ✓	uterus	metrorrhagia _____
		Uterine bleeding occurs at irregular intervals. Ovarian and uterine tumors and foreign bodies such as IUDs can cause metrorrhagia.

menometrorrhagia _____

Excessive uterine bleeding at and between menstrual periods.

perimetrium _____

✓ endometriosis _____

See Section VII, Pathology.

my/o ✓	muscle	myometrium _____
myom/o ✓	muscle tumor	myomectomy _____

Fibroids are removed from the uterus.

nat/i	birth	neonatal _____

The neonatal period is the first 4 weeks of life after birth.

obstetr/o	midwife	obstetric _____
o/o ✓	egg	oogenesis _____
oophor/o	ovary	bilateral oophorectomy _____

Oophor/o means to bear (phor/o) eggs (o/o).

ov/o	egg	ovum _____
ovari/o	ovary	ovarian _____
ovul/o	egg	anovulatory _____
perine/o	perineum	perineorrhaphy _____
phor/o	to bear	oophoritis _____
salping/o ✓	uterine tubes, oviducts, fallopian tubes	salpingectomy _____

Figure 8–9 shows a total hysterectomy with bilateral salpingo-oophorectomy.

uter/o	uterus	uterine prolapse _____
vagin/o	vagina	vaginal orifice _____

Orifice means opening. Colp/o also means vagina.

vaginitis _____

Bacteria and yeast (Candida) are common causes of infection. Use of antibiotics can change the internal environment (pH) of the vagina and destroy normally occurring bacteria, which allows yeast to grow.

vulv/o	vulva	vulvovaginitis _____

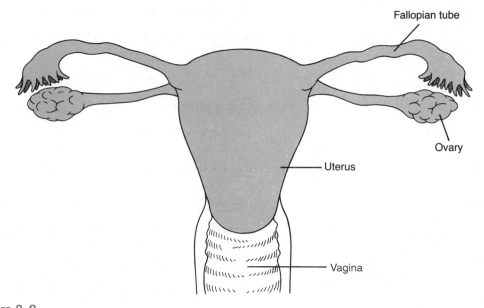

Figure 8–9

Total hysterectomy with bilateral salpingo-oophorectomy.

Suffixes			
Suffix	Meaning	Terminology	Meaning
-arche	beginning	men<u>arche</u> _____	
-cyesis	pregnancy	pseudo<u>cyesis</u> _____	
		Pseudo- means false. No pregnancy occurs, but symptoms such as weight gain and amenorrhea are present.	
-gravida	pregnancy	primi<u>gravida</u> _____	
		A woman during her first pregnancy (primi- means first). Gravida is also used as a noun to describe a pregnant woman, and it may be followed by numbers to indicate the number of pregnancies (gravida 1, 2, 3)	
-parous	to bear, bring forth	primi<u>parous</u> _____	
		An adjective describing a woman who has borne (delivered) one child. Para is also used as a noun and may be followed by numbers to indicate the number of deliveries after the 20th week of gestation (para 1, 2, 3). When a woman arrives on the labor and delivery floor, her gravity and parity are important facts for her medical and surgical history.	
-rrhea	discharge	leuko<u>rrhea</u> _____	
		This is a nonbloody vaginal discharge that may be mucoid or purulent (containing pus) and a sign of infection or cervicitis.	
		men<u>orrhea</u> _____	

-salpinx	uterine tube	pyosalpinx _____	
-tocia	labor, birth	dystocia _____	
		oxytocia _____	

Oxy- means rapid. Oxytocin is a hormone released from the pituitary gland that stimulates the pregnant uterus to induce labor. It also causes milk to be secreted from the mammary glands.

-version	act of turning	cephalic version _____

The fetal head turns or is turned toward the cervix. Presentation is the manner in which the fetus appears to the examiner during delivery. A breech presentation is buttocks first or feet first in a footling breech; a cephalic presentation is head first (Fig. 8–10).

Prefixes			
Prefix	Meaning	Terminology	Meaning
ante-	before, forward	antenatal _____	
		anteversion _____	

The normal position of the uterus—tilted anteriorly.

dys-	painful	dyspareunia _____

Dĭs-pă-ROO-nē-ă. Pareunia means sexual intercourse.

endo-	within	endometritis _____

Placenta

Figure 8–10

Cephalic presentation of the fetus.

IUD

Nylon threads

Figure 8–11

Intrauterine device to prevent implantation of the fertilized egg.

in-	in	<u>in</u>volution of the uterus _____

Vol- means to roll. The uterus returns to its normal nonpregnant size.

intra-	within	<u>intra</u>uterine device _____

Figure 8–11 shows an IUD in place in the uterus.

multi-	many	<u>multi</u>para _____
		<u>multi</u>gravida _____

A woman who has been pregnant at least twice.

nulli-	no, not, none	<u>nulli</u>gravida _____
		<u>nulli</u>para _____

Para O. Figure 8–12 shows the cervix of a nulliparous woman and the cervix of a parous woman (who has had a vaginal delivery).

primi-	first	<u>primi</u>parous _____
retro-	backward	<u>retro</u>flexion _____

Flexion means to bend. The uterus is abnormally bent posteriorly.

Nulliparous

Parous

Figure 8–12

The cervix of a nulliparous woman (the os or opening is small and perfectly round) and the cervix of a parous woman. (From Jacob S, Francone CA: Elements of Anatomy and Physiology, 2nd ed. Philadelphia, WB Saunders, 1989, p 288.)

VIII. Pathology: Gynecological and Breast, Pregnancy, and Neonatal

Gynecological and Breast

Uterus

cervical carcinoma

Malignant tumor of the cervix.

Carcinoma of the cervix ranks with cancers of the lung, colon, and breast as the most common cancers affecting women. Neoplastic changes in the cervix vary from **minimal cervical dysplasia** (abnormal cell growth) to **carcinoma in situ** (localized cancer growth). Tumor cells can later metastasize to lymph nodes and other pelvic organs. The **Papanicolaou test (Pap smear or test)** detects early cervical neoplasia by microscopic examination of cells scraped off the cervical epithelium. **Conization** (biopsy is taken by excising a cone of tissue) is used to diagnose and treat in situ disease. Surgery and/or radiation therapy is used to treat more extensive tumor.

Research has demonstrated that the human papilloma virus (HPV) is important in the etiology of cervical cancer.

cervicitis

Inflammation of the cervix.

This condition can become chronic because the lining of the cervix is not renewed each month as is the uterine lining during menstruation.

Common pathogens infecting the cervix are bacterial *(Chlamydia trachomatis* and *Neisseria gonorrhoeae),* but many infections are nonspecific and the pathogenesis is not understood. **Cervical erosions,** or ulcers, may appear as raw, red patches on the cervical mucosa. **Leukorrhea** (discharge of white or yellow mucoid substance) is a symptom of cervical erosion.

After excluding the presence of malignancy (by Pap smear or biopsy), **cryocauterization** (destroying tissue by freezing) of the eroded area and treatment with antibiotics may be indicated.

endometrial carcinoma

Malignant tumor of the uterus (inner lining).

The major symptom of adenocarcinoma of the uterus (cancer of the lining cells of the uterine cavity) is postmenopausal bleeding. **Dilation** (opening the cervical canal) and **curettage** (scraping the lining of the uterus) is the best method for diagnosing the disease. If the tumor is confined to the uterus, it is curable by surgery and radiotherapy.

endometriosis

Endometrial tissue is found in abnormal locations, including the ovaries, cul-de-sac, pelvic peritoneum, and small intestine.

Endometriosis can be associated with dysmenorrhea, pelvic pain, infertility (inability to become pregnant), and dyspareunia. Most cases develop as a result of bits of menstrual endometrium that pass backward through the **lumen** (opening) of the uterine tube into the peritoneal cavity. Often, when the ovaries are involved, large blood-filled cysts, called chocolate cysts, may develop. Treatment ranges from symptomatic relief of pain and drugs to regulate the menstrual cycle to surgical removal of ectopic endometrial tissue. Figure 8–13 shows sites of endometrial implants.

fibroids

Benign tumors in the uterus.

Fibroids, also called **leiomyomata or leiomyomas** (lei/o = smooth, my/o = muscle, and -oma = tumor), are composed of fibrous tissue and muscle. If they

Fallopian tube

Cul-de-sac

Ovary

Uterus

Urinary bladder

Cervix

Vagina

Figure 8–13

Locations of endometrial implants. (Modified from Swartz MH: Textbook of Physical Diagnosis: History and Examination. Philadelphia, WB Saunders, 1989, p 384.)

grow too large and cause symptoms such as metrorrhagia, pelvic pain, or menorrhagia, hysterectomy or myomectomy is indicated. Figure 8–14 shows uterine fibroids.

Ovaries

ovarian carcinoma

Malignant tumor of the ovary **(adenocarcinoma).** It may be cystic (see below) or solid in consistency.

Carcinomas of the ovary account for more deaths than those of cancers of the cervix or the uterus together. The tumor is usually discovered in an advanced stage as an abdominal mass and may produce few symptoms in its early stages. In most patients, the disease metastasizes within or beyond the pelvic region before diagnosis. Surgery (oophorectomy and salpingectomy), radiotherapy, and more important, chemotherapy are used as therapeutic measures.

ovarian cysts

Collections of fluid within a sac (cyst) in the ovary.

Some cysts are lined by cells that are typical, normal lining cells of the ovary. These cysts originate in unruptured graafian follicles (follicle cysts) or in follicles that have ruptured and have immediately been sealed (luteal cysts). Other cysts may be lined with tumor cells **(cystadenomas** and **cystadenocarcinomas).** Occasionally it is necessary to remove these cysts to distinguish between benign and malignant tumors (Fig. 8–15).

Dermoid cysts are lined with a variety of cell types, including skin, hair, teeth, and cartilage, and arise from immature egg cells in the ovary. They are often called benign cystic teratomas (terat/o = monster) because of the strange assortment of tissue in the tumor (Fig. 8–16). Surgery to remove a dermoid cyst is curative.

Figure 8–14

Fibroids (uterine leiomyomas). (From Ignatavicius DD, Bayne MV: Medical-Surgical
Nursing: A Nursing Process Approach. Philadelphia, WB Saunders, 1991, p 1709.)

Subserosal

Intramural

Submucosal

Figure 8–15

Cystadenoma of the ovary, on cross section.
(From Robbins SL, Cotran RS, Kumar V: Patho-
logic Basis of Disease, 3rd ed. Philadelphia, WB
Saunders, 1984, p 1145.)

Figure 8–16

Dermoid cyst of the ovary with hair,
skin, and teeth. (Courtesy of Dr.
Elizabeth Chabner.)

Fallopian Tubes

pelvic inflammatory disease (PID)

Inflammation in the pelvic region; salpingitis.

The leading causes of PID are gonorrhea and chlamydial infection. They often occur at the same time, and repetitive episodes of these infections can lead to adhesions and scarring within the fallopian tubes. Women have an increased risk of ectopic pregnancies and difficulty getting pregnant after PID. Symptoms are vaginal discharge, pain in the abdomen (LLQ and RLQ), fever, and tenderness on **palpation** (examining by touch) of the cervix. An intrauterine device is the most common iatrogenic cause of PID. Antibiotics are used as treatment.

Breast

carcinoma of the breast

Malignant tumor of the breast that arises from milk glands and ducts.

This tumor first spreads to the lymph nodes located in the axilla (armpit) adjacent to the affected breast and then to the skin and chest wall. From the lymph nodes it may spread to any of the other body organs, including bone, liver, lung, or brain. The tumor is usually removed for purposes of diagnosis and as a primary means of treatment.

There are two objectives in the surgical treatment of breast cancer: first, to remove the tumor; and second, to sample the axillary lymph nodes to determine whether the tumor has spread beyond the breast. Various operations may be performed to accomplish these objectives. For small primary tumors the lump may be removed **(lumpectomy),** with the remainder of the breast left intact. This operation is usually followed by radiotherapy to the breast to kill remaining tumor cells. Alternatively, the surgeon may remove the entire breast (**simple** or **total mastectomy**). With either of these operations a separate incision is made to remove axillary lymph nodes to determine whether spread beyond the breast has taken place. Another surgical procedure is removal of the breast, lymph nodes, and some adjacent chest wall muscles (pectorals) in a single procedure called a **modified radical mastectomy** (Fig. 8–17). If additional tumor is found in the axillary lymph nodes, the patient can then be treated with drugs (adjuvant chemotherapy) to prevent recurrence, and cure is possible.

It is also important to test the tumor for the presence of **estrogen receptors.** These receptors are proteins that indicate that the tumor will respond to hormone therapy. If metastases should subsequently develop, this information will be valuable in selecting further treatment.

Figure 8–17

Surgical scar, modified radical mastectomy, right breast. (Courtesy of Dr. Elizabeth Chabner.)

fibrocystic changes in the breast

Small sacs of tissue and fluid in the breast.

This is a benign and often common condition of the female breast. The patient notices a nodular (lumpy) consistency of the breast, often associated with premenstrual tenderness and fullness. Mammography and then surgical biopsy may be indicated to differentiate fibrocystic changes from carcinoma of the breast.

Pregnancy

abruptio placentae

Premature separation of the implanted placenta.

Abruptio means a breaking or tearing away from, and placentae means of the placenta.

choriocarcinoma

Malignant tumor of the pregnant uterus.

The tumor may appear following pregnancy or abortion. Cure is possible with surgery and chemotherapy.

ectopic pregnancy ✓

Implantation of the fertilized egg in any site other than the normal uterine location.

The condition occurs in up to 1 per cent of pregnancies, and 90 per cent of these occur in the oviducts **(tubal pregnancy).** Rupture of the ectopic pregnancy within the fallopian tube can lead to massive hematosalpinx. Surgery is indicated to remove the implant and preserve the uterine tube before rupture occurs. Other sites of ectopic pregnancies include the ovaries and abdominal cavity, and all are surgical emergencies.

placenta previa

Placental implantation over the cervical opening or the lower region of the uterine wall (Fig. 8–18).

Placenta previa

Figure 8–18

Placenta previa. Previa means before or in the front of.

preeclampsia	A condition during pregnancy or shortly after, marked by high blood pressure, proteinuria, and edema. If seizures occur, the condition is known as **eclampsia** or **toxemia.**
	Mild preeclampsia can be managed by bed rest, but the more serious form of the illness is often more difficult to treat, and women are placed on medications such as magnesium sulfate and Dilantin while in labor to prevent seizures.

Neonatal

The following terms describe a few of the conditions or symptoms that may affect the newborn. The **Apgar score** is a system of scoring an infant's physical condition 1 and 5 minutes after birth. **Heart rate, respiration, color, muscle tone,** and **response to stimuli** are rated 0, 1, or 2. Maximal total score is 10. Infants with low Apgar scores require prompt medical attention (Fig. 8–19).

Down syndrome	Chromosomal abnormality that leads to mental retardation, Oriental appearance of the eyes, low-set ears, and generally dwarfed physique.
erythroblastosis fetalis	**Hemolytic disease in the newborn** caused by a blood group (Rh factor) incompatibility between the mother and the fetus.
hyaline membrane disease	Respiratory problem primarily in the premature neonate; lack of protein in the lining of the lung tissue causes collapse of the lungs.
	This condition is also known as **respiratory distress syndrome.** Hyaline refers to the shiny (hyaline means glassy) membrane that forms in the lung sacs.
hydrocephalus	Accumulation of fluid in the spaces of the brain.
	In an infant the entire head can enlarge because the bones of the skull are never completely fused together at birth. The soft spot, normally present between the cranial bones of the fetus, is called a **fontanelle.** Hydrocephalus occurs because of a problem in the circulation of fluid within the brain and spinal cord.
kernicterus	High levels of bilirubin in the bloodstream of neonates, leading to brain damage and mental retardation.
	Kern- means nucleus, referring to a collection of nerve cells in the brain. Icterus means yellow color or jaundice.
pyloric stenosis	Narrowing of the opening of the stomach to the duodenum (pyloric lumen).
	Surgical repair of the pyloric opening may be necessary.

APGAR SCORING CHART

SIGN	0	1	2
Heart rate	Absent	Below 100	Over 100
Respiratory effort	Absent	Slow, irregular	Good, crying
Muscle tone	Limp	Some flexion of extremities	Active motion
Response to catheter in nostril (tested after oropharynx is clear)	No response	Grimace	Cough or sneeze
Color	Blue, pale	Body pink, extremities blue	Completely pink

Figure 8–19

Apgar scoring chart. (From O'Toole M [ed]: Miller-Keane Encyclopedia of Medicine, Nursing, and Allied Health, 5th ed. Philadelphia, WB Saunders, 1992, p 106.)

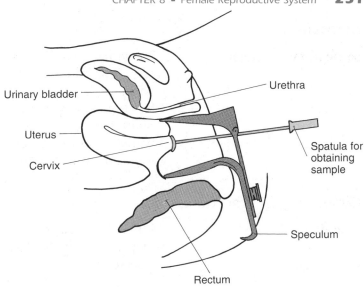

Figure 8–20

Method of obtaining a sample for the Pap test.

VIII. Clinical Tests, Procedures, and Abbreviations

Clinical Tests

Pap smear

The physician, after inserting a vaginal speculum (instrument to hold apart the vaginal walls), uses a spatula and cytobrush to scrape the cervix (Fig. 8–20). Microscopic analysis of the cell smear (spread on a glass slide) can detect the presence of cervical or vaginal carcinoma.

pregnancy test

Blood or urine test to detect the presence of HCG.

Procedures

X-Ray

hysterosalpingography

Contrast material is injected into the uterus and uterine tubes, and x-rays are taken.

mammography

X-rays are taken of the breast. It is recommended that women have a baseline mammogram around the age of 50 for later comparisons if needed. Every 1 to 2 years a mammogram is recommended for women over the age of 50 to screen for breast cancer. Figure 8–21 illustrates mammography.

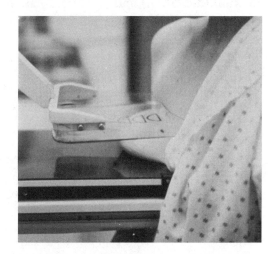

Figure 8–21

Mammography. The breast is compressed and x-rays are taken. (Courtesy of Dr. Elizabeth Chabner.)

Ultrasound

pelvic ultrasonography
A record of sound waves as they bounce off organs in the pelvic region. This technique can evaluate fetal size and maturity and fetal and placental position. Uterine tumors and other pelvic masses, including abscesses, can be diagnosed by ultrasonography. **Transvaginal ultrasound** is a new technique that allows the radiologist a closer, sharper look at normal and pathological structures within the pelvis. The sound probe is placed in the vagina instead of across the pelvis or abdomen.

Gynecological Procedures

aspiration
Fluid is withdrawn by suction from a cavity or sac with a needle. Aspiration biopsy is a valuable technique for the evaluation of a patient with breast disease.

cauterization
Destruction of abnormal tissue with chemicals (silver nitrate) or an electrically heated instrument. It is used to treat cervical dysplasia or cervical erosion.

colposcopy
Visual examination of the vagina and cervix using a colposcope (a lighted, magnifying instrument resembling a small, mounted pair of binoculars). This procedure is more accurate than a Pap smear, since it can identify the specific areas in which abnormal cells are located. A biopsy then can be taken from those areas for accurate diagnosis (Fig. 8–22).

conization
Removal of a cone-shaped section of the cervix for biopsy (diagnosis). The cone is cut out with a cold knife or **laser** (a device that produces a very thin beam of light in which high energies are concentrated) so as not to distort the tissue for histological examination (Fig. 8–23).

cryosurgery
Use of cold temperatures to destroy tissue. The freezing temperature is produced by a probe containing liquid nitrogen. Also called **cryocauterization.**

culdocentesis
Needle aspiration (through the vagina) of fluid from the cul-de-sac. Presence of blood may indicate ruptured ectopic pregnancy.

dilation (dilatation) and curettage (D & C)
Dilation (widening) of the cervical opening is accomplished by inserting a series of probes of increasing size. Curettage (scraping) is then performed using a curette (metal loop at the end of a long, thin handle) to remove the lining of the uterus (Fig. 8–24).

exenteration
Removal of internal organs. Pelvic exenteration is the removal of the uterus, ovaries, uterine tubes, vagina, bladder, rectum, and lymph nodes.

laparoscopy
Visual examination of the abdominal cavity by making a small incision near a woman's navel and introducing a laparoscope (thin tube containing a viewing instrument and light). The procedure is performed for diagnosis of disease or for tubal ligation.

Figure 8–22

Colposcopy. The female being examined is in the dorsal lithotomy position.

Colposcope

Cervix

Figure 8–23

Cone biopsy.

Cone biopsy

Dilator

Cervix

Vagina

Dilation

Uterine cavity

Cervical canal

Curette

Vagina

Curettage

Figure 8–24

Dilation and curettage.

tubal ligation

Blocking of the uterine tubes by burning or cutting and tying them off. This **sterilization** (making an individual incapable of reproduction) technique involves making an small incision into the abdomen and inserting a laparoscope through which the instrument to block the tubes can be introduced.

Procedures During Pregnancy

abortion

Premature termination of pregnancy before the embryo or fetus is able to exist on its own. Major methods for abortion are vaginal evacuation by D & C or vacuum aspiration (suction) and stimulation of uterine contractions by saline (salt) injected into the amniotic cavity (second trimester).

amniocentesis

Surgical puncture (transabdominal) of the amniotic sac to withdraw amniotic fluid for analysis. The cells of the fetus, found in the fluid, are cultured (grown), and cytological and biochemical studies are made.

cesarean section

Removal of the fetus by abdominal incision into the uterus. Indications for cesarean section are cephalopelvic disproportion, hemorrhage from abruptio placentae or placenta previa, fetal distress (fetal hypoxia), and breech or shoulder presentation. The procedure was so named because it was included in the *lex cesarea* under Roman law in 70 BCE.

fetal monitoring

Use of a machine to electronically record the infant's heart rate during labor.

pelvimetry

Measurement of the dimensions of the mother's pelvis to determine its capacity to allow passage of the fetus through the birth canal. Usually this is a part of the prenatal examination, but it is also of vital importance during protracted labor or with breech presentation.

ABBREVIATIONS

AB	Abortion
AFP	Alpha-fetoprotein; high levels in amniotic fluid of fetus or maternal serum indicate increased risk of neurological birth defects in the infant.
C-section	Cesarean section
CIS	Carcinoma in situ
CS	Cesarean section
Cx	Cervix
D & C	Dilation (dilatation) and curettage
DES	Diethylstilbestrol; an estrogen compound used in the treatment of menopausal problems involving estrogen deficiency; if administered during pregnancy, it has been found to be related to subsequent tumors in the daughters (rarely in sons) of mothers so treated.
DUB	Dysfunctional uterine bleeding
ECC	Endocervical curettage
EDC	Estimated date of confinement
EMB	Endometrial biopsy
ERT	Estrogen replacement therapy
FHT	Fetal heart tones
FSH	Follicle-stimulating hormone
G	Gravida (pregnant)
GYN	Gynecology

HCG; hCG	Human chorionic gonadotropin	**Pap smear**	Papanicolaou smear (test for cervical or vaginal cancer)
HSG	Hysterosalpingography	**Path**	Pathology
IUD	Intrauterine device; contraceptive	**peds**	Pediatrics
IUP	Intrauterine pregnancy	**PID**	Pelvic inflammatory disease
LH	Luteinizing hormone	**PMS**	Premenstrual syndrome
LMP	Last menstrual period	**primip**	Primipara; primiparous
multip	Multipara; multiparous	**TAH-BSO**	Total abdominal hysterectomy with bilateral salpingo-oophorectomy
OB	Obstetrics		
OCPs	Oral contraceptive pills	**UC**	Uterine contractions
Para 2-0-1-2	Woman's reproductive history: 2 full-term infants, 0 preterm, 1 abortion, and 2 living children		

IX. Practical Applications

This section contains medical terms that you have studied in this and previous chapters. Explanations of more difficult terms are added in brackets.

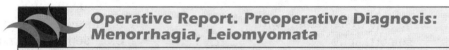

Operative Report. Preoperative Diagnosis: Menorrhagia, Leiomyomata

Anesthetic: General
Material forwarded to laboratory for examination:

    A. Endocervical curettings
    B. Endometrial curettings

Operation performed: Dilation and curettage of the uterus
With the patient in the dorsal lithotomy position [legs are flexed on the thighs, thighs flexed on the abdomen and abducted] and sterilely prepped and draped, manual examination of the uterus revealed it to be 6-8-week size, retroflexed; no adnexal masses noted. The anterior lip of the cervix was then grasped with a tenaculum [hook-like surgical instrument for grasping and holding parts]. The cervix was dilated up to a #20 Hank's dilator. The uterus was sounded [widened] up to 4 inches. A sharp curettage of the endocervix showed only a scant amount of tissue. With a sharp curettage, the uterus was curetted in a clockwise fashion with an irregularity noted in the posterior floor. A large amount of hyperplastic endometrial tissue was removed. The patient tolerated the procedure well.
    Operative diagnosis: Leiomyomata uteri

Sentences Using Medical Terminology

1. Mammogram report: The breast parenchyma [essential tissue] is symmetrical bilaterally. There are no abnormal masses or calcifications in either breast. The axillae are normal.

2. This is a 43-year-old G3P2 with premature ovarian failure and now on ERT. She has history of endocervical atypia [cells are not normal or typical] secondary to chlamydial infection, which is now being treated.

3. The patient is a 40-year-old gravida II, para II, white female admitted for exploratory celiotomy [laparotomy] to remove and evaluate 10-cm left adnexal mass. Discharge diagnosis: (1) endometriosis, left ovary; (2) benign cystic teratoma [dermoid cyst], left ovary.

Operating Schedule: General Hospital

Match the surgery list in column I with a diagnosis or reason for the surgery in column II. Answers can be found at the end of the Answers to Exercises section, page 267.

Column I–Surgery

1. Conization of the cervix _____

2. Vaginal hysterectomy with colporrhaphy _____

3. TAH-BSO, pelvic and periaortic lymphadenectomy _____

4. Exploratory laparotomy for uterine myomectomy _____

5. Excision of bilateral gynecomastia _____

6. Modified radical mastectomy _____

Column II–Diagnosis

A. Persistent, excessive breast tissue in a male
B. Fibroids
C. Endometrial carcinoma
D. Adenocarcinoma of the breast
E. Suspected cervical cancer
F. Uterine prolapse

X. Exercises

Remember to check your answers carefully with those given in Section XI, Answers to Exercises.

A. *Match the following terms for structures or tissues with their meanings below.*

fimbriae	clitoris	perimetrium
chorion	labia	mammary papilla
amnion	vulva	ovaries
areola	perineum	placenta
cervix	uterine tubes	vagina
endometrium		

1. inner lining of the uterus _____

2. area between the anus and the vagina in females _____

3. dark-pigmented area around the breast nipple _____

4. finger-like ends of the fallopian tube _____

5. oviducts; ducts through which the egg travels into the uterus from the ovary

   _____

6. organ of sensitive erectile tissue in females; anterior to urethral orifice _____

7. nipple of the breast _____

8. blood-vessel–filled organ that develops during pregnancy in the uterine wall and serves as a communication between maternal and fetal bloodstreams _____

9. lower, neck-like portion of the uterus _____

10. innermost membrane around the developing embryo _____

11. outermost layer of the membranes around the developing embryo and forming part of the placenta

    _____

12. membrane surrounding the uterus _____

13. lips of the vagina _____

14. female gonads; producing ova and hormones _____

15. includes the perineum, labia, clitoris, and hymen; external genitalia _____

16. muscular tube extending from the uterus to the exterior of the body _____

B. Identify the following terms.

1. fetus _____

2. lactiferous ducts _____

3. gametes _____

4. gonads _____

5. adnexa _____

6. cul-de-sac _____

7. genitalia _____

8. Bartholin's glands _____

9. graafian follicle _____

10. corpus luteum _____

C. Match the terms below with their descriptions.

menarche   coitus   human chorionic gonadotropin
luteinizing hormone   follicle stimulating hormone   progesterone
myometrium   anteversion   fertilization
estrogen

1. a hormone produced by the ovaries; responsible for femaleness and buildup of the uterine lining during

   the menstrual cycle _____

2. a hormone produced by the pituitary gland to stimulate the maturation of the graafian follicle and ovum

   in the ovary _____

3. sexual intercourse _____

4. the normal bending forward of the uterus in the pelvic cavity _____

5. beginning of the first menstrual period during puberty _____

6. hormone produced by the placenta to sustain pregnancy by stimulating the ovaries to produce estrogen

   and progesterone _____

7. muscle layer lining the uterus _____

8. hormone produced by the corpus luteum in the ovary and also the placenta of pregnant women

_____

9. hormone produced by the pituitary gland to promote ovulation _____

10. fusion of the nuclei of the sperm and ovum _____

D. Give meanings for the following.

1. galact/o and lact/o both mean _____

2. colp/o and vagin/o both mean _____

3. mamm/o and mast/o both mean _____

4. metr/o, uter/o, and hyster/o all mean _____

5. oophor/o and ovari/o both mean _____

6. o/o, ov/o, and ovul/o all mean _____

7. in- and endo- both mean _____

8. -cyesis and -gravida both mean _____

9. salping/o and -salpinx both mean _____

10. episi/o and vulv/o both mean _____

E. Complete the terms from the meanings given.

1. inflammation of the cervix: _____ itis

2. suture of the vagina: colp _____

3. surgical puncture to remove fluid from the cul-de-sac: _____ centesis

4. surgical repair of the breast: mammo _____

5. removal of both fallopian tubes: bi _____ _____ ectomy

6. pertaining to newborn: neo _____

7. difficult labor: dys _____

8. first menstrual period: men _____

9. rapid labor: _____ tocia

10. production of milk: lacto _____

F. Give the meanings for the following symptoms.

1. amenorrhea _____

2. dysmenorrhea _____

3. leukorrhea _____

4. metrorrhagia _____

5. galactorrhea _____

6. menorrhagia _____

7. pyosalpinx _____

8. dyspareunia _____

9. menometrorrhagia _____

10. oligomenorrhea _____

G. Answer the following true or false and explain your answer.

1. after a total (complete) hysterectomy, a woman still has regular menstrual periods

_____

2. after a total hysterectomy, a woman may still produce estrogen and progesterone

_____

3. birth control pills prevent pregnancy by reducing the levels of FSH and LH in the bloodstream

_____

4. After a total hysterectomy with bilateral salpingo-oophorectomy, a doctor may advise estrogen

replacement therapy _____

5. a total mastectomy involves removal of the entire breast, axillary nodes, and chest muscles

_____

6. an episiotomy is an incision of the cervix and is part of a Pap smear _____

7. human chorionic gonadotropin is produced by the ovaries during pregnancy

_____

8. gynecomastia is a common condition in pregnant women _____

9. treatment for endometriosis is uterine myomectomy _____

10. a gravida 3, para 2 is a woman who has given birth 3 times _____

11. a nulligravida is a woman who has had several pregnancies _____

12. pseudocyesis is the same condition as a tubal pregnancy _____

13. fibrocystic changes in the breast are a malignant condition _____

14. cystadenomas occur in the ovary _____

15. FSH and LH are ovarian hormones _____

H. Give the meaning for the following terms.

1. parturition _____

2. menopause _____

3. menarche _____

4. ovulation _____

5. gestation _____

6. anovulatory _____

7. sterilization _____

8. lactation _____

9. nulliparous _____

10. oophoritis _____

I. Match the following terms with their meanings below.

abruptio placentae
carcinoma in situ
endometrial carcinoma
placenta previa

cervical carcinoma
cervicitis
endometriosis
leiomyomas

cystadenocarcinoma
choriocarcinoma
preeclampsia

1. a malignant tumor of the ovary _____

2. a chlamydial infection causing inflammation in the lower, neck-like portion of the uterus

   _____

3. cancerous tumor cells are localized in a small area _____

4. a condition during pregnancy or shortly thereafter, marked by hypertension, proteinuria, and edema

   _____

5. uterine tissue located outside the uterus (in the ovaries, cul-de-sac, or attached to the peritoneum)

   _____

6. premature separation of a normally implanted placenta _____

7. placenta implantation over the cervical opening _____

8. a malignant tumor of the pregnant uterus _____

9. a malignant condition that can be diagnosed by a Pap smear, revealing dysplastic changes in cells

   _____

10. a malignant condition of the inner lining of the uterus _____

11. benign muscle tumors in the uterus _____

J. Give the name of the test or procedure described below. Parts of some terms are given.

1. destruction of abnormal tissue with chemicals or an electrically heated instrument:

   _____

2. contrast material is injected into the uterus and uterine tubes, and x-rays are taken:

   _____ graphy

3. cold temperatures are used to destroy tissue:

   _____

4. visual examination of the vagina and cervix:

   _____ scopy

5. widening the cervical opening and scraping the lining of the uterus:

   _____

6. withdrawal of fluid by suction with a needle:

   _____

7. process of recording x-rays of the breast:

   mammo _____

8. a cone-shaped section of the cervix is removed for diagnosis or treatment of cervical dysplasia:

   _____

9. surgical puncture to remove fluid from the cul-de-sac:

   _____

10. echos from sound waves are used to create an image of structures in the region of the hip:

    pelv _____ _____ ography

11. blocking the oviducts by burning or cutting and tying them off:

    _____

12. visual examination of the abdominal cavity:

    _____ scopy

13. HCG is measured in the urine or blood:

    _____ test

14. cells are taken from the cervix or vagina for microscopic analysis:

    _____ smear

15. complete removal of internal organs in the pelvic region:

    _____

K. Match the obstetrical and neonatal terms with their descriptions below.

abortion
Apgar
pelvimetry
kernicterus

fontanelle
cephalic version
erythroblastosis fetalis
pyloric stenosis

hydrocephalus
cesarean section
hyaline membrane disease
fetal monitoring

1. Turning the fetus so that the head is toward the examiner is called _____

2. Measurement of the dimensions of the maternal pelvic bone is called _____

3. The soft spot between the newborn's cranial bones is called a (an) _____

4. The evaluation of the newborn's physical condition is called a (an) _____ score.

5. Premature termination of pregnancy is known as _____ .

6. Removal of the fetus by abdominal incision of the uterus is a (an) _____ .

7. A serious respiratory condition of the fetal lungs leading to collapse of the lungs is

_____ .

8. Use of a machine to electronically record the infant's heart rate during labor is known as

_____ .

9. Narrowing of the opening of the stomach to the small intestine in the infant is called

_____ .

10. Hemolytic disease of the newborn is called _____ .

11. Accumulation of fluid in the spaces of a neonate's brain is called _____ .

12. The condition of high blood levels of bilirubin that can cause brain damage in the neonate is called

_____ .

L. Give medical terms for the following meanings. Pay careful attention to spelling.

1. benign muscle tumors in the uterus: _____

2. no menstrual discharge: _____

3. accessory organs: _____

4. suture of the vagina: _____

5. removal of an ovary: _____

6. condition of female breasts (in a male): _____

7. reproductive organs: _____

8. widening: _____

9. scraping: _____

10. ovarian hormone that sustains pregnancy: _____

11. nipple-shaped elevation: _____

12. inflammation of the vulva and vagina: _____

M. Give the meaning for the following abbreviations.

1. PID _____

2. IUD _____

3. AFP _____

4. DES _____

5. CIS _____

6. ERT _____

7. PMS _____

8. G _____

9. LMP _____

10. OB _____

N. Circle the term in parentheses that best completes the meaning of each sentence.

1. Dr. Hanson felt that it was important to do a **(culdocentesis, Pap smear, amniocentesis)** once yearly on each of her gyn patients to screen for abnormal cells.

2. When Doris missed her period, her doctor checked for the presence of **(LH, IUD, HCG)** in Doris' urine to see if she was pregnant.

3. Ellen was 34 weeks pregnant, experiencing bad headaches, a 10-pound weight gain in 2 days, and blurry vision. Dr. Murphy told her to go to the obstetrical emergency room because she suspected **(preeclampsia, pelvic inflammatory disease, fibroids)**.

4. Dr. Harris felt a breast mass when examining Mrs. Clark. She immediately ordered a (**dilation and curettage, hysterosalpingogram, mammogram**) for her 35-year-old patient.

5. Clara knew that she should not ignore her fevers, yellow vaginal discharge, and pain in her side. She had a previous episode of (**PMS, PID, DES**) that was treated with IV antibiotics and was worried that she might have a recurrence.

XI. Answers to Exercises

A

1. endometrium
2. perineum
3. areola
4. fimbriae
5. uterine tubes
6. clitoris
7. mammary papilla
8. placenta
9. cervix
10. amnion
11. chorion
12. perimetrium
13. labia
14. ovaries
15. vulva
16. vagina

B

1. the embryo from the 3rd month (after 8 weeks) to birth
2. tubes that carry milk within the breast
3. sex cells; the egg and sperm cells
4. organs (ovaries and testes) in the female and male that produce gametes
5. accessory parts of an organ; the adnexa uteri are the ovaries, uterine tubes, and supporting ligaments
6. the region of the abdomen between the rectum and the uterus
7. reproductive organs (genitals)
8. small exocrine glands at the vaginal orifice that secrete a lubricating fluid
9. the developing sac in the ovary that encloses the ovum
10. empty graafian follicle that secretes estrogen and progesterone after ovulation

C

1. estrogen
2. follicle-stimulating hormone
3. coitus
4. anteversion
5. menarche
6. human chorionic gonadotropin
7. myometrium
8. progesterone
9. luteinizing hormone
10. fertilization

D

1. milk
2. vagina
3. breast
4. uterus
5. ovary
6. egg
7. in, within
8. pregnancy
9. fallopian (uterine) tube; oviduct
10. vulva (external female genitalia)

E

1. cervicitis
2. colporrhaphy
3. culdocentesis
4. mammoplasty
5. bilateral salpingectomy
6. neonatal
7. dystocia
8. menarche
9. oxytocia
10. lactogenesis

F

1. no menstrual flow
2. painful menstrual flow
3. white discharge (from the vagina and associated with cervicitis)
4. bleeding from the uterus at irregular intervals
5. abnormal discharge of milk from the breasts
6. profuse or prolonged menstrual bleeding occurring at regular intervals
7. pus in the uterine tubes
8. painful sexual intercourse
9. heavy bleeding at and between menstrual periods
10. scanty menstrual flow

G

1. False. Total hysterectomy means removal of the entire uterus so that menstruation does not occur.
2. True. Total hysterectomy does not mean that the ovaries have been removed.
3. True. Birth control pills contain estrogen and progesterone, which cause negative feedback to the pituitary gland, lowering FSH and LH in the bloodstream and preventing ovulation.
4. True. This may be necessary to treat symptoms of estrogen loss (vaginal atrophy, hot flashes) and prevent bone deterioration (osteoporosis).
5. False. A total (simple) mastectomy is removal of the breast and a sampling of axillary lymph nodes. A radical mastectomy involves removal of the breast, axillary nodes, *and* chest wall muscles.
6. False. An episiotomy is an incision of the perineum and is done during delivery to prevent tearing of the perineum.
7. False. HCG is produced by the *placenta* during pregnancy.

G

8. False. Gynecomastia is a condition of increased breast development in *males*.
9. False. Myomectomy means removal of muscle tumors (fibroids). Endometriosis is abnormal location of uterine tissue outside the uterine lining.
10. False. A gravida 3, para 2 is a woman who has had 3 pregnancies but has given birth (delivered) twice.
11. False. A nulligravida is a woman who has had no pregnancies. A multigravida has had many pregnancies.
12. False. A pseudocyesis is a false pregnancy (no pregnancy occurs), and a tubal pregnancy is an ectopic pregnancy (pregnancy occurs in the uterine tube, not in the uterus).
13. False. Fibrocystic changes in the breast are a benign condition.
14. True. Cystadenomas are glandular sacs lined with tumor cells and occur in the ovaries.
15. False. FSH and LH are pituitary gland hormones. Estrogen and progesterone are secreted by the ovaries.

H

1. act of giving birth
2. gradual ending of menstrual function
3. beginning of the first menstrual period at puberty
4. release of the ovum from the ovary
5. pregnancy
6. pertaining to no ovulation (egg is not released from the ovary)
7. loss of ability to reproduce
8. production of milk
9. a woman who has never given birth
10. inflammation of the ovaries

I

1. cystadenocarcinoma
2. cervicitis
3. carcinoma in situ
4. preeclampsia
5. endometriosis
6. abruptio placentae
7. placenta previa
8. choriocarcinoma
9. cervical carcinoma
10. endometrial carcinoma
11. leiomyomas

J

1. cauterization
2. hysterosalpingography
3. cryosurgery
4. colposcopy
5. dilation (dilatation) and curettage
6. aspiration
7. mammography
8. conization
9. culdocentesis
10. pelvic ultrasonography
11. tubal ligation
12. laparoscopy
13. pregnancy test
14. Pap smear
15. pelvic exenteration

K

1. cephalic version
2. pelvimetry
3. fontanelle
4. Apgar
5. abortion
6. cesarean section
7. hyaline membrane disease
8. fetal monitoring
9. pyloric stenosis
10. erythroblastosis fetalis
11. hydrocephalus
12. kernicterus

L

1. fibroids
2. amenorrhea
3. adnexa
4. colporrhaphy
5. oophorectomy
6. gynecomastia
7. genitalia
8. dilation
9. curettage
10. progesterone
11. papilla
12. vulvovaginitis

M

1. pelvic inflammatory disease (salpingitis)
2. intrauterine device (form of contraception)
3. alphafetoprotein (high levels in amniotic fluid and maternal serum are linked to neurological abnormalities in the fetus)
4. diethylstilbestrol (a form of estrogen that was given to pregnant women to prevent loss of the fetus and that is now found to cause abnormalities in the daughters of women who took the drug)
5. carcinoma in situ
6. estrogen replacement therapy
7. premenstrual syndrome
8. gravida (pregnant woman)
9. last menstrual period
10. obstetrics

N

1. Pap smear
2. HCG
3. preeclampsia
4. mammogram
5. PID

Answers to Practical Applications—Operating Schedule, General Hospital:

1. E
2. F
3. C
4. B
5. A
6. D

XII. Pronunciation of Terms

To test your understanding of the terminology in this chapter, write the meaning of each term in the space provided. In addition, you may wish to cover the terms and write them by looking at your definitions. Make sure your spelling is correct. The page number after each term indicates where it is defined or used in the text so you can easily check your responses. (If you are not sure what the pronunciation symbols mean, refer to page 21.)

Vocabulary and Terminology

Term	Pronunciation	Meaning
adnexa (236)	ăd-NĔK-să	
amenorrhea (240)	ā-mĕn-ō-RĒ-ă	
amniocentesis (239)	ăm-nē-ō-sĕn-TĒ-sĭs	
amniotic fluid (239)	ăm-nē-ŎT-ĭk FLOO-id	
anovulatory (241)	ăn-ŎV-ū-lă-tōr-ē	
antenatal (243)	ăn-tē-NĀ-tăl	
anteversion (243)	ăn-tē-VĔR-shŭn	
areola (236)	ă-RĒ-ō-lă	
Bartholin's glands (236)	BĂR-thō-lĭnz glandz	
bilateral oophorectomy (241)	bī-LĂ-tĕr-ăl ō-ŏf-ō-RĔK-tō-mē or oo-fō-RĔK-tō-mē	
cephalic version (243)	sĕ-FĂL-lĭk VĔR-shŭn	
cervix (236)	SĔR-vĭkz	
choriogenesis (239)	kŏr-ē-ō-JĔN-ĕ-sĭs	
chorion (236)	KŌ-rē-ŏn	
chorionic (239)	kō-rē-ŎN-ĭk	
clitoris (237)	KLĬ-tō-rĭs	
coitus (237)	KŌ-ĭ-tŭs	
colporrhaphy (239)	kŏl-PŎR-ă-fē	
colposcopy (239)	kŏl-PŎS-kō-pē	
corpus luteum (237)	KŎR-pŭs LŪ-tē-ŭm	
cul-de-sac (237)	KŬL-dĕ-săk	

culdocentesis (239)	kŭl-dō-sĕn-TĒ-sĭs	_____
dysmenorrhea (240)	dĭs-mĕn-ō-RĒ-ă	_____
dyspareunia (243)	dĭs-pă-ROO-nē-ă	_____
dystocia (243)	dĭs-TŌ-sē-ă	_____
embryo (237)	ĔM-brē-ō	_____
endocervicitis (239)	ĕn-dō-sĕr-vĭs-SĪ-tĭs	_____
endometritis (243)	ēn-dō-mē-TRĪ-tis	_____
endometrium (237)	ĕn-dō-MĒ-trē-ŭm	_____
episiotomy (239)	ĕ-pĕ-zē-ŎT-ō-mē	_____
estrogen (237)	ĔS-trō-jĕn	_____
fallopian tubes (237)	fă-LŌ-pē-ăn tūbz	_____
fertilization (237)	fĕr-tĭl-ĭ-ZĀ-shŭn	_____
fetus (237)	FĒ-tŭs	_____
fimbriae(237)	FĬM-brē-ē	_____
follicle-stimulating hormone (237)	FŎL-lĭ-k'l STĬM-ū-lā-tĭng HŌR-mōn	_____
galactorrhea (239)	gă-lăk-tō-RĒ-ă	_____
gamete (237)	GĂM-ēt	_____
genitalia (237)	jĕn-ĭ-TĀ-lē-ă	_____
gestation (237)	jĕs-TĀ-shŭn	_____
gonads (237)	GŌ-nădz	_____
graafian follicle (237)	GRĂF-ē-ăn FŎL-lĭ-k'l	_____
gynecomastia (239)	gī-nĕ-kō-MĂS-tē-ă	_____
human chorionic gonadotropin (237)	HŪ-măn kō-rē-ŎN-ĭk gō-nă-dō-TRŌ-pĭn	_____
hymen (237)	HĪ-mĕn	_____
hysterectomy (239)	hĭs-tĕr-ĔK-tō-mē	_____
intrauterine device (244)	ĭn-tră-Ū-tĕ-rĭn dĕ-VĪS	_____
involution (244)	ĭn-vō-LŪ-shŭn	_____

labia (237)	LĀ-bē-ă	_____
lactation (239)	lăk-TĀ-shŭn	_____
lactiferous ducts (237)	lăk-TĬ-fĕ-rŭs dŭkts	_____
lactogenesis (239)	lăk-tō-JĚN-ĕ-sĭs	_____
leukorrhea (242)	loo-kō-RĒ-ă	_____
luteinizing hormone (238)	LŪ-tĕ-nī-zĭng HŎR-mōn	_____
mammary (240)	MĂM-ŏr-ē	_____
mammoplasty (240)	MĂM-ō-plăs-tē	_____
mastectomy (240)	măs-TĒK-tō-mē	_____
mastitis (240)	măs-TĪ-tĭs	_____
menarche (238)	mĕ-NĂR-kē	_____
menometrorrhagia (241)	mĕn-ō-mĕt-rō-RĀ-jă	_____
menopause (238)	MĒN-ō-păwz	_____
menorrhea (242)	mĕn-ō-RĒ-ă	_____
menstruation (238)	mĕn-strū-Ā-shŭn	_____
metrorrhagia (240)	mĕ-trō-RĀ-jă	_____
multigravida (244)	mŭl-tē-GRĂV-ĭ-dă	_____
multipara (244)	mŭl-TĬP-ă-ră	_____
myomectomy (241)	mī-ō-MĚK-tō-mē	_____
myometrium (238)	mī-ō-MĒ-trē-ŭm	_____
neonatal (241)	nē-ō-NĀ-tăl	_____
nullipara (244)	nŭl-LĬP-ă-ră	_____
obstetric (241)	ŏb-STĚT-rĭk	_____
oligomenorrhea (240)	ŏl-ĭ-gō-mĕn-ō-RĒ-ă	_____
oogenesis (241)	ō-ō-JĚN-ĕ-sĭs	_____
oophoritis (241)	ō-ōf-ōr-Ī-tĭs	_____
orifice (238)	ŎR-ĭ-fĭs	_____
ovarian (241)	ō-VĂ-rē-an	_____

ovaries (238)	Ō-vă-rēz	_____
ovulation (238)	ōv-ū-LĀ-shŭn	_____
ovum; ova (238)	Ō-vŭm; Ō-vă	_____
oxytocia (243)	ŏks-ē-TŌ-sē-ă	_____
oxytocin (243)	ŏks-ē-TŌ-sĭn	_____
papilla (238)	pă-PĬL-ă	_____
parturition (238)	păr-tū-RĬSH-ŭn	_____
perimetrium (238)	pĕ-rĭ-MĒ-trē-ŭm	_____
perineorrhaphy (241)	pĕ-rĭ-nē-ŎR-ră-fē	_____
perineum (238)	pĕ-rĭ-NĒ-ŭm	_____
placenta (238)	plă-SĔN-tă	_____
presentation (243)	prē-zĕn-TĀ-shŭn	_____
primigravida (242)	prī-mĭ-GRĂV-ĭ-dă	_____
primiparous (242)	prī-MĬP-ă-rŭs	_____
progesterone (238)	prō-JĔS-tĕ-rōn	_____
pseudocyesis (242)	sū-dō-sī-Ē-sĭs	_____
pyosalpinx (243)	pī-ō-SĂL-pĭnks	_____
retroflexion (244)	rĕ-trō-FLĔK-shŭn	_____
salpingectomy (241)	săl-pĭng-JĔK-tō-mē	_____
salpingitis (248)	săl-pĭng-JĪ-tĭs	_____
uterine tubes (238)	Ū-tĕr-ĭn tūbz	_____
uterus (238)	Ū-tĕr-ŭs	_____
vagina (238)	vă-JĪ-nă	_____
vaginal orifice (241)	vā-jī-năl ŎR-ĭ-fĭs	_____
vaginitis (241)	vă-jĭ-NĪ-tĭs	_____
vulva (238)	VŬL-vă	_____
vulvovaginitis (241)	vŭl-vō-vă-jĭ-NĪ-tĭs	_____

Pathology, Clinical Tests, and Procedures

Term	Pronunciation	Meaning
abortion (254)	ă-BŎR-shŭn	
abruptio placentae (249)	ă-BRŬP-shē-ō plă-SĔN-tē	
Apgar score (250)	ĂP-găr skōr	
aspiration (252)	ăs-pĕ-RĀ-shŭn	
carcinoma in situ (245)	kăr-sĭ-NŌ-mă ĭn SĪ-tū	
carcinoma of the breast (248)	kăr-sĭ-NŌ-mă of the brĕst	
carcinoma of the cervix (245)	kăr-sĭ-NŌ-mă of the SĔR-vĭkz	
carcinoma of the endometrium (245)	kăr-sĭ-NŌ-mă of the ĕn-dō-MĒ-trē-ŭm	
cauterization (252)	kăw-tĕr-ĭ-ZĀ-shŭn	
cervical dysplasia (245)	SĔR-vĭ-kăl dĭs-PLĀ-zē-ă	
cervicitis (245)	sĕr-vĭ-SĪ-tĭs	
cesarean section (254)	sĕ-SĀ-rē-ăn SĔK-shŭn	
Chlamydia (245)	klă-MĬD-ē-ă	
choriocarcinoma (249)	kō-rē-ō-kăr-sĭ-NŌ-mă	
colposcopy (252)	kōl-PŎS-kō-pē	
conization (252)	kō-nĭ-ZĀ-shŭn	
cryocauterization (252)	krī-ō-kăw-tĕr-ĭ-ZĀ-shŭn	
culdocentesis (252)	kŭl-dō-sĕn-TĒ-sĭs	
cystadenocarcinoma (246)	sĭs-tăd-ĕ-nō-kăr-sĭ-NŌ-mă	
cystadenoma (246)	sĭs-tăd-ĕ-NŌ-mă	
dermoid cyst (246)	DĔR-moyd sĭst	
dilatation (252)	dĭ-lă-TĀ-shŭn	
dilation and curettage (252)	dī-LĀ-shŭn and kŭr-ĕ-TĂZH	
ectopic pregnancy (249)	ĕk-TŎP-ĭk PRĔG-năn-sē	
endometriosis (245)	ĕn-dō-mē-trē-Ō-sĭs	

erythroblastosis fetalis (250)	ĕ-rĭth-rō-blăs-TŌ-sĭs fĕ-TĂ-lĭs	_____
exenteration (252)	ĕks-ĕn-tĕ-RĀ-shŭn	_____
fetal monitoring (254)	FĒ-tăl MŎN-ĭ-tĕ-rĭng	_____
fibrocystic (249)	fī-brō-SĬS-tĭk	_____
fibroids (245)	FĪ-broydz	_____
hyaline membrane disease (250)	HĪ-ă-lĭn MĔM-brān dĭ-ZĒZ	_____
hydrocephalus (250)	hī-drō-SĔF-ă-lŭs	_____
hysterosalpingography (251)	hĭs-tĕr-ō-săl-pĭng-ŎG-ră-fē	_____
kernicterus (250)	kĕr-NĬK-tĕr-ŭs	_____
laparoscopy (252)	lă-pă-RŎS-kō-pē	_____
leiomyoma (245)	lī-ō-mī-Ō-mă	_____
mammography (251)	măm-MŎG-ră-fē	_____
ovarian carcinoma (246)	ō-VĂR-ē-an kăr-sĭ-NŌ-mă	_____
ovarian cysts (246)	ō-VĂR-ē-an sĭst	_____
palpation (248)	păl-PĀ-shŭn	_____
Pap smear (251)	Păp smēr	_____
pelvic inflammatory disease (248)	PĔL-vĭk ĭn-FLĂM-mă-tō-rē dĭ-ZĒZ	_____
pelvic ultrasonography (252)	PĔL-vĭk ŭl-tră-sŏn-ŎG-ră-fē	_____
pelvimetry (254)	pĕl-VĬM-ĭ-trē	_____
placenta previa (249)	plă-SĔN-tă PRĒ-vē-ă	_____
preeclampsia (250)	prē-ĕ-KLĂMP-sē-ă	_____
pyloric stenosis (250)	pī-LŎR-ĭk stĕ-NŌ-sĭs	_____
respiratory distress syndrome (250)	RĔS-pĭr-ă-tō-rē dĭs-STRĔS SĬN-drōm	_____
tubal ligation (254)	TŌŌ-băl lī-GĀ-shŭn	_____

XIII. Review Sheet

Write the meanings for each word part in the space provided and test yourself. Check your answers with the information in the chapter or in the Glossary (Medical Terms—English) at the end of the book.

Combining Forms

Combining Form	Meaning	Combining Form	Meaning
amni/o	_____	myom/o	_____
cephal/o	_____	nat/i	_____
cervic/o	_____	obstetr/o	_____
chori/o	_____	olig/o	_____
colp/o	_____	oophor/o	_____
culd/o	_____	ov/o	_____
episi/o	_____	ovari/o	_____
galact/o	_____	ovul/o	_____
gynec/o	_____	perine/o	_____
hyster/o	_____	peritone/o	_____
lact/o	_____	phor/o	_____
mamm/o	_____	py/o	_____
mast/o	_____	salping/o	_____
men/o	_____	uter/o	_____
metr/o	_____	vagin/o	_____
metri/o	_____	vulv/o	_____
my/o	_____		

Suffixes

Suffix	Meaning	Suffix	Meaning
-arche		-ptosis	
-cele		-rrhagia	
-cyesis		-rrhaphy	
-ectasis		-rrhea	
-ectomy		-salpinx	
-flexion		-scopy	
-genesis		-stenosis	
-gravida		-stomy	
-itis		-tocia	
-parous		-tomy	
-pareunia		-tresia	
-plasia		-version	
-plasty			

Prefixes

Prefix	Meaning	Prefix	Meaning
ante-		nulli-	
bi-		oxy-	
dys-		peri-	
endo-		primi-	
in-		pseudo-	
intra-		retro-	
multi-		uni-	

9

Male Reproductive System

This Chapter is divided into the following sections

In this Chapter you will

- Name, locate, and describe the functions of the organs of the male reproductive system;
- Define some abnormal and pathological conditions that affect the male system;
- Differentiate among several types of sexually transmitted diseases;
- Define many combining forms used to describe the structures of this system; and
- Explain various laboratory tests, clinical procedures, and abbreviations that are pertinent to the system.

I. Introduction

The male sex cell, the **spermatozoon** (sperm cell), is microscopic—in volume, only one third the size of a red blood cell, and less than 1/100,000th the size of the female ovum. It is a relatively uncomplicated cell, composed of a head region, which contains nuclear hereditary material (chromosomes), and a tail region, consisting of a **flagellum** (hair-like process) that makes the sperm motile, somewhat resembling a tadpole. The sperm cell contains relatively little food and cytoplasm, for it need live only long enough to travel from its point of release from the male to where the egg cell lies within the female (uterine tube). Only one spermatozoon out of approximately 300 million sperm cells that may be released during a single **ejaculation** (ejection of sperm and fluid from the male urethra) can penetrate a single ovum and produce fertilization of the ovum.

If more than one egg is passing down the uterine tube when sperm are present, multiple fertilizations are possible, and twins, triplets, quadruplets, and so forth may occur. Twins resulting from the fertilization of separate ova by separate sperm cells are called **fraternal twins.** Fraternal twins, developing in utero with separate placentas, can be of the same sex or different sexes and resemble each other no more than ordinary brothers and sisters. Fraternal twinning is hereditary; a gene is carried by the daughters of mothers of twins.

Identical twins are formed from the fertilization of a single egg cell by a single sperm. As the fertilized egg cell divides and forms many cells, it somehow splits and each part continues separately to undergo further division, each producing an embryo. Depending on when the embryo splits (day 1, 2, or 3), the fetuses will share the same gestational sac and/or placenta. Identical twins are always of the same sex and are very similar in form and feature.

The organs of the male reproductive system are designed to produce and release billions of spermatozoa throughout the lifetime of a male from puberty onward. In addition, the male reproductive system secretes a hormone called **testosterone** (-one = hormone). Testosterone is responsible for the production of bodily characteristics of the male (such as beard, pubic hair, voice deepening) and for the proper development of male gonads **(testes)** and accessory organs **(prostate gland** and **seminal vesicles)** that secrete fluids to ensure the lubrication and viability of sperm.

II. Anatomy

Label Figure 9–1 as you study the following description of the anatomy of the male reproductive system.

The male gonads consist of a pair (only one is pictured here) of **testes** (singular: **testis**), also called **testicles** (1), that develop in the abdomen about the level of the kidneys before descending during embryonic development into the **scrotum** (2), a sac enclosing the testes on the outside of the body.

The scrotum, lying between the thighs, exposes the testes to a lower temperature than that of the rest of the body. This lower temperature is necessary for the adequate maturation and development of sperm **(spermatogenesis).** Lying between the anus and the scrotum, at the floor of the pelvic cavity in the male, is the **perineum** (3), which is analogous to the perineal region in the female.

The interior of a testis is composed of a large mass of narrow, coiled tubules called the **seminiferous tubules** (4). These tubules contain cells that manufacture spermatozoa. The seminiferous tubules are the **parenchymal tissue** of the testis, which means that they perform the essential work of the organ (formation of sperm). Other cells in the testis, called **interstitial cells,** manufacture an important male hormone, **testosterone.**

All body organs contain **parenchyma** (parenchymal cells or tissue), which perform the essential functions of the organ. Organs also contain supportive, connective, and framework tissue, such as blood vessels, connective tissues, and sometimes muscle as well. This supportive tissue is called **stroma** (stromal tissue).

As soon as the sperm cells are formed, they move through the seminiferous tubules and are collected in ducts that lead to a large tube at the upper part of each testis. This is the **epididymis** (5). The spermatozoa mature and become motile in the epididymis and are temporarily stored there. The epididymis runs down the length of the testicle (the coiled tube

Kidney

Ureter

Urinary bladder

Pubic bone

(10)

(9)

(6)

(12)

(13)

(7)

(8)

(11)

(3)

(5)

(4)

(1)

(2)

Figure 9–1

Male reproductive system, sagittal view.

is about 16 feet long) and then turns upward again and becomes a narrow, straight tube called the **vas deferens** (6). Figure 9–2 shows the internal structure of a testis and the epididymis. The vas deferens is about 2 feet long and carries the sperm up into the pelvic region, at the level of the urinary bladder, merging with ducts from the **seminal vesicles** (7) to form the **ejaculatory duct** (8) leading toward the urethra. It is the vas deferens that is cut or tied off when a **sterilization** procedure called a **vasectomy** is performed.

The seminal vesicles, two glands (only one is shown in Figure 9–1) located at the base of the bladder, open into the ejaculatory duct as it joins the **urethra** (9). They secrete a thick sugary, yellowish substance that nourishes the sperm cells and forms much of the volume of ejaculated semen. **Semen** is a combination of fluid and spermatozoa (sperm cells account for less than 1 per cent of the semen volume) that is ejected from the body through the urethra. In the male, as opposed to in the female, the genital orifice combines with the urinary (urethral) opening.

At the region where the vas deferens enters the urethra, and almost encircling the upper end of the urethra, is the **prostate gland** (10). The prostate gland secretes a thick fluid that,

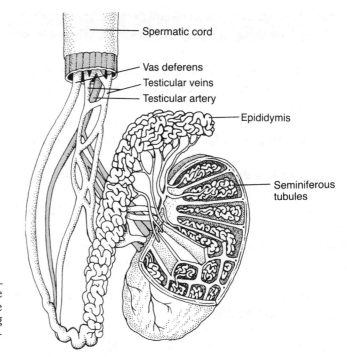

Figure 9–2

The internal structure of a testis and the epididymis. (From Ignatavicius DD, Bayne MV: Medical-Surgical Nursing: A Nursing Process Approach. Philadelphia, WB Saunders, 1991, p 2168.)

as part of semen, aids the motility of the sperm. This gland is also supplied with muscular tissue that aids in the expulsion of sperm during ejaculation. **Cowper's glands (bulbourethral glands)** (11) are just below the prostate gland and also secrete fluid into the urethra.

The urethra passes through the **penis** (12) to the outside of the body. The penis is composed of erectile tissue and at its tip expands to form a soft, sensitive region called the **glans penis** (13). Ordinarily, a fold of skin called the **foreskin (prepuce)** covers the glans penis. Circumcision is the process whereby the foreskin is removed, leaving the glans penis visible at all times.

The flow diagram in Figure 9–3 traces the path of spermatozoa from their formation in the seminiferous tubules of the testes to the outside of the body.

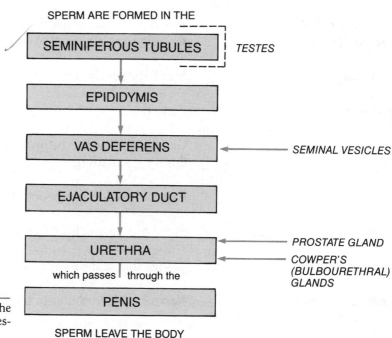

Figure 9–3

The passage of sperm from the seminiferous tubules in the testes to the outside of the body.

III. Vocabulary

This list will help you review many of the new terms introduced in the text. Short definitions will reinforce your understanding of their terms. See Section X of this chapter for help in pronouncing the more difficult terms.

bulbourethral glands	Two exocrine glands near the male urethra.
Cowper's glands	Bulbourethral glands.
ejaculation	Ejection of sperm and fluid from the male urethra.
ejaculatory duct	Tube formed by the union of the vas deferens and the duct of the seminal vesicles, opening into the urethra at the prostate gland.
epididymis (plural: **epididymides**)	Tube located on top of each testis; it carries and stores the sperm cells before they enter the vas deferens. *Didymos* is a Greek word for testis.
flagellum	Hair-like process on a sperm cell that makes it motile (movable).
foreskin	Skin covering the tip of the penis.
fraternal twins	Twins resulting from two separate, concurrent fertilizations.
glans penis	Sensitive tip of the penis.
identical twins	Twins resulting from the separation of one fertilized egg into two distinct embryos.
interstitial cells of the testis	Cells that lie between the seminiferous tubules and produce the hormone testosterone. A pituitary gland hormone (luteinizing hormone [LH]) stimulates the interstitial cells to produce testosterone.
parenchymal tissue (**parenchyma**)	Tissue composed of the essential cells of an organ. In the testes these are the seminiferous tubules that produce sperm.
perineum	Area between the anus and the scrotum in the male.
prepuce	Foreskin.
prostate gland	Gland at the base of the urinary bladder that secretes a fluid into the urethra during ejaculation.
scrotum	External sac (double pouch) that contains the testes.
semen	Spermatozoa and fluid (prostatic and other glandular secretions).
seminal vesicles	Glands that secrete a fluid into the vas deferens.
seminiferous tubules	Narrow, coiled tubules in the testes that produce sperm.

spermatozoon (plural: **spermatozoa**)	Sperm cell.
sterilization	Any procedure rendering an individual incapable of reproduction; vasectomy and salpingectomy are examples.
stroma	Supportive, connective tissue of an organ.
testis (plural: **testes**)	Male gonad that produces spermatozoa and the hormone testosterone; testicle.
testosterone	Hormone secreted by the interstitial tissue of the testes; responsible for male sex characteristics.
vas deferens	Narrow tube that carries sperm from the epididymis into the body and toward the urethra.

IV. Combining Forms and Terminology

Write the meaning of the medical term in the space provided.

Combining Form	Meaning	Terminology	Meaning
andr/o	male	androgen _____	
		Testosterone is an androgen. The testes in males and the adrenal glands in both men and women produce androgens.	
balan/o	glans penis	balanitis _____	
cry/o	cold	cryogenic surgery _____	
		A method used to remove portions of the prostate gland during a transurethral resection of the prostate. See page 287, Section VI, under Clinical Procedures.	
crypt/o	hidden	cryptorchism _____	
		In this congenital condition, one or both testicles remain in the abdominal cavity and have not descended by the time of birth.	
epididym/o	epididymis	epididymitis _____	
gon/o	seed	gonorrhea _____	
		See Sexually Transmitted Diseases, page 286.	

hydr/o	water, fluid	hydrocele _____
		See Pathological Conditions, page 284.
orch/o, orchi/o, orchid/o	testis, testicle (the botanical name for orchid, the flower, is derived from the Greek word *orchis,* meaning testicle; describing the fleshy tubers on the rootstocks of the plant)	orchiectomy _____
		Castration in males.
		anorchism _____
		orchitis _____
		Caused by injury or by mumps (infectious disease of the salivary glands).
prostat/o	prostate gland	prostatitis _____
		Bacterial (E. coli, streptococci) prostatitis is often associated with urethritis and infection of the lower urinary tract.
		prostatectomy _____
semin/i	semen, seed	seminiferous tubules _____
		-ferous means pertaining to bearing or carrying.
		seminal vesicles _____
sperm/o spermat/o	spermatozoa, semen	spermolytic _____
		Noun suffixes ending in -sis, like -lysis, form adjectives by dropping the -sis and adding -tic.
		oligospermia _____
		aspermia _____
		Semen (sperm and fluid) is not formed or emitted.
terat/o	monster	teratoma _____
		A tumor occurring in the testes composed of different types of tissue, such as bone, hair, cartilage, and skin cells. See page 283, Section V under Pathological Conditions (carcinoma of the testes).
test/o	testis, testicle	testicular _____
		The term testis originates from a Latin term meaning witness. In ancient times men would take an oath with one hand on their testes, swearing by their manhood to tell the truth.

varic/o	varicose veins	varicocele _____
		A collection of varicose (swollen, twisted) veins above the testes.
vas/o	vessel, duct (referring to the vas deferens)	vasectomy _____
		See page 287, Section VI, under Clinical Procedures.
zo/o	animal life	azoospermia _____
		No sperm cells are found in the semen.

Suffixes			
Suffix	Meaning	Terminology	Meaning
-genesis	formation	✓spermatogenesis _____	
-one	hormone	testosterone _____	
		ster/o means that this hormone is a type of chemical called a steroid.	
-pexy	fixation, put in place	orchiopexy _____	
		An operation to correct cryptorchism.	
-stomy	new opening	vasovasostomy _____	
		A reversal of vasectomy; the cut ends of the vas deferens are rejoined.	

V. Pathological Conditions; Sexually Transmitted Diseases

Pathological Conditions

Testes

carcinoma of the testes ✓ Malignant tumor of the testicles.

Testicular tumors are rare except in the 15- to 35-year-old age group. The most common tumor is a **seminoma,** which arises from embryonic (also called germ) cells in the testes. Nonseminomatous germ cell tumors are **embryonal carcinoma, teratoma,** and **teratocarcinoma** (combination of embryonal carcinoma and teratoma). Teratomas are composed of tissue such as bone, hair, cartilage, and skin cells (terat/o means monster).

Tumors of the testes are commonly treated with surgery (orchiectomy), radiotherapy, and chemotherapy.

cryptorchism; cryptorchidism ✓ Undescended testicles.

Orchiopexy is performed to bring the testes into the scrotum, if they do not descend on their own before the boy is 2 years old. Undescended testicles put the male at high risk of sterility and testicular cancer.

hydrocele

Sac of clear fluid (-cele means swelling or protrusion) in the scrotum.

Hydroceles may occur as a response to infection or tumors, or they may occur from generalized edema. Often they are idiopathic. They can be differentiated from testicular masses by *transillumination* (shining a light source to the side of a scrotal enlargement). If the hydrocele does not resolve on its own, hydrocelectomy may be necessary. The sac is aspirated via needle and syringe or surgically removed through an incision in the scrotum.

varicocele

Enlarged, swollen veins near the testicle.

This condition is often associated with oligospermia and azoospermia. Oligospermic men with varicoceles and scrotal pain should have a varicocelectomy. In this procedure, the internal spermatic vein is ligated (a segment is cut out and the ends are tied off), leading to a marked increase in fertility. Figure 9–4 shows a hydrocele and a varicocele.

Prostate Gland

carcinoma of the prostate

Malignant tumor of the prostate gland.

This cancer commonly occurs in men who are over 50 years of age. Careful rectal examination by a physician with digital (finger) palpation is a useful method for detection of early prostatic carcinoma (Fig. 9–5). Lymphangiography and computed tomography (CT) scans can detect lymph node metastases. Acid phosphatase (an enzyme) is normally released into the blood in small quantities by the prostate, and elevated levels are found in patients with metastatic disease. Treatment consists of surgery (prostatectomy), radiotherapy, and hormonal chemotherapy. Since prostatic cells need androgens, antiandrogen hormones and estrogens are used to slow tumor growth by depriving the cells of testosterone.

Prostate-specific antigen (PSA) is a protein tumor marker because it is elevated in carcinoma of the prostate.

prostatic hyperplasia

Growth (benign) of nodules (glandular and stromal tissue) within the prostate gland; benign prostatic hyperplasia (BPH).

This condition (which is an increase in numbers of cells) is also called **benign prostatic hypertrophy** because the gland enlarges and overdevelops. However, hyperplasia is the correct pathological term. BPH is a common occurrence in men over 60 years old. Urinary obstruction and inability to empty the bladder completely are symptoms. Figure 9–6 shows the prostate gland with BPH and with carcinoma. Surgical treatment by **transurethral resection (TUR or TURP)** is curative. An endoscope (resectoscope) is passed through the urethra, and prostatic tissue is removed by cauterization (burning) or cryogenic devices.

Penis

epispadias; epispadia

Congenital opening of the male urethra on the upper surface of the penis; -spadia means condition of tearing, cutting, or rending.

hypospadias; hypospadia

Congenital opening of the male urethra on the undersurface of the penis (Fig. 9–7).

Both epispadias and hypospadias can be corrected surgically.

Figure 9–4

Hydrocele and varicocele.

Blood vessels

Vas deferens

Epididymis

Testis

Hydrocele

Dilated spermatic veins (varicocele)

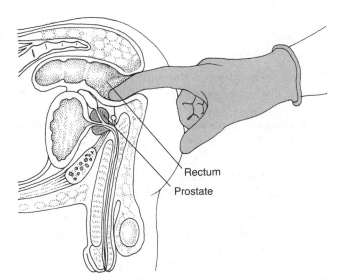

Rectum

Prostate

Figure 9–5

Digital rectal examination of the prostate. (From Ignatavicius DD, Bayne MV: Medical-Surgical Nursing: A Nursing Process Approach. Philadelphia, WB Saunders, 1991, p 1647.)

Figure 9–6

The prostate gland with carcinoma and benign prostatic hyperplasia (BPH). Cancer usually arises around the sides of the gland, whereas BPH occurs in the center of the gland. (Redrawn from Ignatavicius DD, Bayne MV: Medical-Surgical Nursing: A Nursing Process Approach. Philadelphia, WB Saunders, 1991, p 1750.)

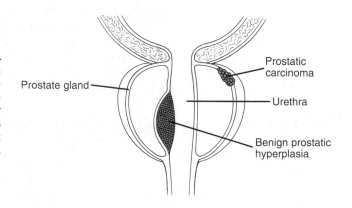

Prostate gland

Prostatic carcinoma

Urethra

Benign prostatic hyperplasia

Figure 9–7

Hypospadias. (From Dorland's Illustrated Medical Dictionary, 27th ed. Philadelphia, WB Saunders, 1988, p 808.)

phimosis

Narrowing of the opening of the foreskin over the glans penis; phim/o means to muzzle.

This condition can interfere with urination and cause secretions to accumulate under the prepuce, leading to infection. Treatment is circumcision (cutting around the prepuce to remove it).

Sexually Transmitted Diseases (STD, Venereal Diseases)

The following conditions, occurring in both men and women, are the most communicable diseases in the world and are transmitted by sexual contact (**vener/o** refers to **sexual intercourse**). AIDS (acquired immuno-deficiency syndrome) is transmitted by sexual contact and is discussed in Chapter 14, under abnormal conditions of the lymphatic and immune systems.

chlamydial infection

Bacteria *(Chlamydia trachomatis)* invade the urethra of men and the vagina and cervix of women.

Within 3 weeks after becoming infected, men may experience dysuria and a white or clear discharge from the penis. The term **nongonococcal urethritis** (NGU) is used to describe this condition in men.

Women may develop a yellowish endocervical discharge, but often the disease is asymptomatic. Treatment with tetracycline (an antibiotic) is curative.

gonorrhea

Inflammation of the genital tract mucous membranes, caused by infection with gonococci (berry-shaped bacteria).

Other areas of the body such as the eye, oral mucosa, rectum, and joints may be affected as well. Symptoms include dysuria and a yellow, muco**purulent** (purulent means pus-filled) discharge from the urethra. The ancient Greeks mistakenly thought that this discharge was a leakage of semen; hence they named the condition **gonorrhea,** meaning discharge of seed (gon/o).

Many women carry the disease asymptomatically, and others have pain, vaginal and urethral discharge, and salpingitis (pelvic inflammatory disease [PID]). As a result of sexual activity, men and women can acquire anorectal and pharyngeal gonococcal infections as well. Chlamydial infection and gonorrhea often occur together. When treating these infections, doctors give antibiotics for both and treat both partners.

herpes genitalis

Infection of the skin and mucosa of the genitals, caused by the herpes simplex virus (HSV).

Most causes of herpes genitalis are caused by HSV type II (although some are caused by HSV I, which is commonly associated with oral infections). Symptoms are reddening of skin with small, fluid-filled blisters and ulcers. Initial episodes can also involve inguinal lymphadenopathy, fever, headache, and malaise. Remissions and relapse periods occur; no drug is known to be effective as a cure. Neonatal herpes is a serious complication that affects infants born to women infected near the time of delivery, and studies suggest that women with herpes genitalis have a higher risk of developing vulval and cervical cancer than do women not infected by HSV II.

syphilis

Chronic infectious disease caused by a spirochete (spiral-shaped bacterium); it can affect any organ of the body.

A **chancre** (hard ulcer) usually appears on the external genitalia a few weeks after bacterial infection. Lymphadenopathy follows as the infection spreads to internal organs. Later stages include damage to the brain, spinal cord, and heart. Syphilis (named after a shepherd in an Italian poem) can be congenital in the fetus if it is transmitted from the mother during pregnancy. Penicillin is the treatment.

trichomoniasis

Infection of the genitourinary tract by *Trichomonas,* a one-celled organism (protozoa).

This condition is more commonly found in women and causes vaginitis, urethritis, and cystitis. Symptoms include a copious, greenish-yellow vaginal discharge. Treatment is administration of metronidazole (Flagyl), and all sexual partners should be examined and treated.

VI. Laboratory Tests, Clinical Procedures, and Abbreviations

Laboratory Tests

semen analysis

This test is done as a part of fertility studies and is also required to establish the effectiveness of vasectomy. The semen specimen is collected in a sterile container and is analyzed microscopically. Sperm cells are counted and examined for motility and shape. Men with fewer than 20 million sperm/ml of semen are usually sterile. Fever or infection of the testes may also cause temporary sterility. In some cases of mumps in adult males, the testes become inflamed and sperm cells deteriorate, resulting in sterility.

Clinical Procedures

castration

Orchiectomy in males, and oophorectomy in females. When a male is castrated before puberty, he becomes a **eunuch.** His sex organs remain childlike and he does not develop secondary sex characteristics.

circumcision

A surgical procedure to remove the prepuce of the penis (Fig. 9–8).

transurethral resection of the prostate (TUR or TURP)

A resectoscope (instrument similar to a cystoscope) is inserted into the urethra, and pieces of the prostate gland are removed by electrocautery (burning) or cryogenic (freezing) techniques (Fig. 9–9).

vasectomy

The vas deferens on each side is cut, a piece is removed, and the free ends are **ligated** (tied) with sutures, **fulgurated** (sealed by means of a high-frequency electric current), or occluded with metal clips. The procedure is done through an incision in the scrotal sac (Fig. 9–10). Vasectomy sterilizes the male, so that sperm are not released with the semen. It does not interfere with nerves or blood vessel supply to the testes or penis, so hormone secretion, sex drive, and **potency** (ability to have an erection) are not impaired. Unexpelled sperm degenerate and are reabsorbed within the epididymis and vas deferens. A small percentage of vasectomies are successfully reversed with vasovasostomy.

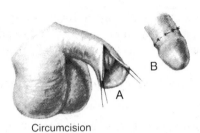

Circumcision

Figure 9–8

Circumcision. *(A)* The prepuce is cut and then removed. *(B)* The wound is sutured (in an adult) after removal of the prepuce. *(A and B,* From Jacob S, Francone CA: Elements of Anatomy and Physiology, 2nd ed. Philadelphia, WB Saunders, 1989, p 283.)

Figure 9–9

Transurethral resection of the prostate (TURP). (From Ignatavicius DD, Bayne MV: Medical-Surgical Nursing: A Nursing Process Approach. Philadelphia, WB Saunders, 1991, p 1746.)

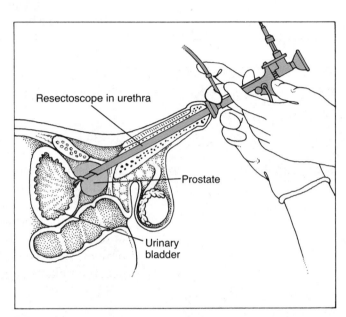

Resectoscope in urethra

Prostate

Urinary bladder

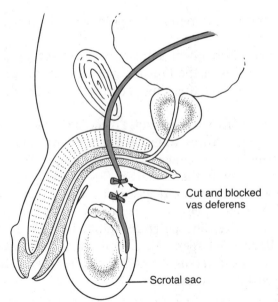

Cut and blocked vas deferens

Scrotal sac

Figure 9–10

Vasectomy.

ABBREVIATIONS

BPH	Benign prostatic hyperplasia	**RPR**	Rapid plasma reagin (test for syphilis)
DRE	Digital rectal examination	**PSA**	Prostate-specific antigen
GU	Genitourinary	**TRUS**	Transrectal ultrasound (test to assess the prostate gland)
HSV	Herpes simplex virus		
NGU	Nongonococcal urethritis	**TUR, TURP**	Transurethral resection of the prostate

VII. Practical Applications

 ### Case Report: A Man with Post-TURP Complaints

The patient is a 70 year-old man who underwent a TURP for BPH 5 years ago and now has severe obstructive urinary symptoms with a large post-void-residual.

On DRE, his prostate was found to be large, bulky, and nodular, with palpable extension to the left seminal vesicle. His PSA level was 120 ng/mL [normal is about 4 ng/mL] and a bone scan was negative. A pelvic sonogram revealed bilateral external iliac adenopathy with lymph nodes measuring 1.5 cm on average [normal lymph node size is less than 1 cm]. A prostatic biopsy revealed a poorly differentiated adenocarcinoma.

This patient most likely has at least stage D1 disease [distant metastases with pelvic lymph node involvement]. Recommendation is hormonal drug treatment to suppress secretion of testosterone, which stimulates prostatic tumor growth.

Questions on the Case Report

Answers are at the end of Answers to Exercises, page 296.

1. Five years previously the patient had which type of surgery?
   (A) Removal of testicles
   (B) Perineal prostatectomy
   (C) Partial prostatectomy (transurethral)
2. What was the reason for the surgery then?
   (A) Cryptorchism
   (B) Benign overgrowth of the prostate gland
   (C) Testicular cancer
3. What symptom does he have now?
   (A) Burning pain on urination
   (B) Urinary retention
   (C) Premature ejaculation
4. What examination allowed the physician to feel the tumor?
   (A) Finger inserted into rectum
   (B) Pelvic sonogram
   (C) Prostate-specific antigen test

5. Where had the tumor spread?
    (A) Pelvic lymph nodes
    (B) Pelvic lymph nodes and left seminal vesicle
    (C) Pelvic bone
6. What is likely to stimulate prostatic adenocarcinoma growth?
    (A) Hormonal drug treatment
    (B) Prostatic biopsy
    (C) Testosterone secretion
7. Stage D1 means that the tumor
    (A) Is localized in the hip area
    (B) Is confined to the prostate gland
    (C) Has spread to lymph nodes and other organs
8. Why is staging of tumors important?
    (A) To classify the extent of spread of the tumor and to plan treatment
    (B) To make the initial diagnosis
    (C) To make an adequate biopsy of the tumor

 FYI: Anabolic Steroids

Anabolic steroids are male hormones (androgens) that increase body weight and muscle size and may be used by doctors to increase growth in boys who do not mature physically as expected for their age. Steroids are also used by athletes in an effort to increase strength and enhance performance. However, there are significant detrimental side effects to their use:

1. High levels of anabolic steroids cause acne, hepatic tumors, and sterility (testicular atrophy and oligospermia).
2. In women, the androgenic effect of anabolic steroids leads to male hair distribution, deepening of voice, amenorrhea, and clitoral enlargement.
3. Anabolic steroid use also causes hypercholesterolemia, hypertension, jaundice (liver abnormalities), and salt and water retention (edema).

VIII. Exercises

Remember to check your answers carefully with those given in Section IX, Answers to Exercises.

A. *Build medical terms.*

1. inflammation of the testes _____

2. inflammation of the tube that carries the spermatozoa to the vas deferens

_____

3. resection of the prostate gland _____

4. inflammation of the prostate gland _____

5. the process of producing (formation of) sperm cells _____

6. fixation of undescended testicle _____

7. inflammation of the glans penis _____

8. condition of scanty sperm _____

9. no sperm or semen is produced _____

10. pertaining to a testicle _____

B. *Give the meanings for the following medical terms.*

1. hypospadias _____

2. parenchyma _____

3. stroma _____

4. cryogenic _____

5. interstitial cells of the testes _____

6. testosterone _____

7. phimosis _____

8. azoospermia _____

9. androgen _____

10. testicular seminoma _____

11. teratocarcinoma _____

C. *Give medical terms for the descriptions below.*

1. tube above each testis; carries and stores sperm _____

2. gland surrounding the urethra at the base of the urinary bladder _____

3. parenchymal tissue of the testes; produces spermatozoa _____

4. sperm cell _____

5. foreskin _____

6. male gonad; produces hormone and sperm cells _____

7. pair of sacs; secrete fluid into ejaculatory ducts _____

8. sac on outside of the body enclosing the testes _____

9. tube carrying sperm from the epididymis into the body toward the urethra

_____

10. pair of glands near the urethra; secrete fluid into the urethra; Cowper's glands

_____

D. Match the term in column I with the letter of its meaning in column II.

Column I

1. castration   _____

2. semen analysis   _____

3. ejaculation   _____

4. purulent   _____

5. vasectomy   _____

6. circumcision   _____

7. ligation   _____

8. cryosurgery   _____

Column II

A. to tie off or bind
B. removal of a piece of the vas deferens
C. orchiectomy
D. removal of the prepuce
E. destruction of tissue by freezing
F. pus-filled
G. test of fertility (reproductive ability)
H. ejection of sperm and fluid from the urethra

E. Give medical terms for the following abnormal conditions.

1. prostatic enlargement, nonmalignant _____

2. opening of the urethra on the undersurface of the penis _____

3. sexually transmitted disease; infection with herpes virus _____

4. malignant tumor of the prostate gland _____

5. enlarged, swollen veins near the testes _____

6. sexually transmitted disease; primary stage marked by chancre _____

7. malignant tumor of the testes (three types) _____ ,

_____ , _____

8. venereal disease (etiologic agent is berry-shaped bacteria) marked by inflammation of genital mucosa

and mucopurulent discharge _____

9. venereal disease caused by infection with Trichomonas _____

10. undescended testicles _____

11. sac of clear fluid in the scrotum _____

F. *Give the meanings for the following abbreviations.*

1. PSA _____

2. TURP _____

3. GU _____

4. D & C _____

5. BPH _____

6. NGU _____

G. *Review exercise. Give the meaning of the following.*

1. -stasis _____   11. -ectasis _____

2. -sclerosis _____   12. -centesis _____

3. -stenosis _____   13. -genesis _____

4. -cele _____   14. balan/o _____

5. -rrhagia _____   15. oophor/o _____

6. -ptosis _____   16. salping/o _____

7. -plasia _____   17. hyster/o _____

8. -phagia _____   18. metr/o _____

9. -rrhaphy _____   19. colp/o _____

10. -pexy _____   20. mast/o _____

H. Match the following surgical procedures with the reasons they would be performed.

hydrocelectomy   vasectomy   varicocelectomy
orchiopexy   vasovasostomy   circumcision
bilateral orchiectomy   radical (complete)
TURP   prostatectomy

1. carcinoma of the prostate gland _____

2. cryptorchism _____

3. sterilization (hormones remain and potency is not impaired) _____

4. benign prostatic hyperplasia _____

5. abnormal collection of fluid in a scrotal sac _____

6. reversal of sterilization procedure _____

7. teratocarcinoma of the testes _____

8. phimosis _____

9. swollen, twisted veins above the testes _____

I. Give the following medical terms from their meanings and partial spelling. Check your answers carefully.

1. gland at the base of the urinary bladder in males: pro _____ gland

2. coiled tube on top of each testis: epi _____

3. the essential cells of an organ: par _____

4. the foreskin: pre _____

5. genus of bacteria that is the major cause of nongonococcal urethritis in males and cervicitis in females:

   Ch _____

6. the ulcer that forms on genital organs after infection with syphilis: ch _____

7. androgen that is produced by the interstitial cells of the testis: test _____

8. fluid secreted by male reproductive gland and ejaculated with sperm: se _____

J. Circle the correct terminology to complete the following sentences.

1. Fred's doctors could only feel one testicle shortly after his birth and suggested close following of his condition of (**gonorrhea, cryptorchism, prostatic hyperplasia**).

2. Bob had many sexual partners, one of whom had been diagnosed with (**testosterone, phimosis, chlamydial infection**), a highly infectious STD.

3. At age 65, Mike had some difficulty with urgency and discomfort when urinating. His doctor did a digital rectal examination to examine his (**prostate gland, urinary bladder, vas deferens**).

4. Just after his birth, Nick's parents had a difficult time deciding whether to have the boy undergo (**TURP, castration, circumcision**).

5. Ted noticed a hard ulcer called a (**eunuch, chancre, trichomoniasis**) on his penis and made an appointment with his doctor, who is a (**gastroenterologist, gynecologist, urologist**). The doctor viewed a specimen of the ulcer under the microscope and did a blood test, which revealed that Bill had contracted (**gonorrhea, herpes genitalia, syphilis**).

IX. Answers to Exercises

A
1. orchitis
2. epididymitis
3. prostatectomy
4. prostatitis
5. spermatogenesis
6. orchiopexy
7. balanitis
8. oligospermia
9. aspermia
10. testicular

B
1. Congenital anomaly in which the urethra opens on the underside of the penis.
2. The distinctive, essential tissue or cells of an organ, as for example, glomeruli and tubules of the kidney, seminiferous tubules of the testis.
3. The supportive and connective tissue of an organ.
4. Pertaining to producing cold or low temperatures.
5. The cells that produce the hormone testosterone. These cells are stimulated by luteinizing hormone from the pituitary gland.
6. A hormone made by the interstitial cells of the testes; responsible for secondary sex characteristics.
7. A narrowing, or stenosis, of the foreskin on the glans penis.
8. Lack of spermatozoa in the semen.
9. Hormone producing male characteristics.
10. Malignant tumor of the testes composed of germ or embryonic cells.
11. Malignant tumor of testes (composed of embryonic tissue forming bone, hair, skin, cartilage).

C
1. epididymis
2. prostate gland
3. seminiferous tubules (semin = semen, fer = to carry)
4. spermatozoon
5. prepuce
6. testis; testicle
7. seminal vesicles
8. scrotum; scrotal sac
9. vas deferens
10. bulbourethral glands

D
1. C
2. G
3. H
4. F
5. B
6. D
7. A
8. E

E
1. benign prostatic hyperplasia (hypertrophy)
2. hypospadias
3. herpes genitalia
4. adenocarcinoma of the prostate
5. varicocele
6. syphilis
7. embryonal carcinoma; seminoma; teratoma or teratocarcinoma
8. gonorrhea
9. trichomoniasis
10. cryptorchism
11. hydrocele

F
1. prostate-specific antigen
2. transurethral resection of the prostate gland
3. genitourinary
4. dilation and curettage
5. benign prostatic hyperplasia (hypertrophy)
6. nongonococcal urethritis

G
1. stopping, controlling
2. hardening
3. narrowing
4. hernia, swelling
5. hemorrhage
6. prolapse
7. formation
8. eating, swallowing
9. suture
10. fixation
11. widening
12. surgical puncture to remove fluid
13. producing
14. penis
15. ovary
16. uterine tube; fallopian tube; oviduct
17. uterus
18. uterus
19. vagina
20. breast

H
1. radical (complete) prostatectomy
2. orchiopexy
3. vasectomy
4. TURP
5. hydrocelectomy
6. vasovasostomy
7. bilateral orchiectomy
8. circumcision
9. varicocelectomy

I
1. prostate
2. epididymis
3. parenchyma
4. prepuce
5. Chlamydia
6. chancre
7. testosterone
8. semen

J
1. cryptorchism
2. chlamydial infection
3. prostate gland
4. circumcision
5. chancre; urologist; syphilis

Answers to Practical Applications

1. C
2. B
3. B
4. A
5. B
6. C
7. C
8. A

X. Pronunciation of Terms

To test your understanding of the terminology in this chapter, write the meaning of each term in the space provided. In addition, you may wish to cover the terms and write them by looking at your definitions. Make sure your spelling is correct. The page number after each term indicates where it is defined or used in the text so you can easily check your responses. (If you are not sure what the pronunciation symbols mean, refer to page 21.)

Term	Pronunciation	Meaning
androgen (281)	ĂN-drō-jĕn	_____
anorchism (282)	ăn-ŎR-kĭzm	_____
aspermia (282)	ā-SPĔR-mē-ă	_____
azoospermia (283)	ā-zō-ō-SPĔR-mē-ă	_____
balanitis (281)	băl-ă-NĪ-tĭs	_____
bulbourethral gland (280)	bŭl-bō-ū-RĒ-thrăl glănd	_____
castration (287)	kăs-TRĀ-shŭn	_____
chancre (286)	SHĂNG-kĕr	_____
chlamydial infection (286)	klă-MĬD-ē-al in-FĔK-shŭn	_____
circumcision (287)	sĕr-kŭm-SĬZH-ŭn	_____
cryogenic surgery (281)	krī-ō-GĔN-ik SŬR-jĕr-ē	_____
cryptorchism (281)	krĭp-TŎR-kĭzm	_____

ejaculation (280)	ē-jăk-ū-LĀ-shŭn	_____
embryonal carcinoma (283)	ĕm-brē-ŎN-ăl kăr-sĭ-NŌ-mă	_____
epididymis (280)	ĕp-ĭ-DĬD-ĭ-mĭs	_____
epididymitis (281)	ĕp-ĭ-dĭd-ĭ-MĪ-tĭs	_____
epispadias (284)	ĕp-ĭ-SPĀ-dē-ăs	_____
eunuch (287)	Ū-nŭk	_____
flagellum (280)	flă-JĔL-ŭm	_____
gonorrhea (281)	gŏn-ō-RĒ-ă	_____
herpes genitalis (286)	HĔR-pēz jĕn-ĭ-TĂL-ĭs	_____
hydrocele (284)	HĪ-drō-sēl	_____
hypospadias (284)	hī-pō-SPĀ-dē-ăs	_____
interstitial cells (280)	ĭn-tĕr-STĬSH-ăl sĕlz	_____
oligospermia (282)	ŏl-ĭ-gō-SPĔR-mē-ă	_____
orchiectomy (282)	ŏr-kē-ĔK-tō-mē	_____
orchiopexy (283)	ŏr-kē-ō-PĔK-sē	_____
orchitis (282)	ŏr-KĪ-tĭs	_____
parenchymal tissue (280)	pă-RĔNG-kĭ-măl TĬSH-ū	_____
perineum (280)	pĕr-ĭ-NĒ-ŭm	_____
phimosis (286)	fi-MŌ-sĭs	_____
prepuce (280)	PRĒ-pŭs	_____
prostatectomy (282)	prŏs-tă-TĔK-tō-mē	_____
prostate gland (280)	PRŎS-tāt glănd	_____
prostatic hyperplasia (284)	prŏs-TĂT-ĭk hĭ-pĕr-PLĀ-zē-ă	_____
prostatitis (282)	prŏs-tă-TĪ-tĭs	_____
purulent (286)	PŪR-ū-lent	_____
scrotum (280)	SKRŌ-tŭm	_____
semen (280)	SĒ-mĕn	_____
seminal vesicles (280)	SĔM-ĭn-ăl VĔS-ĭ-k'lz	_____

seminiferous tubules (280)	sĕ-mĭ-NĬF-ĕr-ŭs TŪB-ūlz	_____
seminoma (283)	sĕ-mĭ-NŌ-mă	_____
spermatogenesis (283)	spĕr-mă-tō-JĔN-ĕ-sĭs	_____
spermatozoa (281)	spĕr-mă-tō-ZŌ-ă	_____
spermatozoon (281)	spĕr-mă-tō-ZŌ-ōn	_____
spermolytic (282)	spĕr-mō-LĬT-ĭk	_____
sterilization (281)	stĕr-ĭ-lĭ-ZĀ-shŭn	_____
stroma (281)	STRŌ-mă	_____
syphilis (286)	SĬF-ĭ-lĭs	_____
teratoma (282)	tĕr-ă-TŌ-mă	_____
testicular (282)	tĕs-TĬK-ŭ-lăr	_____
testis (281)	TĔS-tĭs	_____
testosterone (281)	tĕs-TŎS-tĕ-rōn	_____
trichomoniasis (287)	trĭk-ō-mō-NĪ-ă-sĭs	_____
varicocele (283)	VĂR-ĭ-kō-sēl	_____
vas deferens (281)	văs DĔF-ĕr-ĕnz	_____
vasectomy (283)	vă-SĔK-tō-mē	_____
vasovasostomy (283)	vă-zō-vă-ZŎS-tō-mē	_____
venereal (286)	vĕ-NĒ-rē-ăl	_____

XI. Review Sheet

Write the meanings for each word part in the space provided. Check your answers with the information in the chapter or in the Glossary (Medical Terms—English) at the end of the book.

Combining Forms

Combining Form	Meaning	Combining Form	Meaning
andr/o	_____	prostat/o	_____
balan/o	_____	semin/o	_____
cry/o	_____	sperm/o	_____
crypt/o	_____	spermat/o	_____
epididym/o	_____	terat/o	_____
gon/o	_____	test/o	_____
hydr/o	_____	varic/o	_____
orchid/o	_____	vas/o	_____
orchi/o	_____	vener/o	_____
orch/o	_____	zo/o	_____

Suffixes

Suffix	Meaning	Suffix	Meaning
-cele	_____	-one	_____
-ectomy	_____	-pexy	_____
-gen	_____	-plasia	_____
-genesis	_____	-rrhea	_____
-genic	_____	-stomy	_____
-lysis	_____	-tomy	_____
-lytic	_____	-trophy	_____

10

Nervous System

This Chapter is divided into the following sections

In this Chapter you will

- Name, locate, and describe the functions of the major organs and parts of the nervous system;
- Recognize nervous system combining forms and make terms using them with new and familiar suffixes;
- Define several pathological conditions affecting the nervous system; and
- Describe some laboratory tests, clinical procedures, and abbreviations that pertain to the system.

I. Introduction

The nervous system is one of the most complex of all human body systems. More than 10 billion nerve cells are operating constantly all over the body to coordinate the activities we do consciously and voluntarily, as well as those that occur unconsciously or involuntarily. We speak, we move muscles, we hear, we taste, we see, we think, our glands secrete hormones, we respond to danger, pain, temperature, touch, we have memory, association, discrimination—all of these functions compose only a small number of the many activities controlled by our nervous system.

Microscopic **nerve cells** collected into macroscopic bundles called **nerves** carry electrical messages all over the body. External stimuli, as well as internal chemicals such as **acetylcholine,** activate the cell membranes of nerve cells in order to release stored electrical energy within the cells. This energy, when released and passed through the length of the nerve cell, is called the **nervous impulse.** External **receptors,** like sense organs, as well as internal receptors in muscles and blood vessels receive and transmit these impulses to the complex network of nerve cells in the brain and spinal cord. Within this central part of the nervous system, impulses are recognized, interpreted, and finally relayed to other nerve cells that extend out to all parts of the body, such as muscles, glands, and internal organs.

II. General Structure of the Nervous System

The nervous system can be classified into two major divisions: the **central nervous system (CNS)** and the **peripheral nervous system.** The central nervous system consists of the **brain** and **spinal cord.** The peripheral nervous system consists of 12 pairs of **cranial nerves** and 31 pairs of **spinal nerves.** The cranial nerves carry impulses between the brain and the head and neck. The one exception is the tenth cranial nerve, called the vagus nerve. It carries messages to and from the chest and abdomen, as well as the head and neck regions. Table 10–1 lists the cranial nerves and the parts of the body they affect. The spinal nerves carry messages between the spinal cord and the chest, abdomen, and extremities.

In addition to the spinal and cranial nerves (whose functions are mainly voluntary and involved with sensations of smell, taste, sight, hearing, and muscle movements), the peripheral nervous system consists of a large group of nerves that function involuntarily or automatically without conscious control. These peripheral nerves are those of the **autonomic**

Table 10–1. CRANIAL NERVES AND THEIR FUNCTIONS

A nerve is sensory when it carries messages toward the brain from sense organs and motor when it carries messages from the brain to muscles and internal organs. Mixed nerves carry both sensory and motor fibers.

Cranial Nerve	Function
I. Olfactory (sensory)	Smell
II. Optic (sensory)	Vision
III. Oculomotor (motor)	Eye movement
IV. Trochlear (motor)	Eye movement
V. Trigeminal	
Ophthalmic (sensory)	Face and scalp sensation
Maxillary (sensory)	Mouth and nose sensation
Mandibular (mixed)	Chewing
VI. Abducens (motor)	Eye movement
VII. Facial (mixed)	Face and scalp movement
	Tongue taste sensation
	Ear pain and temperature
VIII. Vestibulocochlear (sensory)	Hearing and equilibrium
IX. Glossopharyngeal (mixed)	Ear pain and temperature
	Tongue and throat sensations
	Throat movement
X. Vagus (mixed)	Throat, voice box, chest, abdominal sensations
	Voice box and throat movement
	Chest and abdominal viscera movement
XI. Accessory (motor)	Neck and back movement
XII. Hypoglossal (motor)	Tongue movement

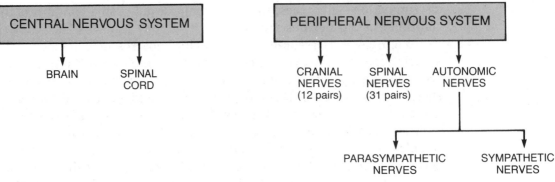

Figure 10–1

Divisions of the central and peripheral nervous systems.

nervous system. This system of nerve fibers carries impulses *from* the central nervous system to the glands, heart, blood vessels, and the involuntary muscles found in the walls of tubes like the intestines and hollow organs like the stomach and urinary bladder. These nerves are called **efferent,** since they carry (-ferent) impulses away from (ef-) the central nervous system.

Some of the autonomic nerves are called **sympathetic** nerves and others are called **parasympathetic** nerves. The sympathetic nerves stimulate the body in times of stress and crisis; that is, they increase heart rate and forcefulness, dilate (relax) airways so more oxygen can enter, increase blood pressure, stimulate the adrenal glands to secrete epinephrine (adrenaline), and inhibit intestinal contractions so that digestion is slower. The parasympathetic nerves normally act as a balance for the sympathetic nerves. Parasympathetic nerves slow down heart rate, contract the pupils of the eye, lower blood pressure, stimulate peristalsis to clear the rectum, and increase the quantity of secretions like saliva.

A **plexus** is a large network of nerves in the peripheral nervous system. The cervical, lumbar, sacral, and coccygeal plexuses are examples.

Figure 10–1 summarizes the divisions of the central and peripheral nervous systems.

III. Neurons, Nerves, and Neuroglia

A **neuron** is an individual nerve cell, a microscopic structure. Impulses are passed along the parts of a nerve cell in a definite manner and direction. The parts of a neuron are pictured in Figure 10–2; label it as you study the following.

A **stimulus** begins a wave of excitability in the receptive branching fibers of the neuron, which are called **dendrites** (1). A change in the electrical charge of the dendrite membranes is thus begun, and the nervous impulse wave moves along the dendrites like the movement of falling dominoes. The impulse, traveling in only one direction, next reaches the **cell body** (2), which contains the **cell nucleus** (3). Extending from the cell body is the **axon** (4), which carries the impulse away from the cell body. Axons are covered with a fatty tissue called a **myelin sheath** (5). The myelin sheath gives a white appearance to the nerve fiber; hence the term white matter, as in parts of the spinal cord, white matter of the brain, and most peripheral nerves. The gray matter of the brain and spinal cord refers to the collections of cell bodies and dendrites that appear gray because they are not covered by a myelin sheath.

Another axon covering, called the **neurilemma,** is a membranous sheath outside the myelin sheath on the nerve cells of peripheral nerves. The nervous impulse passes through the axon to leave the cell via the **terminal end fibers** (6) of the neuron. The space where the nervous impulse jumps from one neuron to another is called the **synapse** (7). The transfer of the impulse across the synapse depends upon the release of a chemical substance, called a

neurotransmitter, by the neuron that brings the impulse to the synapse. Tiny sacs containing the neurotransmitter are located at the ends of neurons, and they release the neurotransmitter into the synapse. Acetylcholine, epinephrine (adrenaline), and dopamine are examples of neurotransmitters.

Whereas a neuron is a microscopic structure within the nervous system, a **nerve** is macroscopic, able to be seen with the naked eye. A nerve consists of a bundle of dendrites and axons that travel together like strands of rope. Peripheral nerves that carry impulses to the brain and spinal cord from stimulus receptors like the skin, eye, ear, and nose are called **afferent (sensory) nerves;** those that carry impulses *from* the CNS to organs that produce responses, for example, muscles and glands, are called **efferent (motor) nerves.**

Neurons and nerves are the parenchymal tissue of the nervous system; that is, they do the essential work of the system by conducting impulses throughout the body. The stromal tissue of the nervous system consists of other cells called **neuroglia.** Neuroglial cells are supportive and connective in function, as well as phagocytic, and are able to help the nervous system ward off infection and injury. Neuroglial cells do not transmit impulses.

There are three types of neuroglial cells. **Astrocytes (astroglia),** as their name suggests, are star-like and are believed to be responsible for transporting water and salts between

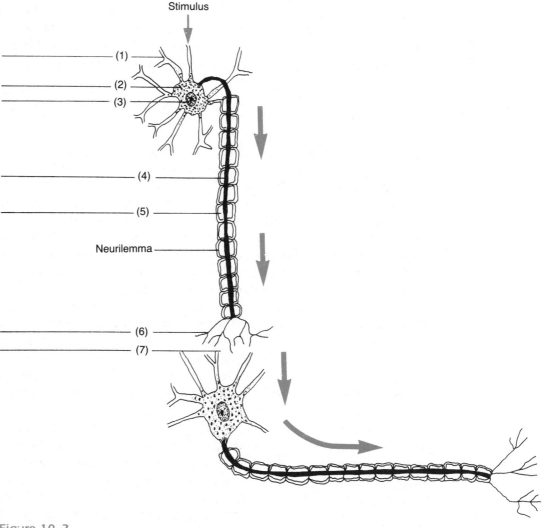

Figure 10–2

Parts of a neuron and the pathway of a nervous impulse.

Astrocyte   Oligodendroglia   Microglia

Figure 10–3

Neuroglial cells—the supporting and connective cells of the nervous system.

capillaries and nerve cells. **Microglial cells (microglia)** are very small and have many branching processes. These cells are phagocytes. **Oligodendroglia,** as their name implies, possess few dendrites. They are responsible for the production of myelin that covers nerve fibers in the central nervous system. They are also associated with blood vessels and can help regulate the passage of potentially harmful substances from the blood into the nerve cells of the brain. This protective barrier between the blood and the brain cells is called the **blood-brain barrier.** Figure 10–3 pictures the different kinds of neuroglia.

IV. The Brain

The brain is the primary center for regulating and coordinating body activities. In the human adult, it weighs about 3 pounds and has many different parts, all of which control different aspects of body functions.

The largest part of the brain is the **cerebrum.** The outer nervous tissue of the cerebrum, known as the **cerebral cortex,** is arranged in folds to form elevated portions known as **convolutions** (also called **gyri**) and depressions or grooves known as **fissures** (also called **sulci**). The **cerebral hemispheres** are the paired halves of the cerebrum. Each hemisphere is subdivided into four major lobes named for the cranial (skull) bones that overlie them. Figure 10–4 shows these areas as well as the gyri and sulci.

The cerebrum has many functions. All thought, judgment, memory, association, and discrimination take place within it. In addition, sensory impulses are received through afferent cranial nerves and when registered in the cortex are the basis for perception. Efferent cranial nerves carry motor impulses from the cerebrum to muscles and glands, and these produce movement and activity. Figure 10–5 shows the location of some of the centers in the cerebral cortex that control speech, vision, smell, movement, hearing, thought processes, and so forth.

Within the middle region of the cerebrum are spaces, or canals, called **ventricles** (pictured in Fig. 10–6). They contain a watery fluid that flows throughout the brain and around the spinal cord. This fluid is called **cerebrospinal fluid (CSF)** and protects the brain and spinal cord from shock as might a cushion. CSF is usually clear and colorless and contains lymphocytes, sugar, chlorides, and protein. Spinal fluid can be withdrawn for diagnosis or relief of pressure on the brain; this is called a **spinal puncture** or **lumbar puncture (LP).** A hollow needle is inserted in the lumbar region of the spinal column below the region where the nervous tissue of the spinal cord ends, and fluid is withdrawn.

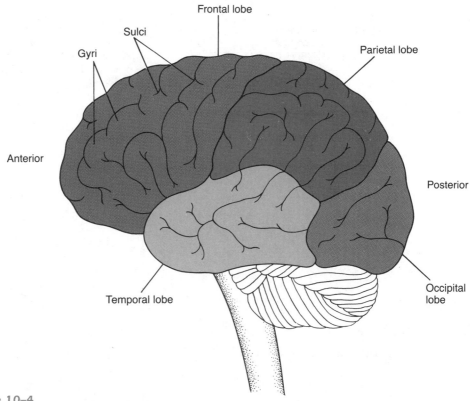

Figure 10–4

Lobes of the cerebrum; gyri (convolutions) and sulci (fissures). This is a lateral view of the left cerebral hemisphere.

Figure 10–5

Some of the functional areas of the cerebral cortex. (From Chabner DE: Medical Terminology: A Short Course. Philadelphia, WB Saunders, 1990.)

Figure 10–6

Circulation of cerebrospinal fluid in brain and spinal cord.

Two other important parts of the brain, the **thalamus** and **hypothalamus,** are below the cerebrum (Fig. 10–7). The thalamus is a large mass of gray matter that acts as a relay center for impulses that travel from receptors such as the eye, ear, and skin to the cerebrum. The thalamus integrates and monitors these sensory impulses, suppressing some and magnifying others. Perception of pain is controlled by this area of the brain. The hypothalamus (below

Figure 10–7

Parts of the brain: cerebrum, thalamus, hypothalamus, cerebellum, pons, and medulla oblongata. Note the location of the pituitary gland below the hypothalamus. The corpus callosum is a mass of tissue in the center of the brain, connecting the two hemispheres.

Table 10–2. FUNCTIONS OF THE PARTS OF THE BRAIN

Part of the Brain	Functions
Cerebrum	Thinking, reasoning, sensations, movements, memory
Thalamus	Relay station for body sensations; pain
Hypothalamus	Body temperature, sleep, appetite, emotions, control of the pituitary gland
Cerebellum	Coordination of voluntary movements
Pons	Connection of nerve fiber tracts
Medulla oblongata	Nerve fibers cross over, left to right and right to left; contains centers to regulate heart, blood vessels, and respiratory system

the thalamus) contains neurons that control body temperature, sleep, appetite, sexual desire, and emotions such as fear and pleasure. The hypothalamus also regulates the release of hormones from the pituitary gland at the base of the brain and integrates the activities of the sympathetic and parasympathetic nervous systems.

The following structures within the brain lie below the posterior portion of the cerebrum and connect the cerebrum with the spinal cord; the cerebellum, pons, and medulla oblongata. The pons and medulla are part of the **brain stem.**

The **cerebellum** is located beneath the posterior part of the cerebrum. Its function is to aid in the coordination of voluntary movements and to maintain balance, posture, and muscular tone.

The **pons** is a part of the brain that literally means bridge. It contains nerve fiber tracts that connect the cerebellum and cerebrum with the rest of the brain.

The **medulla oblongata,** located at the base of the brain, connects the spinal cord with the rest of the brain. Nerve tracts cross over in the medulla oblongata. For example, nerve cells that control the movement of the left side of the body are found in the right half of the cerebrum. These cells send out axons that cross over (decussate) to the opposite side of the brain in the medulla oblongata and then travel down the spinal cord.

In addition, the medulla oblongata contains important vital centers that regulate internal activities of the body. These are:

1. Respiratory center, which controls muscles of respiration in response to chemicals or other stimuli;

2. Cardiac center, which slows the heart rate when the heart is beating too rapidly; and

3. Vasomotor center, which affects (constricts or dilates) the muscles in the walls of blood vessels, thus influencing blood pressure.

Figure 10–7 shows the locations of the thalamus, hypothalamus, cerebellum, pons, and medulla oblongata. Table 10–2 reviews the functions of the parts of the brain.

V. The Spinal Cord and Meninges

Spinal Cord

The **spinal cord** is a column of nervous tissue extending from the medulla oblongata to the second lumbar vertebra within the vertebral column. It ends as the **cauda equina** (horse's tail), a fan of nerve fibers found below the second lumbar vertebra of the spinal column (Fig. 10–8). It carries all the nerves that affect the limbs and lower part of the body, and it is the pathway for impulses going to and from the brain. A cross section of the spinal cord (Fig. 10–9) reveals an inner section of **gray matter** (containing cell bodies and dendrites of peripheral nerves) and an outer region of **white matter** (containing the nerve fiber tracts with myelin sheaths) conducting impulses to and from the brain.

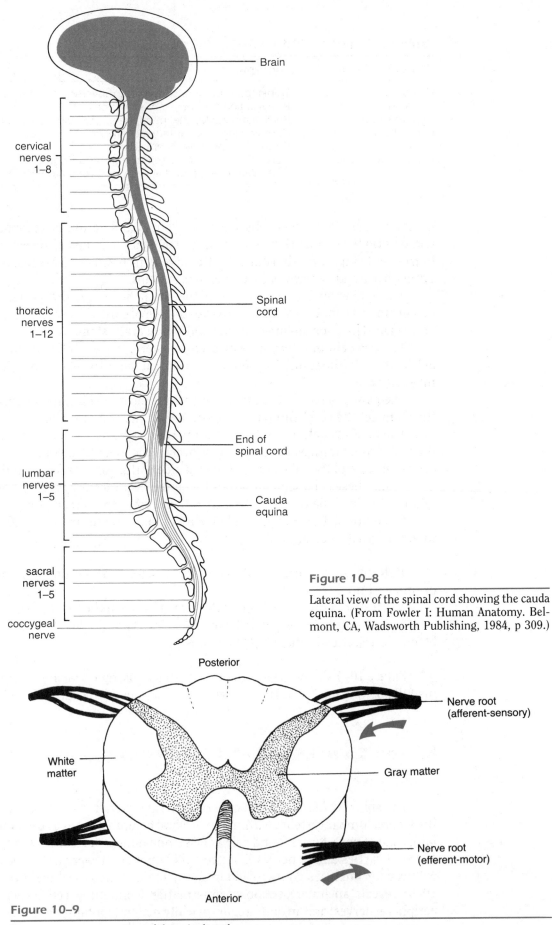

Brain

cervical
nerves
1–8

Spinal
cord

thoracic
nerves
1–12

lumbar
nerves
1–5

End of
spinal cord

Cauda
equina

sacral
nerves
1–5

coccygeal
nerve

Figure 10–8

Lateral view of the spinal cord showing the cauda equina. (From Fowler I: Human Anatomy. Belmont, CA, Wadsworth Publishing, 1984, p 309.)

Posterior

Nerve root
(afferent-sensory)

White
matter

Gray matter

Nerve root
(efferent-motor)

Anterior

Figure 10–9

Transverse or cross section of the spinal cord.

Figure 10–10

The layers of the meninges, frontal view.

Meninges

The **meninges** are three layers of connective tissue membranes that surround the brain and spinal cord. Label Figure 10–10 as you study the following description of the meninges.

The outermost membrane of the meninges is called the **dura mater** (1). It is a thick and tough membrane and contains channels for blood to come into the brain tissue. The **subdural space** (2) is a space below the dura membrane and contains many blood vessels. The second layer around the brain and spinal cord is called the **arachnoid membrane** (3). The arachnoid (spider-like) membrane is loosely attached to the other meninges by web-like fibers so there is a space for fluid between the fibers and the third membrane. This space is called the **subarachnoid space** (4), and it contains the CSF. The third layer of the meninges, closest to the brain and spinal cord, is called the **pia mater** (5). It is made of delicate (pia) connective tissue with a rich supply of blood vessels.

VI. Vocabulary

This list will help you review many of the new terms introduced in the text. Short definitions will reinforce your understanding of the terms. See Section XIII of this chapter for help in pronouncing the more difficult terms.

acetylcholine   Neurotransmitter chemical released at the ends of some nerve cells.

afferent nerves   Nerves that carry impulses *toward* (af- means toward) the brain and spinal cord; sensory nerves.

arachnoid membrane	Middle layer of the three membranes (meninges) that surround the brain and spinal cord; means "spider-like."
astrocyte	A type of neuroglial cell; connective, supporting cell of the nervous system. Astrocytes transport water and salts between capillaries and nerve cells.
autonomic nervous system	Nerves that control involuntary body functions; automatically carry impulses from the brain and spinal cord to muscles, glands, and internal organs.
axon	Microscopic fiber that carries the nervous impulse along a nerve cell.
blood-brain barrier	Blood vessels (capillaries) that selectively let certain substances enter the brain tissue and keep other substances out.
brain stem	Lower portion of the brain that connects the cerebrum with the spinal cord. The pons and medulla oblongata are part of the brain stem.
cauda equina	Horse's tail—a collection of spinal nerves below the end of the spinal cord at the level of the second lumbar vertebra.
cell body	Part of a nerve cell that contains the nucleus.
central nervous system (CNS)	The brain and the spinal cord.
cerebellum	Posterior part of the brain. It is responsible for coordinating voluntary muscle movements and maintaining balance.
cerebral cortex	Outer region of the cerebrum; also called the gray matter of the brain.
cerebrospinal fluid (CSF)	Liquid that circulates throughout the brain and spinal cord.
cerebrum	Largest part of the brain; responsible for voluntary muscular activity, vision, speech, taste, hearing, thought, memory, and many other functions.
convolution	Elevated portion of the cerebral cortex; gyrus.
dendrite	Microscopic branching fiber of a nerve cell that is the first part to receive the nervous impulse.
dura mater	Outermost layer of the meninges surrounding the brain and spinal cord; from the Latin, meaning hard mother.
efferent nerves	Nerves that carry impulses away from the brain and spinal cord to the muscles, glands, and organs; motor nerves.
fissure	Depression, or groove, in the surface of the cerebral cortex; sulcus.
gyrus (plural: **gyri**)	Elevation in the surface of the cerebral cortex; convolution.
hypothalamus	Portion of the brain beneath the thalamus; controls sleep, appetite, body temperature, and the secretions from the pituitary gland.

medulla oblongata	Part of the brain just above the spinal cord; controls breathing, heartbeat, and the size of blood vessels; nerve fibers cross over here.
meninges	Three protective membranes that surround the brain and spinal cord.
microglial cell	One type of neuroglial cell.
motor nerves	Nerves (controlling motion) that carry messages away from the brain and spinal cord to muscles and organs.
myelin sheath	Fatty tissue that surrounds and protects the axon of a nerve cell.
nerve	Macroscopic structure consisting of axons and dendrites in bundles like strands of rope.
neuroglia	Cells in the nervous system that do not carry impulses but are supportive and connective in function. Examples are astrocytes, microglial cells, and oligodendroglia. There are about 100 billion neuroglial cells.
neuron	A nerve cell; carries impulses throughout the body. There are about 10 billion neurons.
neurotransmitter	Chemical messenger, released at the end of a nerve cell, that stimulates or inhibits another cell. The second cell affected may be another nerve cell, a muscle cell, or a gland cell. Examples of neurotransmitters are acetylcholine, epinephrine, and dopamine.
oligodendroglia	A neuroglial cell that produces myelin, which is the fatty tissue that forms a sheath covering the axons.
parasympathetic nerves	Involuntary, autonomic nerves that help regulate body functions like heart rate and respiration.
peripheral nervous system	Nerves outside the brain and spinal cord; cranial, spinal, and autonomic nerves.
pia mater	Thin, delicate, inner membrane of the meninges.
plexus (plural: plexuses)	A large, interlacing network of nerves. Examples are cervical, lumbar, and brachial (brachi/o means arm) plexuses. The term originated from the Indo-European *plek* meaning to weave together.
pons	Bridge—part of the brain anterior to the cerebellum and between the medulla and the rest of the brain.
receptor	An organ that receives a nervous stimulation and passes it on to nerves within the body. The skin, ears, eyes, and taste buds are receptors.
sensory nerves	Nerves that carry messages to the brain and spinal cord from a receptor.
stimulus (plural: stimuli)	A change in the internal or external environment that can evoke a response.

sulcus (plural: **sulci**)	Depression in the surface of the cerebral cortex; fissure.
sympathetic nerves	Autonomic nerves that influence body functions involuntarily in times of stress.
synapse	The space (juncture) through which a nervous impulse is transmitted from one neuron to another or from a neuron to another cell, such as a muscle or gland cell. From the Greek *synapto* meaning I join together.
thalamus	Main relay center of the brain. It conducts impulses between the spinal cord and the cerebrum; incoming sensory messages are relayed through the thalamus to appropriate centers in the cerebrum. The name thalamus, meaning room, comes from the Romans who thought this part of the brain was hollow—therefore resembling a room.
ventricles of the brain	Reservoirs (canals) in the interior of the brain that are filled with cerebrospinal fluid.

VII. Combining Forms and Terminology

This section is divided into terms that describe organs and structures of the nervous system and those that relate to neurological symptoms. Write the meaning of the medical term in the space provided.

Organs and Structures

Combining Form	Meaning	Terminology	Meaning
cerebell/o	cerebellum	cerebellar _____	
		cerebellospinal _____	
cerebr/o	cerebrum	cerebrospinal fluid _____	
		cerebral cortex _____	
		Cortical means pertaining to the cortex or outer area of an organ.	
dur/o	dura mater	subdural hematoma _____	
		epidural hematoma _____	
		Figure 10–11 shows subdural and epidural hematomas.	
encephal/o	brain	encephalitis _____	
		encephalopathy _____	

Figure 10–11

Subdural and epidural hematomas.

		anencephaly _____
		encephalomalacia _____
gli/o	glue, parts of the nervous system that support and connect	neuroglial cells _____
		Stromal or connective tissue of the nervous system.
		glioma _____
lept/o	thin, slender	leptomeningitis _____
		The pia and arachnoid membranes are known as the leptomeninges because of their thin, delicate structure.
mening/o, meningi/o	membranes, meninges	meningeal _____
		meningioma _____
		meningomyelocele _____
		This abnormality occurs in infants born with spina bifida. See Section VIII, Pathological Conditions.
my/o	muscle	myoneural _____
myel/o	spinal cord	myelogram _____
	(means bone marrow in other contexts)	poliomyelitis _____
		Polio means gray matter. This is a viral disease in which the gray matter of the spinal cord is affected, leading to paralysis of the muscles that rely on the damaged neurons.

neur/o	nerve	neuropathy _____	
		polyneuritis _____	
		neuroanastomosis _____	
		neurorrhaphy _____	
pont/o	pons	cerebellopontine _____	
		-ine means pertaining to.	
radicul/o	nerve root (of spinal nerves)	radiculopathy _____	
thalam/o	thalamus	thalamic _____	
thec/o	sheath (refers to the meninges)	intrathecal injection _____	
		Chemicals, such as chemotherapeutic drugs, are delivered into the subarachnoid space.	
vag/o	vagus nerve (tenth cranial nerve)	vagal _____	
		This cranial nerve has branches to the head and neck as well as the chest (larynx, trachea, bronchial tubes, lungs, heart) and abdomen (esophagus, stomach, and intestines).	
		vagotomy _____	

Symptoms			
Combining Form or Suffix	Meaning	Terminology	Meaning
alges/o **-algesia**	excessive sensitivity to pain	analgesia _____	
-algia	pain	neuralgia _____	
caus/o	burning	causalgia _____	
		This is intense burning pain following an injury to a sensory (afferent) nerve.	
		cephalalgia _____	
		Also written cephalgia. Most headaches result from vasodilation (widening) of blood vessels in tissues surrounding the brain, or from tension in neck and scalp muscles. A migraine is a severe (often unilateral) headache sometimes accompanied by nausea and vomiting.	

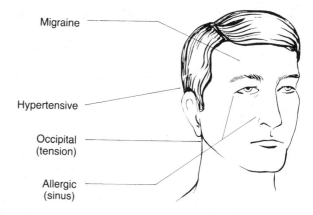

Migraine

Hypertensive

Occipital
(tension)

Allergic
(sinus)

Figure 10–12

Location of pain in some common types of headache. (Modified with permission from Ferguson GG: Pathophysiology: Mechanisms and Expressions. Philadelphia, WB Saunders Company, 1984.)

Figure 10–12 shows the location of pain with some of the more common types of headache.

comat/o	deep sleep (coma)	<u>comat</u>ose _____

A coma is a state of unconsciousness from which the patient cannot be aroused. An irreversible coma is one in which there is complete unresponsivity to stimuli, no spontaneous breathing or movement, and a flat EEG. Also called brain death.

esthesi/o **-esthesia**	feeling, nervous sensation	an<u>esthesia</u> _____

Lack of nervous sensation—for example, absence of sense of touch or pain.

hyper<u>esthesia</u> _____

A light touch with a pin may provoke increased sensation.

par<u>esthesia</u> _____

Par- (from para-) means abnormal here. Examples are sensations such as burning, prickling, tingling, or numbness for no apparent reason.

kines/o **-kinesia**	movement	brady<u>kinesia</u> _____

kinesi/o **-kinesis**	movement	hyper<u>kinesis</u> _____

Amphetamines (CNS stimulants) are used to treat hyperkinesis in children, but the mechanism of their action is not understood.

<u>kinesi</u>ology _____

-lepsy	seizure	epi<u>lepsy</u> _____

See page 319, Section VIII, Pathological Conditions.

narco<u>lepsy</u> _____

Sudden, uncontrollable compulsion to sleep (narc/o = stupor, sleep).

lex/o	word, phrase	dyslexia _____
		Reading, writing, and learning disorders.
-paresis	slight paralysis	hemiparesis _____
		Affects either right or left side (half) of the body. Paresis is also used by itself to mean partial paralysis or weakness of muscles.
-phasia	speech	aphasia _____
		Motor aphasia *is present when a patient knows what she or he wants to say but cannot move muscles properly to speak.* ***Sensory aphasia*** *is present when the patient articulates (pronounces) words easily but uses them inappropriately. The patient has difficulty in understanding written and verbal commands and cannot repeat them.*
-plegia	paralysis (loss or impairment of the ability to move parts of the body)	hemiplegia _____
		Affects right or left half of the body and results from a stroke or other brain injury. The hemiplegia is contralateral to the brain lesion because motor nerve fibers from the right half of the brain cross to the left side of the body (in the medulla oblongata).
		paraplegia _____
		Originally, the term paraplegia meant a stroke (paralysis) on one side (para-). Now, however, the term means paralysis of both legs and the lower part of the body, due to injury or disease of the spinal cord at the lumbar level.
		quadriplegia _____
		Quadri- means four. All four extremities are affected. Injury is at the cervical level of the spinal cord.
-praxia	action	apraxia _____
		Movements and behavior are not purposeful.
-sthenia	strength	neurasthenia _____
		Nervous exhaustion; weakness and irritability. Asthenia is used as a noun to describe loss or lack of bodily strength.
syncop/o	to cut off, cut short	syncopal _____
		Syncope (SĬN-kō-pē) is fainting; sudden and temporary loss of consciousness caused by inadequate flow of blood to the brain. The term syncope comes from a Greek word meaning a cutting into pieces. The implication is that a fainting spell meant one was cut off from strength.
tax/o	order, coordination	ataxia _____
		Persistent unsteadiness on the feet can be caused by a disorder involving the cerebellum.

VIII. Pathological Conditions

The CNS is protected from external injury by the bones of the skull and the vertebral column and by the meninges containing CSF, which provides a cushion around the brain and spinal cord. In addition, neuroglial cells, which surround neurons, help to form a blood-brain barrier that prevents many potentially harmful substances in the bloodstream from gaining access to nerve cells. However, these protective factors are counterbalanced by the sensitivity of nerve cells to oxygen deficiency (brain cells die in a few minutes when deprived of oxygen) and by the inability of neurons to regenerate (adult nerve cells do not undergo cell division and cannot replace themselves).

Neurological diseases may be classified in the following categories of disorders:

1. Congenital
2. Degenerative, Movement, and Seizure
3. Infectious
4. Neoplastic
5. Traumatic
6. Vascular

Congenital Disorders

hydrocephalus

Abnormal accumulation of fluid (CSF) in the brain.

If circulation of CSF in the brain or spinal cord is impaired, it accumulates under pressure in the ventricles of the brain. Characteristic features in infants are enlarged head and small face (Fig. 10–13). To relieve pressure on the brain, a catheter (shunt) is placed from the ventricle of the brain into the peritoneal space (ventriculoperitoneal shunt) so that the CSF is continually drained from the brain.

Hydrocephalus can also occur in an adult as a result of tumors and infections.

Figure 10–13

Child, 4 months old, with hydrocephalus. (From Jacob S, Francone CA: Elements of Anatomy and Physiology, 2nd ed. Philadelphia, WB Saunders, 1989, p 137.)

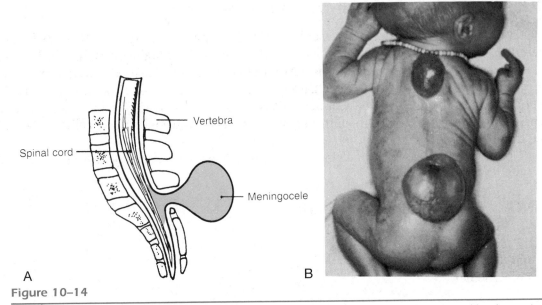

Figure 10–14

(A) Spina bifida with meningocele. *(B)* Spina bifida with meningomyelocele in the thoracic and lumbar regions. *(B,* Courtesy of Dr. Dwight Parkinson, Children's Centre, Winnipeg.)

spina bifida

Congenital defect in the spinal column due to imperfect union of vertebral parts.

Spina bifida (bi- = two, fid = split) usually occurs in the lumbar region and there are several forms:

Spina bifida occulta—The vertebral lesion is covered over with skin and evident only on x-ray examination. In its most minor form, there is no defect in the skin, and the only evidence of its presence may be a small dimple with a tuft of hair.

Spina bifida cystica—These are more severe types of spina bifida, involving protrusion of the meninges **(meningocele)** or protrusion of the meninges and spinal cord **(meningomyelocele)** (Fig. 10–14).

Spina bifida cystica can involve hydrocephalus, paraplegia, and lack of control of bladder and rectum. Surgery may be indicated to remove the herniated tissue.

Degenerative, Movement, and Seizure Disorders

Alzheimer's disease

Brain disorder marked by deterioration of mental capacity **(dementia)** beginning in middle age.

The disorder develops gradually, and early signs are loss of memory for recent events, persons, and places, followed by impairment of judgment, comprehension, and intellect. Anxiety, depression, and emotional disturbances can occur as well. On autopsy of the brain there is cerebral cortex atrophy and widening of the cerebral sulci, especially in the frontal and temporal regions. Microscopic examination shows senile plaques resulting from degeneration of neurons and neurofibrillary tangles (bundles of fibrils in the cytoplasm of a neuron) in the cerebral cortex. There is as yet no effective treatment.

amyotrophic lateral sclerosis (ALS)

Progressive disorder characterized by degeneration of motor neurons in the spinal cord and brain stem; also called **Lou Gehrig's disease.**

Named for a famous baseball player, Lou Gehrig, who became a victim of the disease, ALS presents in adulthood and affects men more often than women. Symptoms are weakness in skeletal muscles, difficulty in swallowing and talking, and dyspnea as the respiratory muscles become affected. Eventually muscles atrophy, and the patient becomes a quadriplegic. Etiology (cause) and cure for ALS are both unknown.

epilepsy

Chronic disorder characterized by recurrent seizure activity.

A seizure is an abnormal, sudden excessive discharge of electrical activity within the brain. Seizures are often symptoms of underlying brain pathological conditions, such as brain tumors, meningitis, vascular disease, or scar tissue from a head injury. **Tonic-clonic seizures (grand mal seizures)** are characterized by a sudden loss of consciousness, falling down, and then tonic contractions (stiffening of muscles) followed by clonic contractions (twitching and jerking movements of the limbs). Often, these convulsions are preceded by an **aura,** which is a peculiar sensation appearing before more definite symptoms. Dizziness, numbness, or visual disturbances are examples of an aura. **Absence seizures (petit mal seizures)** are a minor form of seizure consisting of momentary clouding of consciousness and loss of contact with the environment. Drug therapy (anticonvulsants) is used for control of epileptic seizures.

The term comes from the Greek *epilepsis* meaning a laying hold of. The Greeks thought a victim of a seizure was laid hold of by some mysterious force.

Huntington's chorea

Hereditary nervous disorder due to degenerative changes in the cerebrum and involving bizarre, abrupt, involuntary, dance-like movements.

This condition begins in adulthood (between the ages of 30 and 45) and results in mental decline with choreic (meaning dance) movements (uncontrollable, irregular, jerking movements of the arms, legs, and face).

The recent discovery that the genetic defect in patients with Huntington's disease is located on chromosome 4 has made it possible to test and identify those who will eventually develop the disease. Inheritance is as a dominant trait (the disorder appears when only one of a pair of chromosomes carries the defective gene) and the offspring of a parent with the disease has a 50 per cent chance of eventually manifesting the condition. There is no cure; management is symptomatic.

multiple sclerosis (MS)

Destruction of the myelin sheath on neurons in the CNS and its replacement by plaques of sclerotic (hard) tissue.

One of the leading causes of neurologic disability in persons 20–40 years of age, MS is a chronic disease marked by periods of remission and then relapse. **Demyelination** prevents the conduction of nerve impulses through the axon and causes paresthesias, muscle weakness, unsteady **gait** (manner of walking), and paralysis. Etiology is unknown, and there is no effective treatment, although immunosuppressive agents are often given with some benefit.

myasthenia gravis

Neuromuscular disorder characterized by relapsing weakness (-asthenia) of skeletal muscles (attached to bones).

Myasthenia gravis means grave muscle weakness and is a chronic autoimmune disorder. Antibodies block the ability of *acetylcholine* (a neurotransmitter) to transmit the nervous impulse from nerve to muscle cell, and normal muscle contraction fails to occur. Muscles on the outside of the eye (extraocular) are affected (causing ptosis of the eyelid) as well as those of the face, tongue, and extremities. Therapy to reverse symptoms includes anticholinesterase drugs, which inhibit the enzyme that breaks down acetylcholine. Corticosteroids (prednisone), and immunosuppressive drugs (azathioprine, methotrexate, and cyclophosphamide), are also used in treatment. **Thymectomy** (removal of the thymus gland, the source of antibody-producing white blood cells) is an alternative method of treatment and is beneficial to many patients.

palsy

Paralysis (partial or complete loss of motor function).

Cerebral palsy is partial paralysis and lack of muscular coordination caused by damage to the cerebrum during gestation or in the perinatal period. **Bell's palsy** involves unilateral facial paralysis, which is due to a disorder of the facial nerve. Etiology is unknown, but complete recovery is possible.

Parkinson's disease

Degeneration of nerves in the brain, occurring in later life, leading to tremors, weakness of muscles, and slowness of movement.

This slowly progressive condition is caused by a deficiency of **dopamine** (a neurotransmitter) that is made by cells in the midbrain (below the cerebrum and above the pons and medulla oblongata). Motor disturbances include stooped posture, shuffling gait, muscle stiffness (rigidity), and often a tremor of the hands. Drugs (such as levodopa) that increase dopamine levels in the brain are useful **palliative** (relieving but not curative) measures to control symptoms. Implantation of fetal brain tissue containing dopamine-producing cells is currently being used as an experimental treatment with uncertain results.

Tourette syndrome

Neurological disorder marked by involuntary, spasmodic, twitching movements; uncontrollable vocal sounds; and inappropriate words.

These involuntary movements, usually beginning with twitching of the eyelid and muscles of the face, are called **tics.** Although psychological problems do not cause Tourette syndrome, physicians have had some success in treating it with an antipsychotic drug, haloperidol.

Infectious Disorders

meningitis

Inflammation of the meninges; leptomeningitis.

This condition can be caused by meningococcal or streptococcal bacteria **(pyogenic meningitis)** or viruses **(viral meningitis).** Symptoms are fever and signs of meningeal irritation, such as headache, photophobia (sensitivity to light), and a stiff neck. Antibiotics are used to treat the more serious pyogenic form, and the viral form is treated symptomatically until it runs its course.

shingles

Viral disease affecting peripheral nerves.

Blisters and pain spread in a band-like pattern over the skin, following the peripheral nerves that are affected. Shingles is caused by a herpes virus **(herpes zoster),** the same virus that causes chickenpox. Reactivation of the chickenpox virus (herpes varicella-zoster), which remained in the body after the person had chickenpox, occurs.

Neoplastic Disorders

brain tumors

Abnormal growths of brain tissue and meninges.

Most of the primary intracranial tumors arise from neuroglial cells **(gliomas)** or the meninges **(meningiomas).** Examples of gliomas are **astrocytoma** and **oligodendroglioma.** The most malignant form of the astrocytoma is the **glioblas-**

toma multiforme (-blast means immature). Tumors can cause swelling **(cerebral edema)** and hydrocephalus. If there is increased CSF pressure, swelling can also occur near the optic nerve (at the back of the eye). Gliomas are removed surgically, and radiotherapy is used for those that are not completely resected. Steroids are given to reduce swelling after surgery.

Meningiomas are usually benign and surrounded by a capsule, but they may cause compression and distortion of the brain.

About 25–30 per cent of tumors in the brain are metastatic growths. Most arise in the lung, breast, skin (melanoma), kidney, and gastrointestinal tract.

Traumatic Disorders

cerebral concussion

Temporary brain dysfunction (brief loss of consciousness) after injury, usually clearing within 24 hours.

There is no evidence of structural damage to the brain tissue. Severe concussions may lead to coma.

cerebral contusion

Bruising of brain tissue as a result of direct trauma to the head; neurological deficits persist longer than 24 hours.

A contusion is usually associated with a fracture of the skull. Subdural and epidural hematomas occur and can lead to permanent brain injury or epilepsy.

Vascular Disorders

cerebrovascular accident (CVA)

Disruption in the normal blood supply to the brain.

This condition, also known as **stroke** or **cerebral infarction,** is the result of a localized area of ischemia (and ultimately infarction or necrosis) in the brain. There are three types of strokes (Fig. 10–15):

1. **Thrombotic**—blood clot **(thrombus)** in the arteries leading to the brain, resulting in **occlusion** (blocking) of the vessel. Atherosclerosis leads to this common type of stroke as blood vessels become blocked over time. Before total occlusion occurs, a patient may experience symptoms that point to the gradual occlusion of

Blood flows freely through a normal artery.

Hemorrhagic strokes are caused by cerebral arterial wall rupture.

Embolic (embolitic) strokes are caused by dislodged thrombi (emboli) that occlude cerebral arteries.

Thrombotic strokes are caused by atheromatous plaques that occlude cerebral arteries.

Figure 10–15

Three types of strokes. (From Ignatavicius DD, Bayne MV: Medical-Surgical Nursing: A Nursing Process Approach. Philadelphia, WB Saunders, 1991, p 880.)

blood vessels. These short episodes of neurological dysfunction are known as **TIAs (transient ischemic attacks)**.

2. **Embolic**—an **embolus** (a clot that breaks off from an area of the body) travels to the cerebral arteries and occludes a small vessel. This type of stroke occurs very suddenly.

3. **Hemorrhagic**—bursting forth of blood from a cerebral artery. This type of stroke is often fatal and results from advancing age, atherosclerosis, or high blood pressure—all of which result in degeneration of cerebral blood vessels. If the hemorrhage is small, the blood is reabsorbed and the patient can make a good recovery with only slight disability. In a younger patient, cerebral hemorrhage is usually due to mechanical injury associated with skull fracture or bursting of an arterial **aneurysm** (weakness in the vessel wall that balloons and eventually bursts).

Three major risk factors for stroke are hypertension, diabetes, and heart disease. Other risk factors include smoking, obesity, substance abuse (cocaine), and elevated cholesterol levels.

Thrombotic strokes are treated medically with anticoagulant drug therapy and surgically with endarterectomy (removal of the atherosclerotic plaque from the inner lining of an artery).

STUDY SECTION

The following is a review of new terms used in Section VIII, Pathological Conditions. Practice spelling each term and know its meaning.

absence seizure	Minor (petit mal) form of seizure, consisting of momentary clouding of consciousness and loss of contact with the environment.
aneurysm	Abnormal widening of a blood vessel; can lead to hemorrhage and CVA (stroke).
astrocytoma	Malignant tumor of neuroglial brain cells (astrocytes).
aura	Peculiar sensation appearing before more definite symptoms.
-blast	Immature cells (as in glio*blast*oma).
dementia	Mental decline and deterioration.
demyelination	Destruction of myelin on the axons of nerves (seen in multiple sclerosis).
dopamine	A neurotransmitter that is deficient in Parkinson's disease.
embolus	A mass (clot) of material travels through the bloodstream and suddenly blocks a vessel.
gait	Manner of walking.
herpes zoster	Type of herpes virus that causes shingles—eruption of blisters in a pattern that follows the path of peripheral nerves around the trunk of the body; zoster means girdle.

occlusion	Blockage.
palliative	Relieving symptoms but not curing.
thymectomy	Removal of the thymus gland (a lymphocyte-producing gland in the chest); used as treatment for myasthenia gravis.
TIA	Transient ischemic attack; mini-stroke.
tonic-clonic seizure	Major convulsive seizure marked by sudden loss of consciousness, stiffening of muscles, and twitching and jerking movements.

IX. Laboratory Tests, Clinical Procedures, and Abbreviations

Laboratory Tests

cerebrospinal fluid analysis	Cell counts, bacterial smears, and cultures of samples of CSF are done when disease of the meninges or brain is suspected. Normal constituents of CSF are water, glucose, sodium, chloride, and protein, and changes in their concentrations are helpful in diagnosis of brain disease. CSF normally has more chloride and less glucose than blood.

Clinical Procedures

X-Ray

cerebral angiography	Contrast medium is injected into an artery (usually the femoral) and x-rays are taken of the blood vessel system of the brain. The purpose of the test is to diagnose vascular disease (aneurysm, occlusion, hemorrhage) in the brain.
computed tomography (CT)	X-rays are used to compose a computerized cross-sectional picture of the brain and spinal cord. Contrast medium may also be injected intravenously to see abnormalities. The contrast material leaks through the **blood-brain barrier** from blood vessels into the brain tissue and shows areas of tumor, hemorrhage, and blood clots (Fig. 10–16).

Tumor

Figure 10–16

The CT scan of a 40-year-old woman with carcinoma of the lung, who developed occipital headache and gait unsteadiness. The scan (following contrast agent infusion) shows a round, high-density (white) area in the left cerebellar hemisphere, which is probably a metastatic lung carcinoma in the brain. (From Weisberg LA, Nice C, Katz M: Cerebral Computed Tomography: A Text-Atlas. Philadelphia, WB Saunders, 1978, p 153.)

myelography

Contrast medium (iodine-based solution such as Pantopaque) is injected into the subarachnoid space (via lumbar puncture), and x-rays are taken of the spinal cord. This procedure demonstrates neoplasms of the spinal cord and slipped disks. Myelography may be less commonly performed as CT and magnetic resonance imaging (MRI) replace this more invasive technique.

Ultrasound

echoencephalography

Ultrasonic waves are beamed through the head, and echoes coming from brain structures are recorded as a picture. This is useful in detecting head injuries, brain tumors, and hydrocephalus.

Magnetic Imaging

MRI of the brain

Use of magnetic waves to create an image of the brain (frontal, cross-sectional, and sagittal planes can be viewed). MRI and CT are used to complement each other in diagnosing brain and spinal cord lesions. MRI is excellent for viewing soft tissues.

Radioactive Studies

brain scan

Radioactive chemicals are given intravenously and travel to the brain. Special scanner machines then record the passage and absorption of the

Site of needle puncture

Dura mater

Distal end of spinal cord

Third lumbar vertebra

Subarachnoid space

Figure 10–17

Lumbar puncture. (From Chabner DE: Medical Terminology: A Short Course. Philadelphia, WB Saunders, 1990.)

chemicals into the brain tissue. If there is a brain lesion, the radioactive molecules "leak" across the blood-brain barrier and concentrate in abnormal sites.

positron emission tomography (PET scan)	An isotope (radioactive chemical) that gives off particles called positrons is injected intravenously, combined with a form of glucose. The uptake of the radioactive material is then recorded on a television screen. The cross-sectional images show how the brain uses glucose and give information about brain function. PET scans give valuable information in patients with Alzheimer's disease, stroke, schizophrenia, and epilepsy.

Other Procedures

electroencephalography (EEG)	Recording of the electrical activity of the brain. EEG is used to demonstrate seizure activity in the brain, brain tumors, and other diseases and injury to the brain.
lumbar (spinal) puncture	CSF is withdrawn from between two lumbar vertebrae (Fig. 10–17). A device to measure the pressure of the CSF can be attached to the end of the needle after it has been inserted. Contrast medium for x-ray studies (myelography) or intrathecal medicines may be administered through the lumbar puncture as well. Leakage of CSF around the puncture site can sometimes lead to lower pressure in the subarachnoid space and cause headache.
stereotactic radiosurgery	Use of a stereotactic instrument that, when fixed onto the skull, can locate a target by three-dimensional measurement. **Stereotactic radiosurgery** with a **gamma knife** (high-energy radiation beams) has been used to treat deep and often inaccessible intracranial brain tumors and abnormal blood vessel masses (arteriovenous malformations) without surgical incision.

ABBREVIATIONS

AFP	Alpha-fetoprotein (elevated levels in amniotic fluid and maternal blood are associated with congenital malformations of the nervous system, such as anencephaly and spina bifida)	**ICP**	Intracranial pressure
		LP	Lumbar puncture
		MRI	Magnetic resonance imaging
ALS	Amyotrophic lateral sclerosis	**MS**	Multiple sclerosis
CNS	Central nervous system	**PET**	Positron emission tomography
CSF	Cerebrospinal fluid	**RIND**	Reversible, ischemic neurological deficit
CT	Computed tomography (also CAT—computed axial tomography)	**TENS**	Transcutaneous electrical nerve stimulation (a battery-powered device used to relieve acute and chronic pain)
CVA	Cerebrovascular accident		
EEG	Electroencephalogram	**TIA**	Transient ischemic attack (temporary interference with the blood supply to the brain)

X. Practical Applications

Case Report

This patient was admitted on January 14 with a history of progressive right hemiparesis for the previous 1–2 months, fluctuating numbness of the right arm, thorax, and buttocks, jerking of the right leg, periods of speech arrest, diminished comprehension in reading, and recent development of a spastic hemiplegic gait [partial hemiplegia with spasmodic contractions of muscles when walking]. He is suspected of having a left parietal tumor [the parietal lobes of the cerebrum are on either side under the roof of the skull].

Examinations done prior to hospitalization included skull films, EEG, brain scan, and CSF analysis, which were all normal. After admission, the brain scan was abnormal in the left parietal region, as was the EEG.

Left percutaneous common carotid angiography [the carotid arteries are in the neck and supply the brain with blood] was attempted, but the patient became progressively more restless and agitated after receiving the sedation, so that it was impossible to do the procedure. During the recovery phase from the sedation, the patient was alternately somnolent [sleepy] and violent, but it was later apparent that he had developed almost a complete aphasia and right hemiplegia.

In the next few days, he became more alert although he remained dysarthric [from arthroun—to utter distinctly] and hemiplegic.

Bilateral carotid angiograms under general anesthesia on January 19 showed complete occlusion of the left internal carotid artery with cross-filling of the left anterior and middle cerebral arteries from the right internal carotid circulation.

Final diagnosis: Left cerebral infarction due to left internal carotid artery occlusion.

[Fig. 10–18 shows the common carotid arteries and their branches within the head and brain.]

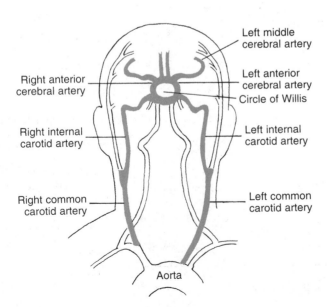

Figure 10–18

Common carotid arteries and their branches.

XI. Exercises

Remember to check your answers carefully with those given in Section XII, Answers to Exercises.

A. Match the following neurological structures with their meanings below.

dendrite	meninges	astrocyte
cauda equina	axon	plexus
myelin sheath	cerebral cortex	neuron
oligodendroglia		

1. microscopic fiber leading from the cell body that carries the nervous impulse along a nerve cell

   _____

2. a large, interlacing network of nerves _____

3. three protective membranes surrounding the brain and spinal cord _____

4. microscopic branching fiber of a nerve cell that is the first part to receive the nervous impulse

   _____

5. outer region of the largest part of the brain; composed of gray matter _____

6. neuroglial cell that transports water and salts between capillaries and nerve cells

   _____

7. neuroglial cell that produces myelin _____

8. a nerve cell that transmits a nervous impulse _____

9. collection of spinal nerves below the end of the spinal cord at the level of the second lumbar vertebra

   _____

10. protective fatty tissue that surrounds the axon of a nerve cell _____

B. Give the meanings for the following terms.

1. dura mater _____

2. central nervous system _____

3. peripheral nervous system _____

4. arachnoid membrane _____

5. hypothalamus _____

6. synapse _____

7. sympathetic nerves _____

8. medulla oblongata _____

9. pons _____

10. cerebellum _____

11. thalamus _____

12. ventricles of the brain _____

13. brain stem _____

14. cerebrum _____

C. *Match the following terms with their meanings or associated terms below.*

convolutions	neuroglial cell	afferent nerves
neurotransmitter	pia mater	efferent nerves
fissures	parenchymal cell	subarachnoid space

1. innermost meningeal membrane _____

2. motor nerves; carry messages away from the brain and spinal cord to muscles and glands (effectors)

_____

3. sensory nerves; carry messages toward the brain and spinal cord from receptors

_____

4. sulci; grooves in the cerebral cortex _____

5. contains cerebrospinal fluid _____

6. gyri; elevations in the cerebral cortex _____

7. acetylcholine is an example of this chemical that is released at the end of a nerve cell and stimulates or

inhibits another cell _____

8. essential cell of the nervous system; neuron _____

9. connective and supportive (stromal) cell _____

D. Choose the correct term to fit the definition given.

1. softening of the brain (encephalopathy, encephalomalacia)

2. pertaining to the part of the brain that controls muscular coordination and balance (cerebral, cerebellar)

3. collection of blood above the dura mater (subdural hematoma, epidural hematoma)

4. inflammation of the pia and arachnoid membranes (leptomeningitis, causalgia)

5. condition of no brain (vagotomy, anencephaly)

6. inflammation of the gray matter of the spinal cord (poliomyelitis, polyneuritis)

7. pertaining to the membranes around the brain and spinal cord (cerebellopontine, meningeal)

8. disease of nerve roots (of spinal nerves) (neuropathy, radiculopathy)

9. hernia of the meninges and the spinal cord (meningomyelocele, meningioma)

10. suture of a nerve (neuroanastomosis, neurorrhaphy)

E. Give the meanings for the following terms.

1. cerebral cortex _____

2. intrathecal _____

3. polyneuritis _____

4. thalamic _____

5. cerebellopontine _____

6. vagotomy _____

7. myelogram _____

8. meningioma _____

9. glioma _____

10. subdural hematoma _____

F. Match the following neurological symptoms with their meanings below.

causalgia   bradykinesia   ataxia
hyperesthesia   neurasthenia   apraxia
paraplegia   narcolepsy   hemiparesis
aphasia   dyslexia   syncope

1. reading, writing, or learning disorder _____

2. condition of no coordination _____

3. condition of slow movement _____

4. condition of increased nervous sensation _____

5. seizure of sleep; uncontrollable compulsion to sleep _____

6. inability to speak _____

7. movements and behavior are not purposeful _____

8. slight paralysis in the right or left half of the body _____

9. burning pain _____

10. paralysis in the lower part of the body (damage to the lower part of the spinal cord)

_____

11. fainting _____

12. nervous exhaustion (lack of strength) and irritability _____

G. Give the meanings for the following terms.

1. analgesia _____

2. motor aphasia _____

3. paresis _____

4. quadriplegia _____ _____

5. asthenia _____

6. comatose _____

7. paresthesia _____

8. hyperkinesis _____

9. anesthesia _____

10. causalgia _____

H. Match the following terms with their descriptions below. The terms in boldface should give you a clue to the pathological condition described.

spina bifida cystica   Alzheimer's disease   myasthenia gravis
amyotrophic lateral sclerosis   epilepsy   Parkinson's disease
hydrocephalus   Huntington's chorea   multiple sclerosis
Bell's palsy

1. Destruction of myelin sheaths (demyelination) and their replacement by plaques of **hard** tissue lead to this condition. _____

2. Sudden, transient disturbances of brain function cause **seizures** in this abnormal condition.

   _____

3. The **spinal** column is imperfectly joined (a **split** in a vertebra occurs), and part of the meninges and spinal cord can herniate out of the spinal cavity in this congenital condition. _____

4. This condition involves **atrophy** of muscles and paralysis because of damage to motor neurons in the spinal cord and brain stem. _____

5. In this hereditary condition, the patient displays bizarre, abrupt, involuntary, **dance**-like movements, as well as decline in mental functions. _____

6. Cerebrospinal **fluid** accumulates in the **head** (in the ventricles of the brain) in this condition.

   _____

7. This neuromuscular disorder is marked by **loss of muscle strength** because of the inability of a neurotransmitter (acetylcholine) to transmit impulses from nerve cells to muscle cells.

   _____

8. Degeneration of nerves in the brain occur in later life, leading to tremors, shuffling gait, and muscle stiffness; **dopamine** (neurotransmitter) is deficient in the brain. _____

9. This condition begins in middle age and is marked by deterioration of mental capacity **(dementia);** autopsy shows cerebral cortex atrophy, widening of cerebral sulci, and microscopic neurofibrillary tangles. _____

10. Unilateral facial **paralysis** characterizes this condition. _____

I. Give the meanings for the following abnormal conditions.

1. astrocytoma _____

2. pyogenic meningitis _____

3. Tourette syndrome _____

4. cerebral contusion _____

5. cerebrovascular accident _____

6. cerebral concussion _____

7. shingles _____

8. cerebral embolus _____

9. cerebral thrombosis _____

10. cerebral hemorrhage _____

11. cerebral aneurysm _____

J. Match the term in column I with the letter of its associated term or meaning in column II.

Column I

1. ataxia   _____

2. aura   _____

3. transient ischemic attack _____

4. tonic-clonic seizure   _____

5. herpes zoster   _____

6. palliative   _____

7. dopamine   _____

8. occlusion   _____

9. absence seizure   _____

10. glioblastoma multiforme _____

Column II

A. relieving, but not curing
B. virus that causes chickenpox and shingles
C. uncoordinated gait
D. neurotransmitter
E. peculiar symptoms appearing before more definite symptoms
F. malignant brain tumor of immature neuroglial cells
G. major convulsive epileptic seizure; grand mal
H. interruption of blood supply to the cerebrum; mini-stroke
I. minor form of epileptic seizure; petit mal
J. blockage

K. Identify the following clinical procedures.

1. lumbar puncture _____

2. CT scan of the brain _____

3. echoencephalography _____

4. electroencephalography _____

5. brain scan _____

6. stereotactic radiosurgery _____

7. CSF analysis _____

8. cerebral angiography _____

L. Give the meanings for the following abbreviations.

1. PET scan _____

2. MRI of the brain _____

3. TIA _____

4. CNS _____

5. LP _____

M. Select the term that completes the meaning of the sentence.

1. Suzy had such severe headaches that she could only find relief with strong analgesics. Her condition of (spina bifida, migraine, epilepsy) was debilitating.

2. Paul was in a coma after his high-speed car accident. His physicians were concerned that he had suffered a (palsy, meningomyelocele, concussion and subdural hematoma) as a result of the accident.

3. Dick went to the ER complaining of dizziness, nausea, and headache. The physician, suspecting ICP (intracranial pressure), prescribed corticosteroids, and Dick's symptoms disappeared. Symptoms returned when the steroids were removed. (MRI of the brain, electroencephalography, CSF analysis) revealed a lesion that was removed surgically and proved to be a(an) (hydrocele, astrocytoma, herpes zoster).

4. Dorothy felt tingling sensations in her hands, and noticed blurred vision and numbness in her arm, all signs of (shingles, meningitis, TIA). Her physician requested (myelography, cerebral angiography, lumbar puncture) to assess any damage to cerebral blood vessels and possible stroke.

5. When Bill noticed ptosis and muscle weakness in his face, he reported these symptoms to his doctor. The doctor diagnosed his condition as (Tourette syndrome, Huntington's chorea, myasthenia gravis) and prescribed (dopamine, anticonvulsants, immunosuppressants), which relieved his condition.

N. Complete the spelling of the following terms from their meanings.

1. part of the brain that controls sleep, appetite, temperature, and secretions of the pituitary gland:

   hypo _____

2. pertaining to fainting: syn _____

3. abnormal sensations: par _____

4. slight paralysis: par _____

5. inflammation of a spinal nerve root: _____ itis

6. inability to speak: a _____

7. movements and behavior are not purposeful: a _____

8. lack of muscular coordination: a _____

9. reading, writing, and learning disorders: dys _____

10. excessive movement: hyper _____

11. paralysis in one half (right or left) of the body: _____ plegia

12. paralysis in the lower half of the body: _____ plegia

13. paralysis in all four limbs: _____ plegia

14. nervous exhaustion and weakness: neur _____

XII. Answers to Exercises

A

1. axon
2. plexus
3. meninges
4. dendrite
5. cerebral cortex
6. astrocyte
7. oligodendroglia
8. neuron
9. cauda equina
10. myelin sheath

B

1. outermost meningeal layer surrounding the brain and spinal cord
2. the brain and the spinal cord
3. nerves outside the brain and spinal cord; cranial, spinal, and autonomic nerves
4. middle meningeal membrane surrounding the brain and spinal cord
5. part of the brain below the thalamus; controls sleep, appetite, body temperature, and secretions from the pituitary system
6. space through which a nervous impulse is transmitted from a nerve cell to another nerve cell or to a muscle or gland cell
7. autonomic nerves that influence body functions involuntarily in times of stress
8. part of the brain just above the spinal cord that controls breathing, heartbeat, and the size of blood vessels
9. part of the brain anterior to the cerebellum and between the medulla and the upper parts of the brain; connects these parts of the brain
10. posterior part of the brain that coordinates voluntary muscle movements
11. part of the brain below the cerebrum; relay center that conducts impulses between the spinal cord and the cerebrum
12. canals in the interior of the brain that are filled with CSF

B

13. lower portion of the brain that connects the cerebrum with the spinal cord (includes the pons and the medulla)
14. largest part of the brain; controls voluntary muscle movement, vision, speech, hearing, thought, memory

C

1. pia mater
2. efferent nerves
3. afferent nerves
4. fissures
5. subarachnoid space
6. convolutions
7. neurotransmitter
8. parenchymal cell
9. neuroglial cell

D

1. encephalomalacia
2. cerebellar
3. epidural hematoma
4. leptomeningitis
5. anencephaly
6. poliomyelitis
7. meningeal
8. radiculopathy
9. meningomyelocele
10. neurorrhaphy

E

1. the outer region of the cerebrum (contains gray matter)
2. pertaining to within a sheath—through the meninges and into the subarachnoid space
3. inflammation of many nerves
4. pertaining to the thalamus
5. pertaining to the cerebellum and the pons
6. incision of the vagus nerve
7. record (x-ray) of the spinal cord (after contrast is injected via lumbar puncture)
8. tumor of the meninges
9. tumor of neuroglial cells (a brain tumor)
10. mass of blood below the dura mater (outermost meningeal membrane)

F

1. dyslexia
2. ataxia
3. bradykinesia
4. hyperesthesia
5. narcolepsy
6. aphasia
7. apraxia
8. hemiparesis
9. causalgia
10. paraplegia
11. syncope
12. neurasthenia

G

1. lack of sensitivity to pain
2. inability to speak (cannot articulate words, but can understand speech and know what she or he wants to say)
3. slight paralysis
4. paralysis in all four extremities (damage is to the cervical part of the spinal cord)
5. no strength (weakness)
6. pertaining to coma (loss of consciousness from which the patient cannot be aroused)
7. condition of abnormal sensations (prickling, tingling, numbness, burning) for no apparent reason
8. excessive movement
9. condition of no sensation or nervous feeling
10. intense burning pain

H

1. multiple sclerosis
2. epilepsy
3. spina bifida cystica
4. amyotrophic lateral sclerosis
5. Huntington's chorea
6. hydrocephalus
7. myasthenia gravis
8. Parkinson's disease
9. Alzheimer's disease
10. Bell's palsy

I

1. tumor of neuroglial brain cells (astrocytes)
2. inflammation of the meninges (bacterial infection with pus formation)
3. involuntary spasmodic, twitching movements (tics), uncontrollable vocal sounds, and inappropriate words
4. bruising of brain tissue as a result of direct trauma to the head
5. disruption of the normal blood supply to the brain; stroke or cerebral infarction
6. temporary brain dysfunction; loss of consciousness that usually clears within 24 hours
7. neurological condition caused by infection with herpes zoster virus; blisters form along the course of peripheral nerves
8. blockage of a blood vessel in the cerebrum from material that suddenly occludes the vessel from another part of the body
9. blockage of a blood vessel in the cerebrum from the formation of a clot within the vessel
10. bursting forth of blood from a cerebral artery (can cause a stroke)
11. a widening of a blood vessel (artery) in the cerebrum; the aneurysm can burst and lead to a CVA

J

1. C
2. E
3. H
4. G
5. B
6. A
7. D
8. J
9. I
10. F

K

1. CSF is withdrawn from the subarachnoid space between two lumbar vertebrae
2. computed tomography; x-ray pictures are taken in the transverse plane (cross sections)
3. process of recording the echoes from sound waves that are beamed at the brain
4. process of recording the electricity produced within the brain
5. radioactive substance is injected intravenously, and its uptake in brain tissue is recorded with a scanner device
6. an instrument (stereotactic) is fixed onto the skull and locates a target by three dimensional measurement; gamma radiation beams are used to treat deep brain lesions
7. laboratory examination of the cerebrospinal fluid
8. process of recording the blood vessels of the cerebrum after dye has been injected into arteries

L

1. positron emission tomography (a radioactive test that shows uptake of radioactive material indicating the functioning of brain cells)
2. magnetic resonance imaging (magnetic waves are beamed at the brain and pictures are made of brain structure—in frontal, transverse, and sagittal planes)
3. transient ischemic attack (stroke symptoms appear and disappear within 24 hours)
4. central nervous system (brain and spinal cord)
5. lumbar puncture

M

1. migraine
2. concussion and subdural hematoma
3. MRI of the brain; astrocytoma
4. TIA; cerebral angiography
5. myasthenia gravis; immunosuppressants

N

1. hypothalamus
2. syncopal
3. paresthesias
4. paresis
5. radiculitis
6. aphasia
7. apraxia
8. ataxia
9. dyslexia
10. hyperkinesis
11. hemiplegia
12. paraplegia
13. quadriplegia
14. neurasthenia

XIII. Pronunciation of Terms

To test your understanding of the terminology in this chapter, write the meaning of each term in the space provided. In addition, you may wish to cover the terms and write them by looking at your definitions. Make sure your spelling is correct. The page number after each term indicates where it is defined or used in the text so you can easily check your responses. (If you are not sure what the pronunciation symbols mean, refer to page 21.)

Vocabulary and Combining Forms and Terminology

Term	Pronunciation	Meaning
acetylcholine (309)	ăs-ĕ-tĭl-KŌ-lēn	_____
afferent nerves (309)	ĂF-ĕr-ĕnt nervz	_____
analgesia (314)	ăn-ăl-JĒ-zē-ă	_____
anencephaly (313)	ăn-ĕn-SĔF-ă-lē	_____
anesthesia (315)	ăn-ĕs-THĒ-zē-ă	_____
aphasia (316)	ă-FĀ-zē-ă	_____
apraxia (316)	ā-PRĂK-sē-ă	_____
arachnoid membrane (310)	ă-RĂK-noyd MĔM-brān	_____
astrocyte (310)	ĂS-trō-sīt	_____
ataxia (316)	ă-TĂK-sē-ă	_____
autonomic nervous system (310)	ăw-tō-NŌM-ĭk NĔR-vŭs SĬS-tĕm	_____
axon (310)	ĂK-sŏn	_____

blood-brain barrier (310)	blŭd-brān BĂ-rē-ĕr	_____
bradykinesia (315)	brā-dē-kĭ-NĒ-zē-ă	_____
brain stem (310)	brān stĕm	_____
cauda equina (310)	KĂW-dă ĕ-QUĪ-nă	_____
causalgia (314)	kăw-ZĂL-jē-ă	_____
cephalalgia (cephalgia) (314)	sēf-ăl-ĂL-jē-ă (sĕ-FĂL-jă)	_____
cerebellar (312)	sĕr-ĕ-BĔL-ăr	_____
cerebellopontine (314)	sĕr-ĕ-bĕl-ō-PŎN-tēn	_____
cerebellospinal (312)	sĕr-ĕ-bĕl-ō-SPĪ-năl	_____
cerebellum (310)	sĕr-ĕ-BĔL-ŭm	_____
cerebral cortex (310)	sĕ-RĒ-brăl (or SĔR-ĕ-brăl) KŎR-tĕks	_____
cerebrospinal fluid (310)	sĕ-rē-brō-SPĪ-năl FLŪ-ĭd	_____
cerebrum (310)	sĕ-RĒ-brŭm	_____
coma (315)	KŌ-mă	_____
comatose (315)	KŌ-mă-tōs	_____
convolution (310)	kŏn-vō-LŪ-shŭn	_____
dendrite (310)	DĔN-drīt	_____
dura mater (310)	DŪ-ră MĀ-tĕr	_____
dyslexia (316)	dĭs-LĔK-sē-ă	_____
efferent nerves (310)	ĔF-ĕr-ĕnt nervz	_____
encephalitis (312)	ĕn-sĕf-ă-LĪ-tĭs	_____
encephalomalacia (313)	ĕn-sĕf-ă-lō-mă-LĀ-shē-ă	_____
encephalopathy (312)	ĕn-sĕf-ă-LŎP-ă-thē	_____
epidural hematoma (312)	ĕp-ĕ-DŪ-răl hē-mă-TŌ-mă	_____
epilepsy (319)	ĔP-ĭ-lĕp-sē	_____
fissure (310)	FĬSH-ŭr	_____
glioma (313)	glī-Ō-mă	_____

gyrus; gyri (310)	JĪ-rŭs; JĪ-rē	_____
hemiparesis (316)	hĕm-ē-pă-RĒ-sĭs	_____
hemiplegia (316)	hĕm-ē-PLĒ-jă	_____
hyperesthesia (315)	hī-pĕr-ĕs-THĒ-zē-ă	_____
hyperkinesis (315)	hī-pĕr-kĭ-NĒ-sĭs	_____
hypothalamus (310)	hī-pō-THĂL-ă-mŭs	_____
intrathecal (314)	ĭn-tră-THĒ-kăl	_____
leptomeningitis (313)	lĕp-tō-mĕn-ĭn-JĪ-tĭs	_____
medulla oblongata (311)	mĕ-DŪL-ă (or mĕ-DŬL-ă) ŏb-lŏn-GĂ-tă	_____
meningeal (313)	mĕ-NĬN-jē-ăl or mĕ-nĭn-JĒ-ăl	_____
meninges (311)	mĕ-NĬN-jēz	_____
meningioma (313)	mĕ-nĭn-jē-Ō-mă	_____
meningomyelocele (313)	mĕ-nĭng-gō-MĪ-ĕ-lō-sēl	_____
microglial cell (311)	mĭ-krō-GLĒ-ăl or mī-KRŎG-lē-ăl sĕl	_____
motor nerves (311)	MŌ-tĕr nervz	_____
myelin sheath (311)	MĪ-ĕ-lĭn shēth	_____
myelogram (313)	MĪ-ĕ-lō-grăm	_____
myoneural (313)	mī-ō-NŪ-răl	_____
narcolepsy (315)	NĂR-kō-lĕp-sē	_____
neuralgia (314)	nū-RĂL-jă	_____
neurasthenia (316)	nū-răs-THĒ-nē-ă	_____
neuroanastomosis (314)	nū-rō-ă-nă-stō-MŌ-sĭs	_____
neuroglia (311)	nū-rō-GLI-ă or nū-RŎG-lē-ă	_____
neuron (311)	NŪ-rŏn	_____
neuropathy (314)	nū-RŎP-ă-thē	_____
neurorrhaphy (314)	nū-RŎR-ră-fē	_____

neurotransmitter (311)	nū-rō-trăns-MĬ-těr	_____
paraplegia (316)	păr-ă-PLĒ-jă	_____
parasympathetic nerves (311)	păr-ă-sĭm-pă-THĔT-ĭk nervz	_____
paresis (316)	pă-RĒ-sĭs	_____
paresthesia (315)	păr-ĕs-THĒ-zē-ă	_____
peripheral nervous system (311)	pĕ-RĬF-ĕr-ăl NĔR-vŭs SĬS-tĕm	_____
pia mater (311)	PĒ-ă MĂ-tĕr	_____
plexus (311)	PLĔK-sŭs	_____
poliomyelitis (313)	pō-lē-ō-mī-ĕ-LĪ-tĭs	_____
polyneuritis (314)	pōl-ē-nū-RĪ-tĭs	_____
pons (311)	pŏnz	_____
quadriplegia (316)	kwŏd-rĭ-PLĒ-jă	_____
radiculopathy (314)	ră-dĭk-ū-LŎP-ă-thē	_____
sensory nerves (311)	SĔN-sō-rē nervz	_____
stimulus (311)	STĬM-ū-lŭs	_____
subdural hematoma (312)	sŭb-DŪ-răl hē-mă-TŌ-mă	_____
sulcus; sulci (312)	SŬL-kŭs; SŬL-sī	_____
sympathetic nerves (312)	sĭm-pă-THĔT-ĭk nervz	_____
synapse (312)	SĬN-ăps	_____
syncopal (316)	SĬN-kō-păl	_____
syncope (316)	SĬN-kō-pē	_____
thalamic (314)	THĂL-ă-mĭk or thă-LĂM-ĭk	_____
thalamus (312)	THĂL-ă-mŭs	_____
vagal (314)	VĀ-găl	_____
vagotomy (314)	vā-GŎT-ō-mē	_____
ventricles of the brain (312)	VĔN-trĭ-k'lz of the brān	_____

Pathological Conditions, Laboratory Tests, and Clinical Procedures

Term	Pronunciation	Meaning
absence seizures (319)	ĂB-sĕns SĒ-zhŭrz	_____
Alzheimer's disease (318)	ĂLZ-hī-mĕrz dĭ-ZĒZ	_____
amyotrophic lateral sclerosis (318)	ā-mī-ō-TRŌ-fĭk LĂ-tĕr-ăl sklĕ-RŌ-sĭs	_____
aneurysm (322)	ĂN-ūr-ĭ-zĭm	_____
astrocytoma (320)	ăs-trō-sī-TŌ-mă	_____
aura (319)	ĂW-ră	_____
Bell's palsy (320)	bĕlz PĂL-zē	_____
cerebral angiography (323)	sĕ-RĒ-brăl ăn-jē-ŌG-ră-fē	_____
cerebral concussion (321)	sĕ-RĒ-brăl kŏn-KŬS-shŭn	_____
cerebral contusion (321)	sĕ-RĒ-brăl kŏn-TŪ-shŭn	_____
cerebral hemorrhage (322)	sĕ-RĒ-brăl HĔM-ŏr-ĭj	_____
cerebral palsy (320)	sĕ-RĒ-brăl (or SĔR-ĕ-brăl) PĂL-zē	_____
cerebrospinal fluid analysis (323)	sĕ-rē-brō-SPĪ-năl FLOO-ĭd ă-NĂL-ĭ-sĭs	_____
cerebrovascular accident (321)	sĕ-rē-brō-VĂS-kū-lăr ĂK-sĭ-dĕnt	_____
dementia (318)	dĕ-MĔN-shē-ă	_____
demyelination (319)	dē-mĭ-ĕ-lĭ-NĀ-shun	_____
dopamine (320)	DŌ-pă-mēn	_____
echoencephalography (324)	ĕk-ō-ĕn-sĕ-fă-LŎG-ră-fē	_____
electroencephalography (325)	ĕ-lĕk-trō-ĕn-sĕf-ă-LŎG-ră-fē	_____
embolus (322)	ĔM-bō-lŭs	_____
gait (319)	GĀT	_____
glioblastoma multiforme (320)	glī-ō-blăs-TŌ-mă mŭl-tē-FŎR-mă	_____
grand mal seizure (319)	grăn măl SĒ-zhŭr	_____

herpes zoster (320)   HĔR-pēz ZŎS-tĕr   _____

Huntington's chorea (319)   HŬN-ting-tŏnz Kō-RĒ-ă   _____

hydrocephalus (317)   hī-drō-SĔF-ă-lŭs   _____

lumbar puncture (325)   LŬM-băr PŬNK-shŭr   _____

magnetic resonance imaging (324)   măg-NĔT-ĭk rĕ-zō-NĂNCE ĬM-ă-jĭng   _____

meningitis (320)   mĕn-ĭn-JĪ-tĭs   _____

migraine (314)   MĪ-grān   _____

multiple sclerosis (319)   mŭl-tĭ-p'l sklĕ-RŌ-sĭs   _____

myasthenia gravis (319)   mī-ăs-THĒ-nē-ă GRĂ-vĭs   _____

palliative (320)   PĂ-lē-ă-tĭv   _____

palsy (320)   PĂWL-zē   _____

Parkinson's disease (320)   PĂR-kĭn-sŭnz dĭ-ZĒZ   _____

petit mal seizures (319)   pĕ-TĒ măl SĒ-zhŭrz   _____

positron emission tomography (325)   PŎS-ĭ-trŏn ē-MĬ-shŭn tō-MŎG-ră-fē   _____

shingles (320)   SHĬNG-ălz   _____

spina bifida (318)   SPĪ-nă BĬF-ĭ-dă   _____

stereotactic radiosurgery (325)   stĕ-rē-ō-TĂK-tĭk rā-dē-ō SŬR-gĕr-ē   _____

thrombosis (321)   thrŏm-BŌ-sĭs   _____

tonic-clonic seizures (319)   TŎN-ĭk-KLŌ-nĭk SĒ-zhŭrz   _____

Tourette syndrome (320)   Tŭ-RĔT SĬN-drōm   _____

transient ischemic attack (322)   TRĂN-zē-ĕnt ĭs-KĒ-mĭk ă-TĂK   _____

XIV. Review Sheet

Write the meanings for each word part in the space provided. Check your answers with the information in the chapter or in the Glossary (Medical Terms—English) at the end of the book.

Combining Forms

Combining Form	Meaning	Combining Form	Meaning
alges/o	_____	lex/o	_____
angi/o	_____	mening/o	_____
caus/o	_____	meningi/o	_____
cephal/o	_____	my/o	_____
cerebell/o	_____	myel/o	_____
cerebr/o	_____	narc/o	_____
comat/o	_____	neur/o	_____
crani/o	_____	pont/o	_____
cry/o	_____	radicul/o	_____
dur/o	_____	spin/o	_____
encephal/o	_____	syncop/o	_____
esthesi/o	_____	tax/o	_____
gli/o	_____	thalam/o	_____
hydr/o	_____	thec/o	_____
kines/o	_____	troph/o	_____
kinesi/o	_____	vag/o	_____
lept/o	_____		

Prefixes

Prefix	Meaning	Prefix	Meaning
a-,an-	_____	micro-	_____
dys-	_____	para-	_____
epi-	_____	polio-	_____
hemi-	_____	poly-	_____
hyper-	_____	quadri-	_____
hypo-	_____	sub-	_____
intra-	_____		

Suffixes

Suffix	Meaning	Suffix	Meaning
-algesia	_____	-ose	_____
-algia	_____	-paresis	_____
-blast	_____	-pathy	_____
-cele	_____	-phagia	_____
-esthesia	_____	-phasia	_____
-gram	_____	-plegia	_____
-graphy	_____	-praxia	_____
-ine	_____	-ptosis	_____
-itis	_____	-rrhaphy	_____
-kinesia	_____	-sclerosis	_____
-kinesis	_____	-sthenia	_____
-lepsy	_____	-tomy	_____
-oma	_____	-trophy	_____

Cardiovascular System

This Chapter is divided into the following sections

In this Chapter you will

- Name the parts of the heart and associated blood vessels and their functions in the circulation of blood;
- Trace the pathway of blood through the heart;
- List the meanings of major pathological conditions affecting the heart and blood vessels;
- Define combining forms that relate to the cardiovascular system; and
- Recognize the meaning of many laboratory tests, clinical procedures, and abbreviations pertaining to the cardiovascular system.

I. Introduction

In previous chapters we have discussed the diverse and important functions of many organs of the body. These functions include conduction of nerve impulses, production of hormones and reproductive cells, excretion of waste materials, and digestion and absorption of food substances into the bloodstream. In order to perform these functions reliably and efficiently, the body organs are powered by a unique energy source. The cells of each organ receive energy from the food substances that reach them after being taken into the body. Food contains stored energy that can be converted into the energy of movement and work. This conversion of stored energy into the active energy of work occurs when food and oxygen combine in cells during the chemical process of catabolism. It is obvious then that each cell of each organ is dependent on a constant supply of food and oxygen in order to receive sufficient energy to work well.

How does the body assure that oxygen and food will be delivered to all its cells? The cardiovascular system, consisting of a fluid called blood, vessels to carry the blood, and a hollow, muscular pump called the heart, transports food and oxygen to all organs and cells of the body. Blood vessels in the lungs absorb the oxygen that has been inhaled from the air, and blood vessels in the small intestine absorb food substances from the digestive tract. In addition, blood vessels carry cellular waste materials such as carbon dioxide and urea and transport these substances to the lungs and kidneys, respectively, where they can be eliminated from the body.

The heart and blood vessels and the terminology related to their anatomy, physiology, and disease conditions will be explored in this chapter. The nature of blood and another body fluid called lymph will be discussed in a later chapter.

II. Blood Vessels and the Circulation of Blood

Blood Vessels

There are three major types of blood vessels in the body. These are called arteries, veins, and capillaries.

Arteries are the large blood vessels that lead blood away from the heart. Their walls are made of connective tissue, elastic fibers, and an innermost layer of epithelial cells called **endothelium.** Endothelial cells, which line all blood vessels, secrete substances that affect the size (dilation) of blood vessels, blood clotting, and the growth of blood vessels. Because arteries carry blood away from the heart, they must be strong enough to withstand the high pressure of the pumping action of the heart. Their elastic walls allow them to expand as the heartbeat forces blood into the arterial system throughout the body. Smaller branches of arteries are called **arterioles.** Arterioles are thinner than arteries and carry the blood to the tiniest of blood vessels, the capillaries.

Capillaries have walls that are only one endothelial cell thick. These delicate, microscopic vessels carry nutrient-rich, oxygenated blood from the arteries and arterioles to the body cells. Their walls are thin enough to allow passage of oxygen and nutrients out of the bloodstream and into the tissue fluid surrounding the cells. Once inside the cells, the nutrients are burned in the presence of oxygen (catabolism) to release needed energy within the cell. At the same time, waste products such as carbon dioxide and water pass out of the cells and into the thin-walled capillaries. The waste-filled blood then flows back to the heart in small veins called **venules,** which branch to form larger vessels called veins.

Veins are thinner-walled than arteries. They conduct blood (that has given up most of its oxygen) toward the heart from the tissues. Veins have little elastic tissue and less

Figure 11-1

Blood vessels. Note the difference in wall thickness of the artery, vein, and capillary.

Endothelium

ARTERY   VEIN   CAPILLARY

Valve

connective tissue than arteries, and blood pressure in veins is extremely low compared with pressure in arteries. In order to keep blood moving back toward the heart, veins have valves that prevent the backflow of blood and keep the blood moving in one direction. Muscular action also helps the movement of blood in veins. Figure 11–1 illustrates the differences in blood vessels.

Circulation of Blood

Arteries, arterioles, veins, venules, and capillaries, together with the heart, form a circulatory system for the flow of blood. Figure 11–2 is a schematic representation of this circulatory system. Refer to it as you read the following paragraphs. (Note that the numbers in the following paragraphs correspond with those in Fig. 11–2.)

Blood deficient in oxygen flows through two large veins, the **venae cavae** (1), on its way from the tissue capillaries to the heart. The blood became oxygen-poor at the tissue capillaries when oxygen left the blood and entered the body cells.

Oxygen-poor blood enters the **right side of the heart** (2) and travels through that side and into the **pulmonary artery** (3), a vessel that divides in two, one branch leading to the left lung, the other to the right lung. The arteries continue dividing and subdividing within the **lungs** (4), forming smaller and smaller vessels (arterioles) and finally reaching the lung capillaries. The pulmonary artery is unusual in that it is the only artery in the body that carries blood deficient in oxygen.

While passing through the lung (pulmonary) capillaries, blood absorbs the oxygen that entered the body during inhalation. The newly oxygenated blood next returns immediately to the heart through **pulmonary veins** (5). The pulmonary veins are unusual in that they are the only veins in the body that carry oxygen-rich **(oxygenated)** blood. The circulation of blood through the vessels from the heart to the lungs and then back to the heart again is known as the **pulmonary circulation.**

Oxygen-rich blood enters the **left side of the heart** (6) from the pulmonary veins. The muscles in the left side of the heart pump the blood out of the heart through the largest single artery in the body, the **aorta** (7). The aorta moves up at first (ascending aorta) but then arches over dorsally and runs downward (descending aorta) just in front of the vertebral column. The aorta divides into numerous branches called **arteries** (8) that carry the oxygenated blood to all parts of the body. The names of some of these arterial branches will be familiar to you: brachial (brachi/o means arm), axillary, splenic, gastric, and renal arteries. The **carotid** arteries supply blood to the head and neck.

The relatively large arterial vessels branch further to form smaller **arterioles** (9). The arterioles, still containing oxygenated blood, branch into smaller **tissue capillaries** (10), which are near the body cells. Oxygen leaves the blood and passes through the thin capillary walls to enter the body cells. There, food is broken down, in the presence of oxygen, and energy is released.

One metabolic product of this chemical process is **carbon dioxide** (CO_2). CO_2 is produced in the cell but is harmful to the cell if it remains. It must thus pass out of the cells and into the capillary bloodstream at the same time that oxygen is entering the cell. As the blood makes its way back from the tissue capillaries toward the heart in **venules** (11) and **veins** (12), it is full of CO_2 and is oxygen-poor.

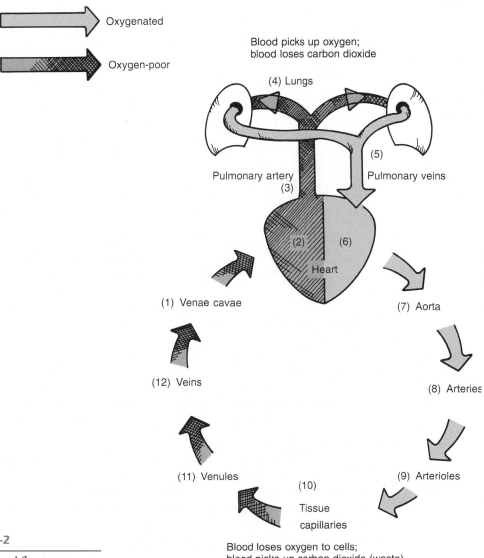

Figure 11–2

Circuit of blood flow.

Figure 11–3

The aorta and arteries that branch from it.

The circuit is thus completed when oxygen-poor blood enters the heart from the venae cavae. This circulation of blood from the body organs (except the lungs) to the heart and back again is called the **systemic circulation.** Figure 11–3 shows the aorta and its arterial branches.

III. Anatomy of the Heart

The human heart weighs less than a pound, is roughly the size of an adult fist, and lies in the thoracic cavity, just behind the breastbone in the mediastinum (between the lungs).

The heart is a pump, consisting of four chambers: two upper chambers called **atria** (singular: **atrium**), and two lower chambers called **ventricles.** It is actually a double pump, bound into one organ and synchronized very carefully. Blood passes through each pump in a definite pattern. Pump station number one, on the right side of the heart, sends oxygen-deficient blood to the lungs, where the blood picks up oxygen and releases its carbon dioxide. The newly oxygenated blood returns to the left side of the heart to pump station number two and does not mix with the oxygen-poor blood in pump station number one. Pump station number two then forces the oxygenated blood out to all parts of the body. At the body tissues, the blood loses its oxygen and on returning to the heart, to pump station number one, blood poor in oxygen (rich in carbon dioxide) is sent out to the lungs to begin the cycle anew.

Label Figure 11–4 as you learn the names of the parts of the heart and the vessels that carry blood to and from it.

Oxygen-poor blood enters the heart through the two largest veins in the body, the **venae cavae.** The **superior vena cava** (1) drains blood from the upper portion of the body, and the **inferior vena cava** (2) carries blood from the lower part of the body.

The venae cavae bring oxygen-poor blood that has passed through all of the body to the **right atrium** (3), the thin-walled upper right chamber of the heart. The right atrium contracts to force blood through the **tricuspid valve** (4) (cusps are the flaps of the valves) into the **right ventricle** (5), which is the lower right chamber of the heart. The cusps of the tricuspid valve form a one-way passage designed to keep the blood flowing in only one direction. As the right ventricle contracts to pump oxygen-poor blood through the **pulmonary valve** (6) into the **pulmonary artery** (7), the tricuspid valve stays shut, thus preventing blood from pushing back into the right atrium. The pulmonary artery then branches to carry oxygen-deficient blood to each lung.

The blood that enters the lung capillaries from the pulmonary artery soon loses its large quantity of carbon dioxide into the lung tissue, and the carbon dioxide is expelled. At the same time, oxygen enters the capillaries of the lungs and is brought back to the heart within the **pulmonary vein** (8). There are several pulmonary veins that transport oxygen-rich blood back to the left side of the heart from both lungs. The newly oxygenated blood enters the **left atrium** (9) of the heart from the pulmonary veins. The walls of the left atrium contract to force blood through the **mitral valve** (10) into the **left ventricle** (11).

The left ventricle has the thickest walls of all four heart chambers (three times the thickness of the right ventricle). It must pump blood with great force so that the blood travels through arteries to all parts of the body. The blood is pumped out of the left ventricle through the **aortic valve** (12) and into the **aorta** (13), which branches to carry blood all over the body. The aortic valve prevents the return of aortic blood to the left ventricle once it has been pumped out.

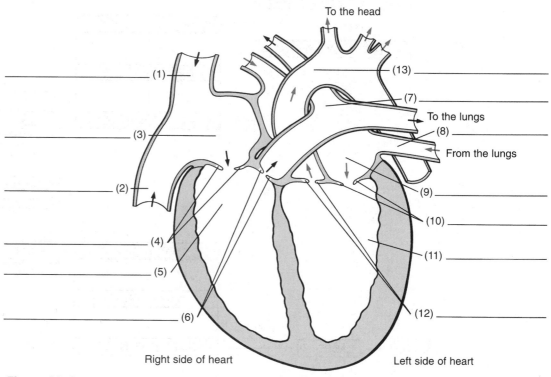

Figure 11–4

Structure of the heart. *Black arrows* indicate oxygen-poor blood flow. *Colored arrows* show oxygenated blood flow.

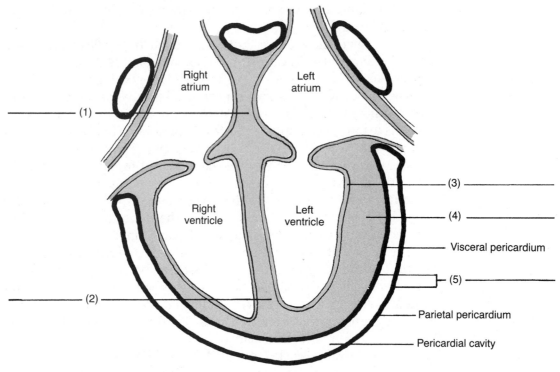

Figure 11–5

The heart wall and pericardium.

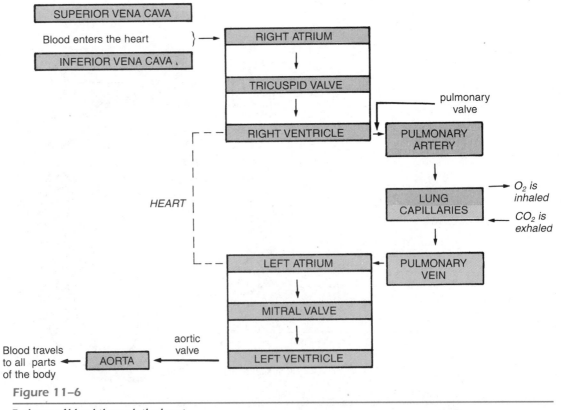

Figure 11–6

Pathway of blood through the heart.

In Figure 11–5 it can be seen that the four chambers of the heart are separated by partitions called **septa** (singular: **septum**). (Label Fig. 11–5 as you read these paragraphs.) The **interatrial septum** (1) separates the two upper chambers (atria), and the **interventricular septum** (2) is a muscular wall that comes between the two lower chambers (ventricles).

The heart wall is composed of three layers as shown in Figure 11–5. The **endocardium** (3) is a smooth layer of endothelial cells that lines the interior of the heart and the heart valves. The **myocardium** (4) is the middle, muscular layer of the heart wall and is its thickest layer. The **pericardium** (5) is a fibrous and membranous sac surrounding the heart. It is composed of two layers, the **visceral pericardium,** which adheres to the heart, and the **parietal** (parietal means wall) **pericardium,** which lines the outer fibrous coat. The **pericardial cavity** (between the visceral and the parietal pericardia) normally contains 10–15 ml of fluid, which lubricates the membranes as the heart beats.

Figure 11–6 traces the flow of blood through the heart.

IV. Physiology of the Heart

Heartbeat and Heart Sounds

There are two phases of the heartbeat. These phases are called **diastole** (relaxation) and **systole** (contraction). Diastole occurs when the ventricle walls relax and blood flows into the heart from the venae cavae and the pulmonary veins. The tricuspid and mitral valves are open in diastole, as blood passes from the right and left atria into the ventricles. The pulmonary and aortic valves are closed during diastole (Fig. 11–7).

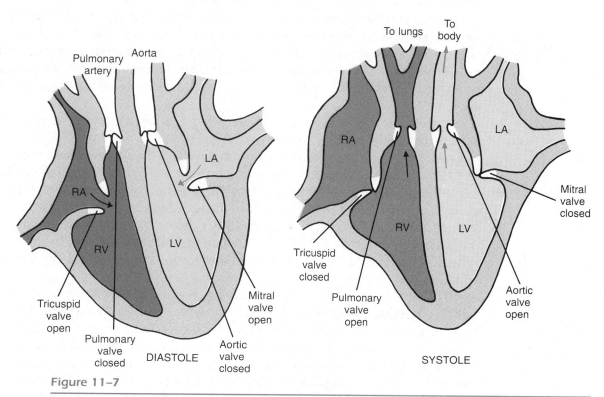

Figure 11–7

Phases of the heartbeat: diastole and systole. During diastole, tricuspid and mitral valves are open. During systole, pulmonary and aortic valves are open. (RA = right atrium; RV = right ventricle; LV = left ventricle; LA = left atrium.)

Systole occurs next, as the walls of the right and left ventricles contract to pump blood into the pulmonary artery and the aorta. Both the tricuspid and the mitral valves are closed during systole, thus preventing the flow of blood back into the atria (see Fig. 11–7).

This diastole-systole cardiac cycle occurs between 70 and 80 times per minute (100,000 times a day). The heart pumps about 3 ounces of blood with each contraction. This means that about 5 quarts of blood are pumped by the heart in 1 minute (75 gallons an hour and about 2000 gallons a day).

The beat of the heart as felt through the walls of the arteries is called the **pulse.** What is felt is a shock wave that travels along the fibers of the arteries as the heart contracts in systole. The pulse is usually felt just inside the wrist below the thumb at the radial artery (the radius is one of the two bones in the lower arm). Other sites of pulsation include the side of the neck (carotid artery), the elbow (brachial artery), and the anterior side of the hip (femoral artery).

Closure of the heart valves is associated with audible sounds, such as "lub, dub, lub, dub" that can be heard when listening to a normal heart with a stethoscope. The "lub" is associated with closure of the tricuspid and mitral valves at the beginning of systole and the "dub" with the closure of the aortic and pulmonary valves at the end of systole. The "lub" sound is called the first heart sound and the "dub" is the second heart sound because the normal cycle of the heartbeat starts with the beginning of systole. An abnormal heart sound is known as a **murmur.**

Conduction System of the Heart

What keeps the heart at its perfect rhythm? Although the heart does have nerves that can affect its rate, they are not primarily responsible for its beat. It is known that the heart starts beating in the embryo before the heart is supplied with nerves, and it will continue to beat in experimental animals even when the nerve supply is cut.

Primary responsibility for initiating the heartbeat rests with a small region of specialized muscle tissue in the posterior portion of the right atrium, where an electrical impulse originates. This region of the right atrium is called the **sinoatrial node (SA node).** The SA node is also called the **pacemaker** of the heart. The current of electricity generated by the pacemaker causes the walls of the atria to contract and force blood into the ventricles (ending diastole).

Almost like ripples in a pond of water when a stone is thrown, the wave of electricity passes from the pacemaker to another region of the myocardium. This region is at the posterior portion of the interatrial septum and is called the **atrioventricular node (AV node).** The AV node immediately sends the excitation wave to a bundle of specialized muscle fibers called the **bundle of His** (pronounced hiss). Within the interventricular septum, the bundle of His divides into right and left bundle branches, which carry the impulse to the right and left ventricles, causing them to contract. Thus, systole occurs and blood is pumped away from the heart. A short rest period follows, and then the pacemaker begins the wave of excitation across the heart again. Figure 11–8 shows the location of the SA node, the AV node, and the bundle of His.

The record used to detect these electrical changes in heart muscle as the heart beats is called an **electrocardiogram** (EKG or ECG, from the Greek root *kardia*). The normal EKG shows five waves, or deflections, that represent the electrical changes as a wave of excitation spreads through the heart. The deflections are called P, QRS, and T waves. The P wave represents electrical activity of the SA node impulse formation and the change in the electrical activity in the wall of the atria (atrial depolarization). The QRS wave is ventricular depolarization as electricity passes through the bundle of His and the ventricular wall. This is the largest wave because the ventricle contains the most muscle. The T wave represents

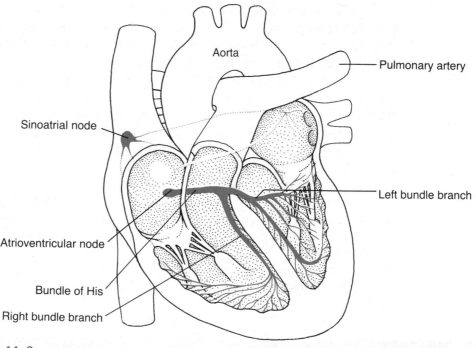

Figure 11–8

Conduction system of the heart. (From Ignatavicius DD, Bayne MV: Medical-Surgical Nursing: A Nursing Process Approach. Philadelphia, WB Saunders, 1991.)

ventricular repolarization, which is when the ventricular wall relaxes and recovers from contraction. Figure 11–9 illustrates P, QRS, and T waves in a normal EKG. The EKG is used to diagnose a heart attack (myocardial infarction), which causes abnormal deflections.

Normal heart rhythm (originating in the SA node and traveling through the heart) is called **sinus rhythm.** Sympathetic nerves speed up the heart rate during conditions of emotional stress or vigorous exercise. Parasympathetic nerves slow the heart rate when the need for extra pumping is past.

V. Blood Pressure

Blood pressure is the force that the blood exerts on the arterial walls. This pressure is measured by a device called a **sphygmomanometer.**

The sphygmomanometer consists of a rubber bag inside a cloth cuff that is wrapped around the upper arm, just above the elbow. The rubber bag is inflated with air by means of a rubber bulb. As the bag is pumped up, the pressure within it increases and is measured on a recording device attached to the cuff.

Figure 11–9

An ECG. P wave = spread of excitation wave over the atria; QRS wave = spread of excitation wave over the ventricle; T wave = electrical recovery and relaxation of the ventricles.

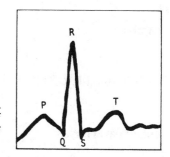

The vessels in the upper arm are compressed by the air pressure in the bag. When there is sufficient air pressure in the bag to stop the flow of blood in the main artery of the arm (brachial artery), the pulse in the lower arm (where the observer is listening with a stethoscope) obviously drops.

Air is then allowed to escape from the bag and the pressure is lowered slowly, allowing the blood to begin to make its way through the gradually opening artery. At the point when the person listening with the stethoscope first hears the sounds of the pulse beats, the reading on the device attached to the cuff shows the higher, systolic, blood pressure (pressure in the artery when the left ventricle is contracting to force the blood into the aorta and other arteries).

As air continues to escape, the sounds become progressively louder. Finally, when a change in sound from loud to soft occurs, the observer makes note of the pressure on the recording device. This is called the diastolic blood pressure (pressure in the artery when the ventricles are relaxing and the heart is filling, receiving blood from the venae cavae and pulmonary veins).

Blood pressure is usually expressed as a fraction: for example, 120/80, in which 120 represents the systolic pressure and 80 the diastolic pressure.

VI. Vocabulary

This list will help you review many of the new terms introduced in the text. Short definitions will reinforce your understanding of the terms. See Section XIII of this chapter for help in pronouncing the more difficult terms.

aorta	Largest artery in the body.
arteriole	Small artery.
artery	Largest type of blood vessel; carries blood away from the heart to all parts of the body.
atrioventricular node (AV node)	Specialized tissue at the base of the wall between the two upper heart chambers. Electrical impulses pass from the pacemaker (SA node) through the AV node to the bundle of His.
atrium (plural: **atria**)	Upper chamber of the heart.
bundle of His	Specialized muscle fibers in the wall between the ventricles that carry the electric impulses to the ventricles.
capillary	Smallest blood vessel. Materials pass to and from the bloodstream through the thin capillary walls.
carbon dioxide (CO_2)	A gas (waste) released by body cells and transported via veins to the heart and then to the lungs to be expelled.
coronary arteries	The blood vessels that branch from the aorta and carry oxygen-rich blood to the heart muscle.

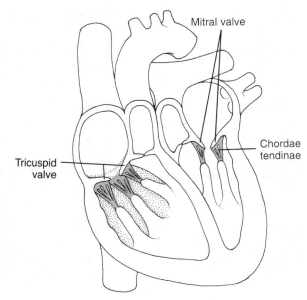

Figure 11–10

Tricuspid and mitral valves. These valves work like parachutes. The chordae tendinae are the strings that attach to the lining of the ventricles and anchor the valve in place. As blood rushes into the ventricles, it strikes the valves (parachute), which swing up, meet in the midline, and fit together so that the valve is shut watertight.

deoxygenated blood	Blood that is oxygen-poor.
diastole	Relaxation phase of the heartbeat.
endocardium	Inner lining of the heart.
endothelium	Innermost lining of blood vessels.
mitral valve	Valve found between the left atrium and the left ventricle of the heart (Fig. 11–10).
murmur	An abnormal heart sound caused by improper closure of heart valves.
myocardium	Muscle layer of the heart.
oxygen	Gas that enters the blood through the lungs and travels to the heart to be pumped via arteries to all body cells.
pacemaker	Sensitive tissue in the right atrium that begins the heartbeat; also called the **sinoatrial node.**
pericardium	Sac-like membrane surrounding the heart.
pulmonary artery	An artery carrying oxygen-poor blood from the heart to the lungs.
pulmonary circulation	The flow of blood from the heart to the lungs and back to the heart.
pulmonary valve	Valve between the right ventricle and the pulmonary artery.
pulmonary vein	A vein carrying oxygenated blood from the lungs to the heart.

pulse   The beat of the heart as felt through the walls of the arteries.

septum (plural: **septa**)   A partition; in the cardiovascular system, a partition between the right and the left sides of the heart.

sinoatrial node (SA node)   The pacemaker of the heart.

sphygmomanometer   Instrument to measure blood pressure.

systemic circulation   The flow of blood from the body cells to the heart and then back out from the heart to the cells.

systole   The contraction phase of the heartbeat.

tricuspid valve   Valve located between the right atrium and the right ventricle; it has three (tri) leaflets, or cusps (see Fig. 11–10).

valve   A structure in veins or in the heart that temporarily closes an opening so that blood flows in only one direction.

vein   Thin-walled blood vessel that carries blood from the body tissues and lungs to the heart.

vena cava (plural: **venae cavae**)   Largest vein in the body. The superior and inferior venae cavae bring blood into the right atrium of the heart.

ventricle   Lower and larger chamber of the heart.

venule   Small vein.

VII. Combining Forms and Terminology

Write the meaning of the medical term in the space provided.

Combining Form	Meaning	Terminology	Meaning
angi/o	vessel	angiogram _____	
		angioplasty _____	
		Percutaneous transluminal coronary angioplasty is described in Section IX, page 373, under Clinical Procedures.	
aort/o	aorta	aortic stenosis _____	
arter/o **arteri/o**	artery	arteriosclerosis _____	

arterial anastomosis _____

arteriography _____

endarterectomy _____

See Section IX, page (372), under Clinical Procedures.

ather/o   yellowish   atherosclerosis _____
                     plaque, fatty
                     substance   *The major form of arteriosclerosis in which deposits of yellow plaque*
                                        containing cholesterol and lipids are found within the lining of the
                                        artery (Fig. 11–11).

atherectomy _____

atheroma _____

The suffix -oma means mass or collection.

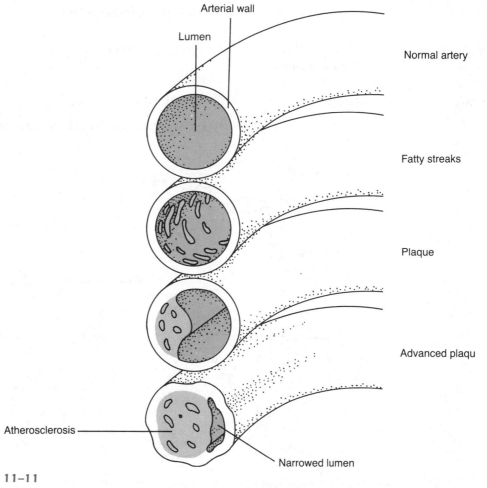

Figure 11–11

Atherosclerosis and narrowing of the lumen of an artery. (From Miller BF, Keane CB: Encyclopedia and Dictionary of Medicine, Nursing, and Allied Health, 4th ed. Philadelphia, WB Saunders, 1987, p 122.)

atri/o	atrium, upper heart chamber	atrial _____
		atrioventricular _____
brachi/o	arm	brachial artery _____
cardi/o	heart	cardiomegaly _____
		cardiomyopathy _____

Toxic or infectious agents may be the cause, but often the etiology is unknown (idiopathic). Hypertrophic cardiomyopathy is an increase in heart muscle weight, especially along the septum, which causes narrowing (stenosis) of the aortic valve.

bradycardia _____

Slower than 60 beats per minute. Normal pulse is about 60–80 beats per minute.

tachycardia _____

Faster than 100 beats per minute.

cholesterol/o	cholesterol (a lipid substance)	hypercholesterolemia _____
coron/o	heart	coronary arteries _____

These arteries come down over the top of the heart like a crown (corona) (Fig. 11–12).

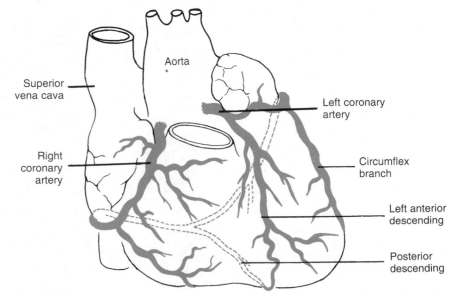

Figure 11–12

Coronary arteries supplying the heart.

cyan/o	blue	cyanosis _____

This bluish discoloration of the skin indicates diminished oxygen content of the blood.

ox/o	oxygen	hypoxia _____
pericardi/o	pericardium	pericardiocentesis _____
phleb/o	vein	phlebotomy _____
		phlebitis _____
rrhythm/o	rhythm	arrhythmia _____
sphygm/o	pulse	sphygmomanometer _____

A manometer measures pressure.

steth/o	chest	stethoscope _____

A misnomer because the examination is by ear, not by eye. Auscultation means listening to sounds within the body using a stethoscope.

thromb/o	clot	thrombolysis _____
valvul/o **valv/o**	valve	valvuloplasty _____
		mitral valvulitis _____
		valvotomy _____
vas/o	vessel	vasoconstriction _____

Constriction means to tighten or narrow.

		vasodilation _____
vascul/o	vessel	vascular _____
ven/o	vein	venous _____
ventricul/o	ventricle, lower heart chamber	ventriculotomy _____
		interventricular septum _____

VIII. Pathological Conditions: The Heart and Blood Vessels

Heart

arrhythmias

Abnormal heart rhythms.

Examples of cardiac arrhythmias are:

1. heart block (atrioventricular block)

Failure of proper conduction of impulses through the AV node to the bundle of His.

Damage to the SA node may cause its impulses to be too weak to activate the AV node and impulses fail to reach the ventricles. If the failure occurs only occasionally, the heart will miss a beat in a rhythm at regular intervals (partial heart block). If no impulses reach the AV node from the SA node, the ventricles contract slower than the atria and are not coordinated. This is complete heart block.

Implantation of a **cardiac pacemaker** can overcome heart block and establish a normal rhythm. Most pacemakers are powered with batteries that will function at a normal heart rate for 5–10 years (Fig. 11–13).

2. flutter

Rapid but regular contractions of atria or ventricles.

This condition can occur in patients with heart disease. The heart rhythm may reach up to 300 beats per minute.

3. fibrillation

Rapid, random, ineffectual, and irregular contractions of the heart (350 beats or more per minute).

In atrial fibrillation, the wave of excitation passes through the atrial myocardium even more quickly than in atrial flutter. In order to restore normal heart rhythm, an electrical device called a **defibrillator** is applied to the chest wall. The electric shock stops the heart and reverses its abnormal rhythm. This is also called

Figure 11–13

Permanent pacemaker is placed within the chest.

Aorta
Postductal coarctation

Figure 11–14

Coarctation of the aorta. (From Tackett JJM, Hunsberger M: Family-Centered Care of Children and Adolescents: Nursing Concepts in Child Health. Philadelphia, WB Saunders, 1981, p 545.)

cardioversion. Drugs, such as **digitalis,** are also used to convert fibrillation into regular rhythm.

Cardiac arrest is the sudden and often unexpected stoppage of heart movement, caused by heart block or ventricular fibrillation (resulting from underlying heart disease).

Palpitations are uncomfortable sensations in the chest associated with different types of arrhythmias. Palpitations do not necessarily indicate serious heart disease (smoking, caffeine, and drugs, such as antidepressants, can produce palpitations). Two cardiac causes of palpitations are **premature ventricular contractions (PVCs)** and **premature atrial contractions (PACs).**

congenital heart disease

Abnormalities in the heart at birth.

The following conditions are congenital anomalies resulting from some failure in the development of the fetal heart.

1. coarctation of the aorta

Narrowing (coarctation) of the aorta.

Figure 11–14 shows one form of coarctation of the aorta. Surgical treatment consists of removal of the constricted region and end-to-end anastomosis of the aortic segments.

2. patent ductus arteriosus

A small duct (ductus arteriosus) between the aorta and the pulmonary artery, which normally closes soon after birth, remains open **(patent).**

This condition, illustrated in Figure 11–15, means that oxygenated blood flows from the aorta to the pulmonary artery. The anomaly occurs most often in females and is commonly associated with intrauterine rubella (German measles) infection, prematurity, and infantile respiratory distress syndrome. Treatment is surgery to close the ductus arteriosus.

3. septal defects

Small holes in the septa between the atria **(atrial septal defects [ASDs])** or the ventricles **(ventricular septal defects [VSDs]).**

Septal defects can be closed while maintaining a general circulation by means of a **heart-lung machine.** This machine is connected to the patient's circulatory system and relieves the heart and lungs of pumping and oxygenation functions during heart surgery.

Many VSDs present at birth will close spontaneously.

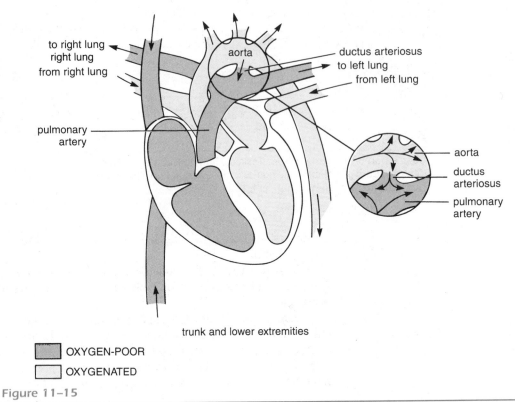

head and upper extremities

to right lung
right lung
from right lung

aorta

ductus arteriosus
to left lung
from left lung

pulmonary
artery

aorta
ductus
arteriosus
pulmonary
artery

trunk and lower extremities

■ OXYGEN-POOR

□ OXYGENATED

Figure 11–15

Patent ductus arteriosus.

---

4. tetralogy of Fallot (fă-LŌ)

A congenital malformation of the heart involving four (tetra-) distinct defects.

The condition, named for Etienne Fallot, the French physician who described it in 1888, is illustrated in Figure 11–16. The four defects are:

1. **Pulmonary artery stenosis.** This means that blood is not adequately passed to the lungs for oxygenation.
2. **Ventricular septal defect.** The gap in the septum allows deoxygenated blood to pass into the left ventricle, and from there to the aorta.
3. **Shift of the aorta to the right,** so that the aorta overrides the interventricular septum. Oxygen-poor blood passes even more easily from the right ventricle to the aorta.
4. **Hypertrophy of the right ventricle.** The myocardium has to work harder to pump blood through a narrowed pulmonary artery.

An infant with this condition is described as a "blue baby" because of the extreme degree of **cyanosis** present at birth (other congenital conditions that involve a shunt of blood from the right to the left without passing through the lungs and receiving proper oxygenation can lead to cyanosis as well). Surgery is required to repair the various heart defects.

congestive heart failure

The heart is unable to pump its required amount of blood (more blood enters the heart from the veins than leaves through the arteries).

Blood accumulates in the lungs (left-sided heart failure) causing **pulmonary edema** (fluid seeps out of capillaries into the tiny air sacs of the lungs). Damming back of blood resulting from right-sided heart failure results in accumulation of fluid in the abdominal organs (liver and spleen) and subcutaneous tissue of the legs. Congestive heart failure often develops gradually over several years, although it can be acute. It is treated with drugs, such as digitalis (digoxin), to strengthen the heart and diuretics to promote loss of fluid.

coronary artery disease

Disease of the arteries surrounding the heart.

The coronary arteries are three large vessels that arise from the aorta and supply oxygenated blood to the heart. It is interesting that the blood that constantly flows through the four hollow chambers of the heart does not itself nourish the myocardial tissue. Instead, after blood leaves the heart via the aorta, a portion is at once led back over the surface of the heart through the coronary arteries, so that the heart muscle receives blood before any other organ. This seems logical because the energy requirements of the heart are greater than those of any other organ. Figure 11–13 shows the right and left coronary arteries as they branch from the aorta.

Coronary artery disease is usually the result of **atherosclerosis.** This is the deposition of fatty compounds on the inner lining of the coronary arteries (any other artery can be similarly affected). The ordinarily smooth lining of the artery becomes roughened as the atherosclerotic plaque collects in the artery.

Atherosclerosis is dangerous for two important reasons. First, narrowing of the vessel due to atherosclerosis can cause inflexibility and plugging up of the vessel. Second, the roughened lining of the artery may rupture or cause abnormal clotting of blood, leading to a **thrombotic occlusion** (blocking of the coronary artery by a

Figure 11–16

Tetralogy of Fallot.

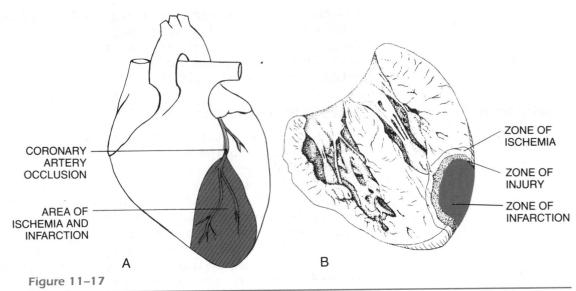

CORONARY
ARTERY
OCCLUSION

AREA OF
ISCHEMIA AND
INFARCTION

A

ZONE OF
ISCHEMIA

ZONE OF
INJURY

ZONE OF
INFARCTION

B

Figure 11–17

(A) Ischemia and infarction produced by coronary artery occlusion. *(B)* Myocardial infarction shown in cross section of heart (ventricles only).

clot). In both cases, blood flow is decreased **(ischemia)** or stopped entirely, leading to death **(necrosis)** of a part of the myocardium. The area of dead myocardial tissue is known as an **infarction.** The infarcted area is eventually replaced by scar tissue. Figure 11–17 illustrates coronary artery occlusion leading to ischemia and infarction of heart muscle.

The severity of a **myocardial infarction** (also known as a **heart attack**) depends on the size of the artery that is blocked and the extent of the blockage. If the blocked artery is small, the result may be death of only a small portion of the heart immediately fed by the artery. After scar tissue forms, the patient may be able to resume completely normal activity.

Angina pectoris is an episode of chest pain resulting from a temporary difference between the supply and the demand of oxygen to the heart muscle. Angina can be the result of low oxygen levels in the blood (from smoking or respiratory disease), restricted blood flow to the heart (coronary artery disease), or an increase in the work of the heart beyond normal levels. For acute attacks of angina, **nitroglycerin** is given sublingually. This drug, one of several called **nitrates,** is a powerful vasodilator and muscle relaxant. Other drugs, called **beta-blockers,** slow the heartbeat and the force of contraction. They block sympathetic nerve stimulation to the myocardium. Examples of beta-blockers are propranolol (Inderal), nadolol (Corgard), and atenolol (Tenormin).

Calcium channel blockers cause dilation of blood vessels, making it easier for the heart to pump blood through the vessels. Examples of calcium channel blockers are nifedipine (Procardia) and verapamil (Isoptin, Calan).

endocarditis

Inflammation of the inner lining of the heart caused by bacteria (also called **bacterial endocarditis**).

This condition may be a complication of another infectious disease, an operation, or an injury. Damage to the heart valves can produce lesions called **vegetations** (named because they looked like cauliflower) that may break off into the bloodstream as **emboli** (material that travels through the bloodstream). When the emboli lodge in the small vessels of the skin, multiple pinpoint hemorrhages known as **petechiae** (from the Italian *petechio,* meaning a fleabite) form. Antibiotics are effective in curing bacterial endocarditis.

hypertensive heart disease

High blood pressure affecting the heart.

This condition is caused by the contraction of arterioles of the body leading to increased pressure in arteries. The heart itself is affected because it has to pump more vigorously to overcome the increased resistance in the arteries. The vessels lose their elasticity, become like solid pipes, and place increased burden on the heart to pump blood through the body.

mitral valve prolapse (MVP)

Improper closure of the mitral valve when the heart is pumping blood (Fig. 11–18).

This condition, found most frequently in otherwise healthy young women, occurs because the mitral valve enlarges and prolapses into the left atrium during systole. The physician hears a midsystolic click upon auscultation (listening with a stethoscope). Most people with MVP live normal lives, but because prolapsed valves can on rare occasions become infected, persons with MVP are advised to have preventive antibiotics at the time of dental procedures if the murmur is present.

murmur

An extra heart sound, heard between normal beats.

Murmurs are heard with the aid of a stethoscope and are usually caused by a valvular defect or disease that disrupts the smooth flow of blood in the heart. They can also be heard in cases of interseptal defects where blood is flowing abnormally between chambers through holes in the septa. A functional murmur is one that is not caused by a valve or septal defect and is not a serious danger to the patient's health.

pericarditis

Inflammation of the membrane (pericardium) surrounding the heart.

In most instances, pericarditis is secondary to disease elsewhere in the body (such as pulmonary infection). Bacteria and viruses can cause the condition, or the etiology may be idiopathic. Malaise, fever, and chest pain occur, as well as accumulation of fluid within the pericardial cavity. Compression of the heart due to collection of fluid is called cardiac tamponade (tăm-pŏ-NĀD). If a considerable amount of fluid is present, pressure on the pulmonary veins may slow the return of blood from the lungs. Excess fluid is drained by pericardiocentesis.

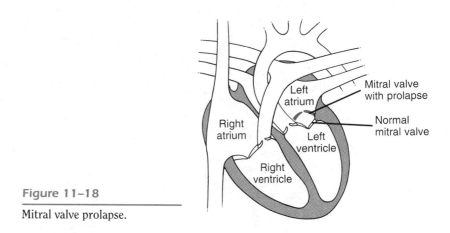

Figure 11–18

Mitral valve prolapse.

rheumatic heart disease Heart disease caused by rheumatic fever.

Rheumatic fever is a disease, usually occurring in childhood, that can follow a few weeks after a streptococcal infection. Damage may be done to the heart, particularly the heart valves, by one or more attacks of rheumatic fever. The valves, especially the mitral valve, become inflamed and scarred (with vegetations), so that they do not open and close normally. **Mitral stenosis,** atrial fibrillation, and congestive heart failure, due to weakening of the myocardium, can occur. Treatment consists of reduced activity, drugs to control arrhythmia, surgery to repair a damaged valve, and anticoagulant therapy to prevent emboli from forming. Mechanical or porcine (pig) valve implants are also used to replace deteriorated heart valves. Figure 11–19 shows types of artificial valves.

Blood Vessels

aneurysm Local widening (ballooning out of a small area) of an artery caused by weakness in the arterial wall or breakdown of the wall owing to atherosclerosis.

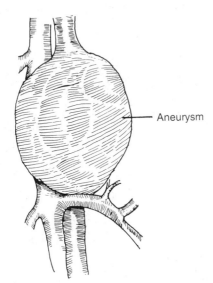

Aneurysm

Figure 11–20

Aneurysm of the aorta.

Aneurysm literally means to widen (-eurysm) up (ana-). It may occur anywhere in the body but most commonly in the aorta. The danger of an aneurysm is that as the wall of the artery pushes outward it becomes progressively thinner and may eventually rupture. Figure 11-20 shows an aneurysm of the aorta. Treatment of an aneurysm depends on the particular vessel involved, the site, and the health of the patient. In aneurysms of small vessels in the brain, treatment is occlusion of the vessel with small clips. For larger arteries, such as the aorta, a synthetic graft is sewn within the aneurysm.

hypertension

High blood pressure.

Most high blood pressure is **essential hypertension,** in which the cause of the increased pressure is idiopathic. In adults, a blood pressure equal to or greater than 140/90 mmHg is considered high. Diuretics, beta-blockers, and other drugs are used as treatment for essential hypertension. Losing weight, limiting sodium (salt) intake, stopping smoking, and reducing fat in the diet are also important in therapy.

In **secondary hypertension,** there is always some associated lesion, such as glomerulonephritis, pyelonephritis, or disease of the adrenal glands, that is responsible for the elevated blood pressure.

peripheral vascular disease

Blockage of blood vessels (arteries) in the lower extremities due to atherosclerosis.

When arteries in the groin or upper leg narrow or become blocked, blood flow to the lower leg and feet is reduced. Often, the **femoral** (thigh) **artery** or the **popliteal** (back of the knee) **artery** is involved. An early sign of the problem is **intermittent claudication** (absence of pain or discomfort in a leg at rest, but pain, tension, and weakness after walking has begun). Treatment is exercise, avoidance of nicotine, which causes vessel constriction, and control of risk factors such as hypertension, hyperlipidemia, and diabetes. Surgical treatment includes endarterectomy and bypass grafting (from the normal proximal vessel around the diseased area to a normal vessel distally).

Raynaud's phenomenon

Short episodes of pallor and numbness in the fingers and toes due to temporary constriction of arterioles in the skin.

This condition is usually idiopathic, but it may also be secondary to some other, more serious disorder. The episodes can be triggered by cold temperatures, emotional stress, or cigarette smoking. Protecting the body from cold and use of vasodilators are effective treatment.

varicose veins

Abnormally swollen and twisted veins, usually occurring in the legs.

This condition is due to damaged valves that fail to prevent the backflow of blood (Fig. 11–21). The blood then collects in the veins, which distend to many times their normal size. Because of the slow flow of blood in the varicose veins and frequent injury to the vein, thrombosis may occur as well. **Hemorrhoids** (piles) are varicose veins near the anus (Fig. 11–22). Surgical treatment of hemorrhoids includes injection of sclerosing solutions, ligation with rubber bands, and cryosurgery.

Treatment of varicose veins includes wearing elastic stockings, elevation of the legs if edema occurs, and surgery to ligate (tie off) and strip (remove) the twisted swollen veins. The surgical procedure is called vein stripping.

NORMAL VEINS

Functional valves
aid in flow of venous
blood back to heart

(see enlargement at left)

VARICOSE VEINS

Failure of valves and
pooling of blood in
superficial veins

Figure 11–21

Normal and varicose veins. (From O'Toole M [ed]: Miller-Keane Encyclopedia and Dictionary of Medicine, Nursing, and Allied Health, 5th ed. Philadelphia, WB Saunders, 1992, p 1575.)

Figure 11–22

Hemorrhoids (internal, external, and prolapsed). (From Ignatavicius DD, Bayne MV: Medical-Surgical Nursing: A Nursing Process Approach. Philadelphia, WB Saunders, 1991, p 1403.)

Internal

External

Prolapsed

STUDY SECTION

Practice spelling each term and know its meaning.

angina pectoris

Chest pain resulting from a temporary difference between the supply and the demand of oxygen to the heart muscle.

auscultation

Listening with a stethoscope.

beta-blockers

Drugs used to treat angina, hypertension, and arrhythmias. They block the action of epinephrine (Adrenalin) at receptor sites on cells so that the heart beats more slowly and with less force and requires less oxygen.

calcium channel blockers

Drugs used to treat angina and hypertension. They dilate blood vessels by blocking the influx of calcium into muscles that line the vessels.

claudication

Pain, tension, and weakness in a leg after walking has begun, but absence of pain at rest.

digitalis

Drug that increases the strength and regularity of the heartbeat.

emboli (singular: **embolus**)

Collections of material (clots or other substances) that travel to and suddenly block a blood vessel.

infarction

Area of dead tissue.

nitrates

Drugs used in the treatment of angina pectoris. They dilate blood vessels, so that a patient is less likely to develop myocardial oxygen deficit.

nitroglycerin

A nitrate drug used in the treatment of angina pectoris.

occlusion

Closure of a blood vessel.

palpitations

Uncomfortable sensations in the chest related to cardiac arrhythmias.

patent

Open.

petechiae

Small, pinpoint hemorrhages.

vegetations

Collections of platelets, clotting proteins, microorganisms, and red blood cells that attach to the endocardium in conditions such as bacterial endocarditis and rheumatic heart disease.

IX. Laboratory Tests, Clinical Procedures, and Abbreviations

Laboratory Tests

lipid tests

Lipids are fatty substances found in foods and in the body. Examples of lipids are **cholesterol** and **triglycerides.** Lipid tests measure the amounts of these substances in a blood sample. High levels of triglycerides and cholesterol in the blood are associated with a greater risk of atherosclerosis. A cholesterol level in a middle-aged adult below 200 mg/dL is associated with a relatively low risk for coronary artery disease (CAD). A diet high in **saturated fat** (solid fats of animal origin, such as in milk, butter, and meats) tends to increase the amount of cholesterol in the blood. **Polyunsaturated fats** (such as corn oil and safflower oil) do not raise blood cholesterol.

The mainstay of treatment for people with hyperlipidemia is proper diet (low fat and high fiber intake with fresh fruits and vegetables) and exercise. Niacin (a vitamin) is also helpful in reducing lipids. Drug therapy is sometimes administered and includes cholestyramine (Questran), gemfibrozil (Lopid), and lovastatin (Mevacor), all of which lower blood cholesterol.

lipoprotein electrophoresis

Lipoproteins are proteins that carry lipids (fats) in the bloodstream. Protein electrophoresis is the process of physically separating lipoproteins from a blood sample. High levels of **low-density lipoproteins (LDL)** and **very low density lipoproteins (VLDL)** are associated with atherosclerosis. High levels of **high-density lipoproteins (HDL),** which remove cholesterol and transport it to the liver, protect adults from the development of atherosclerosis. Factors that increase HDL are estrogen, exercise, and alcohol in moderation.

serum enzyme tests

During a myocardial infarction, enzymes are released into the bloodstream from the dying heart muscle. These enzymes can be measured and are useful as evidence of an infarction. The enzymes tested for are **creatine phosphokinase (CPK)** and **lactate dehydrogenase (LDH).** Newer blood tests measure levels of muscle proteins, myoglobin and troponin-T.

Clinical Procedures

X-Ray Tests

angiography

Dye is injected into the bloodstream or heart chamber, and x-rays are taken of the heart and large blood vessels in the chest. If dye is injected into the aorta or an artery in the groin the procedure is called **arteriography.**

digital subtraction angiography (DSA)

Video equipment and a computer are used to produce x-ray pictures of blood vessels. First, an x-ray is taken of the area to be studied, and the results are stored in a computer. Next, contrast material is injected into a vein, and a second image is produced that is also recorded in the computer. The computer then compares the two images and subtracts the first image from the second (removing parts not being studied such as bone, muscle, and fat), leaving nothing but an image of the contrast medium and vessels.

Ultrasound Tests

Doppler ultrasound An instrument is used to focus sound waves on a blood vessel; blood flow is measured as echoes bounce off of red blood cells. Velocity of blood flow increases in areas of stenosis. Arteries or veins in the arms, neck, or legs are examined to detect vascular occlusion (blockage due to clots or atherosclerosis).

echocardiography (ECHO) Pulses of high-frequency sound waves (ultrasound) are transmitted into the chest, and echoes returning from the valves, chambers, and surfaces of the heart are electronically plotted and recorded. This procedure can show the structure and movement of the heart.

Radioactive Tests

cardiac scan A radioactive substance is injected intravenously, and its accumulation in heart muscle is measured with a special detection device (scanner). The presence of ischemia and myocardial infarction can be demonstrated as areas of decreased movement during the contraction of the heart.

Magnetic Resonance Imaging (MRI)

cardiac MRI Magnetic waves are beamed at the heart, and an image is produced. The procedure is used to obtain detailed information about congenital heart disease, cardiac masses, and lesions of large blood vessels prior to surgery.

Other Procedures

cardiac catheterization A thin, flexible tube (catheter) is introduced into a vein or artery and is guided into the heart for purposes of detecting pressures and patterns of blood flow. Dye can also be injected and x-rays taken (angiography). Figure 11–23 shows catheterization of the heart.

Catheter inserted in femoral artery

Figure 11–23

Cardiac catheterization.

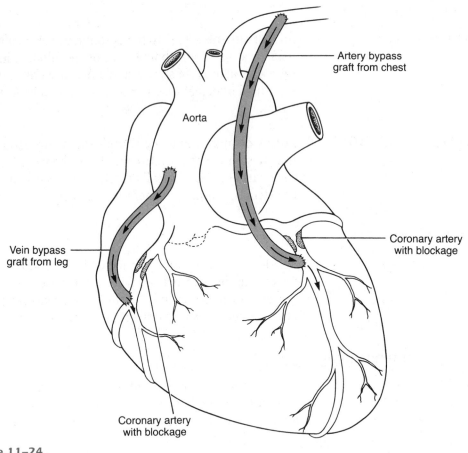

Aorta

Artery bypass
graft from chest

Coronary artery
with blockage

Vein bypass
graft from leg

Coronary artery
with blockage

Figure 11–24

Coronary artery bypass surgery with anastomosis of vein and arterial grafts.

cardioversion (defibrillation)	Very brief discharges of electricity are applied across the chest to stop a cardiac arrhythmia and to allow a more normal rhythm to begin.
coronary bypass surgery (CABG)	Vessel grafts, consisting of veins taken from other parts of the body, are anastomosed (connected) to existing coronary arteries to detour around blockages in the coronary arteries and keep the myocardium supplied with oxygenated blood (Fig. 11–24).
electrocardiography (EKG, ECG)	Process of recording the electricity flowing through the heart.
endarterectomy	This procedure involves surgical removal of the innermost (end-) lining of an artery when it is thickened by fatty deposits (atheromas) and thromboses.
extracorporeal circulation	A heart-lung machine is used as a bypass to divert blood from the heart and lungs while the heart is being repaired. Blood leaves the body, enters the heart-lung machine, where it is oxygenated, and then returns to a blood vessel (artery) to circulate through the bloodstream. Extracorporeal means outside (extra-) the body (corpor/o).
heart transplantation	A donor heart is tranferred to a recipient. The surgery consists of removal of the diseased heart (from cardiomyopathy or heart failure), leaving the

Figure 11–25

Heart transplantation. (From Ignatavicius DD, Bayne MV: Medical-Surgical Nursing: A Nursing Process Approach. Philadelphia, WB Saunders, 1991, p 2170.)

posterior walls of the recipient's atria, and anastomosis of the atria, aorta, and pulmonary arteries (Fig. 11–25).

Holter monitoring

A compact version (about the size of a portable tape player) of an electrocardiograph (instrument to measure the electricity flowing through the heart) is worn during a 24-hour period to detect cardiac arrhythmias.

percutaneous transluminal coronary angioplasty (PTCA)

In this procedure, also called **balloon catheter dilation,** a catheter equipped with a small balloon on the end is inserted via the femoral (thigh) artery and threaded up the aorta into a coronary artery. The balloon is then carefully inflated, compressing fatty deposits or plaque against the side of the artery and opening the artery to allow for the passage of blood. **Balloon valvuloplasty** is used to open narrowed cardiac valves and is seen as a possible alternative to surgery for valvular stenosis.

Plaque is removed (atherectomy) using devices such as low-speed rotating catheters. Lasers and stents (expandable slotted tubes) are used to create wider lumens and may make restenosis less likely. Figure 11–26 illustrates PTCA.

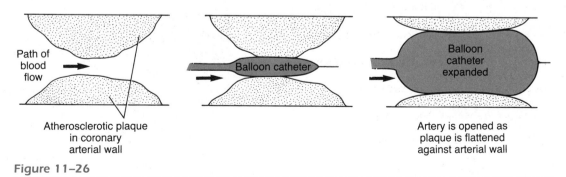

Figure 11–26

Percutaneous transluminal coronary angioplasty.

stress test	Also known as exercise tolerance test (ETT), this procedure determines the heart's response to physical exertion (stress). An EKG and other measurements (blood pressure and heart rate) are taken while the patient is exercising on a treadmill. Changes in the EKG during increasing workload or stress indicate the presence and severity of ischemia.
thrombolytic therapy	Drugs, such as **tPA** (tissue-type plasminogen activator) and **streptokinase,** that dissolve clots are injected into the bloodstream in patients diagnosed as having a coronary thrombosis. This technique, which restores blood flow to the heart and limits irreversible damage to heart muscle, must be undertaken within 12 hours after the onset of a heart attack. Thrombolytic agents reduce mortality in patients with myocardial infarction by 25 per cent.

ABBREVIATIONS

AF	Atrial fibrillation	**HDL**	High-density lipoproteins; high blood levels are associated with lower incidence of coronary artery disease
AS	Aortic stenosis		
ASD	Atrial septal defect	**LDH**	Lactate dehydrogenase (enzyme released from dying heart muscle)
AV, A-V	Atrioventricular		
BP	Blood pressure	**LDL**	Low-density lipoproteins
CABG	Coronary artery bypass graft	**LV**	Left ventricle
CAD	Coronary artery disease	**LVH**	Left ventricular hypertrophy
CCU	Coronary care unit	**MI**	Myocardial infarction
Cath	Catheterization	**MR**	Mitral regurgitation
CHD	Coronary heart disease	**MUGA**	Multiple-gated acquisition scan; a radioactive test of heart function
CHF	Congestive heart failure	**MVP**	Mitral valve prolapse
CPK	Creatine phosphokinase; released into bloodstream following injury to heart or skeletal muscles	**PAC**	Premature atrial contraction
		PDA	Patent ductus arteriosus
CVP	Central venous pressure (measured with catheter in the superior vena cava)	**PND**	Paroxysmal (sudden) nocturnal dyspnea (difficult breathing); often a symptom of congestive heart failure
DOE	Dyspnea on exertion		
DSA	Digital subtraction angiography	**PTCA**	Percutaneous transluminal coronary angioplasty
DVT	Deep venous thrombosis	**PVC**	Premature ventricular contraction
ECC	Extracorporeal circulation	**SA, S-A**	Sinoatrial
ECG	Electrocardiogram	**tPA**	Tissue-type plasminogen activator; a drug used to prevent thromboses
ECHO	Echocardiography		
EKG	Electrocardiogram	**VLDL**	Very low density lipoproteins
ETT	Exercise tolerance test	**VSD**	Ventricular septal defect
		VT	Ventricular tachycardia

X. Practical Applications

Operating Schedule: General Hospital

Match the operation in column I with a diagnosis in column II. Answers are found at the end of Answers to Exercises, page 387.

COLUMN I—Operation

1. Coronary artery bypass _____

2. Left carotid endarterectomy _____

3. Varicose vein bilateral ligation and stripping _____

4. LV aneurysmectomy _____

5. Atrial septal defect repair _____

6. Pulmonary balloon valvuloplasty _____

7. Pericardiocentesis _____

8. Aortic valve replacement _____

9. Pacemaker implantation _____

10. Femoral-popliteal bypass graft _____

COLUMN II — Diagnosis

A. stenosis of the pulmonary valve

B. cardiac tamponade (fluid in the space surrounding the heart)

C. atherosclerotic occlusion of a main artery leading to the head

D. congenital hole in the wall of the upper chamber of the heart

E. disabling angina pectoris and extensive coronary atherosclerosis despite medical therapy

F. peripheral vascular disease

G. heart block

H. swollen, twisted blood vessels in the leg

I. protrusion of the wall of a lower heart chamber

J. aortic stenosis

Medical Language As Written

1. The main determinants of death after acute MI are the extent of left ventricular damage and occurrence of arrhythmias.

2. Evaluation of risk factors for sudden cardiac death is important in patients with coronary artery disease. Risk factors include a family history of sudden cardiac death and early MI (before age 50), hypertension and left ventricular hypertrophy, smoking, diabetes mellitus, and markedly elevated serum cholesterol levels.

3. A 24-year-old woman with a history of palpitations [heartbeat is unusually strong, rapid, or irregular, so that patient is aware of it] and vague chest pains enters the hospital. With the patient supine, you hear a midsystolic click that is followed by a grade 3/6 [moderately loud—6/6 is loud and 1/6 is quiet] honking murmur. Your diagnosis: mitral valve prolapse (click-murmur syndrome).

4. A 47-year-old man had a myocardial infarction in November 1984. On March 3, 1985, he was readmitted to the hospital with an acute inferior myocardial infarction,

> documented by electrocardiograms and blood enzyme elevations. On April 8, the patient developed a loud systolic murmur and his blood pressure fell sharply. A diagnosis of rupture of the ventricular septum was made, and he was transferred to the surgical service. Right cardiac catheterization confirmed the presence of a left-to-right shunt [of blood] at the ventricular level. Emergency surgery was attempted, but the patient died suddenly. Autopsy diagnosis: ruptured ventricular septum secondary to myocardial infarction.

XI. Exercises

Remember to check your answers carefully with those given in Section XII, Answers to Exercises.

A. *Match the following terms with their meanings below.*

arteriole   venule   tricuspid valve
aorta   atrium   pulmonary artery
mitral valve   superior vena cava pulmonary vein
capillary   inferior vena cava ventricle

1. valve that lies between the right atrium and the right ventricle _____

2. smallest blood vessel _____

3. carries oxygenated blood from the lungs to the heart _____

4. largest artery in the body _____

5. brings oxygen-poor blood into the heart from the upper parts of the body

   _____

6. upper chamber of the heart _____

7. carries oxygen-poor blood to the lungs from the heart _____

8. small artery _____

9. valve that lies between the left atrium and the left ventricle _____

10. brings blood from the lower half of the body to the heart _____

11. a small vein _____

12. lower chamber of the heart _____

B. *Trace the path of blood through the heart. Begin as the blood enters the right atrium from the venae cavae (and include the valves within the heart).*

1. _____   7. _____

2. _____   8. _____

3. _____   9. _____

4. _____   10. _____

5. _____   11. _____

6. capillaries of the lung   12. aorta

C. *Complete the following sentences.*

1. The pacemaker of the heart is the _____ .

2. The sac-like membrane surrounding the heart is the _____ .

3. The wall of the heart between the right and the left atria is the _____ .

4. The relaxation phase of the heartbeat is called _____ .

5. Specialized conductive tissue in the wall between the ventricles is the _____ .

6. The inner lining of the heart is the _____ .

7. The contractive phase of the heartbeat is called _____ .

8. A gas released as a metabolic product of catabolism is _____ .

9. Specialized conductive tissue at the base of the wall between the two upper heart chambers is the _____ .

10. The inner lining of the pericardium, adhering to the outside of the heart, is the

   _____ .

11. An abnormal heart sound caused by improper closure of heart valves is a

   _____ .

12. The beat of the heart as felt through the walls of arteries is called the _____ .

D. Complete the following terms from their definitions.

1. hardening of arteries: arterio _____

2. disease condition of heart muscle: cardio _____

3. enlargement of the heart: cardio _____

4. inflammation of a vein: phleb _____

5. condition of rapid heartbeat: _____ cardia

6. condition of slow heartbeat: _____ cardia

7. high levels of cholesterol in the blood: hyper _____

8. surgical repair of a valve: valvulo _____

9. condition of deficient oxygen: hyp _____

10. pertaining to an upper heart chamber: _____ al

11. narrowing of the mitral valve: mitral _____

12. breakdown of a clot: thrombo _____

E. Give the meanings for the following terms.

1. cyanosis _____

2. phlebotomy _____

3. arterial anastomosis _____

4. aneurysmorrhaphy _____

5. atheroma _____

6. arrhythmia _____

7. sphygmomanometer _____

8. stethoscope _____

9. mitral valvulitis _____

10. atherosclerosis _____

11. vasoconstriction _____

12. vasodilation _____

F. Match the following pathological conditions of the heart with their meanings below.

fibrillation	tetralogy of Fallot	endocarditis
hypertensive heart disease	atrial septal defect	pericarditis
coarctation of the aorta	congestive heart failure	mitral valve prolapse
patent ductus arteriosus	coronary artery disease	flutter

1. inflammation of the inner lining of the heart _____

2. rapid but regular atrial or ventricular contractions _____

3. small hole between the upper heart chambers; congenital anomaly

   _____

4. improper closure of the valve between the left atrium and ventricle during systole

   _____

5. blockage of the arteries surrounding the heart leading to ischemia _____

6. high blood pressure affecting the heart _____

7. rapid, random, ineffectual, and irregular contractions of the heart _____

8. inflammation of the sac surrounding the heart _____

9. inability of the heart to pump its required amount of blood _____

10. congenital malformation involving four separate heart defects _____

11. congenital narrowing of the large artery leading from the heart _____

12. a small duct between the aorta and the pulmonary artery, which normally closes soon after birth,

    remains open _____

G. Give the meanings for the following terms.

1. heart block _____

2. cardiac arrest _____

3. palpitations _____

4. artificial cardiac pacemaker _____

5. thrombotic occlusion _____

6. angina pectoris _____

7. myocardial infarction _____

8. necrosis _____

9. infarction _____

10. ischemia _____

11. nitroglycerin _____

12. digitalis _____

H. Match the following terms with their descriptions.

rheumatic heart disease	vegetations	emboli
Raynaud's phenomenon	essential hypertension	secondary hypertension
petechiae	auscultation	peripheral vascular disease
aneurysm	claudication	murmur

1. lesions that form on heart valves after damage by infection _____

2. clots that travel to and suddenly block a blood vessel _____

3. small, pinpoint hemorrhages _____

4. an extra heart sound, heard between normal beats and caused by a valvular defect or condition that

   disrupts the smooth flow of blood through the heart _____

5. listening with a stethoscope _____

6. heart disease caused by rheumatic fever _____

7. high blood pressure in arteries when the etiology is idiopathic _____

8. high blood pressure related to kidney disease _____

9. short episodes of pallor and numbness in fingers and toes due to a temporary constriction of arterioles

   in the skin _____

10. local widening of an artery _____

11. pain, tension, and weakness in a limb after walking has begun _____

12. blockage of arteries in the lower extremities; etiology is atherosclerosis _____

I. Give short answers for the following.

1. Name three types of drugs used to treat angina _____

   _____ .

2. When damaged valves in veins fail to prevent the backflow of blood the condition that results is called

   _____ .

3. If veins are swollen and twisted in the rectal region, the condition is known as

   _____ .

4. Name the four defects in tetralogy of Fallot from their descriptions:

   A. Narrowing of the artery leading to the lungs from the heart

   _____ .

   B. Gap in the wall between the ventricles _____ .

   C. The large vessel leading from the left ventricle moves over the interventricular septum

   _____ .

   D. Excessive development of the wall of the right lower heart chamber _____ .

J. **Select from the following terms to complete the definitions below.**

lipid test   angiography   cardiac MRI
lipoprotein electrophoresis   echocardiography   cardioversion
serum enzyme test   cardiac scan   coronary bypass surgery
electrocardiography   endarterectomy   stress test

1. surgical removal of the innermost lining of an artery when it is thickened with fatty deposits

   _____

2. very brief discharges of electricity are applied across the chest to stop a cardiac arrhythmia; defibrillation _____

3. measurement of levels of fatty substances (cholesterol and triglycerides) in the bloodstream

   _____

4. measurement of the heart's response to physical exertion (patient is monitored while jogging on a treadmill) _____

5. blood measurement of creatine phosphokinase (CPK) and lactate dehydrogenase (LDH) after myocardial infarction _____

6. contrast material is injected into vessels and x-rays are taken _____

7. process of recording the electricity in the heart _____

8. a radioactive substance is injected intravenously, and its accumulation in heart muscle is measured with a special detection device _____

9. pulses of high-frequency sound waves are transmitted into the chest, and echoes are electronically recorded to show the structure and movement of the heart _____

10. process of physically separating HDL, VLDL, and LDL from a blood sample

    _____

11. vessel grafts are anastomosed to existing coronary arteries to keep the myocardium supplied with oxygenated blood _____

12. magnetic waves are beamed at the heart, and an image is produced to show the structure of the heart

    _____

K. *Give the meanings for the following terms and abbreviations.*

1. digital subtraction angiography _____

2. HDL _____

3. CAD _____

4. heart transplantation _____

5. balloon catheter dilation _____

6. Doppler ultrasound _____

7. Holter monitoring _____

8. thrombolytic therapy _____

9. extracorporeal circulation _____

10. cardiac catheterization _____

L. *The figure below shows a congenital heart defect characterized by a murmur (up to grade 5 in intensity) and an associated thrill (a vibration in the chest felt by the examiner on palpation).*

What is your diagnosis? _____

M. *Give the meanings for the following abbreviations.*

1. CCU _____

2. SA _____

3. ECHO _____

4. MI _____

5. MVP _____

6. PAC _____

7. ECG _____

8. tPA _____

9. VSD _____

10. AS _____

N. Spell the term correctly from its definition below.

1. pertaining to the heart: _____ary

2. not a normal heart rhythm: arr _____

3. abnormal condition of blueness: _____osis

4. relaxation phase of the heart beat: _____tole

5. chest pain: _____ pectoris

6. inflammation of a vein: _____itis

7. widening of a vessel: vaso _____

8. enlargement of the heart: cardio _____

9. hardening of arteries with fatty plaque: _____sclerosis

10. swollen veins in the rectal region: _____oids

O. Match the following surgical terms with their meanings below.

CABG   atherectomy   PTCA
embolectomy   valvotomy   aneurysmorrhaphy
endarterectomy   pericardiocentesis

1. incision of a heart valve _____

2. removal of a clot that has traveled into a blood vessel and suddenly caused occlusion

_____

3. coronary bypass surgery (to relieve ischemia) _____

4. surgical puncture to remove fluid from the pericardial space _____

5. percutaneous transluminal coronary angioplasty _____

6. removal of the inner lining of an artery to make it wider _____

7. suture (repair) of a ballooned out portion of an artery _____

8. removal of plaque from an artery (using rotating catheters, lasers, and stents)

_____

P. Select the term that best completes each sentence.

1. Simon was having pain in his chest that radiated up his neck and down his arm. He called Dr. Dan who thought Simon should report to the emergency room immediately. The first test they performed was a (stress test, EKG, balloon angioplasty).

2. Dr. Kelly explained to family that their observation about the bluish color of baby Charles' skin helped him make the diagnosis of a (thrombotic, aneurysmal, septal) defect in the baby's heart, which needed immediate attention.

3. Mr. Duggan had a fever of unknown origin. When the doctors completed an echocardiogram and saw vegetations on his mitral valve, they suspected (bacterial endocarditis, hypertensive heart disease, angina pectoris).

4. Claudia's hands turned red, almost purple, whenever she went out into the cold or became stressed. Her physician thought it might be wise to work her up for (varicose veins, Raynaud's phenomenon, intermittent claudication).

5. Daisy's heart felt like it was skipping beats every time she drank coffee. Her physician suggested that she wear a (Holter monitor, PTCA, CABG) for 24 hours to assess the nature of the arrhythmia.

XII. Answers to Exercises

A

1. tricuspid valve	5. superior vena cava	9. mitral valve
2. capillary	6. atrium	10. inferior vena cava
3. pulmonary vein	7. pulmonary artery	11. venule
4. aorta	8. arteriole	12. ventricle

B

1. right atrium	5. pulmonary artery	9. mitral valve
2. tricuspid valve	6. capillaries of the lung	10. left ventricle
3. right ventricle	7. pulmonary veins	11. aortic valve
4. pulmonary valve	8. left atrium	12. aorta

C

1. sinoatrial (SA) node	6. endocardium	10. visceral pericardium (the outer lining is
2. pericardium	7. systole	the parietal pericardium)
3. interatrial septum	8. carbon dioxide (CO_2)	11. murmur
4. diastole	9. atrioventricular (AV) node	12. pulse
5. bundle of His		

D

1. arteriosclerosis
2. cardiomyopathy
3. cardiomegaly
4. phlebitis
5. tachycardia
6. bradycardia
7. hypercholesterolemia
8. valvuloplasty
9. hypoxia
10. atrial
11. mitral stenosis
12. thrombolysis

E

1. bluish discoloration of the skin owing to deficient oxygen in the blood
2. incision of a vein
3. new connection between arteries
4. suturing (repair) of an aneurysm
5. mass of yellowish plaque (fatty substance)
6. abnormal heart rhythm
7. instrument to measure blood pressure
8. instrument to listen to sounds within the chest
9. inflammation of the mitral valve
10. hardening of arteries with a yellowish, fatty substance (plaque)
11. narrowing of a vessel
12. widening of a vessel

F

1. endocarditis
2. flutter
3. atrial septal defect
4. mitral valve prolapse
5. coronary artery disease
6. hypertensive heart disease
7. fibrillation
8. pericarditis
9. congestive heart failure
10. tetralogy of Fallot
11. coarctation of the aorta
12. patent ductus arteriosus

G

1. failure of proper conduction of impulses through the AV node to the bundle of His
2. sudden stoppage of heart movement
3. uncomfortable sensations in the chest associated with arrhythmias
4. battery-operated device that is placed in the chest and wired to send electrical current to the heart to establish a normal rhythm
5. blockage of a vessel by a clot
6. chest pain resulting from insufficient oxygen being supplied to the heart muscle
7. area of necrosis (dead tissue) in the heart muscle; heart attack
8. abnormal condition of death (dead tissue)
9. tissue that dies because of deprivation of oxygen
10. blood is held back from an area of the body
11. a nitrate drug used in the treatment of angina pectoris
12. a drug that increases the strength and regularity of the heartbeat

H

1. vegetations
2. emboli
3. petechiae
4. murmur
5. auscultation
6. rheumatic heart disease
7. essential hypertension
8. secondary hypertension
9. Raynaud's phenomenon
10. aneurysm
11. claudication
12. peripheral vascular disease

I

1. nitrates, beta-blockers, calcium channel blockers
2. varicose veins
3. hemorrhoids
4. A. pulmonary artery stenosis
   B. ventricular septal defect
   C. shift of the aorta to the right
   D. hypertrophy of the right ventricle

J

1. endarterectomy
2. cardioversion
3. lipid test
4. stress test
5. serum enzyme test (-ase means enzyme)
6. angiography (arteriography)
7. electrocardiogram
8. cardiac scan
9. echocardiography
10. lipoprotein electrophoresis
11. coronary bypass surgery
12. cardiac MRI

K

1. Video equipment and a computer produce x-ray pictures of blood vessels by taking two pictures (without dye and with dye) and subtracting the first image (without dye) from the second.
2. High-density lipoproteins (high levels of these protect adults from atherosclerosis).
3. Coronary artery disease.
4. A donor heart is transferred to a recipient.
5. A catheter is threaded into a coronary artery, and a balloon is inflated that compresses the fatty deposits and opens the artery so that more blood can pass through (also called percutaneous transluminal coronary angioplasty).
6. An instrument that focuses sound waves on a blood vessel to measure blood flow.
7. A compact version of an electrocardiograph is worn during a 24-hour period to detect cardiac arrhythmias.
8. Treatment with drugs (streptokinase and tPA) to dissolve clots after a heart attack.
9. A heart-lung machine is used to divert blood from the heart and lungs during surgery. The machine oxygenates the blood and sends it back into the bloodstream.
10. A catheter (tube) is inserted into an artery or vein and threaded into the heart chambers. Dye can be injected to take x-ray pictures, patterns of blood flow can be detected, and blood pressures can be measured.

L

1. ventricular septal defect

M

1. coronary care unit
2. sinoatrial
3. echocardiography
4. myocardial infarction (heart attack)
5. mitral valve prolapse
6. premature atrial contractions
7. electrocardiogram
8. tissue plasminogen activator (used in thrombolytic therapy)
9. ventricular septal defect
10. aortic stenosis

N

1. coronary
2. arrhythmia
3. cyanosis
4. diastole

5. angina pectoris
6. phlebitis
7. vasodilation

8. cardiomegaly
9. atherosclerosis
10. hemorrhoids

O

1. valvotomy
2. embolectomy
3. CABG
4. pericardiocentesis

5. PTCA
6. endarterectomy
7. aneurysmorrhaphy
8. atherectomy

P

1. EKG
2. septal
3. bacterial endocarditis

4. Raynaud's phenomenon
5. Holter monitor

Answers to Practical Applications

1. E
2. C
3. H
4. I

5. D
6. A
7. B

8. J
9. G
10. F

XIII. Pronunciation of Terms

To test your understanding of the terminology in this chapter, write the meaning of each term in the space provided. In addition, you may wish to cover the terms and write them by looking at your definitions. Make sure your spelling is correct. The page number after each term indicates where it is defined or used in the text so you can easily check your responses. (If you are not sure what the pronunciation symbols mean, refer to page 21.)

Vocabulary and Terminology

Term	Pronunciation	Meaning
angiogram (356)	ĂN-jē-ō-grăm	
angioplasty (356)	ĂN-jē-ō-plăs-tē	
aorta (354)	ā-ŎR-tă	
aortic stenosis (356)	ā-ŎR-tĭk stĕ-NŌ-sĭs	
arrhythmia (359)	ā-RĬTH-mē-ă	
arterial anastomosis (357)	ăr-TĒ-rē-ăl ă-năs-tō-MŌ-sĭs	
arteriography (357)	ăr-tē-rē-ŎG-ră-fē	
arteriole (354)	ăr-TĒ-rē-ōl	
arteriosclerosis (356)	ăr-tē-rē-ō-sklĕ-RŌ-sĭs	
artery (354)	ĂR-tĕ-rē	

atherectomy (357)	ă-thĕ-RĔK-tō-mē	
atheroma (357)	ăth-ĕr-Ō-mă	
atherosclerosis (357)	ăth-ĕr-ō-sklĕ-RŌ-sĭs	
atrial (358)	Ā-trē-ăl	
atrioventricular node (354)	ā-trē-ō-vĕn-TRĬK-ū-lăr nōd	
atrium (plural: atria) (354)	Ā-trē-ŭm (Ā-trē-ă)	
brachial artery (358)	BRĀ-kē-ăl ĂR-tĕ-rē	
bradycardia (358)	brād-ē-KĂR-dē-ă	
bundle of His (354)	BŬN-d'l of Hĭs	
capillary (354)	KĂP-ĭ-lăr-ē	
carbon dioxide (354)	kăr-bŏn dī-ŎK-sīd	
cardiomegaly (358)	kăr-dē-ō-MĔG-ă-lē	
cardiomyopathy (358)	kăr-dē-ō-mī-ŎP-ă-thē	
coronary arteries (354)	KŎR-ō-năr-ē ĂR-tĕ-rēz	
cyanosis (359)	sī-ă-NŌ-sĭs	
deoxygenated blood (355)	dē-ŎK-sĭ-jĕ-NĀ-tĕd blŭd	
diastole (355)	dī-ĂS-tō-lē	
endocardium (355)	ĕn-dō-KĂR-dē-ŭm	
endothelium (355)	ĕn-dō-THĒ-lē-um	
hypercholesterolemia (358)	hī-pĕr-kō-lĕs-tĕr-ŏl-Ē-mē-ă	
hypoxia (359)	hī-PŎK-sē-ă	
interventricular septum (359)	ĭn-tĕr-vĕn-TRĬK-ū-lăr SĔP-tŭm	
mitral valve (355)	MĪ-trăl vălv	
mitral valvulitis (359)	MĪ-trăl văl-vū-LĪ-tĭs	
myocardium (355)	mī-ō-KĂR-dē-ŭm	
oxygen (355)	ŎK-sĭ-jĕn	
pacemaker (355)	PĀS-mā-kĕr	
pericardiocentesis (359)	pĕr-ĭ-kăr-dē-ō-sĕn-TĒ-sĭs	
pericardium (355)	pĕr-ĭ-KĂR-dē-ŭm	

phlebitis (359)	flē-BĪ-tĭs	_____
phlebotomy (359)	flĕ-BŎT-ō-mē	_____
pulmonary artery (355)	PŬL-mō-nĕr-ē ĂR-tĕr-ē	_____
pulmonary circulation (355)	PŬL-mō-nĕr-ē sĕr-kŭ-LĀ-shŭn	_____
pulmonary valve (355)	PŬL-mō-nĕr-ē vălv	_____
pulmonary vein (355)	PŬL-mō-nĕr-ē vān	_____
septum (plural: septa) (356)	SĔP-tŭm (SĔP-tă)	_____
sinoatrial node (356)	sī-nō-Ā-trē-ăl nōd	_____
sphygmomanometer (356)	sfĭg-mō-mă-NŌM-ĕ-tĕr	_____
stethoscope (359)	STĔTH-ō-skōp	_____
systemic circulation (356)	sĭs-TĔM-ĭk sĕr-kŭ-LĀ-shŭn	_____
systole (356)	SĬS-tō-lē	_____
tachycardia (358)	tăk-ē-KĂR-dē-ă	_____
thrombolysis (359)	thrŏm-BŎL-ĭ-sĭs	_____
tricuspid valve (356)	trī-KŬS-pĭd -vălv	_____
valvotomy (359)	văl-VŎT-ō-mē	_____
valvuloplasty (359)	văl-vū-lō-PLĂS-tē	_____
vascular (359)	VĂS-kū-lăr	_____
vasoconstriction (359)	văz-ō-kŏn-STRĬK-shŭn	_____
vasodilation (359)	văz-ō-dī-LĀ-shŭn	_____
vein (356)	vān	_____
vena cava (plural: venae cavae) (356)	VĒ-nă KĀ-vă (VĒ-nē KĀ-vē)	_____
venous (359)	VĒ-nŭs	_____
ventricle (356)	VĔN-trĭ-k'l	_____
ventriculotomy (359)	vĕn-trĭk-ū-LŎT-ō-mē	_____
venule (356)	VĔN-u'l	_____

Pathology, Laboratory Tests, and Clinical Procedures

Term	Pronunciation	Meaning
aneurysm (366)	ĂN-ū-rĭzm	_____
angina pectoris (369)	ăn-JĪ-nă PĔK-tŏr-ĭs or ĂN-jĭ-nă PĔK-tŏr-ĭs	_____
angiography (370)	ăn-jē-ŎG-ră-fē	_____
atrioventricular block (360)	ā-trē-ō-vĕn-TRĬK-ū-lăr blŏk	_____
auscultation (369)	ăw-skŭl-TĀ-shŭn	_____
beta-blocker (369)	BĀ-tă-BLŎK-ĕr	_____
calcium channel blocker (369)	KĂL-sē-ŭm CHĂ-nĕl BLŎK-ĕr	_____
cardiac arrest (361)	KĂR-dē-ăk ā-RĔST	_____
cardiac catheterization (371)	KĂR-dē-ăk kăth-ĕ-tĕr-ĭ-ZĀ-shŭn	_____
cardiac scan (371)	KĂR-dē-ăk skăn	_____
cardioversion(361)	kăr-dē-ō-VĔR-zhŭn	_____
claudication (369)	klăw-dĕ-KĀ-shŭn	_____
coarctation of the aorta (361)	kō-ărk-TĀ-shŭn of the ā-ŎR-tă	_____
congenital heart disease (361)	kŏn-GĔN-ĭ-tăl hărt dĭ-ZĒZ	_____
congestive heart failure (362)	kŏn-GĔS-tĭv hărt FĀL-ŭr	_____
coronary artery disease (363)	kŏr-ō-NĂR-ē ĂR-tĕ-rē dĭ-ZĒZ	_____
coronary bypass surgery (372)	kŏr-ō-NĂR-ē BĪ-păs SŬR-jĕr-ē	_____
digitalis (369)	dĭj-ĭ-TĂL-ĭs	_____
digital subtraction angiography (370)	DĬJ-ĭ-tăl sŭb-TRĂK-shŭn ăn-jē-ŎG-ră-fē	_____
Doppler ultrasound (371)	DŎP-lĕr ŬL-tră-sŏnd	_____
echocardiography (371)	ĕk-ō-kăr-dē-ŌG-ră-fē	_____
electrocardiography (372)	ē-lĕk-trō-kăr-dē-ŎG-ră-fē	_____

embolus (plural: emboli) (369)   ĔM-bō-lŭs (ĔM-bō-lī)   _____

endarterectomy (372)   ĕnd-ăr-tĕr-ĔK-tō-mē   _____

endocarditis (364)   ĕn-dō-kăr-DĪ-tĭs   _____

extracorporeal circulation (372)   ĕks-tră-kŏr-PŎR-ē-ăl sĕr-kū-LĀ-shŭn   _____

fibrillation (360)   fĭb-rĭ-LĀ-shŭn   _____

flutter (360)   FLŬ-tĕr   _____

hemorrhoids (367)   HĔM-ō-roydz   _____

Holter monitoring (373)   HŎL-tĕr MŎN-ĭ-tĕ-rĭng   _____

hypertension (367)   hī-pĕr-TĔN-shŭn   _____

infarction (369)   ĭn-FĂRK-shŭn   _____

ischemia (364)   ĭs-KĒ-mē-ă   _____

lipid tests (370)   LĬ-pĭd tĕsts   _____

lipoprotein electrophoresis (370)   lī-pō-PRŌ-tēn ē-lĕk-trō-fŏr-Ē-sĭs   _____

mitral stenosis (366)   MĪ-trăl stĕ-NŌ-sĭs   _____

mitral valve prolapse (365)   MĪ-trăl vălv PRŌ-laps   _____

murmur (365)   MŬR-mĕr   _____

myocardial infarction (364)   mī-ō-KĂR-dē-ăl ĭn-FĂRK-shŭn   _____

nitroglycerin (369)   nī-trō-GLĬS-ĕr-ĭn   _____

peripheral vascular disease (367)   pĕ-RĬ-fĕr-ăl VĂS-kū-lăr dĭ-ZĒZ   _____

palpitations (369)   păl-pĭ-TĀ-shŭnz   _____

patent ductus arteriosus (361)   PĀ-tĕnt DŬK-tŭs ăr-tĕr-ē-Ō-sŭs   _____

percutaneous transluminal coronary angioplasty (373)   pĕr-kū-TĀ-nē-ŭs trăns-LŪ-mĭ-năl KŎR-ō-năr-ē ĂN-jē-ō-plăs-tē   _____

pericarditis (365)   pĕr-ĭ-kăr-DĪ-tĭs   _____

petechiae (369)   pĕ-TĒ-kē-ē   _____

Raynaud's phenomenon (367)	rā-NŌZ fĕ-NŎM-ĕ-nŏn
rheumatic heart disease (366)	roo-MĂT-ik hărt dĭ-ZĒZ
septal defects (361)	SĔP-tăl DĒ-fĕks
stress test (374)	STRĔS tĕst
tetralogy of Fallot (362)	tĕ-TRĂL-ō-jē of fă-LO
thrombolytic therapy (374)	thrŏm-bō-LĬ-tĭk THĔ-ră-pē
thrombotic occlusion (363)	thrŏm-BŎT-ĭk ō-KLŪ-zhŭn
varicose veins (367)	VĂR-ĭ-kōs vānz
vegetations (369)	vĕj-ĕ-TĀ-shŭnz

XIV. Review Sheet

Write the meanings of each word part in the space provided. Check your answers with the information in the chapter or in the Glossary (Medical Terms—English) at the end of the book.

Combining Forms

Combining Form	Meaning	Combining Form	Meaning
aneurysm/o	_____	ox/o	_____
angi/o	_____	pericardi/o	_____
aort/o	_____	phleb/o	_____
arter/o	_____	pulmon/o	_____
arteri/o	_____	rrhythm/o	_____
ather/o	_____	sphygm/o	_____
atri/o	_____	steth/o	_____
axill/o	_____	thromb/o	_____
brachi/o	_____	valv/o	_____
cardi/o	_____	valvul/o	_____
cholesterol/o	_____	vas/o	_____
coron/o	_____	vascul/o	_____
cyan/o	_____	ven/o	_____
isch/o	_____	ventricul/o	_____
my/o	_____		

Suffixes

Suffix	Meaning	Suffix	Meaning
-constriction	_____	-emia	_____
-dilation	_____	-graphy	_____

Continued on following page

-lysis	_____	-plasty	_____
-megaly	_____	-sclerosis	_____
-meter	_____	-stenosis	_____
-oma	_____	-tomy	_____
-osis	_____		

Prefixes

Prefix	Meaning	Prefix	Meaning
brady-	_____	inter-	_____
de-	_____	peri-	_____
endo-	_____	tachy-	_____
hyper-	_____	tetra-	_____
hypo-	_____	tri-	_____

Respiratory System

This Chapter is divided into the following sections

In this Chapter you will

- Name the organs of the respiratory system and describe their location and function;
- Identify various pathological conditions that affect the system;
- Recognize medical terms that pertain to respiration; and
- Identify clinical procedures and abbreviations related to the system.

I. Introduction

We usually think of **respiration** as the mechanical process of breathing, that is, the repetitive and, for the most part, unconscious exchange of air between the lungs and the external environment. This exchange of air at the lungs is also called **external respiration.** In external respiration, oxygen is inhaled (air inhaled contains about 21 per cent oxygen) into the air spaces (sacs) of the lungs and immediately passes into tiny capillary blood vessels surrounding the air spaces. Simultaneously, carbon dioxide, a gas produced when oxygen and food combine in cells, passes from the capillary blood vessels into the air spaces of the lungs to be exhaled (exhaled air contains about 16 per cent oxygen).

While external respiration occurs between the outside environment and the capillary bloodstream of the lungs, another form of respiration is occurring simultaneously between the individual body cells and the tiny capillary blood vessels that surround them. This process is called **internal (cellular) respiration.** Internal respiration is the exchange of gases not at the lungs but at the cells within all the organs of the body. In this process, oxygen passes out of the bloodstream and into the tissue cells. At the same time, carbon dioxide passes from the tissue cells into the bloodstream and is carried by the blood back to the lungs to be exhaled.

II. Anatomy and Physiology of Respiration

Label Figure 12–1 as you read the following paragraphs.

Air enters the body through the **nose** (1) and passes through the **nasal cavity** (2), which is lined with a mucous membrane and fine hairs **(cilia)** to help filter out foreign bodies, as well as to warm and moisten the air. **Paranasal sinuses** (3) are hollow, air-containing spaces within the skull that communicate with the nasal cavity. They, too, have a mucous membrane

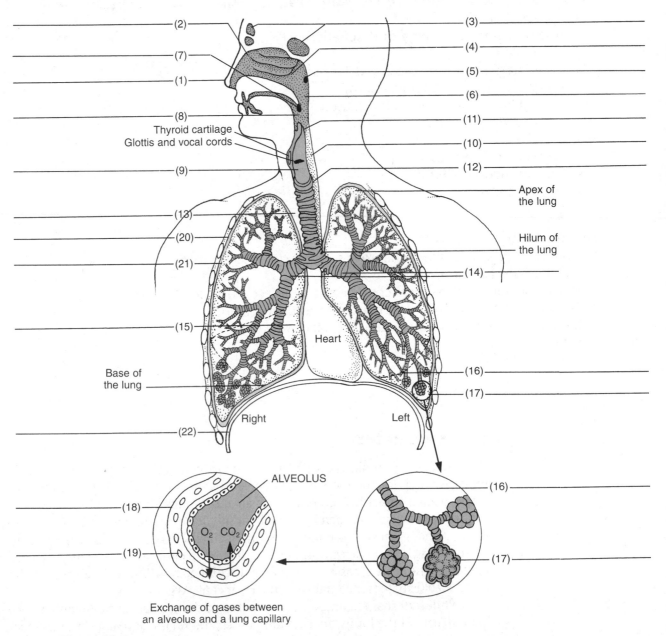

Figure 12–1

Organs of the respiratory system.

Posterior aspect
of tongue

Epiglottis

Aryepiglottic fold

Vocal folds
abducted

Vocal folds
adducted

Cartilage

Cartilage

A   Open   B   Closed

Figure 12–2

The larynx from a superior view. (From Jacob SW, Francone CA, Lossow WJ: Structure and Function in Man, 5th ed. Philadelphia, WB Saunders, 1982, p 448.)

lining and function to provide the lubricating fluid mucus, as well as to lighten the bones of the skull and help produce sound.

After passing through the nasal cavity, the air next reaches the **pharynx (throat).** There are three divisions of the pharynx. The **nasopharynx** (4) is the first division, and it is nearest to the nasal cavities. It contains the **adenoids** (5), which are collections of lymphatic tissue. The adenoids (also known as the **pharyngeal tonsils**) are more prominent in children, and if enlarged, they can obstruct air passageways. Below the nasopharynx and closer to the mouth is the second division of the pharynx, the **oropharynx** (6). The **palatine tonsils** (7), two rounded masses of lymphatic tissue, are located in the oropharynx. The third division of the pharynx is the **hypopharynx** (also called the **laryngopharynx**) (8). It is in the hypopharyngeal region that the pharynx, serving as a common passageway for food from the mouth and air from the nose, divides into two branches, the **larynx (voice box)** (9) and the **esophagus** (10).

The esophagus leads into the stomach and carries food to be digested. The larynx contains the vocal cords and is surrounded by pieces of cartilage for support. The thyroid cartilage is the largest and is commonly referred to as the Adam's apple. Sounds are produced as air is expelled past the vocal cords, and the cords vibrate. The tension of the vocal cords determines the high or low pitch of the voice.

Since food entering from the mouth and air entering from the nose mix in the pharynx, what prevents the passing of food or drink into the larynx and respiratory system after it has been swallowed? Even with a small quantity of solid or liquid matter finding its way into the air passages, breathing could be seriously blocked and the aspirated food can cause a chemical irritation in the lungs. A special deterrent to this event is provided for by a flap of cartilage attached to the root of the tongue that acts like a lid over the larynx. This flap of cartilage is called the **epiglottis** (11). It covers the **glottis,** which is the opening to the larynx. In the act of swallowing, when food and liquid move through the throat, the epiglottis closes off the larynx, so that these cannot enter. Figure 12-2 shows the larynx from a superior view.

On its way to the lungs, air passes from the larynx to the **trachea (windpipe)** (12), a vertical tube about 4½ inches long and 1 inch in diameter. The trachea is kept open by 16–20 C-shaped rings of cartilage separated by fibrous connective tissue that stiffen the front and sides of the tube.

In the region of the **mediastinum** (13), the trachea divides into two branches called **bronchi** (14) (singular, **bronchus**). Each bronchus leads to a separate **lung** (15) and divides and subdivides into smaller and finer tubes, somewhat like the branches of a tree.

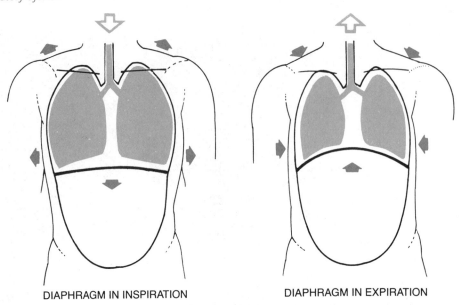

DIAPHRAGM IN INSPIRATION   DIAPHRAGM IN EXPIRATION

Figure 12–3

Position of the diaphragm during inspiration and expiration. During inspiration air flows in as the chest cavity enlarges. During expiration air flows out as the chest cavity becomes smaller.

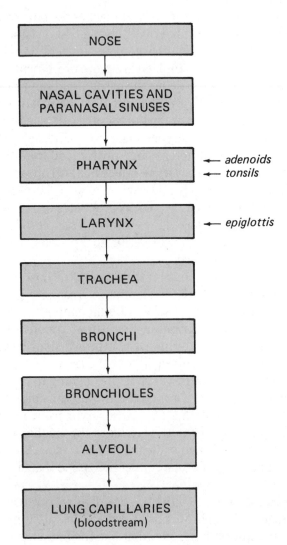

Figure 12–4

Pathway of air from the nose to the capillaries of the lungs.

The smallest of the bronchial branches are called **bronchioles** (16). At the end of the bronchioles are clusters of air sacs called **alveoli** (17) (singular: **alveolus**). Each alveolus is made of a one-cell layer of epithelium. The very thin wall allows for the exchange of gases between the alveolus and the **capillaries** (18) that surround and come in close contact with it. The blood that flows through the capillaries accepts the oxygen from the alveolus and deposits carbon dioxide into the alveolus to be exhaled. Oxygen is bound to a protein (hemoglobin) in **erythrocytes** (19) and carried to all parts of the body.

Each lung is enveloped in a double-folded membrane called the **pleura.** The outer layer of the pleura, nearest the ribs, is the **parietal pleura** (20), and the inner layer, closest to the lung, is the **visceral pleura** (21). The pleura is moistened with a serous (thin, watery fluid) secretion that facilitates the movements of the lungs within the chest (thorax).

The two lungs are not quite mirror images of each other. The right lung, which is the slightly larger of the two, is divided into three **lobes** and the left lung is divided into two lobes. It is possible for one lobe of the lung to be removed without damage to the rest, which can continue to function normally. The uppermost part of the lung is called the **apex,** and the lower area is the **base.** The **hilum** or **hilus** of the lung is the midline region where blood vessels, nerves, lymphatic tissue, and bronchial tubes enter and exit the organ.

The lungs extend from the collarbone to the **diaphragm** (22) in the thoracic cavity. The diaphragm is a muscular partition that separates the thoracic from the abdominal cavity and aids in the process of breathing. The diaphragm contracts and descends with each **inhalation (inspiration).** The downward movement of the diaphragm enlarges the area in the thoracic cavity and reduces the internal air pressure, so that air flows into the lungs to equalize the pressure. When the lungs are full, the diaphragm relaxes and elevates, making the area in the thoracic cavity smaller, and thus increasing the air pressure in the thorax. Air then is expelled out of the lungs to equalize the pressure; this is called **exhalation (expiration).** Figure 12–3 shows the position of the diaphragm in inspiration and expiration.

Figure 12–4 is a flow diagram reviewing the pathway of air from the nose, where air enters the body, to the capillaries of the lungs, where air enters the bloodstream.

III. Vocabulary

This list will help you review many of the new terms introduced in the text. Short definitions will reinforce your understanding of the terms. See Section X of this chapter for help in pronouncing the more difficult terms.

adenoids	Collections of lymph tissue in the nasopharynx. Also called pharyngeal tonsils.
alveolus (plural: **alveoli**)	Air sac in the lung.
apex of the lung	Uppermost portion of the lung. **Apical** means pertaining to the apex.
base of the lung	Lower portion of the lung.
bronchioles	Smallest branches of the bronchi.
bronchus (plural: **bronchi**)	Branch of the trachea (windpipe) that acts as a passageway into the air spaces of the lung; bronchial tube.
carbon dioxide (CO$_2$)	A gas produced by body cells when oxygen and food combine; exhaled through the lungs.

cilia	Thin hairs attached to the mucous membrane epithelium lining the respiratory tract.
diaphragm	Muscle separating the chest and abdomen.
epiglottis	Lid-like piece of cartilage that covers the larynx.
exhalation	Breathing out (expiration).
external respiration	Exchange of gases in the lungs.
glottis	The opening to the larynx.
hilum (of lung)	Midline region where the bronchi, blood vessels, and nerves enter and exit the lungs. **Hilar** means pertaining to the hilum.
inhalation	Breathing in (inspiration).
internal respiration	Exchange of gases at the tissue cells.
larynx	Voice box.
lobes	Divisions of the lungs.
mediastinum	Region between the lungs in the chest cavity. It contains the trachea, heart, aorta, esophagus, and bronchial tubes.
oxygen (O$_2$)	Gas that passes into the bloodstream at the lungs and travels to all body cells.
palatine tonsils	Rounded masses of lymph tissue in the oropharynx (*palatine* means roof of the mouth).
paranasal sinuses	Air-containing cavities in the bones near the nose.
parietal pleura	The outer fold of pleura lying closest to the ribs and wall of the thoracic cavity.
pharynx	Throat; composed of the nasopharynx, oropharynx, and laryngopharynx.
pleura	Double-folded membrane surrounding each lung.
pleural cavity	Space between the folds of the pleura.
pulmonary parenchyma	The essential cells of the lung, those performing its main function; the air sacs (alveoli) and small bronchioles.
trachea	Windpipe.
visceral pleura	The inner fold of pleura lying closest to the lung tissue.

IV. Combining Forms, Suffixes, and Terminology

Write the meaning of the medical term in the space provided.

Combining Forms

Combining Form	Meaning	Terminology	Meaning
adenoid/o	adenoids	<u>adenoid</u>ectomy _____	
		<u>adenoid</u> hypertrophy _____	
alveol/o	alveolus, air sac	<u>alveol</u>ar _____	
bronch/o **bronchi/o**	bronchial tube, bronchus	<u>bronch</u>ospasm _____	
		<u>bronchi</u>ectasis _____	
		Caused by weakening of the bronchial wall by infection.	
bronchiol/o	bronchiole, small bronchus	<u>bronchiol</u>itis _____	
		Figure 12–5 shows the relationship among bronchioles, alveoli, and the blood vessels surrounding them.	
capn/o	carbon dioxide	hyper<u>capn</u>ia _____	

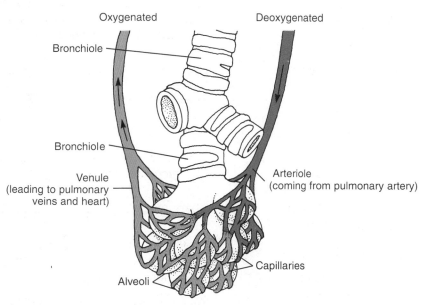

Figure 12–5

Bronchioles, alveoli, and blood vessels.

coni/o	dust	pneumo<u>coni</u>osis _____
		See page 407, Section V, under Pathological Terms.
cyan/o	blue	<u>cyan</u>osis _____
		Caused by deficient oxygen in the blood; hemoglobin in red blood cells is deoxygenated.
epiglott/o	epiglottis	<u>epiglott</u>itis _____
laryng/o	larynx, voice box	<u>laryng</u>eal _____
		<u>laryng</u>ospasm _____
		<u>laryng</u>itis _____
lob/o	lobe of the lung	<u>lob</u>ectomy _____
mediastin/o	mediastinum	<u>mediastin</u>oscopy _____
nas/o	nose	para<u>nas</u>al sinuses _____
		Para- means near in this term.
		<u>nas</u>ogastric tube _____
orth/o	straight, upright	<u>orth</u>opnea _____
		Breathing (-pnea) is easier in the upright position. A major cause of orthopnea is congestive heart failure (the lungs fill with fluid when the patient is lying flat). Physicians assess the degree of orthopnea by the number of pillows a patient requires to sleep comfortably (e.g., two-pillow orthopnea).
ox/o	oxygen	hyp<u>ox</u>ia _____
		Tissues have a decreased amount of oxygen, and cyanosis can result.
pector/o	chest	ex<u>pector</u>ation _____
		Expectorated sputum can contain mucus, blood, cellular debris, pus, and microorganisms.
pharyng/o	pharynx, throat	<u>pharyng</u>eal _____
		naso<u>pharyng</u>itis _____
phon/o	voice	dys<u>phon</u>ia _____
		Hoarseness or other voice impairment.
phren/o	diaphragm	<u>phren</u>ic nerve _____
		<u>phren</u>ohepatic _____

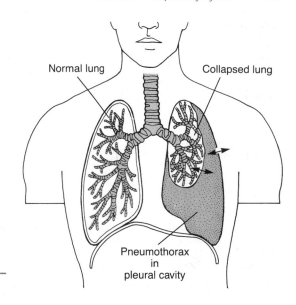

Figure 12–6

Pneumothorax.

pleur/o	pleura	pleuritic _____
		pleurodynia _____
		-dynia means pain.
pneum/o **pneumon/o**	air, lung	pneumothorax _____
		-thorax means chest. Air accumulates in the pleural cavity, between the pleura (Fig. 12–6). This condition can occur with lung disease or may follow trauma to and perforation of (a hole through) the chest wall.
		pneumonitis _____
		pneumonectomy _____
pulmon/o	lung	pulmonary _____
rhin/o	nose	rhinorrhea _____
		rhinoplasty _____
sinus/o	sinus, cavity	sinusitis _____
spir/o	breathing	spirometer _____
		expiration _____
		Note that the s is omitted.
tel/o	complete	atelectasis _____
		Incomplete expansion (-ectasis) of a lung; collapsed lung. Atelectasis may occur after surgery when a patient experiences pain and does not take deep breaths.

thorac/o	chest	thoracotomy _____	
		thoracic _____	
tonsill/o	tonsils	tonsillectomy _____	
		The oropharyngeal (palatine) tonsils are removed.	
trache/o	trachea, windpipe	tracheotomy _____	
		tracheal _____	

Suffixes			
Suffix	Meaning	Terminology	Meaning
-ema	condition	empyema _____	
		Em- means in. Empyema is a collection of pus, and it most commonly occurs in the pleural cavity as pyothorax.	
-osmia	smell	anosmia _____	
-pnea	breathing	apnea _____	
		dyspnea _____	
		Paroxysmal (sudden) nocturnal (at night) dyspnea may occur in patients with congestive heart failure when they recline in bed. Patients often describe the sensation as air hunger.	
		hyperpnea _____	
		An increase in the depth of breathing.	
		tachypnea _____	
		Excessively rapid and shallow breathing; hyperventilation.	
-ptysis	spitting	hemoptysis _____	
-sphyxia	pulse	asphyxia _____	
		Interference with respiration can ultimately lead to absence of pulse.	
-thorax	pleural cavity, chest	hemothorax _____	
		pyothorax _____	
		Empyema of the chest.	

V. Diagnostic and Pathological Terms

Diagnostic Terms

auscultation

Listening to sounds within the body.

This procedure, performed with a stethoscope, is used chiefly for diagnosing conditions of the lungs, pleura, heart, and abdomen, as well as to determine the condition of the fetus during pregnancy.

percussion

Tapping on a surface to determine the difference in the density of the underlying structure.

Tapping over a solid organ produces a dull sound without resonance. Percussion over an air-filled structure, such as the lung, produces a resonant, hollow note. As the lungs are filled with fluid and become more dense, as in pneumonia, resonance is replaced by dullness.

pleural rub

Grating sound produced by the motion of pleural surfaces rubbing each other.

Pleural rub occurs when the pleura are thickened by inflammation or by neoplastic cells. It is heard by auscultation or can be felt by placing the fingers on the chest wall.

rales (crackles)

Abnormal crackling sounds heard during inspiration when there is fluid in alveoli.

Rales are heard (on auscultation) when a patient has pulmonary edema or heart failure.

rhonchi

Abnormal, rumbling sounds heard during expiration.

Rhonchi are heard when secretions have accumulated in narrowed airways. They are commonly associated with spasm of the bronchial tubes due to asthma or infection. **Wheezes** are a type of rhonchi whose sound is of a more musical nature.

sputum

Material expelled from the chest by coughing or clearing the throat.

Purulent (containing pus) sputum results from infection and is often green in color. Blood-tinged sputum makes physicians suspicious of tuberculosis.

stridor

A strained, high-pitched, noisy breathing associated with obstruction of the larynx or a bronchus.

Pathological Terms

Upper Respiratory Disorders

croup

Acute respiratory syndrome in children and infants; characterized by obstruction of the larynx, barking cough, and stridor.

Croup may result from infection, allergy, or foreign body in the larynx.

diphtheria

Acute infection of the throat and upper respiratory tract caused by diphtheria bacteria *(Corynebacterium)*.

Inflammation occurs, and a leathery, opaque membrane forms in the pharynx and respiratory tract.

Immunity to diphtheria (by production of antibodies) is induced by the administration of weakened toxins (antigens) beginning between the 6th and the 8th week of life. These injections are usually given in combination with pertussis and tetanus toxins and are called **DPT** injections.

epistaxis

Nosebleed.

Epistaxis (from the Greek meaning to let fall, drop by drop) results from traumatic or spontaneous rupture of blood vessels in the mucous membrane of the nose.

pertussis

Bacterial infection of the pharynx, larynx, and trachea caused by *Bordetella pertussis,* a highly contagious bacterium. Also known as **whooping cough.**

Bronchial Tube Disorders

asthma

Spasm and narrowing of bronchi leading to bronchial airway obstruction.

Associated symptoms are **paroxysmal** (sudden) dyspnea, wheezing, and cough. Etiology may involve allergy or infection, and asthma may be aggravated by anxiety, cold, and exercise. Asthma (the term comes from a Greek word meaning panting) is treated with drugs including inhaled agents that dilate the bronchi.

bronchogenic carcinoma

Cancerous tumors arising from a bronchus; lung cancer.

This group of malignant tumors, caused by smoking, is responsible for 34 per cent of cancer deaths in males and 11 per cent of cancer deaths in females. There are several forms, including **squamous cell carcinoma** (derived from the lining of the bronchus), **adenocarcinoma** (derived from the mucus-secreting cells), and **small (oat) cell carcinoma** (of uncertain origin). All types of lung cancer readily spread to the liver, brain, and bones.

chronic bronchitis

Inflammation of the bronchi persisting for a long time.

This disease is often caused by infection or cigarette smoking and is characterized by increased secretion from the bronchial mucosa and obstruction of the respiratory passages. Chronic bronchitis, asthma, and emphysema (see Lung Disorders) are known as **chronic obstructive pulmonary diseases (COPD).**

cystic fibrosis

Inherited disease of exocrine glands (pancreas, sweat glands, and mucous membranes of the respiratory tract) leading to airway obstruction.

Chronic respiratory infections are common, as is pancreatic insufficiency (fats are improperly digested). Therapy involves replacement of pancreatic enzymes and treatment of pulmonary obstruction and infection. The gene responsible for the condition has been found, and persons carrying the gene can be identified.

Lung Disorders

atelectasis

Incomplete (atel/o) expansion (-ectasis) of alveoli; collapsed, functionless, airless lung or portion of a lung.

In atelectasis, the bronchioles and alveoli (pulmonary parenchyma) resemble a collapsed balloon. Common causes of atelectasis include poor inspiration effort in the postoperative period, blockage of a bronchus or smaller bronchial tube by secretions, tumor or a chest wound that permits air, fluid, or blood to accumulate in the pleural cavity. Acute atelectasis requires removal of the underlying cause (tumor, foreign body, excessive mucous secretions) and therapy to open airways.

emphysema

Hyperinflation of air sacs with destruction of alveolar walls.

Loss of elasticity and breakdown of the alveoli walls result in loss of air movement in the air sacs. There is a strong association between cigarette smoking and emphysema. Chronic bronchitis is often associated with emphysema. As a result of dyspnea and hypoxemia, the heart must work harder to pump blood and this leads to right ventricular hypertrophy in the heart and heart failure **(cor pulmonale).**

pneumoconiosis

Abnormal condition caused by dust in the lungs, with chronic inflammation, infection, and bronchitis.

Various forms are named according to the type of dust particle inhaled: **anthracosis**—coal (anthrac/o) dust (black lung disease); **asbestosis**—asbestos (asbest/o) particles (in shipbuilding and construction trades); **silicosis**—silica (silic/o = rocks) or glass (grinder's disease).

pneumonia

Acute inflammation and infection of alveoli, which fill with pus or products of the inflammatory reaction.

Etiological agents are most often pneumococci and less frequently staphylococci, fungi, or viruses. Infection damages alveolar membranes, so that fluid, blood cells, and debris consolidate in the alveoli. **Lobar pneumonia** involves one or more lobes of a lung, and **bronchopneumonia** begins in the terminal bronchioles. Bed rest, antibiotics, and respiratory therapy are needed.

pulmonary abscess

Large collection of pus (bacterial infection) in the lungs.

pulmonary edema

Swelling and fluid in the air sacs and bronchioles.

This condition is often caused by inability of the heart to pump blood (congestive heart failure). Blood then backs up in the pulmonary blood vessels, and fluid seeps out into the alveoli and bronchioles. This is a condition that requires immediate medical attention with drugs (diuretics, vasodilators, digitalis), oxygen in high concentrations, and keeping the patient in a sitting position (to decrease venous return to the heart).

pulmonary embolism

Clot or other material lodges in vessels of the lung.

The clot can travel from distant veins or develop idiopathically in branches of the pulmonary artery. Occlusion produces an area of dead (necrotic) lung tissue called a **pulmonary infarction.**

tuberculosis

An infectious disease caused by *Mycobacterium tuberculosis;* lungs are usually involved, but any organ in the body may be affected.

Rod-shaped bacteria called **bacilli** invade the lungs, producing small tubercles (from the Latin word *tuber* meaning a swelling) of infection. Early tuberculosis (TB) is usually asymptomatic and is detected on routine chest x-ray. Symptoms of advanced disease are cough, weight loss, night sweats, hemoptysis, and pleuritic pain. Antituberculous chemotherapy (isoniazid, rifampin) is effective in most cases. Immunocompromised patients are particularly susceptible to antibiotic-resistant tuberculosis. It is important and often necessary to treat TB with many drugs at the same time to prevent drug resistance.

The PPD skin test (see p. 413, Section VI, under Clinical Procedures) is done on most hospital or medical employees because TB can be transmitted very easily.

Pleural Disorders

mesothelioma

A malignant tumor arising in the pleura; composed of mesothelium, which is epithelium that covers the surfaces of membranes such as the pleura, peritoneum, and pericardium.

This is a rare tumor and is associated with exposure to asbestos.

pleural effusion

Escape of fluid into the pleural cavity.

Pleural effusions are typically categorized on the basis of whether they are transudates (fluid that has passed through a membrane or tissue) or exudates (fluid, high in protein, that oozes from blood vessels and wounds). Exudates composed of pus are frequently due to a staphylococcal infection. Figure 12–7 shows a chest x-ray of a patient with empyema.

pleurisy (pleuritis)

Inflammation of the pleura.

This condition causes pleurodynia and dyspnea and, in chronic cases, escape of fluid into the pleural cavity.

pneumothorax

Accumulation of air or gas in the pleural cavity.

Pneumothorax may occur in the course of a pulmonary disease (emphysema, carcinoma, tuberculosis, or lung abscess) when rupture of any pulmonary lesions

Figure 12–7

Staphylococcal empyema. *Left,* Normal x-ray when patient was admitted with high fever. *Right,* Chest x-ray 3 days after admission. (Reproduced with permission from Way LW: Current Surgical Diagnosis and Treatment, 9th ed, 1988 by Appleton & Lange, Norwalk, CT, and San Mateo, CA.)

near the pleural surface allows communication between an alveolus or bronchus and the pleural cavity. It may also follow trauma and perforation of the chest wall, or prolonged high flow oxygen delivered by a respirator in an intensive care unit (ICU).

STUDY SECTION

Practice spelling each term and know its meaning.

anthracosis	Coal dust accumulation in the lungs; a pneumoconiosis.
asbestosis	Asbestos particles accumulate in the lungs.
bacilli (singular: **bacillus**)	Rod-shaped bacteria.
chronic obstructive pulmonary disease (COPD)	A chronic condition of persistent obstruction of air flow through the bronchial tubes and lungs. Chronic bronchitis and emphysema are the two conditions mainly associated with COPD. Patients with COPD are referred to as *blue bloaters* (bronchitic, cyanotic, stocky build) or *pink puffers* (emphysemic, no change in skin color, short of breath).
cor pulmonale	Failure of the right side of the heart to pump sufficient amount of blood to the lungs; occurs as a complication of lung disease.
hydrothorax	Collection of fluid in the pleural cavity.
paroxysmal	Pertaining to a sudden occurrence, such as a spasm or seizure; oxysm/o means sudden.
pulmonary infarction	An area of dead (necrotic) tissue in the lung.
purulent	Pertaining to containing pus.
silicosis	Silica or glass dust in the lungs; occurs in mining occupations.

VI. Clinical Procedures and Abbreviations

Clinical Procedures

X-Ray Tests

chest x-ray	X-ray picture of the chest can be taken in the frontal (coronal) plane (anteroposterior view) or in the sagittal plane (lateral view). **Chest tomograms** are a series of x-rays that show pictures of the chest region at various depths; tomograms are able to detect small masses not seen on a regular film.
CT scan of the chest	A computerized reconstruction of a series of x-ray pictures of the chest taken as slices in a transverse (axial or cross-sectional) plane (Fig. 12–8).

Lesion

Lung

Trachea

Vertebra

R

L

Figure 12–8

CT scan of the chest. Note lesion in the right upper lobe of the patient's lung. (From Line BR, Armstrong MR, Hendrick WJ Jr, Killam DA: Radiographic studies of lung cancer. *In* Roth JA, Ruckdeschel JC, Weisenburger TH [eds]: Thoracic Oncology. Philadelphia, WB Saunders, 1989, p 115.)

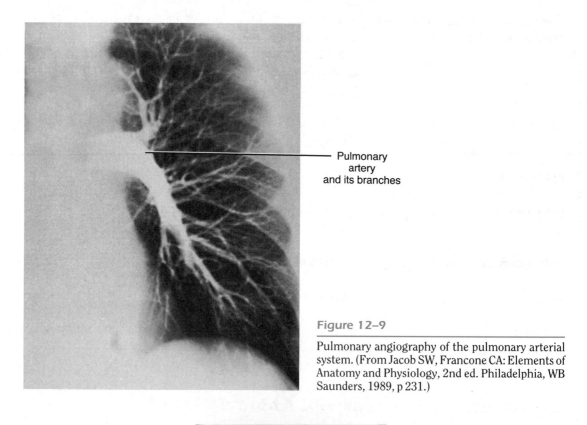

Pulmonary artery and its branches

Figure 12–9

Pulmonary angiography of the pulmonary arterial system. (From Jacob SW, Francone CA: Elements of Anatomy and Physiology, 2nd ed. Philadelphia, WB Saunders, 1989, p 231.)

Lesion

Lung

Aorta

Figure 12–10

MRI scan of the chest, transverse (axial) view. (From Line BR, Armstrong MR, Hendrick WJ Jr, Killam DA: Radiographic studies of lung cancer. *In* Roth JA, Ruckdeschel JC, Weisenburger TH [eds]: Thoracic Oncology. Philadelphia, WB Saunders, 1989, p 115.)

pulmonary angiography	Dye is injected into a blood vessel, and x-rays are taken of the arteries or veins in the lung (Fig. 12-9).

MRI Test

MRI scan of the chest	Magnetic resonance imaging of the chest. Magnetic waves are used to create detailed images of the chest in the frontal, sagittal, and transverse planes. Figure 12–10 shows an MRI of the same patient as that in the CT scan in Figure 12–8. Note that the MRI scan brings the abnormal lesion into sharper focus.

Radioactive Test

lung scan or V/Q scan	Radioactive material is injected intravenously or inhaled, and images are recorded of its distribution in lung tissue, to show air flow (ventilation) and blood supply (perfusion) to the lung.

Other Procedures

bronchoscopy	Examination of the bronchial tubes by passing a lighted, flexible fiberoptic tube through the nose, throat, larynx, and trachea into the bronchi. Specimens can be obtained through the tube for cytological and bacterial studies by aspiration of bronchial secretions or by injecting fluid and retrieving fluid **(bronchial alveolar lavage).** Biopsies can be performed on suspicious areas by means of a forceps (instrument that can grasp tissue) or brush **(bronchial brushing)** inserted through the bronchoscope (Fig. 12–11).
endotracheal intubation	A tube is placed through the nose or mouth, through the pharynx and larynx, and into the trachea to establish an airway (Fig. 12–12). This typically occurs during surgery or in the ICU.
laryngoscopy	Visual examination of the larynx. A lighted flexible tube is passed through the mouth or nose into the larynx.

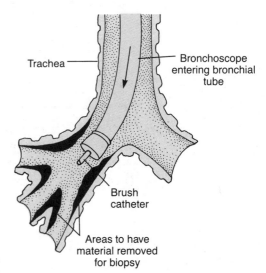

Figure 12–11

Bronchoscope with brush catheter.

Figure 12–12

Endotracheal intubation.

Pharynx

Endotracheal tube

Trachea

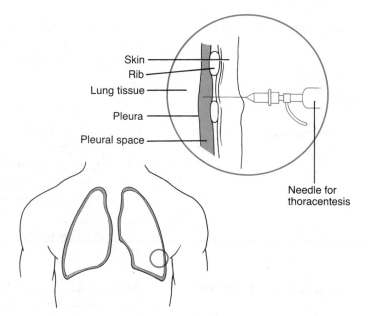

Skin

Rib

Lung tissue

Pleura

Pleural space

Needle for
thoracentesis

Figure 12–13

Thoracentesis. (Modified from O'Toole
M [ed]: Miller-Keane Encyclopedia and
Dictionary of Medicine, Nursing, and
Allied Health, 5th ed. Philadelphia, WB
Saunders, 1992, p 1485.)

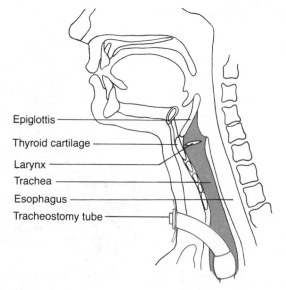

Epiglottis

Thyroid cartilage

Larynx

Trachea

Esophagus

Tracheostomy tube

Figure 12–14

Tracheostomy with tube in place. (Modified from
O'Toole M [ed]: Miller-Keane Encyclopedia and Dic-
tionary of Medicine, Nursing, and Allied Health, 5th ed.
Philadelphia, WB Saunders, 1992, p 1511.)

mediastinoscopy	Visual examination of the mediastinum. This procedure is done in the operating room with local or general anesthesia. A suprasternal (above the breastbone) incision is made and the procedure is used to remove biopsy samples of lymph nodes, tumors, and tuberculosis.
pulmonary function tests	This group of tests measures ventilation (breathing) mechanics of the lungs, i.e., the quantity of air moved into and out of the lungs under normal conditions. A **spirometer** measures the air taken in and out of the lungs. The **forced vital capacity (FVC)** of the lungs is measured by asking the patient to inspire to the maximum and then exhale into the spirometer as forcefully and rapidly as possible.
thoracentesis	Insertion of a needle or catheter through the skin and between the ribs into the pleural space in order to obtain fluid from the pleural cavity for analysis, to drain pleural effusions, or to re-expand a collapsed lung (Fig. 12–13).
thoracotomy	A major surgical procedure in which the chest is opened by an incision for diagnostic or therapeutic procedures, thoracotomy is necessary for **lung biopsy** and lung resections (lobectomy, pneumonectomy).
tracheostomy	Creation of an opening into the trachea through the neck and insertion of a tube to create an airway. Tracheostomy tube insertion may be a permanent as well as an emergency device (Fig. 12–14).
tuberculin tests	Agents such as **PPD** (purified protein derivative) are applied to the surface of the skin with multiple punctures (*Heaf's* and *tine tests*) or by intradermal injection *(Mantoux's test)*. A local cutaneous inflammatory reaction (redness, swelling) is observed in persons who are sensitive to the test substance; a positive test indicates prior or present infection with tuberculosis.
tube thoracostomy	A chest tube is passed through a small incision in the skin to continuously drain pleural spaces after thoracotomy.

ABBREVIATIONS

AFB	Acid-fast bacillus (organism causing tuberculosis)	**CPR**	Cardiopulmonary resuscitation (three basic steps: airway opened by tilting the head, breathing restored by mouth-to-mouth breathing, circulation restored by external cardiac compression)
ARDS	Adult (or acute) respiratory distress syndrome (a group of symptoms—tachypnea, dyspnea, tachycardia, hypoxemia, cyanosis—resulting in acute respiratory failure)		
		CTA	Clear to auscultation
		CXR	Chest x-ray
Bronch	Bronchoscopy	**DPT**	Diphtheria, pertussis, tetanus (injection in an infant to provide immunity to these diseases)
COPD	Chronic obstructive pulmonary disease (airway obstruction associated with emphysema and chronic bronchitis)		
		FVC	Forced vital capacity

ICU	Intensive care unit
IMV	Intermittent mandatory ventilation
LLL	Left lower lobe (of lung)
LUL	Left upper lobe (of lung)
PaCO$_2$, pCO$_2$	Carbon dioxide partial pressure; amount of carbon dioxide in arterial blood
PaO$_2$, pO$_2$	Oxygen partial pressure; amount of oxygen in arterial blood
PCP	*Pneumocystis carinii* pneumonia (a type of pneumonia seen in patients with AIDS)
PEEP	Positive end expiratory pressure (a common mechanical ventilator setting in which airway pressure is maintained above atmospheric pressure)
PFT	Pulmonary function tests
PPD	Purified protein derivative (substance used in a tuberculosis test)
RDS	Respiratory distress syndrome (condition of the newborn marked by dyspnea and cyanosis and related to absence of surfactant, a substance that permits normal expansion of lungs); also called hyaline membrane disease
RLL	Right lower lobe (of lung)
RUL	Right upper lobe (of lung)
SOB	Shortness of breath
TB	Tuberculosis
URI	Upper respiratory infection
V/Q scan	Ventilation-perfusion scan. Radioactive test of lung ventilation space and blood perfusion throughout the lung capillaries (lung scan).

VII. Practical Applications

This section contains actual medical reports using terms that you have studied in this and previous chapters. Explanations of more difficult terms are added in brackets.

Case Report

A 22-year-old known heroin abuser was admitted to an emergency room comatose with shallow respirations. Routine laboratory studies and chest x-rays were done after the patient was aroused. He was then transferred to the ICU. He complained of left-sided chest pain. Examination of the chest x-ray showed three fractured ribs on the right and a large right pleural effusion. Further questioning of a friend revealed that he had fallen and struck the corner of a table after injecting heroin.

The diagnosis was traumatic hemothorax secondary to fractured ribs, and a thoracotomy tube was inserted into the right pleural space. No blood could be obtained despite maneuvering of the tube. Another chest x-ray showed that the tube was correctly placed in the right pleural space but the fractured ribs and pleural effusion were on the left. The radiologist then realized that he had reversed the first film. A second tube was inserted into the left pleural space, and 1500 ml (6–7 cups) of blood was evacuated.

Necropsy Report and Questions

(Answers are found at the end of Answers to Exercises.)

Adenocarcinoma, bronchogenic, left lung, with extensive mediastinal, pleural, and pericardial involvement. Metastasis to tracheobronchial lymph nodes, liver, lumbar vertebrae. Pulmonary emboli, multiple, recent, with recent infarct of left lower lobe. The tumor apparently originated at the left main bronchus and extends peripherally. Parenchyma (alveoli) is particularly atelectatic with a centrally located area of hemorrhage in the lower lobe.

Questions

1. What was the patient's primary disease?
   (A) blood clots in the lung
   (B) mediastinal, pleural, and pericardial inflammation
   (C) lung cancer

2. Which was *not* an area of metastasis?
   (A) backbones
   (B) bone marrow
   (C) hepatocytes

3. What event was probably the cause of death?
   (A) infarction of lung tissue due to pulmonary emboli
   (B) COPD
   (C) myocardial infarction

4. What best describes the pulmonary parenchyma in the lower left lobe?
   (A) alveoli are filled with tumor
   (B) alveoli are collapsed with central area of bleeding
   (C) alveoli are filled with pus and blood

X-Ray Reports and Bronchoscopy

1. CXR: Complete opacification of left hemithorax with deviation of mediastinal structures of right side. Massive pleural effusion.

2. Chest tomograms: Mass most compatible with LUL bronchogenic carcinoma. Possible left paratracheal adenopathy or direct involvement of mediastinum.

3. Bronchoscopy: Larynx, trachea, carina [area of bifurcation or forking of the trachea], and left lung all within normal limits. On the right side there was irregularity and roughening of the bronchial mucosa on the lateral aspect of the bronchial wall. This irregularity extended into the RUL, and the apical and posterior segments [divisions of lobes of the lung] each contained inflamed irregular mucosa. Conclusion: suspicious for infiltrating tumor, but may be nonspecific inflammation. Bronchial washings, brushings, and bxs [biopsies] taken. Bronchial biopsy diagnosis: squamous cell carcinoma. Washings and brushings showed no malignant cells.

VIII. Exercises

Remember to check your answers carefully with those given in Section IX, Answers to Exercises.

A. *Select from the following anatomical structures to complete the sentences below.*

mediastinum	cilia	paranasal sinuses
alveoli	bronchioles	palatine tonsils
larynx	parietal pleura	visceral pleura
pharynx	hilum	adenoids
trachea	epiglottis	bronchi

1. The outer fold of pleura lying closest to the ribs is called _____ .

2. Collections of lymph tissue in the nasopharynx are the _____ .

3. The windpipe is known as the _____ .

4. The lid-like piece of cartilage that covers the voice box is the _____ .

5. Branches of the windpipe that lead into the lungs are the _____ .

6. The region between the lungs in the chest cavity is the _____ .

7. Air-containing cavities in the bones around the nose are the _____ .

8. Thin hairs attached to the mucous membrane lining the respiratory tract are called

    _____ .

9. The inner fold of pleura closest to lung tissue is called _____ .

10. The throat is known as the _____ .

11. Air sacs of the lung are called _____ .

12. The voice box is called the _____ .

13. Smallest branches of bronchi are the _____ .

14. Collections of lymph tissue in the oropharynx are the _____ .

15. The midline region where the bronchi, blood vessels, and nerves enter and exit the lungs is called the

    _____ .

B. *Complete the following sentences.*

1. The apical part of the lung is the _____ .

2. The gas that passes into the bloodstream at the lungs is _____ .

3. Breathing in air is called _____ .

4. Divisions of the lungs are known as _____ .

5. The gas produced by cells and exhaled through the lungs is called _____ .

6. The space between the visceral and the parietal pleura is called the _____ .

7. Breathing out air is called _____ .

8. The essential cells of the lung performing its main function are known as the pulmonary

   _____ .

9. The exchange of gases in the lung is called _____ respiration.

10. The exchange of gases at the tissue cells is called _____ respiration.

C. *Give the meanings for the following medical terms.*

1. rhinoplasty _____

2. thoracotomy _____

3. bronchiectasis _____

4. pleuritis _____

5. pneumothorax _____

6. anosmia _____

7. laryngectomy _____

8. nasopharyngitis _____

9. phrenic _____

10. alveolar _____

11. glottis _____

D. Complete the medical terms for the following respiratory symptoms.

1. excessive carbon dioxide in the blood: hyper _____

2. breathing is possible only in an upright position: _____ pnea

3. difficult breathing: _____ pnea

4. condition of blueness of skin: _____ osis

5. spitting up blood: hemo _____

6. deficiency of oxygen: hyp _____

7. condition of pus in the pleural cavity: pyo _____ or

   em _____

8. high-pitched, strained, noisy breathing associated with laryngeal or bronchial obstruction:

   stri _____

9. hoarseness; voice impairment: dys _____

10. blood in the pleural cavity: hemo _____

11. nosebleed: epi _____

E. Give the meanings for the following medical terms.

1. rales (crackles) _____

2. auscultation _____

3. sputum _____

4. percussion _____

5. rhonchi _____

6. pleural rub _____

7. purulent _____

8. paroxysmal nocturnal dyspnea _____

9. hydrothorax _____

10. pulmonary infarction _____

F. Match the following terms with their descriptions below.

chronic bronchitis   atelectasis   diphtheria
pertussis   emphysema   asthma
asbestosis   croup   bronchogenic carcinoma
cystic fibrosis

1. acute infectious disease of the throat caused by *Corynebacterium* _____

2. acute respiratory syndrome in children and infants marked by obstruction of the larynx and stridor

   _____

3. hyperinflation of air sacs with destruction of alveolar walls _____

4. inflammation of tubes that lead from the trachea; lasts for a long period of time

   _____

5. spasm and narrowing of bronchi leading to obstruction _____

6. lungs or a portion of lung is collapsed _____

7. malignant neoplasm originating in a bronchus _____

8. whooping cough _____

9. inherited disease of exocrine glands leading to airway obstruction _____

10. type of pneumoconiosis; dust particles are inhaled _____

G. Give the meanings for the following medical terms.

1. pulmonary abscess _____

2. pulmonary edema _____

3. pneumoconiosis _____

4. pneumonia _____

5. pulmonary embolism _____

6. small (oat) cell carcinoma _____

7. tuberculosis _____

8. pleural effusion _____

9. pleurisy _____

10. anthracosis _____

11. mesothelioma _____

12. adenoid hypertrophy _____

13. pleurodynia _____

14. expectoration _____

15. tachypnea _____

H. Match the clinical procedure or abbreviation with its description.

pulmonary function tests   mediastinoscopy   tube thoracostomy
tuberculin tests   bronchial alveolar lavage   thoracentesis
endotracheal intubation   bronchoscopy   lung scan (V/Q scan)
tracheostomy   laryngoscopy   pulmonary angiography

1. tube is placed through the mouth into the trachea to establish an airway _____

2. radioactive material is injected or inhaled, and images are recorded of its distribution in the lungs

_____

3. PPD, tine, and Mantoux's tests _____

4. chest wall is punctured with a needle to obtain fluid from the pleural cavity

_____

5. tests that measure the ventilation mechanics of the lung _____

6. an opening is made into the trachea through the neck to establish an airway

_____

7. visual examination of the bronchi _____

8. fluid is injected into the bronchi and then removed for examination _____

9. tube is inserted through the nose into the larynx to view the voice box _____

10. contrast material is injected into a blood vessel; x-rays are taken of arteries or veins in the lung

_____

11. visual examination of the area between the lungs _____

12. a chest tube is passed through a small skin incision to continuously drain the pleural spaces

_____

I. Give the meanings for the following abbreviations.

1. COPD _____

2. CXR _____

3. ARDS _____

4. CPR _____

5. URI _____

6. TB _____

7. Bronch _____

8. PFT _____

9. DPT _____

10. SOB _____

J. Match the surgical procedures with their meanings.

pneumonectomy   thoracotomy   thoracentesis
rhinoplasty   tonsillectomy   tube thoracostomy
laryngectomy   lobectomy

1. removal of lymph tissue in the oropharynx _____

2. surgical puncture of the chest to remove fluid from the pleural space _____

3. surgical repair of the nose _____

4. incision of the chest for lung biopsy _____

5. removal of the voice box _____

6. removal of a region of a lung _____

7. opening into the chest for insertion of drainage tube _____

8. pulmonary resection _____

K. Complete the term from the meaning given. Pay close attention to spelling.

1. muscular wall between the chest and abdomen: dia _____

2. listening for sounds in the chest: aus _____

3. flap of tissue covering the mouth of the larynx: epi _____

4. part of the throat near the nose: naso _____

5. removal of lymphatic tissue in the nasopharynx: aden _____

6. absence of pulse: a _____

7. incomplete expansion of a lung: atel _____

8. visual examination of the space between the lung: _____ scopy

9. hyperinflation of air sacs and breakdown of alveolar walls: em _____

10. swelling and collection of fluid in the lungs: pulmonary _____

11. spasm of bronchi leading to airway obstruction: _____

L. Circle the term that best completes the meaning of the sentence.

1. Ruth was having difficulty taking a deep breath and her chest x-ray showed accumulation of fluid in her pleural spaces. Dr. Smith ordered (PPD, tracheotomy, thoracentesis) to relieve the pressure on her lungs.

2. Dr. Wong used her stethoscope to perform (percussion, auscultation, thoracentesis) on the patient's chest.

3. Before surgery on Mrs. Hope, an 80-year-old-woman with lung cancer, her physicians ordered (COPD, bronchoscopy, PFTs) to determine the functioning of her lungs.

4. Sylvia was bringing up yellow-colored sputum and had a high fever. Her physician told her that she had (pneumonia, pulmonary embolism, pneumothorax) and needed antibiotics.

5. The night before her thoracotomy for lung biopsy, Mrs. White was told by her anesthesiologist that he would place a (an) (thoracostomy tube, laryngoscope, endotracheal tube) down her throat to keep her airways open during surgery.

IX. Answers to Exercises

A

1. parietal pleura	6. mediastinum	11. alveoli
2. adenoids	7. paranasal sinuses	12. larynx
3. trachea	8. cilia	13. bronchioles
4. epiglottis	9. visceral pleura	14. palatine tonsils
5. bronchi	10. pharynx	15. hilum

B

1. uppermost part	5. carbon dioxide	8. parenchyma
2. oxygen	6. pleural cavity	9. external
3. inspiration; inhalation	7. expiration; exhalation	10. internal
4. lobes		

C

1. surgical repair of the nose	5. air in the chest (pleural cavity)	9. pertaining to the diaphragm
2. incision of the chest	6. lack of sense of smell	10. pertaining to an air sac
3. dilation, widening of bronchi	7. removal of the voice box	11. opening to the larynx
4. inflammation of pleura	8. inflammation of the nose and throat	

D

1. hypercapnia
2. orthopnea
3. dyspnea
4. cyanosis
5. hemoptysis
6. hypoxia
7. pyothorax; empyema
8. stridor
9. dysphonia
10. hemothorax
11. epistaxis

E

1. abnormal crackling sounds heard on inspiration (usually indicates fluid inside a bronchus)
2. listening to sounds within the body
3. material expelled from the chest by coughing or clearing the throat
4. tapping on the surface to determine the underlying structure
5. abnormal rumbling sounds on expiration (caused by a narrowed secretion-filled bronchus)
6. abnormal grating sound produced by the motion of pleural surfaces rubbing against each other (caused by inflammation or tumor cells)
7. pertaining to pus-filled
8. sudden attack of difficult breathing associated with lying down at night (caused by congestive heart failure and pulmonary edema as the lungs fill with fluid)
9. fluid in the pleural cavity
10. area of dead tissue in the lung

F

1. diphtheria
2. croup
3. emphysema
4. chronic bronchitis
5. asthma
6. atelectasis
7. bronchogenic carcinoma
8. pertussis
9. cystic fibrosis
10. asbestosis

G

1. collection of pus in the lungs
2. swelling, fluid collection in the air sacs and bronchioles
3. abnormal condition of dust in the lungs
4. acute inflammation and infection of alveoli; they become filled with fluid and blood cells
5. floating clot or other material blocking the blood vessels of the lung
6. type of bronchogenic carcinoma; malignant lung tumor of uncertain origin
7. an infectious disease caused by rod-shaped bacilli and producing tubercules (nodes) of infection
8. collection of fluid in the pleural cavity
9. inflammation of pleura
10. abnormal condition of coal dust in the lungs (black-lung disease)
11. malignant tumor arising in the pleura; composed of mesothelium (epithelium that covers the surfaces of membranes such as pleura and peritoneum)
12. excessive growth of cells in the adenoids (lymph tissue in the nasopharynx)
13. pain of the pleura (irritation of pleural surfaces leads to intercostal pain)
14. coughing up of material from the chest
15. rapid breathing; hyperventilation

H

1. endotracheal intubation
2. lung scan
3. tuberculin tests
4. thoracentesis
5. pulmonary function tests
6. tracheostomy
7. bronchoscopy
8. bronchial alveolar lavage
9. laryngoscopy
10. pulmonary angiography
11. mediastinoscopy
12. tube thoracostomy

I

1. chronic obstructive pulmonary disease
2. chest x-ray
3. acute respiratory distress syndrome
4. cardiopulmonary resuscitation
5. upper respiratory infection
6. tuberculosis
7. bronchoscopy
8. pulmonary function tests
9. diphtheria, pertussis, tetanus
10. shortness of breath

J

1. tonsillectomy
2. thoracentesis
3. rhinoplasty
4. thoracotomy
5. laryngectomy
6. lobectomy
7. tube thoracostomy
8. pneumonectomy

K

1. diaphragm
2. auscultation
3. epiglottis
4. nasopharynx
5. adenoidectomy
6. asphyxia
7. atelectasis
8. mediastinoscopy
9. emphysema
10. pulmonary edema
11. asthma

L

1. thoracentesis
2. auscultation
3. PFTs
4. pneumonia
5. endotracheal tube

Answers to Practical Applications Questions

1. C
2. B
3. A
4. B

X. Pronunciation of Terms

To test your understanding of the terminology in this chapter, write the meaning of each term in the space provided. In addition, you may wish to cover the terms and write them by looking at your definitions. Make sure your spelling is correct. The page number after each term indicates where it is defined or used in the text so you can easily check your responses. (If you are not sure what the pronunciation symbols mean, refer to page 21.)

Vocabulary and Terminology

Term	Pronunciation	Meaning
adenoidectomy (401)	ăd-ĕ-noyd-ĔK-tō-mē	_____
adenoid hypertrophy (401)	ĂD-ĕ-noyd hī-PĔR-trō-fē	_____
adenoids (399)	ĂD-ĕ-noydz	_____
alveolar (401)	ăl-VĒ-ō-lăr	_____
alveolus (alveoli) (399)	ăl-VĒ-ō-lŭs (ăl-VĒ-ō-lī)	_____
anosmia (404)	ăn-ŎS-mē-ă	_____
apex of the lung (399)	Ā-pĕkz of the lŭng	_____
apical (399)	Ā-pĭ-kăl	_____
apnea (404)	ăp-NĒ-ă	_____
asphyxia (404)	ăs-FĬK-sē-ă	_____
atelectasis (403)	ă-tĕ-LĔK-tă-sĭs	_____
bronchiectasis (401)	brŏng-kē-ĔK-tă-sĭs	_____
bronchiole (399)	BRŎNG-kē-ŏl	_____
bronchiolitis (401)	brŏng-kē-ō-LĪ-tĭs	_____
bronchospasm (401)	BRŎNG-kō-spăzm	_____
carbon dioxide (399)	KĂR-bŏn dī-ŎK-sīd	_____
cilia (400)	SĬL-ē-ă	_____
cyanosis (402)	sī-ă-NŌ-sĭs	_____
diaphragm (400)	DĪ-ă-frăm	_____
dysphonia (402)	dĭs-FŌ-nē-ă	_____
dyspnea (404)	DĬSP-nē-ă	_____
empyema (404)	ĕm-pī-Ē-mă	_____

epiglottis (400)	ĕp-ĭ-GLŎT-ĭs
epiglottitis (402)	ĕp-ĭ-glŏ-TĪ-tĭs
expectoration (402)	ĕk-spĕk-tō-RĀ-shŭn
glottis (400)	GLŎ-tĭs
hemoptysis (404)	hē-MŎP-tĭ-sĭs
hemothorax (404)	hē-mŏ-THŌ-răks
hilum of the lung (400)	HĪ-lŭm of the lŭng
hypercapnia (401)	hī-pĕr-KĂP-nē-ă
hyperpnea (404)	hī-PĔRP-nē-ă
hypoxia (402)	hī-PŎK-sē-ă
laryngeal (402)	lă-RĬN-jē-ăl or lăr-ĭn-JĒ-ăl
laryngospasm (402)	lă-RĬNG-gō-spăzm
laryngitis (402)	lă-rĭn-JĪ-tĭs
larynx (400)	LĂR-ĭnks
lobectomy (402)	lō-BĔK-tō-mē
mediastinum (400)	mē-dē-ă-STĪ-nŭm
nasogastric tube (402)	nā-zō-GĂS-trĭk toob
nasopharyngitis (402)	nā-zō-făr-ĭn-JĪ-tĭs
orthopnea (402)	ŏr-thŏp-NĒ-ă
oxygen (400)	ŎKS-ĭ-jĕn
palatine tonsils (400)	PĂL-ĭ-tīn TŎN-sĭlz
paranasal sinuses (400)	pă-ră-NĀ-zăl SĪ-nĭ-sĕz
parietal pleura (400)	pă-RĪ-ĕ-tăl PLOO-răh
pharyngeal (402)	fă-RĬN-jē-ăl or făr-ĭn-JĒ-ăl
pharynx (400)	FĂR-ĭnkz
phrenic nerve (402)	FRĔN-ĭk nĕrv
phrenohepatic (402)	frĕn-ō-hĕ-PĂT-ĭk
pleura (400)	PLOOR-ă

pleural cavity (400)	PLOOR-ăl KĂ-vĭ-tē	_____
pleuritis (408)	ploo-RĪ-tĭs	_____
pneumoconiosis (402)	nū-mō-kō-nē-Ō-sĭs	_____
pneumonectomy (403)	nū-mō-NĔK-tō-mē	_____
pneumonitis (403)	nū-mō-NĪ-tĭs	_____
pneumothorax (403)	nū-mō-THŌ-răks	_____
pulmonary (403)	PŬL-mō-năr-ē	_____
pulmonary parenchyma (400)	pŭl-mō-NĂR-ē pă-RĔN-kă-mă	_____
pyothorax (404)	pī-ō-THŌ-răks	_____
rhinoplasty (403)	RĪ-nō-plăs-tē	_____
rhinorrhea (403)	rī-nō-RĒ-ăh	_____
sinusitis (403)	sī-nū-SĪ-tĭs	_____
spirometer (403)	spī-RŎM-ĕ-tĕr	_____
tachypnea (404)	tăk-ĭp-NĒ-ă	_____
thoracic (404)	thōr-RĂ-sĭk	_____
thoracotomy (404)	thōr-ră-KŎT-ō-mē	_____
tonsillectomy (404)	tŏn-sĭ-LĔK-tō-mē	_____
trachea (400)	TRĀ-kē-ă	_____
tracheal (404)	TRĀ-kē-ăl	_____
tracheotomy (404)	trā-kē-ŎT-ō-mē	_____
visceral pleura (400)	VĬ-sĕr-ăl PLOO-ră	_____

Pathology, Laboratory Tests, and Clinical Procedures

Term	Pronunciation	Meaning
anthracosis (409)	ăn-thră-KŌ-sĭs	_____
asbestosis (409)	ăs-bĕs-TŌ-sĭs	_____
asthma (406)	ĂZ-mă	_____
atelectasis (406)	ă-tĕ-LĔK-tă-sĭs	_____

auscultation (405)	ăw-skŭl-TĀ-shŭn	
bacilli (409)	bă-SĬL-ī	
bronchial alveolar lavage (411)	BRŎNG-kē-ăl ăl-vē-Ō-lar lă-VĂJ	
bronchogenic carcinoma (406)	brŏng-kō-JĔN-ĭk kăr-sĭ-NŌ-mă	
bronchoscopy (411)	brŏng-KŎS-kō-pē	
chest tomograms (409)	chĕst TŌ-mō-grămz	
chronic bronchitis (406)	KRŎ-nĭk brŏng-KĪ-tĭs	
chronic obstructive pulmonary disease (409)	KRŎ-nĭk ŏb-STRŬK-tĭv PŬL-mō-nă-rē dĭ-ZĒZ	
cor pulmonale (409)	kŏr pŭl-mō-NĂ-lē	
croup (405)	kroop	
cystic fibrosis (406)	SĬS-tĭk fī-BRŌ-sĭs	
diphtheria (405)	dĭf-THĔR-ē-ă	
emphysema (407)	ĕm-fĭ-ZĒ-mă	
endotracheal intubation (411)	ĕn-dō-TRĀ-kē-ăl ĭn-tū-BĀ-shŭn	
epistaxis (406)	ĕp-ĭ-STĂK-sĭs	
hydrothorax (409)	hī-drō-THŎR-ăks	
laryngoscopy (411)	lăr-ĭng-GŎS-kō-pē	
lung scan (411)	lŭng skăn	
mediastinoscopy (413)	mē-dē-ă-stī-NŎS-kō-pē	
mesothelioma (408)	mĕz-ō-thē-lē-Ō-mă	
paroxysmal (409)	păr-ŏk-SĬZ-măl	
percussion (405)	pĕr-KŬSH-ŭn	
pertussis (406)	pĕr-TŬS-ĭs	
pleural effusion (408)	PLOOR-ăl ĕ-FŪ-zhŭn	
pleurisy (408)	PLOOR-ă-sē	
pneumonia (407)	nū-MŌ-nē-ă	

pulmonary abscess (407)	PŬL-mō-nă-rē ĂB-sĕs	
pulmonary angiography (411)	PŬL-mō-nă-rē ăn-jē-ŎG-ră-fē	
pulmonary edema (407)	PŬL-mō-nă-rē ĕ-DĒ-mă	
pulmonary embolism (407)	PŬL-mō-nă-rē ĔM-bō-lĭzm	
pulmonary function tests (413)	PŬL-mō-nă-rē FŬNK-shŭn tĕstz	
pulmonary infarction (409)	PŬL-mō-nă-rē ĭn-FĂRK-shŭn	
purulent (409)	PŪ-roo-lĕnt	
rales (405)	răhlz	
rhonchi (405)	RŎNG-kī	
silicosis (409)	sĭ-lĭ-KŌ-sĭs	
sputum (405)	SPŬ-tŭm	
stridor (405)	STRĪ-dŏr	
thoracentesis (413)	thō-ră-sĕn-TĒ-sĭs	
tracheostomy (413)	trā-kē-ŎS-tō-mē	
tuberculin tests (413)	too-BĔR-kū-lĭn tĕstz	
tuberculosis (407)	too-bĕr-kū-LŌ-sĭs	
tube thoracostomy (413)	tūb thŏr-ă-KŎS-tō-mē	

XI. Review Sheet

Write the meanings of each word part in the space provided. Check your answers with the Glossary (Medical Terms—English) at the end of the book.

Combining Forms

Combining Form	Meaning	Combining Form	Meaning
adenoid/o		pector/o	
alveol/o		pharyng/o	
bronch/o		phon/o	
bronchi/o		phren/o	
bronchiol/o		pleur/o	
capn/o		pneum/o	
coni/o		pneumon/o	
cyan/o		pulmon/o	
epiglott/o		py/o	
hydr/o		rhin/o	
laryng/o		sinus/o	
lob/o		spir/o	
mediastin/o		tel/o	
nas/o		thorac/o	
or/o		tonsill/o	
orth/o		trache/o	
ox/o			

Continued on following page

Suffixes

Suffix	Meaning	Suffix	Meaning
-algia	_____	-pnea	_____
-capnia	_____	-ptysis	_____
-centesis	_____	-rrhea	_____
-dynia	_____	-scopy	_____
-ectasis	_____	-sphyxia	_____
-ectomy	_____	-stenosis	_____
-lysis	_____	-stomy	_____
-osmia	_____	-thorax	_____
-oxia	_____	-tomy	_____
-phonia	_____	-trophy	_____
-plasty	_____		

Prefixes

Prefix	Meaning	Prefix	Meaning
a-, an-	_____	hyper-	_____
brady-	_____	hypo-	_____
dys-	_____	para-	_____
em-	_____	per-	_____
eu-	_____	re-	_____
ex-	_____	tachy-	_____

Blood System

This Chapter is divided into the following sections

In this Chapter you will
- Identify terms relating to the composition, formation, and function of blood;
- Differentiate among the different types of blood groups;
- Identify terms related to blood clotting;
- Build words and recognize combining forms used in the blood system;
- Describe various pathological conditions affecting blood; and
- Differentiate among various laboratory tests, clinical procedures, and abbreviations used in connection with the blood system.

I. Introduction

The primary function of blood is to maintain a constant environment for the other living tissues of the body. Thus, blood is the transport system for foods, gases, and wastes throughout the body. Food that is digested in the stomach and small intestine passes into the bloodstream through the lining cells of the small intestine and is carried by the blood to all body cells. Oxygen enters the body through the air sacs of the lungs and is transported by the blood to cells throughout the body. Gaseous waste, such as carbon dioxide, and solid, nitrogen-containing wastes, such as urea, uric acid, and creatinine, are released by cells and travel through the blood to the lungs (where carbon dioxide is expelled) and kidneys (where nitrogenous wastes and salts are excreted in the urine).

Chemical messengers called hormones are also carried by the blood from their site of secretion in glands, such as the thyroid or pituitary, to distant sites where they regulate growth, reproduction, and energy production. These hormones will be discussed later in the endocrine chapter.

Finally, blood contains proteins and white blood cells that fight infection, and platelets (thrombocytes) that help the blood to clot.

II. Composition and Formation of Blood

Blood is composed of **cells,** or formed elements, suspended in a clear, straw-colored liquid called **plasma.** The cells include **erythrocytes** (red blood cells), **leukocytes** (white blood cells), and **platelets** or **thrombocytes** (clotting cells) and constitute about 45 per cent of the total blood volume. The remaining 55 per cent of blood is plasma, a solution of water, proteins, sugar, salts, hormones, and vitamins.

Cells

Most blood cells originate in the marrow cavity of bones. Both the red blood cells that carry oxygen and the white blood cells that fight infection arise from the same immature cells called **stem cells (hemocytoblasts).** Under the influence of proteins found in the bloodstream and bone marrow, the primitive stem cells change their size and shape and assume a specialized, or **differentiated,** form. In this process, the cells change in size from large (immature cells) to small (mature forms) and the cell nucleus shrinks (in red cells, the nucleus actually disappears). Figure 13–1 illustrates these changes in the formation of blood cells. Use Figure 13–1 as a reference as you learn about the names of mature blood cells and their earlier forms.

Erythrocytes

As a red blood cell matures (from the primitive erythroblast to normoblast to reticulocyte and finally to erythrocyte), its nucleus is pushed out and the cell assumes the shape of a disk. This shape (a depressed or hollow surface on each side of the cell, resembling a cough drop with a thin central portion) allows for a large surface area on the erythrocyte so that absorption and release of gases (oxygen and carbon dioxide) can take place. Red cells contain the unique protein **hemoglobin,** which consists of an iron-containing pigment called **heme** and a protein part called **globin.** Hemoglobin in the erythrocyte enables the cell to carry oxygen. The combination of oxygen and hemoglobin (oxyhemoglobin) produces the bright red color of blood.

Erythrocytes originate in the bone marrow, and their production is stimulated by a hormone called **erythropoietin (-poiesis** means formation). Erythropoietin is secreted by the

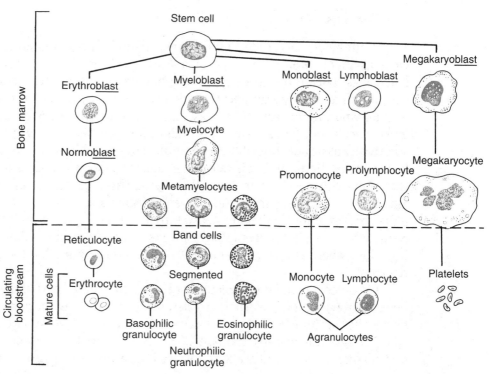

Figure 13-1

Stages in blood cell development. Notice that the suffix -blast is used to indicate immature forms of all cells. Band cells are identical to **segmented** granulocytes except that the nucleus is U-shaped and its lobes are connected by a band rather than a thin thread as in segmented cell forms.

kidney. Erythrocytes live for about 120 days in the circulating bloodstream. After this time, cells (called **macrophages**) in the spleen, liver, and bone marrow destroy the worn-out erythrocytes.

Macrophages break the hemoglobin down into its heme and protein portions. The heme releases iron and decomposes into a dark green pigment called **bilirubin.** The iron in hemoglobin is reutilized to form new red cells or is stored in the spleen, liver, or bone marrow. Bilirubin is excreted into the bile by the liver, and from the bile it enters the small intestine where it can be excreted in the stool. It imparts the dark brown color to stool. Two to 10 million red cells are destroyed each second, but because they are constantly being replaced, the number of circulating cells remains constant (4–6 million per cu mm) (Fig. 13–2).

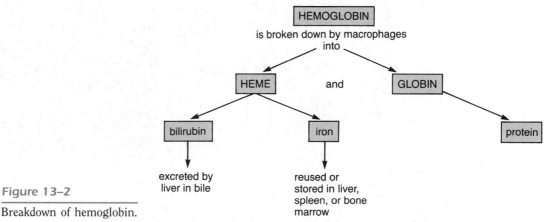

Figure 13–2

Breakdown of hemoglobin.

Leukocytes

White blood cells (7000–9000 cells per cu mm) are less numerous than erythrocytes, but whereas there is only one type of mature erythrocyte, there are five types of mature leukocytes. Locate the three types of granulocytic leukocytes (basophil, neutrophil, and eosinophil) and two agranulocytic leukocytes (monocyte and lymphocyte) in Figure 13–1.

Polymorphonuclear leukocytes, also known as **granulocytes,** are the most numerous leukocytes (about 60 per cent). **Basophils** contain dark-staining cytoplasmic granules that stain with a basic (alkaline) dye. The granules contain heparin (an anticlotting substance) and histamine (a chemical that is released in allergic responses). **Eosinophils** contain granules that stain with a red acidic dye called eosin. These granulocytes increase in numbers in allergic responses and are thought to engulf substances that trigger the allergies. **Neutrophils** contain granules that are neutral; that is, they do not stain intensely with either dye. Neutrophils are **phagocytes (phag/o** means to eat or swallow) that accumulate at sites of infection, where they ingest and destroy bacteria. Figure 13–3 shows phagocytosis by a neutrophil.

Granulocytes and their precursor cells are considered part of the **myeloid** (derived from bone marrow) line of cells. Their growth and proliferation in the bone marrow are stimulated by specific proteins called colony-stimulating factors (CSFs). G-CSF (granulocyte CSF), GM-CSF (granulocyte macrophage CSF), interleukin-1, and interleukin-3 have been produced commercially and are administered to promote or restore myeloid proliferation in cancer patients.

All granulocytes are **polymorphonuclear;** that is, they have multilobed nuclei. The term **polymorphonuclear leukocyte (poly)** is used most often to describe the **neutrophil,** which is the most numerous of the granulocytes.

Figure 13–3

Ingestion (phagocytosis) of a bacterium by a neutrophil. (From Hirsch JG: Cinemicrophotographic observations of granule lysis in polymorphonuclear leucocytes during phagocytosis. J Exp Med 116:827, 1962, by copyright permission of Rockefeller University Press.)

Table 13–1. LEUKOCYTES

Leukocyte	Percentage in Blood	Function
GRANULOCYTE		
Basophil	0–1	Contains heparin (prevents blood from clotting) and histamine (involved in allergic responses)
Eosinophil	1–4	Phagocytic cell involved in allergic reactions
Neutrophil	50–70	Phagocytic cell that accumulates at sites of infection
AGRANULOCYTE		
Lymphocyte	20–40	Controls the immune response; makes antibodies to destroy antigens
Monocyte	3–8	Phagocytic cell that becomes a macrophage and digests bacteria and tissue debris

Agranulocytes are **mononuclear** (containing one large nucleus) leukocytes that do not have dark-staining granules in their cytoplasm. These are the **lymphocytes** and **monocytes** (see Fig. 13–1). Lymphocytes arise in lymph nodes and circulate both in the bloodstream and in the parallel circulating system, the lymphatic system. They will be discussed in greater detail in Chapter 14, Lymphatic and Immune Systems.

Lymphocytes play an important role in the **immune** response that protects the body against infection. They are able to directly attack foreign matter and, in addition, make **antibodies,** which neutralize and destroy foreign **antigens** (bacteria and viruses). Monocytes are phagocytic cells that also fight disease. They move from the bloodstream into tissues (then they are called **macrophages**) and dispose of dead and dying cells and other tissue debris by phagocytosis.

Table 13–1 reviews the different types of leukocytes, their numbers in the blood, and their function.

Platelets

Platelets, or thrombocytes, are formed in the red bone marrow from giant multinucleated cells called **megakaryocytes** (see Fig. 13–1). Tiny fragments of the megakaryocyte break off from the cell to form platelets. The main function of platelets is to help in the clotting of blood. The specific terms related to blood clotting will be discussed in a later section of this chapter.

Plasma

Plasma is the liquid part of the blood and consists of water, dissolved proteins, sugar, wastes, salts, hormones, and other substances. The four major plasma proteins are **albumin, globulin, fibrinogen,** and **prothrombin** (the last two proteins are clotting proteins).

Albumin maintains the proper water content of the blood. Since albumin cannot pass easily through capillary walls, it remains in the blood and carries smaller molecules bound to its surface. It attracts water from the tissues back into the bloodstream and thus opposes the water's tendency to leave the blood and leak out into tissue spaces, which would cause **edema** (swelling). If albumin escapes from the capillaries as a result of injury, such as severe burn, water cannot be held in the blood and the blood volume drops. Shock can result if the loss of water is too great.

The **globulin** portion of plasma contains antibodies, which, as part of the body's immune system, destroy foreign substances called antigens. There are three different kinds of globulins in plasma. They are called **alpha, beta,** and **gamma,** and they can be separated by the process of **electrophoresis.** This technique involves placing the plasma in a special solution and passing an electric current through the solution. The different protein molecules in the plasma separate out as they migrate at different speeds to the source of the electricity.

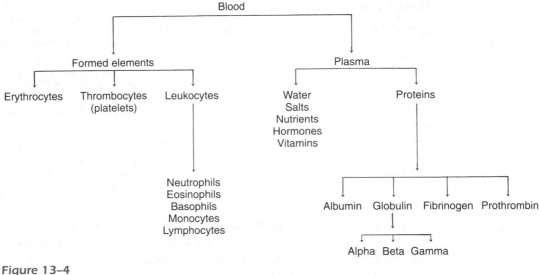

Figure 13–4

Composition of blood.

Immunoglobulins are a specific type of gamma globulin that are capable of acting as antibodies. Examples of immunoglobulin antibodies are **IgG** (found in high concentration in the plasma) and **IgA** (found in breast milk, saliva, tears, and respiratory mucus). Other immunoglobulins are **IgM, IgD,** and **IgE.**

Plasmapheresis (**-apheresis** means to remove) is the process of separating plasma from the formed elements in the blood. This separation is mechanical, not electrical, as electrophoresis is. In plasmapheresis, the entire blood sample is spun in a centrifuge machine, and the plasma, being lighter in weight than the blood cells, moves to the top of the sample.

Figure 13–4 reviews the composition of blood.

III. Blood Groups

Transfusions of "whole blood" (cells and plasma) are used to replace blood lost after injury, during surgery, or in severe shock. If a patient is anemic and needs only red blood cells, a transfusion of packed red cells (whole blood with most of the plasma removed) is given. A transfusion cannot be made between any two people at random, however. Human blood falls into four main groups called A, B, AB, and O, and there are harmful effects of transfusing blood from a donor of one blood group into a recipient who has blood of another blood group.

Each of the blood groups has a specific combination of factors (**antigens** and **antibodies**) that are inherited. These antigen and antibody factors of the various blood types are:

Type A, containing **A antigen** and **anti-B antibody**

Type B, containing **B antigen** and **anti-A antibody**

Type AB, containing **A and B antigens** and **no anti-A or anti-B antibodies**

Type O, containing **no A or B antigens** and **both anti-A and anti-B antibodies**

The problem in transfusing blood from a type A donor into a type B recipient is that A antigens (from the A donor) will react adversely with the anti-A antibodies in the recipient's type B bloodstream. The adverse reaction is called **agglutination,** or clumping of the recipient's blood. The agglutination is fatal to the recipient because it stops the flow of blood. Similar problems can occur in other transfusions if the donor's antigens are incompatible with the recipient's antibodies.

Table 13–2. BLOOD GROUPS

Type	Percentage in Population	Red Cell Antigens	Plasma Antibodies
A	41	A	Anti-B
B	10	B	Anti-A
AB	4	A and B	Neither anti-A nor anti-B
O	45	Neither A nor B	Anti-A and anti-B
Rh positive	85	Rh factor	No anti-Rh
Rh negative	15	No Rh factor	Anti-Rh (occurs if an Rh-negative person is given Rh-positive blood)

People with type O blood are known as universal donors because their blood contains neither A nor B antigens. The anti-A and anti-B antibodies in O blood do not have an effect in the recipient because the antibodies are diluted in the recipient's bloodstream. Those with type AB blood are known as universal recipients because their blood contains neither anti-A nor anti-B antibodies, so that neither the A nor the B group antigens will cause agglutination in their blood.

Besides A and B antigens, there are many other antigens located on the surface of red blood cells. One of these is called the **Rh factor** (named because it was first found in the blood of a rhesus monkey). The term Rh-positive refers to a person who is born with the Rh antigen on her or his red blood cells. An Rh-negative person does not have the Rh antigen. There are no anti-Rh antibodies normally present in the blood of an Rh-positive or an Rh-negative person. However, if Rh-positive blood is transfused into an Rh-negative person, the recipient will begin to develop antibodies that would agglutinate any Rh-positive blood if another transfusion were to occur subsequently.

The same reactions occur during pregnancy if the fetus of an Rh-negative woman happens to be Rh-positive. This situation is described in Chapter 4 as an example of an antigen-antibody reaction.

Table 13–2 shows the blood group types, their frequency of occurrence in the population, and their antigens and antibodies.

IV. Blood Clotting

Blood clotting, or **coagulation,** is a complicated process involving many different substances and chemical reactions. The final result (usually taking less than 15 minutes) is the formation of a **fibrin clot** from the plasma protein **fibrinogen.** Platelets are important in beginning the process following injury to tissues or blood vessels. The platelets clump or aggregate at the site of injury, releasing a protein, **thromboplastin,** which in combination with **calcium** and the sequential release of clotting factors (I–V and VII–XIII) promotes the formation of a fibrin clot. One of the clotting factors is a protein known as clotting factor VIII. It is missing in people who are born with hemophilia. Figure 13–5 reviews the basic sequence of events in the clotting process.

After the fibrin threads form the clot (trapping red blood cells and platelets and plasma), the clot retracts into a tight ball, leaving behind a clear fluid called **serum.** Normally, clots (thrombi) do not form in blood vessels unless the vessel is damaged or the flow of blood is impeded. Anticoagulant substances in the bloodstream inhibit blood clotting, so thrombi and emboli (floating clots) do not form. **Heparin,** produced by tissue cells (especially liver cells), is an example of an anticoagulant. Other drugs (such as dicumarol) are given to patients with thromboembolic diseases to prevent the formation of clots.

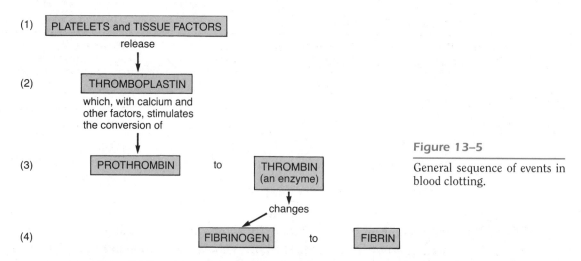

Figure 13–5

General sequence of events in blood clotting.

Vocabulary

This list will help you review many of the new terms introduced in the text. Short definitions will reinforce your understanding of the terms. See Section XII of this chapter for help in pronouncing the more difficult terms.

agglutination   Clumping of recipient's blood cells when incompatible bloods are mixed.

albumin   Protein found in blood; maintains the proper amount of water in the blood. Also called **serum albumin.**

antibodies   Protein substances whose formation by lymphocytes is stimulated by the presence of antigens in the body. An antibody then helps neutralize or inactive the antigen that stimulated its formation.

antigens   Foreign materials that cause the production of an antibody. Naturally occurring antigens are the blood type factors A and B that are present at birth in some individuals.

basophil   White blood cell with large, dark-staining granules that has an affinity for basic dyes.

bilirubin   Dark green pigment produced from hemoglobin when red blood cells are destroyed. Bilirubin is concentrated in bile by the liver and excreted in the feces.

coagulation   The process of blood clotting.

corpuscle   Little body—refers to a blood cell.

differentiation   Change in structure and function of a cell as it matures; specialization.

electrophoresis   Method of separating substances (such as proteins) by electrical charge.

eosinophil	White blood cell with dense, reddish granules having an affinity for the red acid dye eosin; associated with allergic reactions.
erythrocyte	A red blood cell. There are about 5 million in a speck of blood the size of a pinhead.
erythropoietin	A hormone secreted by the kidney to stimulate bone marrow to make red blood cells.
fibrin	Protein threads that form the basis of a blood clot.
fibrinogen	Plasma protein that is converted to fibrin in the clotting process.
formed elements	The cellular elements in blood.
globin	The protein part of hemoglobin.
globulin	Plasma protein; separates into alpha, beta, and gamma types by electrophoresis.
granulocytes	White blood cells with granules: eosinophils, neutrophils, and basophils.
heme	Iron-containing nonprotein portion of the hemoglobin molecule.
hemoglobin	Blood protein found in red blood cells; enables the red blood cell to carry oxygen.
heparin	An anticoagulant produced by liver cells and found in blood and tissues.
immune reaction	Reaction between an antigen and an antibody in which the antigen is neutralized or inactivated by the antibody.
immunoglobulin	A protein (globulin) with antibody activity; examples are IgG, IgM, IgA, IgE, IgD. Immun/o means protection.
leukocyte	A white blood cell.
lymphocyte	White blood cell (agranulocyte) found in lymph tissue; produces antibodies.
macrophages	Large phagocytes that destroy worn-out red blood cells and engulf foreign material in body tissues. They are monocytes that have left the blood and entered tissue spaces.
megakaryocyte	Platelet precursor (forerunner) formed in the bone marrow.
monocyte	White blood cell (agranulocyte) formed in lymph tissue; phagocyte. Monocytes become macrophages as they leave the blood and enter body tissues.
myeloid	Derived from (-oid) bone marrow cells.

neutrophil	White blood cell (granulocyte) formed in bone marrow; a phagocyte with neutral-staining granules; also called a **polymorphonuclear leukocyte.**
plasma	Liquid portion of blood; contains water, proteins, salts, nutrients, hormones, and vitamins.
plasmapheresis	Process of using a centrifuge to separate (-apheresis) or remove the formed elements from the blood plasma. Formed elements are retransfused into the donor, and fresh frozen plasma is used to replace withdrawn plasma. The procedure may be done to collect plasma for analysis or therapy.
platelet	Smallest formed element in the blood; a thrombocyte.
prothrombin	Plasma protein; converted to thrombin in the clotting process.
reticulocyte	Developing red blood cell with a network of granules in its cytoplasm.
Rh factor	An antigen normally found on red blood cells of Rh-positive individuals.
serum	Plasma minus clotting proteins and cells.
stem cell	A cell in bone marrow that gives rise to different types of blood cells.
thrombin	An enzyme that helps to convert fibrinogen to fibrin during coagulation.
thrombocyte	Platelet.
thromboplastin	A clotting factor that, in combination with calcium, promotes the formation of the fibrin clot.

VI. Combining Forms, Suffixes, and Terminology

Write the meaning of the medical term in the space provided.

Combining Forms			
Combining Form	Meaning	Terminology	Meaning
agglutin/o	clumping, sticking together	agglutination _____ *-ation means process.*	
baso/o	base (*alkaline,* the opposite of acid)	basophil _____ *-phil means attraction to.*	

chrom/o	color	hypo<u>chrom</u>ia _____
		Reduction in hemoglobin in red blood cells.
coagul/o	clotting	anti<u>coagul</u>ant _____
cyt/o	cell	<u>cyt</u>ology _____
eosin/o	red, dawn, rosy	<u>eosin</u>ophil _____
erythr/o	red	<u>erythr</u>ocytopenia _____
		-penia means deficiency.
granul/o	granules	<u>granul</u>ocyte _____
hem/o	blood	<u>hem</u>olysis _____
		Destruction of red blood cells. See hemolytic anemia, page 444, Section VII, Pathological Conditions.
hemat/o	blood	<u>hemat</u>ocrit _____
		-crit means to separate. The hematocrit gives the percentage of red blood cells in a volume of blood. See page 448, Section VIII, under Laboratory Tests.
hemoglobin/o	hemoglobin	<u>hemoglobin</u>opathy _____
is/o	same, equal	an<u>is</u>ocytosis _____
		This term refers to an abnormality of red blood cells; they are of unequal (anis/o) size; -cytosis means a slight increase in numbers of cells.
kary/o	nucleus	mega<u>kary</u>ocyte _____
leuk/o	white	<u>leuk</u>ocytopenia _____
		Can be shortened to leukopenia.
mon/o	one, single	<u>mon</u>ocyte _____
		The cell has a single, rather than multilobed, nucleus.
morph/o	shape, form	<u>morph</u>ology _____
myel/o	bone marrow	<u>myel</u>oblast _____
		-blast indicates an immature cell.
neutr/o	neutral (neither base nor acid)	<u>neutr</u>openia _____
		This term refers to neutrophils.

nucle/o	nucleus	mono<u>nuclear</u> _____
		polymorpho<u>nuclear</u> _____
phag/o	eat, swallow	<u>phag</u>ocyte _____
poikil/o	varied, irregular	<u>poikil</u>ocytosis _____

Irregularity in the shape of red blood cells. Poikilocytosis occurs in certain types of anemia.

sider/o	iron	<u>sider</u>openia _____
spher/o	globe, round	<u>spher</u>ocytosis _____

In this condition, the erythrocyte has a round shape, making the cell very fragile and easily destroyed.

thromb/o	clot	<u>thromb</u>ocytopenia _____

Suffixes

Suffix	Meaning	Terminology	Meaning
-apheresis	removal, carry away	plasm<u>apheresis</u> _____	

A centrifuge is used to spin blood to separate or remove plasma from the other parts of blood.

		leuk<u>apheresis</u> _____	
		platelet<u>pheresis</u> _____	

Note that the a of apheresis is dropped in this term. Platelets are removed from the donor's blood (and used in a patient), and the remainder of the blood is retransfused into the donor.

-blast	immature, embryonic	mono<u>blast</u> _____	
		erythro<u>blast</u> _____	
-cytosis	abnormal condition of cells (slight increase in cell numbers)	macro<u>cytosis</u> _____	

This term refers to red blood cells (macrocytes) that are larger (macro-) than normal size.

micro<u>cytosis</u> _____

This term refers to red blood cells that are smaller (micro-) than normal size. Table 13–3 reviews terms related to abnormalities of red blood cell morphology.

Table 13–3. ABNORMALITIES OF RED BLOOD CELL MORPHOLOGY

Abnormality	Description
anisocytosis	Cells are **unequal** in size
hypo**chrom**ia	**Color** of cells is reduced (less hemoglobin)
macrocytosis	Cells are **large**
microcytosis	Cells are **small**
poikilocytosis	Cells are **irregularly shaped**
spherocytosis	Cells are **rounded**

-emia	blood condition	leukemia _____
		See page 446, Section VII, Pathological Conditions.
-globin	protein	hemoglobin _____
-globulin	protein	gamma globulin _____
-lytic	pertaining to destruction	thrombolytic therapy _____
-oid	resembling, derived from	myeloid _____
-osis	abnormal condition	thrombosis _____
-penia	deficiency	granulocytopenia _____
		pancytopenia _____
-phage	eat, swallow	macrophage _____
-philia	attraction for (an increase in cell numbers)	eosinophilia _____
		neutrophilia _____
-phoresis	carrying, transmission	electrophoresis _____
-poiesis	formation	hematopoiesis _____
		erythropoiesis _____
		Erythropoietin is produced by the kidney to stimulate red blood cell formation.
		myelopoiesis _____
-stasis	stop, control	hemostasis _____

VII. Pathological Conditions

Any abnormal or pathological condition of the blood is generally referred to as a blood **dyscrasia** (disease). The blood dyscrasias discussed in this section are organized in the following manner: diseases of red blood cells, disorders of blood clotting, diseases of white blood cells, and bone marrow disease.

Diseases of Red Blood Cells

anemia

Deficiency in erythrocytes or hemoglobin.

The most common type of anemia is **iron-deficiency anemia** caused by a lack of iron, which is required for hemoglobin production (Fig. 13–6). Other types of anemia include:

1. aplastic anemia

Failure of blood cell production due to aplasia (absence of development, formation) of bone marrow cells.

The cause of most cases of aplastic anemia is often unknown (idiopathic), but some cases have been linked to benzene exposure and to antibiotics such as chloramphenicol. **Pancytopenia** occurs as stem cells fail to produce leukocytes, platelets, and erythrocytes. Blood transfusions prolong life until the marrow resumes its normal functioning, and antibiotics are used to control infections. Bone marrow transplants (see Section VIII, under Clinical Procedures) have been successful, particularly those conducted with marrow from an identical twin.

2. hemolytic anemia

Reduction in red cells due to excessive destruction.

One example of hemolytic anemia is **congenital spherocytic anemia** (also called **hereditary spherocytosis**). Instead of their normal biconcave shape, erythrocytes are spheroidal. This shape makes them very fragile and easily destroyed (hemolysis), leading to anemia. The spherocytosis causes increased numbers of reticulocytes in

Figure 13–6

Blood smear from a patient with advanced iron-deficiency anemia *(right)* and from a normal subject *(left)*. Red cells from the iron-deficient subject are poorly hemoglobinized (hypochromic), smaller than normal (microcytic), and vary in size and shape (anisocytosis and poikilocytosis). (From Wyngaarden JB, Smith LH Jr [eds]: Cecil Textbook of Medicine, 19th ed. Philadelphia, WB Saunders, 1992, p 844.)

Figure 13–7

Scanning electron micrographs of oxygenated *(A)* and deoxygenated *(B)* sickle-cell erythrocytes. *(A* and *B,* Courtesy of Dr. James White.)

the circulating blood as the bone marrow attempts to compensate for the hemolysis of mature erythrocytes. The excessive hemolysis leads to jaundice because of accumulation of bilirubin in the circulating bloodstream. Since the spleen is an organ in which red cells are destroyed, it may be removed with helpful results. In some cases, hemolytic anemia is due to production of **autoimmune** antibodies that destroy the red cells.

3. pernicious anemia

Lack of mature erythrocytes owing to inability to absorb vitamin B_{12} into the body. (**Pernicious** means ruinous or hurtful.)

Vitamin B_{12} is necessary for the proper development and maturation of erythrocytes. Although vitamin B_{12} is a common constituent of food matter (liver, kidney, sardines, egg yolks, oysters), it cannot be absorbed into the bloodstream without the aid of a special substance called **intrinsic factor** that is normally found in gastric juice. Individuals with pernicious anemia lack this factor in their gastric juice, and the result is unsuccessful maturation of red blood cells, with an excess of large, immature, nucleated, and poorly functioning cells (**megaloblasts)** in the circulation. Treatment is administration of vitamin B_{12} for life.

4. sickle cell anemia

Hereditary condition characterized by abnormal shape of erythrocytes and by hemolysis.

The crescent or sickle shape of the erythrocyte is caused by an abnormal type of hemoglobin (hemoglobin S) in the red cell (see Fig. 13–7). The distorted, fragile erythrocytes are poorly oxygenated and clump together, blocking blood vessels, leading to thrombosis and infarction (dead tissue). Symptoms include arthralgias, acute attacks of abdominal pain, and ulcerations of the extremities. The genetic defect (presence of the hemoglobin S gene) is particularly prevalent in black persons of African or Afro-American ancestry and appears with different degrees of severity depending on the presence of one or two inherited genes for the trait.

5. thalassemia

An inherited defect in the ability to produce hemoglobin, usually seen in persons of Mediterranean (*thalassa* is a Greek word meaning sea) background.

This condition, consisting of various forms and degrees of severity (the most severe form is called **Cooley's anemia**), usually leads to hypochromic anemia (diminished hemoglobin content in red cells).

hemochromatosis

Excessive deposits of iron throughout the body.

Hepatomegaly occurs and the skin is pigmented, so that it has a bronze hue; diabetes can occur and frequently cardiac failure develops. The condition is usually seen in men over 40 years of age.

polycythemia vera

General increase in red blood cells **(erythremia).**

Blood consistency is viscous (sticky) because of greatly increased numbers of erythrocytes. The bone marrow is hyperplastic, and leukocytosis and thrombocytosis accompany the increase in red blood cells. Treatment consists of reduction of red cell volume to normal levels by phlebotomy (removal of blood from a vein) and by suppressing production with myelotoxic drugs.

Disorders of Blood Clotting

hemophilia

Excessive bleeding caused by a congenital (hereditary) lack of one of the protein substances **(factor VIII)** necessary for blood clotting.

Although the platelet count of a hemophiliac patient is normal, there is a marked deficiency in a plasma clotting factor (factor VIII), which results in a very prolonged coagulation time. Treatment consists of administration of the deficient factor.

purpura

Multiple pinpoint hemorrhages and accumulation of blood under the skin.

Purpura means purple, and in this bleeding condition, hemorrhages into the skin and mucous membranes produce red-purple discoloration of the skin. The bleeding is caused by a fall in the number of platelets (thrombocytopenia). The etiology of the disorder may be immunological, meaning the body produces an antiplatelet factor that harms its own platelets. **Idiopathic thrombocytopenic purpura** is a condition in which a patient makes an antibody that destroys his or her own platelets. Bleeding time is prolonged and the cause is unknown. Splenectomy (spleen is the site of platelet destruction) and drug therapy with corticosteroids to discourage antibody synthesis are methods of treatment. Purpura is also seen in any other condition associated with a low platelet count, such as leukemia and drug reactions.

Diseases of White Blood Cells

leukemia

Excessive increase in cancerous white blood cells.

This is a disease of the bone marrow with malignant leukocytes filling the marrow and bloodstream. There are several types of leukemia, depending on the particular leukocyte involved. The terms **acute** and **chronic** are used to refer to a large number of immature (in acute forms) or mature, differentiated (in chronic forms) leukocytes in the blood. Four types of leukemia are:

acute myelogenous (myelocytic) leukemia (AML)—Immature granulocytes (myeloblasts) predominate. Platelets and erythrocytes are diminished because of infiltration and replacement of the bone marrow by large numbers of myeloblasts (Fig. 13–8).

acute lymphocytic leukemia (ALL)—Immature lymphocytes (lymphoblasts) predominate. This form is seen most often in children and adolescents; onset is sudden.

chronic myelogenous (myelocytic) leukemia (CML)—Both mature and immature granulocytes are present in the marrow and bloodstream. This is

Figure 13-8

(A) A normal blood smear. Note the many erythrocytes, polymorphonuclear lymphocytes, and monocytes. *(B)* Blood smear in acute myelogenous leukemia. Note the many immature granulocytes (myeloblasts).

a slowly progressive illness in which patients may live for many years without encountering life-threatening problems. Also called **chronic granulocytic leukemia.**

chronic lymphocytic leukemia (CLL)—Abnormal numbers of relatively mature lymphocytes predominate in the marrow, lymph nodes, and spleen. This form of leukemia occurs later in life and follows a slowly progressive course.

All forms of leukemia are treated with chemotherapy, using drugs that prevent cell division and selectively injure rapidly dividing cells. Effective treatment can lead to a **remission** (disappearance of signs of disease). **Relapse** occurs when leukemia cells reappear in the blood and bone marrow, necessitating further treatment.

Transplantation of normal bone marrow from closely related donors is successful in restoring normal bone marrow function in some patients with acute leukemia; this procedure is performed following high-dose chemotherapy given to eliminate the leukemic cells.

granulocytosis

Abnormal increase in granulocytes in the blood.

An increase in granulocytes in the blood may occur in response to infection or inflammation of any type. **Eosinophilia** is an increase in eosinophilic granulocytes, which is seen in certain allergic conditions, such as asthma, or in parasitic infections (tapeworm, pinworm). **Basophilia** is an increase in basophilic granulocytes seen in certain types of leukemia.

Diseases of Bone Marrow Cells

multiple myeloma

Malignant tumor of bone marrow.

This is a progressive tumor of antibody-producing cells (called **plasma cells**). The malignant cells invade the bone marrow and destroy bony structures. The tumors lead to overproduction of immunoglobulins and **Bence Jones protein,** an immunoglobulin fragment found in urine. Often, the condition leads to osteolytic lesions, hypercalcemia, anemia, renal damage, and increased susceptibility to infection. Treatment is with analgesics, radiotherapy, **palliative** (relieving, not curing) doses of chemotherapy, and special orthopedic supports.

VIII. Laboratory Tests, Clinical Procedures, and Abbreviations

Laboratory Tests

antiglobulin test (Coombs' test) Demonstrates whether the patient's erythrocytes are coated with antibody and is useful in determining the presence of antibodies in infants of Rh– women or in patients with autoimmune hemolytic anemia.

bleeding time Time it takes for a small puncture wound to stop bleeding. Normal time is 8 minutes or less. Bleeding time is prolonged with use of aspirin and in platelet disorders such as thrombocytopenia. There are several testing methods, but the most widely used is the Simplate (incision is made while constant pressure is applied using a sphygmomanometer). Normal bleeding will stop in 2–9 minutes.

complete blood count (CBC) This usually includes the following studies: red blood cell count, white blood cell count (with differential), platelet count, hemoglobin test, hematocrit, and red cell indices—MCH, MCV, MCHC (see Abbreviations). These routine tests are performed by automatic machines.

coagulation (clotting) time Time required for venous blood to clot in a test tube. Normal time is less than 15 minutes.

erythrocyte sedimentation rate (sed rate) Speed at which erythrocytes settle out of plasma. Venous blood is collected, anticoagulant is added, and the blood is placed in a tube in a vertical position. The distance that the erythrocytes fall in a given period of time is the sedimentation rate. The rate is altered in disease conditions, such as infections, joint inflammation, and tumor, that increase the immunoglobulin content of the blood.

hematocrit (Hct) Percentage of erythrocytes in a volume of blood. A sample of blood is spun in a centrifuge so that the erythrocytes fall to the bottom of the sample.

hemoglobin test (Hb) Total amount of hemoglobin in a sample of peripheral blood.

partial thromboplastin time Measures the presence of factors that act at early points in the coagulation pathway.

platelet count Number of platelets per cubic millimeter. Platelets normally average between 200,000 and 400,000 per cu mm.

prothrombin time This is a test of the ability of blood to clot. It measures the time elapsed between the addition of calcium to a plasma sample and the appearance of a visible clot. The test is used to follow patients taking blood thinners (anticoagulants).

red blood cell count (RBC) Number of erythrocytes per cubic millimeter of blood. The normal number is 4–6 million per cu mm.

red blood cell morphology   A stained blood smear is examined to determine the shape or form of individual red cells. The presence of anisocytosis, poikilocytosis, sickle cells, and hypochromia can be noted.

white blood cell count   This is the number of leukocytes per cubic millimeter. Automatic counting devices can record the numbers within seconds. Leukocytes normally average between 5000 and 10,000 per cu mm.

white blood cell differential   This test determines the numbers of different types of leukocytes (immature and mature forms). The cells are stained and counted under a microscope by a technician. A minimum of 100 cells is counted, and the percentages for neutrophils, lymphocytes, monocytes, basophils, and eosinophils are given.

The term **shift to the left** is used to describe a condition in which there is an increase in immature neutrophils and a decrease in mature forms in the blood.

Clinical Procedures

apheresis   Separation of blood into its parts. It is performed to remove toxic substances or autoantibodies from the blood or to harvest blood cells. Leukapheresis, plateletpheresis, and plasmapheresis are examples.

blood transfusion   In this procedure, whole blood or cells are taken from a donor, and after appropriate testing to assure a close match of red cell or platelet type, the whole blood or cells are infused into a patient. Prior to transfusion, tests are performed to assure that the specimen is free from hepatitis or acquired immunodeficiency syndrome (AIDS) virus. **Autologous transfusion** is the collection and later reinfusion of a patient's own (auto- means self) blood or blood components.

bone marrow biopsy   A needle is introduced into the bone marrow cavity, and a small amount of marrow is aspirated. The marrow is then examined under the microscope. This procedure is helpful in the diagnosis of blood disorders such as anemia, cytopenias, and leukemia.

bone marrow transplant   Bone marrow cells from a donor whose tissue and blood cells closely match those of the recipient are infused into a patient with leukemia or aplastic anemia. First the patient is given total-body irradiation or aggressive chemotherapy to kill all diseased cells. The donor's marrow is then intravenously infused into the patient, and it repopulates the patient's marrow space with normal cells. Problems encountered subsequently may be serious infection, graft versus host disease (immune reaction of the donor's cells to the recipient's), and relapse of the original disease (such as leukemia) despite the treatment (Fig. 13–9).

Figure 13–9

Bone marrow transplantation.

ABBREVIATIONS

ABO	Three main blood types	**G-CSF**	Granulocyte colony-stimulating factor
ALL	Acute lymphocytic leukemia	**GM-CSF**	Granulocyte macrophage colony-stimulating factor
AML	Acute myelogenous leukemia		
baso	Basophils	**Hct**	Hematocrit
BMT	Bone marrow transplant	**Hgb**	Hemoglobin
CBC	Complete blood count	**IgA, IgD, IgE, IgG, IgM**	Immunoglobulins
CLL	Chronic lymphocytic leukemia	**lymphs**	Lymphocytes
CML	Chronic myelogenous leukemia	**MCH**	Average amount of hemoglobin per cell (mean corpuscular hemoglobin)
diff.	Differential count (white blood cells)		
eos	Eosinophils	**MCHC**	Average concentration of hemoglobin in a single red cell (mean corpuscular hemoglobin concentration). When MCHC is low, the cell is hypochromic.
ESR	Erythrocyte sedimentation rate		

MCV	Average volume or size of a single red blood cell (mean corpuscular volume). When MCV is high, the cells are macrocytic and when low, the cells are microcytic.	PT	Prothrombin time
		PTT	Partial thromboplastin time
		RBC	Red blood cell (red blood cell count)
mono	Monocyte	sed rate	Erythrocyte sedimentation rate
poly	Polymorphonuclear leukocyte	segs	Segmented, mature white blood cells
PMN, PMNL	Polymorphonuclear leukocyte	WBC	White blood cell (white blood cell count)

IX. Practical Applications

 Normal Laboratory Values

WBC 5000–10,000/cu mm
Differential:
    Segs (polys) 54–62%
    Lymphs   20–40%
    Eos   1–3%
    Baso   0–1%
    Mono   3–7%
RBC   (M) 4.5–6.0 million
       (F) 4.0–5.5 million

Hct   (M) 40–50%
       (F) 37–47%
Hgb (M) 14–16 gm/dL
       (F) 12–14 gm/dL
Platelets 200,000–400,000/cu mm

Three Short Cases

Answers are at the end of the Answers to Exercises section.

1. A 65-year-old Swedish lady visits her doctor complaining of shortness of breath and swollen ankles. Lab tests reveal that her hematocrit is 18.0 and hemoglobin 5.8. Her blood smear shows megaloblasts and her blood level of vitamin B_{12} is very low. What is your diagnosis?
   (A) aplastic anemia
   (B) hemochromatosis
   (C) pernicious anemia
   (D) polycythemia vera

2. A 22-year-old college student visits the clinic with a fever and complaining of a sore throat. Blood tests show a WBC of 28,000 with 95% myeloblasts (polys are 5%). Platelet count is 15,000, hemoglobin is 10, hematocrit is 32.5. What is your diagnosis?
   (A) Chronic lymphocytic leukemia
   (B) Acute myelogenous leukemia
   (C) Thalassemia
   (D) Multiple myeloma

3. A 35-year-old female comes to her doctor complaining of spots on her legs and bleeding gums. On examination she has minute purple spots covering her legs and evidence of dried blood in her mouth. Her CBC shows hemoglobin 14, hematocrit 42, WBC 5000 with normal differential, platelet count 4000 (with megakaryocytes in bone marrow). What is your diagnosis?

(A) sickle cell anemia
(B) hemolytic anemia
(C) acute lymphocytic leukemia
(D) idiopathic thrombocytopenic purpura

Multiple Myeloma

Multiple myeloma is a neoplastic proliferation of plasma cells. The clinical manifestations of the disease result from the effects of the myeloma tumor cell mass in the bone marrow as well as from the myeloma proteins produced by the malignant cells. The effects of the tumor cell mass include lytic skeletal lesions, hypercalcemia, anemia, leukopenia, and thrombocytopenia. Clinical features related to the myeloma proteins include hyperviscosity [excessive stickiness], coagulopathy, and renal insufficiency [tubules get plugged with protein material].

X. Exercises

Remember to check your answers carefully with those given in Section XI, Answers to Exercises.

A. *Match the following cells with their meanings below.*

eosinophil   lymphocyte   monocyte
stem cell   platelet   neutrophil
basophil   erythrocyte

1. white blood cell (agranulocyte) formed in lymph tissue; it is a phagocyte and the precursor of a

   macrophage _____

2. thrombocyte or cell that helps blood clot _____

3. cell in the bone marrow that gives rise to different types of blood cells

   _____

4. leukocyte formed in lymph tissue; produces antibodies

   _____

5. leukocyte with dense, reddish granules having an affinity for red acid dye; associated with allergic

   reactions _____

6. red blood cell _____

7. leukocyte (polymorphonuclear granulocyte) formed in the bone marrow and having neutral-staining

   granules _____

8. leukocyte (granulocyte) whose granules have an affinity for basic dye; releases histamine and heparin

   _____

B. Give the meanings for the following terms that relate to blood cells.

1. corpuscle _____

2. granulocyte _____

3. mononuclear _____

4. polymorphonuclear _____

5. agranulocyte _____

6. erythroblast _____

7. megakaryocyte _____

8. macrophage _____

9. hemoglobin _____

10. myeloid _____

11. reticulocyte _____

12. myeloblast _____

C. Give the medical terms for the following descriptions.

1. liquid portion of blood _____

2. dark green pigment produced from hemoglobin when red blood cells are destroyed

   _____

3. iron-containing nonprotein part of hemoglobin _____

4. protein in plasma; can be separated into alpha, beta, and gamma types _____

5. hormone secreted by the kidney to stimulate bone marrow to produce red blood cells

   _____

6. foreign material that stimulates the production of an antibody _____

7. plasma protein that maintains the proper amount of water in the blood _____

8. proteins made by lymphocytes in response to antigens in the blood _____

D. Give short answers for the following.

1. Name four plasma proteins. _____

2. What is the RH factor? _____

3. What is agglutination? _____

4. A person with type A blood has _____

   antigens and _____ antibodies in his or her blood.

5. A person with type B blood has _____

   antigens and _____ antibodies in her or his blood.

6. A person with type O blood has _____

   antigens and _____ antibodies in his or her blood.

7. A person with type AB blood has _____ antigens and _____

   antibodies in her or his blood.

8. Can you transfuse blood from an A type donor into a B type recipient? _____

   Why? _____

9. Can you transfuse blood from an AB type donor into an O type recipient? _____

   Why? _____

10. What is electrophoresis? _____

11. What is an immunoglobulin? _____

12. What is differentiation? _____

13. What is plasmapheresis? _____

E. Match the following terms related to clotting with their meanings below.

coagulation   heparin   prothrombin
serum   thrombin   fibrin
fibrinogen   thromboplastin

1. an anticoagulant substance produced by liver cells and found in the bloodstream and tissues

_____

2. protein threads that form the basis of a blood clot _____

3. a plasma protein that is converted to thrombin in the clotting process _____

4. plasma minus clotting proteins and cells _____

5. a clotting factor that, in combination with calcium, promotes the clotting process

_____

6. a plasma protein converted to fibrin in the clotting process _____

7. the process of clotting _____

8. an enzyme that helps convert fibrinogen to fibrin _____

F. Divide the following terms into component parts and give the meaning of the entire term.

1. anticoagulant _____

2. hemoglobinopathy _____

3. cytology _____

4. leukocytopenia _____

5. morphology _____

6. megakaryocyte _____

7. sideropenia _____

8. phagocyte _____

9. myeloblast _____

10. plateletpheresis _____

11. monoblast _____

12. myelopoiesis _____

13. hemostasis _____

14. thrombolytic _____

15. hematopoiesis _____

G. Match the following terms concerning red blood cells with their meanings below.

hematocrit	erythropoiesis	hemoglobin
hemolysis	polycythemia vera	anisocytosis
erythrocytopenia	poikilocytosis	macrocytosis
hypochromia	spherocytosis	microcytosis

1. irregularity in the shape of red blood cells _____

2. oxygen-containing protein in red blood cells _____

3. formation of red blood cells _____

4. deficiency in numbers of red blood cells _____

5. destruction of red blood cells _____

6. reduction of hemoglobin in red blood cells _____

7. variation in size of red blood cells _____

8. abnormal numbers of round, rather than normally biconcave-shaped, red blood cells

   _____

9. increase in number of small red blood cells _____

10. general increase in numbers of red blood cells; erythremia _____

11. increase in numbers of large red blood cells _____

12. separation of blood so that the percentage of red blood cells in relation to the volume of a blood sample

   is measured _____

H. Describe the problem in each of the following forms of anemia.

1. iron-deficiency anemia _____

2. pernicious anemia _____

3. sickle cell anemia _____

4. aplastic anemia _____

5. thalassemia _____

I. Give the meanings for the following abbreviations that describe different types of leukemias.

1. CLL _____

2. AML _____

3. ALL _____

4. CML _____

J. Give the meanings for the following blood dyscrasias.

1. idiopathic thrombocytopenic purpura _____

2. granulocytosis _____

3. hemophilia _____

4. hemochromatosis _____

5. multiple myeloma _____

K. Match the term in column I with its meaning in column II. Write the letter of the meaning in the space provided.

Column I

1. relapse   _____

2. remission   _____

3. palliative   _____

4. Bence Jones protein _____

5. purpura   _____

6. pancytopenia   _____

7. apheresis   _____

8. eosinophilia   _____

Column II

A. deficiency of all blood cells.

B. immunoglobulin fragment found in the urine of patients with multiple myeloma

C. increase in numbers of granulocytes; seen in allergic conditions

D. relieving, but not curing

E. symptoms of the disease return

F. multiple pinpoint hemorrhages with accumulation of blood under the skin

G. symptoms of disease disappear

H. separation of blood into its parts

L. Match the following laboratory test or clinical procedure with its description.

coagulation time   hematocrit   bleeding time
red blood cell morphology   erythrocyte sedimentation rate   bone marrow transplant
bone marrow biopsy   Coombs' test   RBC count
autologous transfusion   WBC differential   platelet count

1. stained blood smear is examined to determine the shape (form) of individual red blood

   cells _____

2. measures the percentage of red blood cells in a volume of blood _____

3. determines the number of clotting cells per cubic millimeter _____

4. ability of venous blood to clot in a test tube _____

5. measures the speed at which erythrocytes settle out of plasma _____

6. determines the numbers of different types of white blood cells (immature and mature

   forms) _____

7. determines the presence of antibodies in infants of Rh-negative women or patients with autoimmune

   hemolytic anemia _____

8. bone marrow cells from a donor are infused into a patient with leukemia or aplastic

   anemia _____

9. time it takes for a small puncture wound to stop bleeding _____

10. needle is introduced into the bone marrow cavity; small amount of marrow is aspirated and then

    examined under a microscope _____

11. gives the number of erythrocytes per cubic millimeter of blood _____

12. blood is collected from and later reinfused into the same patient _____

M. Give the meanings for the following abbreviations.

1. Hct _____

2. Hgb _____

3. PTT _____

4. CBC _____

5. segs _____

6. IgA, IgD, IgG, IgM, IgE _____

N. Select the term that best completes the meaning of the sentences.

1. Gary, a 1-year-old African-American baby, was failing to gain weight normally. He seemed pale and without energy. His blood tests showed a decreased hemoglobin (5.0) and decreased hematocrit (16.5). After a blood smear revealed abnormally shaped red cells, the doctor told Gary's mother that her son had (iron-deficiency anemia, hemophilia, sickle cell anemia).

2. While in the hospital, Mr. Klein was told he had an elevated (red blood cell, white blood cell, platelet) count with a shift to the left. This was information that confirmed his diagnosis of a systemic infection.

3. While taking Coumadin, a blood thinner, Mr. Ratzan's physician made sure to check his (prothrombin time, hematocrit, sed rate).

4. When they checked Babette's blood type during her prenatal examination, she was (B^+, O^+, AB^-). Her physician told her that she and her baby might have condition of (Rh incompatibility, multiple myeloma, pernicious anemia). They gave her a medicine called RhoGAM.

5. Bobby was diagnosed at a very early age with a bleeding disorder called (hemophilia, thalassemia, eosinophilia). He needed factor VIII regularly, especially after even the slightest traumatic injury.

6. Teddy was a 9-year-old boy who suddenly noticed many black and blue marks all over his legs. He had a fever and was tired all the time. The doctor did a blood test that revealed pancytopenia. A bone marrow biopsy confirmed the diagnosis of (acute lymphocytic leukemia, polycythemia vera, aplastic anemia).

XI. Answers to Exercises

A

1. monocyte
2. platelet
3. stem cell (hemocytoblast)
4. lymphocyte
5. eosinophil
6. erythrocyte
7. neutrophil
8. basophil

B

1. blood cell (little body)
2. white blood cell with dense, dark-staining granules (neutrophil, basophil, and eosinophil)
3. pertaining to (having) one (prominent) nucleus (monocytes and lymphocytes are mononuclear leukocytes)
4. pertaining to (having) a many-shaped nucleus (neutrophils are polymorphonuclear leukocytes)
5. white blood cell without dense, dark-staining granules in its cytoplasm (monocyte and lymphocyte)
6. immature red blood cell
7. forerunner (precursor) of platelets (formed in the bone marrow)
8. large phagocytes formed from monocytes and found in tissues; they destroy worn-out red blood cells and engulf foreign material
9. blood protein found in red blood cells; enables the erythrocyte to carry oxygen
10. derived from bone marrow cells
11. immature, developing red blood cell with a network of granules in its cytoplasm
12. immature bone marrow cell that is the forerunner of granulocytes

C

1. plasma
2. bilirubin
3. heme
4. globulin
5. erythropoietin
6. antigen
7. albumin
8. antibodies

D

1. albumin, globulin, fibrinogen, and pro-thrombin
2. an antigen normally found on red blood cells of Rh-positive individuals
3. clumping of recipient's blood cells when incompatible bloods are mixed
4. A antigens; anti-B antibodies
5. B antigens; anti-A antibodies
6. no A or B antigens; anti-A and anti-B antibodies
7. A and B antigens; no anti-A and no anti-B antibodies
8. no; the A antigens will agglutinate with the anti-A antibodies in the B person's bloodstream
9. no; the A and B antigens will agglutinate with the anti-A and anti-B antibodies in the O person's bloodstream
10. a method of separating substances (such as proteins) by electrical charge
11. a type of gamma globulin (blood protein) that contains antibodies
12. change in structure and function (specialization) of a cell as it matures
13. process of using a centrifuge to separate or remove blood cells from plasma.

E

1. heparin
2. fibrin
3. prothrombin
4. serum
5. thromboplastin
6. fibrinogen
7. coagulation
8. thrombin

F

1. anti/coagul/ant—a substance that prevents clotting
2. hemoglobin/o/pathy—disease (abnormality) of hemoglobin
3. cyt/o/logy—study of cells
4. leuk/o/cyt/o/penia—deficiency of white (blood) cells
5. morph/o/logy—study of the shape or form (of cells)
6. mega/kary/o/cyte—cell with a large (mega-) nucleus (kary); platelet precursor
7. sider/o/penia—deficiency of iron
8. phag/o/cyte—cell that eats or swallows other cells
9. myel/o/blast—immature bone marrow cell (gives rise to granulocytes)
10. platelet/pheresis—separation of platelets from the rest of the blood
11. mon/o/blast—immature monocyte
12. myel/o/poiesis—formation of bone marrow cells
13. hem/o/stasis—controlling or stopping the flow of blood
14. thromb/o/lytic—pertaining to destruction of clots
15. hemat/o/poiesis—formation of blood

G

1. poikilocytosis
2. hemoglobin
3. erythropoiesis
4. erythrocytopenia
5. hemolysis
6. hypochromia
7. anisocytosis
8. spherocytosis
9. microcytosis
10. polycythemia vera
11. macrocytosis
12. hematocrit

H

1. lack of iron leading to insufficient hemoglobin production
2. lack of mature erythrocytes due to inability to absorb vitamin B_{12} into the bloodstream (gastric juice lacks a factor that helps absorb B_{12})
3. abnormal shape (cresent-shape) of erythrocytes caused by an abnormal type of hemoglobin (hereditary disorder)
4. lack of all types of blood cells due to lack of development of bone marrow cells
5. defect in the ability to produce hemoglobin leading to hypochromia

I

1. chronic lymphocytic leukemia
2. acute myelogenous (myelocytic or granulocytic) leukemia
3. acute lymphocytic leukemia
4. chronic myelogenous (myelocytic or granulocytic) leukemia

J

1. multiple pinpoint hemorrhages due to a deficiency of platelets (patient makes an antibody that destroys her or his own platelets); cause unknown (idiopathic)
2. abnormal condition of excess numbers of granulocytes (eosinophilia and basophilia)
3. excessive bleeding caused by a lack (hereditary and congenital) of one of the protein factors necessary for clotting
4. excessive deposits of iron in tissues of the body
5. malignant tumor of bone marrow (antibody-producing plasma cells are produced in large numbers)

K

1. E
2. G
3. D
4. B
5. F
6. A
7. H
8. C

L

1. red blood cell morphology
2. hematocrit
3. platelet count
4. coagulation time
5. erythrocyte sedimentation rate
6. white blood cell differential
7. antiglobulin (Coombs') test
8. bone marrow transplantation
9. bleeding time
10. bone marrow biopsy
11. red blood cell count
12. autologous blood transfusion

M

1. hematocrit
2. hemoglobin
3. partial thromboplastin time (test of clotting factors)
4. complete blood count
5. segmented white blood cells (neutrophils)
6. immunoglobulins

N

1. sickle cell anemia
2. white blood cell
3. prothrombin time
4. AB⁻; Rh incompatibility
5. hemophilia
6. aplastic anemia

Answers to Practical Applications

1. C
2. B
3. D

XII. Pronunciation of Terms

To test your understanding of the terminology in this chapter, write the meaning of each term in the space provided. In addition, you may wish to cover the terms and write them by looking at your definitions. Make sure your spelling is correct. The page number after each term indicates where it is defined or used in the text so you can easily check your responses. (If you are not sure what the pronunciation symbols mean, refer to page 21.)

Vocabulary and Terminology

Term	Pronunciation	Meaning
agglutination (438)	ă-glōo-tĭ-NĀ-shŭn	
albumin (438)	ăl-BŪ-mĭn	
anisocytosis (441)	ăn-ī-sō-sī-TŌ-sĭs	
antibody (438)	ĂN-tĭ-bŏd-ē	
anticoagulant (441)	ăn-tĭ-cō-ĂG-ū-lănt	
antigen (438)	ĂN-tĭ-jĕn	
basophil (438)	BĀ-sō-fĭl	
bilirubin (438)	bĭl-ĭ-RŌŌ-bĭn	
coagulation (438)	kō-ăg-ū-LĀ-shŭn	
corpuscle (438)	KŎR-pŭs'l	
cytology (441)	sī-TŎL-ō-jē	
differentiation (438)	dĭf-ĕr-ĕn-shē-Ā-shŭn	

electrophoresis (438)	ē-lĕk-trō-fō-RĒ-sĭs	_____
eosinophil (439)	ē-ō-SĬN-ō-fĭl	_____
eosinophilia (443)	ē-ō-sĭn-ō-FĬL-ē-ă	_____
erythroblast (442)	ĕ-RĬTH-rō-blăst	_____
erythrocytopenia (441)	ĕ-rĭth-rō-PĒ-nē-ă	_____
erythropoiesis (443)	ĕ-rĭth-rō-poy-Ē-sĭs	_____
erythropoietin (439)	ĕ-rĭth-rō-POY-ĕ-tĭn	_____
fibrin (439)	FĪ-brĭn	_____
fibrinogen (439)	fī-BRĬN-ō-jĕn	_____
globulin (439)	GLŎB-ū-lĭn	_____
gamma globulin (443)	GĂ-mă GLŎB-ū-lĭn	_____
granulocyte (434)	GRĂN-ū-lō-sīt	_____
granulocytopenia (443)	grăn-ū-lō-sī-tō-PĒ-nē-ă	_____
hemoglobin (439)	HĒ-mō-glō-bĭn	_____
hemoglobinopathy (441)	hē-mō-glō-bĭn-ŎP-ă-thē	_____
hemolysis (441)	hē-MŎL-ĭ-sĭs	_____
hemostasis (443)	hē-mŏ-STĀ-sĭs	_____
heparin (439)	HĔP-ă-rĭn	_____
hypochromia (441)	hī-pō-KRŌ-mē-ă	_____
immunoglobulin (439)	ĭm-ū-nō-GLŎB-ū-lĭn	_____
leukapheresis (442)	lōō-kă-fĕ-RĒ-sĭs	_____
leukocytopenia (441)	lōō-kō-sī-tō-PĒ-nē-ă	_____
lymphocyte (439)	LĬM-fō-sīt	_____
macrocytosis (442)	măk-rō-sī-TŌ-sĭs	_____
macrophage (439)	MĂK-rō-făj	_____
megakaryocyte (439)	mĕg-ă-KĀR-ē-ō-sīt	_____
microcytosis (442)	mī-krō-sī-TŌ-sĭs	_____

monoblast (442)	MŎN-ō-blăst	
monocyte (439)	MŎN-ō-sīt	
mononuclear (442)	mŏn-ō-NŪ-klē-ăr	
morphology (441)	mŏr-FŎL-ō-Jē	
myeloblast (441)	MĪ-ĕ-lō-blăst	
myeloid (439)	MĪ-ĕ-loyd	
myelopoiesis (443)	mī-ĕ-lō-poy-Ē-sĭs	
neutropenia (441)	nū-trō-PĔ-nē-ă	
neutrophil (440)	NŪ-trō-fĭl	
neutrophilia (443)	nū-trō-FĬL-ē-ă	
pancytopenia (443)	păn-sī-tō-PĒ-nē-ă	
phagocyte (442)	FĂG-ō-sīt	
plasma (440)	PLĂZ-mă	
plasmapheresis (440)	plăz-mă-fĕ-RĒ-sĭs	
plateletpheresis (442)	plăt-lĕt-fĕ-RĒ-sĭs	
poikilocytosis (442)	poy-kĭ-lō-sī-TŌ-sĭs	
polymorphonuclear (442)	pŏl-ē-mŏr-fō-NŪ-klē-ăr	
prothrombin (440)	prō-THRŎM-bĭn	
reticulocyte (440)	rĕ-TĬK-ū-lō-sīt	
serum (440)	SĔ-rŭm	
sideropenia (442)	sĭd-ĕr-ō-PĒ-nē-ă	
spherocytosis (442)	sphĕr-ō-sī-TŌ-sĭs	
stem cell (440)	stĕm sĕl	
thrombin (440)	THRŎM-bĭn	
thrombocyte (440)	THRŎM-bō-sīt	
thrombolytic therapy (443)	thrŏm-bō-LĬ-tĭk THĔR-ă-pē	
thromboplastin (440)	thrŏm-bō-PLĂS-tĭn	
thrombosis (443)	thrŏm-BŌ-sĭs	

Pathology, Laboratory Tests, and Clinical Procedures

Term	Pronunciation	Meaning
acute lymphocytic leukemia (446)	ă-KŪT lĭm-fō-SĬ-tĭk lōō-KĒ-mē-ă	_____
acute myelogenous leukemia (446)	ă-KŪT mī-ĕ-LŎJ-ĕ-nŭs lōō-KĒ-mē-ă	_____
antiglobulin test (448)	ăn-tē-GLŎB-ū-lĭn tĕst	_____
apheresis (449)	ă-fĕ-RĒ-sĭs	_____
aplastic anemia (444)	ā-PLĂS-tĭk ă-NĒ-mē-ă	_____
autologous transfusion (449)	ăw-TŎL-ō-gŭs trăns-FŪ-zhŭn	_____
bleeding time (448)	BLĒ-dĭng tīm	_____
blood transfusion (449)	blŭd trăns-FŪ-zhŭn	_____
bone marrow biopsy (449)	bōn MĂ-rō BĪ-ŏp-sē	_____
bone marrow transplant (449)	bōn MĂ-rō TRĂNS-plănt	_____
chronic lymphocytic leukemia (447)	KRŎ-nĭk lĭm-fō-SĬ-tĭk lōō-KĒ-mē-ă	_____
chronic myelogenous leukemia (446)	KRŎ-nĭk mī-ĕ-LŎJ-ĕ-nŭs lōō-KĒ-mē-ă	_____
coagulation time (448)	kō-ăg-ū-LĀ-shŭn tīm	_____
dyscrasia (444)	dĭs-KRĀ-zē-ă	_____
erythrocyte sedimentation rate (448)	ĕ-RĬTH-rō-sīt sĕd-ĕ-mĕn-TĀ-shŭn răt	_____
granulocytosis (447)	grăn-ū-lō-sī-TŌ-sĭs	_____
hematocrit (448)	hē-MĂT-ō-krĭt	_____
hemochromatosis (446)	hē-mō-krō-mă-TŌ-sĭs	_____
hemoglobin test (448)	HĒ-mō-glō-bĭn tĕst	_____
hemolytic anemia (444)	hē-mō-LĬ-tĭk ă-NĒ-mē-ă	_____
hemophilia (446)	hē-mō-FĬL-ē-ă	_____
multiple myeloma (447)	MŬL-tĭ-p'l mī-ĕ-LŌ-mă	_____

palliative (447)	PĂL-ē-ă-tĭv	_____
partial thromboplastin time (448)	PĂR-shŭl thrŏm-bō-PLĂS-tĭn tīm	_____
pernicious anemia (448)	pĕr-NĬSH-ŭs ă-NĒ-mē-ă	_____
polycythemia vera (446)	pŏl-ē-sī-THĒ-mē-ă VĔR-ă	_____
prothrombin time (448)	prō-THRŎM-bĭn tīm	_____
purpura (446)	PŬR-pū-ră	_____
relapse (447)	RĒ-lăps	_____
remission (447)	rē-MĬSH-ŭn	_____
sickle cell anemia (445)	SĬK'l sĕl ă-NĒ-mē-ă	_____
thalassemia (445)	thăl-ă-SĒ-mē-ă	_____

XIII. Review Sheet

Write the meanings for each word part in the space provided. Check your answers with the information in the chapter or in the Glossary (Medical Terms—English) at the end of the book.

Combining Forms

Combining Form	Meaning	Combining Form	Meaning
agglutin/o	_____	kary/o	_____
bas/o	_____	leuk/o	_____
chrom/o	_____	mon/o	_____
coagul/o	_____	morph/o	_____
cyt/o	_____	myel/o	_____
eosin/o	_____	neutr/o	_____
erythr/o	_____	nucle/o	_____
granul/o	_____	phag/o	_____
hem/o	_____	poikil/o	_____
hemat/o	_____	sider/o	_____
hemoglobin/o	_____	spher/o	_____
is/o	_____	thromb/o	_____

Suffixes

Suffix	Meaning	Suffix	Meaning
-apheresis	_____	-penia	_____
-blast	_____	-phage	_____
-cytosis	_____	-philia	_____
-emia	_____	-phoresis	_____
-globin	_____	-plasia	_____
-globulin	_____	-poiesis	_____
-lytic	_____	-stasis	_____
-oid	_____		

Prefixes

Prefix	Meaning	Prefix	Meaning
a-, an-	_____	micro-	_____
anti-	_____	mono-	_____
hypo-	_____	pan-	_____
macro-	_____	poly-	_____
mega-	_____		

14

Lymphatic and Immune Systems

In this Chapter you will

■ Identify the structures and analyze terms related to the lymphatic system;
■ Learn terms that describe basic elements of the immune system;
■ Recognize terms that describe various pathological conditions affecting the lymphatic and immune systems; and
■ Identify laboratory tests, clinical procedures, and abbreviations that are pertinent to the lymphatic and immune systems.

I. INTRODUCTION

Lymph is a clear, watery fluid (the term lymph comes from the Latin, meaning clear spring water) that surrounds body cells and flows in a system of lymph vessels that extends throughout the body.

Lymph differs from blood, but it has a close relationship with the blood systems. Lymph fluid does not contain erythrocytes or platelets, but it is rich in two types of leukocytes: lymphocytes and monocytes. The liquid part of lymph is similar to blood plasma in that it contains water, salts, sugar, and wastes of metabolism such as urea and creatinine, but it

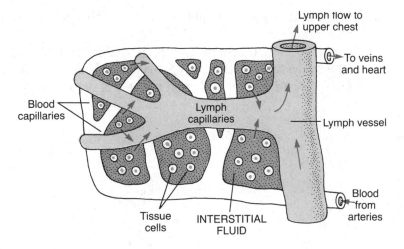

Figure 14–1

Interstitial fluid and lymph capillaries.

differs in that it contains less protein. Lymph actually originates from the blood as fluid filters out of tiny blood vessels into the spaces between cells. This fluid that surrounds the cells of the body is called **interstitial fluid.** Interstitial fluid passes continuously into specialized thin-walled vessels called **lymph capillaries,** which are found at tissue spaces (Fig. 14–1). The fluid in the lymph capillaries, now called **lymph** instead of interstitial fluid, passes through larger lymphatic vessels and through deposits of lymph tissues (called **lymph nodes**), finally to reach large lymph vessels in the upper chest. Lymph enters these large lymphatic vessels, which then empty into the bloodstream. Figure 14–2 illustrates the relationship between the blood and the lymphatic systems.

There are several functions of the lymphatic system. One is to act as a drainage system to transport needed proteins and fluid that have leaked out of the blood capillaries (and into the interstitial fluid) back to the bloodstream via the veins. In addition, the lymphatic vessels

Figure 14–2

Relationship between the circulatory systems of blood and lymph.

in the intestines absorb lipids (fats) from the small intestine and transport them to the bloodstream.

Another function of the lymphatic system is related to the **immune system:** the defense of the body against foreign organisms such as bacteria and viruses. Lymphocytes and monocytes, originating in lymph nodes and organs such as the spleen and thymus gland,

Figure 14–3

Lymphatic system.

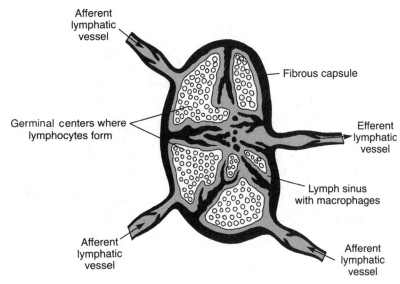

Afferent lymphatic vessel

Fibrous capsule

Germinal centers where lymphocytes form

Efferent lymphatic vessel

Lymph sinus with macrophages

Afferent lymphatic vessel

Afferent lymphatic vessel

Figure 14–4

A lymph node.

protect the body by producing antibodies or by phagocytosis (engulfing and destroying foreign matter).

II. Lymphatic System

Anatomy

Label Figure 14–3 as you read the following paragraphs.

Lymph capillaries (1) begin at the spaces around cells throughout the body. Like blood capillaries, they are thin-walled tubes. Lymph capillaries carry lymph from the tissue spaces to larger **lymph vessels** (2). Lymph vessels have thicker walls than those of lymph capillaries and, like veins, contain valves so that lymph flows only in one direction, toward the thoracic cavity. Collections of stationary lymph tissue, called **lymph nodes** (3), are located along the path of the lymph vessels. These masses of lymph tissue are surrounded by a fibrous, connective tissue capsule (Fig. 14–4). The function of lymph nodes is not only to produce lymph cells (lymphocytes) but also to filter lymph and trap substances from inflammatory and cancerous lesions. Special cells, called **macrophages,** are located in lymph nodes (as well as in the spleen, liver, lungs, brain, and spinal cord), and they can phagocytose (engulf and destroy) foreign substances. When bacteria are present in lymph nodes that drain a particular area of the body, the nodes became swollen with collections of cells and their engulfed debris and become tender. Lymph nodes also fight disease when lymphocytes, present in the nodes, produce antibodies.

Label the major sites of lymph node concentration on Figure 14–3. These are the **cervical** (4), **axillary** (armpit) (5), **mediastinal** (6), and **inguinal** (groin) (7) regions of the body. Remember that the **tonsils** are masses of lymph tissue in the throat near the mouth (oropharynx) and the **adenoids** are enlarged lymph tissue in the part of the throat near the nasal passages (nasopharynx).

Lymph vessels all lead toward the thoracic cavity and empty into two large ducts in the upper chest. These are the **right lymphatic duct** (8) and the **thoracic duct** (9). The thoracic duct drains the lower body and left chest, whereas the right lymphatic duct drains the right chest (a much smaller area). Both ducts carry the lymph into **large veins** (10) in the neck where lymph then merges with the blood system.

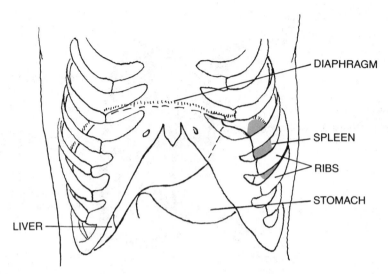

Figure 14–5

The spleen and adjacent organs.

Spleen and Thymus Gland

The spleen and the thymus gland are organs composed of lymph tissue.

The **spleen** (Fig. 14–5) is located in the left upper quadrant of the abdomen, adjacent to the stomach. Although the spleen is not essential to life, it has several important functions:

1. Destruction of old erythrocytes by macrophages. Because of hemolytic activity in the spleen, bilirubin is formed there and added to the bloodstream.

2. Filtration of microorganisms and other foreign material from the blood.

3. Activation of lymphocytes as it filters out antigens from the blood. Activated lymphocytes produce antibodies and engulf the antigens.

4. Storage of blood, especially platelets.

The spleen is an organ that is easily and frequently injured. A sharp blow or injury to the upper abdomen (as from the impact of a car's steering wheel) may cause rupture of the spleen. Massive hemorrhage can occur when the spleen is ruptured, and immediate surgical removal (splenectomy) may be necessary. After splenectomy, the liver, bone marrow, and lymph nodes take over the functions of the spleen.

The **thymus gland** (Fig. 14–6) is a lymphatic organ located in the upper mediastinum between the lungs. During fetal life and childhood it is quite large, but it becomes smaller

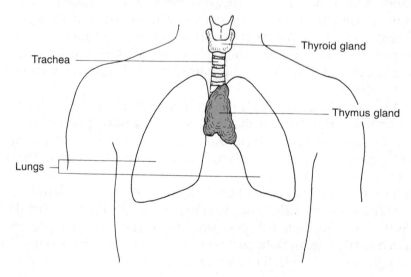

Figure 14–6

The thymus gland.

with age. The thymus gland plays an important role in the body's ability to protect itself from disease (immunity), especially in fetal life and the early years of growth. It is known that a thymectomy (removal of the thymus gland) performed in an animal during the first weeks of life impairs the ability of the animal to make antibodies and to produce immune cells that fight against foreign antigens, such as bacteria and viruses.

III. Immune System

The immune system is the body's special defense response against foreign organisms. This system includes the **lymphoid organs** (lymph nodes, spleen, and thymus gland) and their products (**lymphocytes** and **antibodies**) and **macrophages** (phagocytes that are found in the blood, brain, liver, lymph nodes, and spleen).

Immunity is the capacity to resist all types of organisms and toxins (poisons) that will damage tissues and organs. **Natural** (innate) **immunity** is one's own ability to fight off disease. It is a genetic characteristic protecting a person of a certain race or species from disease. For example, humans are resistant to distemper, which is a viral disease that affects dogs. In addition, when bacteria enter the body, natural immunity protects the body as phagocytes (neutrophils) migrate to the site of infection and ingest the bacteria. They release proteins that attract other immune cells and cause local heat and inflammation. Macrophages from local tissues and from the bloodstream move in to clear away the dead cells and debris as the infection subsides.

Besides having natural immunity, a person may acquire immunity through active or passive means. **Acquired immunity** is important for protection against invading organisms to which the body does not have innate or natural immunity. In this way, the body develops powerful, specific immunity (antibodies and cells) against invading agents such as lethal bacteria, viruses, toxins, and even foreign tissues from other organisms. Acquired **active** immunity occurs in two ways: by **having a disease** (antibodies are made against the foreign organisms and then remain in the body to protect against subsequent infection) or by receiving a **vaccination** containing a modified pathogen or toxin, which stimulates production of antibodies (without having an attack of the disease).

When it is necessary to provide "ready made" immune bodies and immediate protection, acquired **passive** immunity is administered. In this case, the patient receives immune serum, containing antibodies produced in another animal, such as **antitoxins** for a poisonous snake bite or tetanus and diphtheria injections. Injections of **gamma globulin,** containing antibodies, also give protection against disease or lessen its severity. Figure 14–7 reviews the different types of immunity.

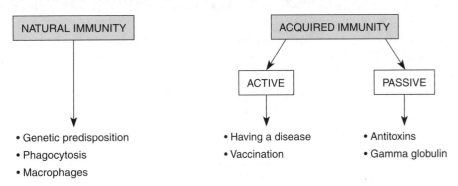

Figure 14–7

Types of immunity.

Figure 14–8

Functions of T cell and B cell lymphocytes.

Acquired active immunity involves two major disease fighters, **B cell lymphocytes (humoral immunity)** and **T cell lymphocytes (cell-mediated immunity).** B cells originate from bone marrow stem cells and migrate to lymph nodes and other lymphoid tissue. When a B cell is confronted with a specific type of antigen, it transforms into an antibody-producing cell called a **plasma cell.** The antibodies that are made by plasma cells are **immunoglobulins,** such as IgM, IgG, IgD, IgE, and IgA. Immunoglobulins travel to the site of an infection to react with and neutralize antigens.

T cell lymphocytes originate from stem cells in the bone marrow and are processed in the thymus gland where they are acted upon by thymic hormones. Then they migrate to lymph nodes and lymphoid organs. When an antigen encounters a T cell, the T cell multiplies rapidly and can engulf and digest the antigen (bacterium, virus, cancer cell, or fungus). T cells also react to foreign tissues, such as skin grafts and transplanted organs.

Some T cells are **cytotoxic** or **killer cells** (called **T8 cells**), whereas other T cells produce chemicals (**interferons** and **interleukins**) that destroy cells or bacteria. One special class of T cells, called **helper cells** or **T4 cells,** stimulate antibody production. CD4+ T cells (CD4+ is the name of the protein on the cell) are attacked by the HIV (human immunodeficiency virus) in AIDS. **Suppressor cells** are other T cells that regulate the amount of antibody produced by inhibiting the activity of the B cell lymphocytes. Figure 14–8 summarizes the functions of T and B cell lymphocytes.

IV. Vocabulary

This list will help you review many of the new terms introduced in the text. Short definitions will reinforce your understanding of the terms. See Section XI of this chapter for help in pronouncing the more difficult terms.

acquired immunity   Formation of antibodies and lymphocytes after exposure to an antigen.

adenoids   Masses of lymph tissue in the nasopharynx.

antibodies   Proteins, produced by plasma cells, that destroy antigens.

axillary nodes   Lymph nodes in the armpit (under arm).

B cells	Lymphocytes that transform into plasma cells and secrete antibodies. The B refers to the bursa of Fabricius, an organ in birds in which B cell differentiation and growth were first noted to occur.
cell-mediated immunity	An immune response involving T cell lymphocytes; antigens are destroyed by direct action of cells.
cervical nodes	Lymph nodes in the neck region.
cytotoxic cells	T cells (killer cells) that directly kill foreign cells; also called **T8 cells.**
helper cells	T cells that aid B cells in recognizing antigens and stimulating antibody production; also called **T4 cells.**
humoral immunity	Immune response in which B cells transform into plasma cells and secrete antibodies.
immune response or immunity	The body's capacity to resist all types of organisms and toxins that can damage tissue and organs.
immunoglobulins	Antibodies (gamma globulins) such as IgA, IgE, IgG, IgM, and IgD that are secreted by plasma cells in humoral immunity.
inguinal nodes	Lymph nodes in the groin region (area where the legs join the trunk of the body).
interferons	Antiviral proteins secreted by T cells; they also stimulate macrophages to ingest bacteria.
interleukins	Proteins that stimulate the growth of T cell lymphocytes and activate immune responses.
interstitial fluid	Fluid in the spaces between cells. This fluid becomes lymph when it enters lymph capillaries.
killer cells	T cells (cytotoxic cells) that engulf foreign cells, tumor cells, and bacteria; also called **T8 cells.**
lymph	Fluid found within lymphatic vessels and collected from tissues throughout the body.
lymph capillaries	Tiniest lymphatic vessels.
lymphoid organs	Lymph nodes, spleen, and thymus gland.
lymph nodes	Stationary lymph tissue along lymph vessels.
lymph vessels	Carriers of lymph throughout the body; lymph vessels empty lymph into veins in the upper part of the chest.
macrophage	A large phagocyte found in lymph nodes and other tissues of the body.

mediastinal nodes	Lymph nodes in the area between the lungs in the thoracic (chest) cavity.
natural immunity	One's own genetic ability to fight off disease.
plasma cell	A cell that secretes antibody and originates from B cell lymphocytes.
right lymphatic duct	A large lymph vessel in the chest that receives lymph from the upper right part of the body.
spleen	Organ near the stomach that produces, stores, and eliminates blood cells.
suppressor cells	T cell lymphocytes that inhibit the activity of B cell lymphocytes.
T cells	Lymphocytes formed in the thymus gland; they act directly on antigens to destroy them or produce chemicals such as interferons and interleukins that are toxic to antigens.
thoracic duct	Large lymph vessel in the chest that receives lymph from below the diaphragm and from the left side of the body above the diaphragm; it empties the lymph into veins in the upper chest.
thymus gland	Organ in the mediastinum that produces T cell lymphocytes and aids in the immune response.
tonsils	Masses of lymph tissue in the back of the oropharynx.
toxin	A poison; a protein produced by certain bacteria, animals, and plants.
vaccination	Introduction of altered antigens (viruses or bacteria) to produce an immune response and protection against disease. The term comes from the Latin *vacca*, meaning cow, and was used when the first inoculations were given with organisms that caused the mild disease cow pox to produce immunity against smallpox.

V. Combining Forms, Prefixes, and Terminology

Write the meaning of the medical term in the space provided.

Combining Forms			
Combining Form	Meaning	Terminology	Meaning
immun/o	protection	immunology _____	
		immunoglobulin _____	
lymph/o	lymph	lymphopoiesis _____	

lymphedema _____

Interstitial fluid collects within the spaces between cells secondary to obstruction of lymph vessels and nodes.

lymphocytopenia _____

lymphocytosis _____

lymphoid _____

-oid means resembling or derived from. Lymphoid organs include lymph nodes, spleen, and thymus gland.

lymphaden/o	lymph node (gland)	lymphadenopathy _____
		lymphadenitis _____
lymphangi/o	lymph vessel	lymphangiogram _____
splen/o	spleen	splenomegaly _____
		splenectomy _____
thym/o	thymus gland	thymoma _____
		thymectomy _____
tox/o	poison	toxic _____

Prefix			
Prefix	Meaning	Terminology	Meaning
inter-	between	interstitial fluid _____

-stitial means pertaining to standing or positioned.

VI. Pathological Conditions

acquired immunodeficiency syndrome (AIDS)

Suppression or deficiency of the immune response caused by exposure to **HIV (human immunodeficiency virus).**

A proper definition of AIDS now includes all HIV-infected people who have fewer than 200 CD4+ T cells. Healthy adults usually have CD4+ T cell counts of 1000 or more.

HIV destroys T cell helper lymphocytes (CD4+ T cells) and thus affects the body's cell-mediated immune response. The patient is predisposed to infections and malignancies that are life-threatening.

The infectious diseases associated with AIDS are often called **opportunistic infections** because the AIDS virus lowers resistance and allows opportunity for infection by bacteria and parasites that are easily contained by normal defenses. Table 14–1 lists many of these opportunistic infections and should be used as a reference.

Malignancies associated with AIDS are **Kaposi's sarcoma** (a cancer arising from the lining cells of capillaries, which produces bluish-red skin nodules usually at first on the legs and feet) and **lymphoma** (cancer of the lymph nodes).

Table 14–1. OPPORTUNISTIC INFECTIONS WITH AIDS

Infection	Description
Candidiasis	Yeast-like fungus *(Candida)* normally present in the mouth, skin, intestinal tract, and vagina overgrows, causing infections of the mouth (thrush), respiratory tract, and skin.
Cryptococcus (Crypto)	Yeast-like fungus *(Cryptococcus)* causes lung, brain, and blood infections. Pathogen is found in pigeon droppings, nesting places, air, water, and soil.
Cryptosporidiosis	One-celled parasitic *(Cryptosporidium)* infection of the gastrointestinal tract, causing diarrhea, fever, and weight loss. Organism is commonly found in farm animals.
Cytomegalovirus (CMV)	Virus causes colitis, pneumonitis, and retinitis (inflammation of the retina at the back of the eye). Found in saliva, semen, cervical secretions, urine, feces, blood, and breast milk, but usually causes disease only when the immune system is compromised.
Herpes simplex	Viral infection causes small blisters on the skin of the lips or nose or on the genitals.
Histoplasmosis (Histo)	Fungal infection due to inhalation of dust contaminated with *Histoplasma capsulatum;* causes fever, chills, and lung infection. Pathogen is found in bird and bat droppings.
Mycobacterium avium-intracellulare (MAI)	Bacterial disease with fever, malaise, night sweats, anorexia, diarrhea, weight loss, and lung and blood infections. Bacterium is found in soil, water, and unpasteurized dairy products.
Pneumocystis carinii pneumonia (PCP)	One-celled organism causes lung infection, with fever, cough, chest pain, and sputum production. Pathogen is found in air, water, and soil and is carried by animals. It is treated with trimethoprim and sulfamethoxazole (Bactrim), an antibiotic, or with pentamidine. Aerosolized pentamidine, which is inhaled, can prevent recurrence of PCP.
Toxoplasmosis (Toxo)	Parasitic infection involving the brain, lungs, and other organs and causing fever, chills, visual disturbances, confusion, hemiparesis (slight paralysis in one-half of the body), and seizures. Pathogen is acquired by eating uncooked lamb or pork, unpasteurized dairy products, raw eggs, or vegetables.

Table 14–2. AIDS VIRUS—COMMON ROUTES OF TRANSMISSION

Route	People Affected
Receptive anal intercourse	Men and women
Receptive vaginal intercourse	Women
Sharing of needles and equipment (users of IV drugs)	Men and women
Contaminated blood (hemophiliacs)	Men and women
From mother in utero	Neonates

Over 1 million people in the U.S. are **HIV-positive**, which means they have been exposed to the virus and they have antibodies in their blood against HIV. HIV is found in blood, semen, vaginal and cervical secretions, in minute quantities in saliva, and in other body fluids (breast milk, urine, and cerebrospinal fluid). It can be transmitted by blood and sexual secretions of an infected person, but there is no evidence of transmission by saliva. Those who are at highest risk for developing AIDS are intravenous drug users, male homosexuals, prostitutes, and hemophiliacs. Table 14–2 summarizes the common routes of transmission of AIDS.

HIV-infected patients may remain asymptomatic for 10 years or more. Symptoms associated with HIV are lymphadenopathy, neurological disease, oral thrush (fungal infection), night sweats, fatigue, and evidence of bacterial or viral infection.

Drugs that are used to treat AIDS are **zidovudine** (ZDV, formerly know as AZT) and **ddI** (dideoxyinosine). These drugs work by blocking the growth of virus after it enters the helper T cell lymphocyte. HIV is called a **retrovirus** because its life cycle requires that its own genetic material, RNA, be copied into the DNA (of the lymphocyte) in a reverse **(retro-)** fashion. New viral particles, containing RNA, are then made from the DNA of the lymphocyte.

For HIV-positive patients, **CD4+ lymphocytes** (helper T4 cells carrying the CD4+ protein antigen on their surface) are monitored to evaluate immune function and track the results of antiretroviral therapy. HIV binds to CD4+ and infects and kills the helper T cells bearing this protein. Patients with CD4+ counts of less than 500 usually require drug treatment. Prophylactic therapy against *Pneumocystis carinii* pneumonia (PCP) with trimethoprim-sulfamethoxazole (TMP-SMX) is recommended for all HIV-positive patients whose CD4+ counts are under 200, who have had previous episodes of PCP, oral candidiasis (thrush), or unexplained fevers.

hypersensitivity

Conditions in which the body reacts with an exaggerated immune response; the immune system produces tissue damage and disordered function rather than immunity.

Commonly known as **allergy,** hypersensitivity reactions occur when a person is exposed to a sensitizing agent **(allergen),** and the immune response that follows on reexposure to the allergen is damaging to the body. These reactions can vary from allergic rhinitis (caused by pollen or animal dander) to systemic **anaphylaxis (ana-** means backward, **-phylaxis** means protection), in which an extraordinary hypersensitivity reaction occurs throughout the body, leading to hypotension, shock, respiratory distress, and edema of the larynx.

Anaphylaxis can be life-threatening, but the patient will usually survive if the airways are kept open and she or he is treated immediately with epinephrine (Adrenalin) and antihistamines.

hypersplenism

A syndrome marked by enlargement of the spleen; it occurs in various disorders. **Splenomegaly** is often associated with destruction of blood cells resulting in anemia, leukopenia, and thrombocytopenia.

lymphoma

Malignant tumor of lymph nodes and lymph tissue.

There are many forms of lymphoma depending on the particular cell type and its degree of differentiation. Some examples are:

Hodgkin's disease—Malignant tumor of lymph tissue in the spleen and lymph nodes; also called **Hodgkin's lymphoma.** This disease is characterized by lymphadenopathy (lymph nodes enlarge), splenomegaly, fever, weakness, and loss of weight and appetite. The diagnosis is often made by identifying a malignant cell (Reed-Sternberg cell) in the lymph nodes. If disease is localized, the treatment of choice is radiotherapy (using high-dose radiation). If the disease is more widespread, chemotherapy is given alone or in combination with radiotherapy. There is a very high probability of cure with available treatments.

Non-Hodgkin's lymphoma—Types of this disease include **lymphocytic lymphoma** (composed of lymphocytes) and **histiocytic lymphoma** (composed of large lymphocytes that resemble histiocytes or large macrophages). Chemotherapy and radiation are used to cure and stop the progress of this disease.

mononucleosis

Acute infectious disease with enlarged lymph nodes and increased numbers of lymphocytes and monocytes in the bloodstream.

This disease is caused by the Epstein-Barr virus (EBV). Lymphadenopathy is present, with fatigue, asthenia (weakness), pharyngeal inflammation, and enlarged, tender nodes in the cervical and sometimes axillary and inguinal regions. Hepatomegaly, splenomegaly, and jaundice may occur as well.

The disease is usually transmitted by direct oral contact (salivary exchange during kissing) and primarily affects young adults. No treatment is necessary for most EBV infections. Antibiotics are not effective in self-limiting viral illnesses. Rest during the period of acute symptoms and slow return to normal activities are advised.

sarcoidosis

Inflammatory disease in which small nodules, or tubercles, form in lymph nodes and other organs.

Lesions develop on the skin and in the spleen, lungs, lymph nodes, and liver. The disease process resembles the tubercles of tuberculosis, but the etiology of this condition is unknown. Many patients are asymptomatic and retain adequate pulmonary function. Others have more active disease and impaired pulmonary function. Corticosteroid drugs must be used to prevent progression in these patients.

thymoma

Malignant tumor of the thymus gland.

Some symptoms of thymoma are cough, dyspnea, dysphagia, fever, chest pain, weight loss, and anorexia. Often, the tumor is associated with other disorders, such as myasthenia gravis and cytopenias.

Surgery is the principal method of treating thymoma; postoperative radiation therapy is used for patients with evidence of spread of the tumor.

STUDY SECTION

Practice spelling each term and know its meaning.

allergen
A substance capable of causing a specific hypersensitivity in the body; a type of antigen.

allergy
A state of abnormal hypersensitivity acquired through exposure to a particular allergen (antigen); the reaction is increased by reexposure to the allergen.

anaphylaxis
An exaggerated or unusual hypersensitivity to foreign protein or other substance.

CD4+ lymphocytes
Helper T cells that carry the CD4+ protein antigen on their surface. HIV binds to CD4+ and infects and kills T cells bearing this protein.

human immunodeficiency virus
The virus (retrovirus) that causes AIDS; HIV.

Kaposi's sarcoma
A malignant (cancerous) condition associated with AIDS; arises from the lining of capillaries and appears as bluish-red skin nodules.

opportunistic infections
Infectious diseases associated with AIDS; they occur because AIDS lowers the body's resistance and allows infection by bacteria and parasites that are normally easily contained.

retrovirus
An RNA virus that makes copies of itself by using the host cell's DNA; this is in reverse (retro-) fashion because the regular method is for DNA to copy itself onto RNA. A retrovirus (like HIV) carries an enzyme, called reverse transcriptase, that enables it to reproduce within the host cell.

zidovudine (ZDV)
Drug (formerly known as AZT) used to treat AIDS.

VII. Laboratory Tests, Clinical Procedures, and Abbreviations

Laboratory Tests

ELISA
Enzyme-linked immunosorbent assay. This test is used to screen blood for antibody to AIDS virus. A positive result indicates probable exposure to the virus and possibly that the virus is in the blood. Since false-positive results can occur with this test, a back-up test (Western blot) is used to confirm positive findings.

Western blot
This test detects the presence of HIV (AIDS virus) in serum.

Clinical Procedures

CT (CAT) scan   Computed tomography (x-ray views in a transverse plane) is used to diagnose abnormalities of lymphoid organs, such as lymph nodes, spleen, and thymus gland.

lymphangiogram   Contrast medium is injected into lymph vessels in the foot, and x-rays are taken to show the path of lymph flow as it moves into the chest region. This test is often used in the staging and diagnosis of lymphoma.

ABBREVIATIONS

AIDS	Acquired immunodeficiency syndrome	**HSV**	Herpes simplex virus
AZT	Azidothymidine (drug used to treat AIDS)	**IgA, IgD, IgE, IgG, IgM**	Immunoglobulins
CD4+	Protein on T cell helper lymphocyte that is infected with HIV in AIDS	**KS**	Kaposi's sarcoma
CMV	Cytomegalovirus (causes opportunistic AIDS-related infection)	**MAI**	*Mycobacterium avium-intracellulare* (causes bacterial disease seen in AIDS patients)
Crypto	Cryptococcus (causes opportunistic AIDS-related infection)	**PCP**	*Pneumocystis carinii* pneumonia (opportunistic AIDS-related infection)
ddI	Dideoxyinosine (drug used to treat AIDS)	**T4**	T cell lymphocyte that is destroyed by the AIDS virus
EBV	Epstein-Barr virus		
ELISA	Enzyme-linked immunosorbent assay (test for presence of antibodies to AIDS virus in serum)	**T8**	T cell lymphocyte (cytotoxic or killer cell)
Histo	Histoplasmosis (fungal infection seen in AIDS patients)	**Toxo**	Toxoplasmosis (parasitic infection associated with AIDS)
HIV	Human immunodeficiency virus (causes AIDS)	**ZDV**	Zidovudine (drug used to treat AIDS)

VIII. Practical Applications

 Medical Terminology in Sentences

Questions are provided below. Answers are found at the end of Answers to Exercises section.

1. In addition to the opportunistic infections and malignancies that typically characterize AIDS, pathology of the central nervous system (CNS) occurs with some regularity. Specifically, CNS tumors, encephalitis, meningitis, progressive leukoencephalopathy, and myelitis have been reported in patients with HIV infection. Cases of dementia and delirium [clouding of consciousness] have also been reported as psychiatric complications.

2. ZDV significantly slows HIV disease when given to HIV-positive asymptomatic persons whose CD4+ counts are below 500.

3. Lymph nodes that are nontender and rock-hard are suspicious for metastatic carcinoma.

4. Infectious mononucleosis and Hodgkin's disease are more common in young adults, whereas non-Hodgkin's lymphoma and chronic lymphocytic leukemia are more common in middle-aged and elderly people.

5. Oral candidiasis (thrush) presenting without a history of recent antibiotic therapy, chemotherapy, or immunosuppression often indicates the possibility of HIV infection.

Questions

1. What parts of the body are often regularly affected by the AIDS virus?
   (A) kidney and urinary bladder
   (B) brain and spinal cord
   (C) pancreas and thyroid glands

2. Which CNS condition is often seen in AIDS patients?
   (A) inflammation of the brain and membranes around the brain
   (B) fluid collection in the brain
   (C) disk impinging on the spinal cord

3. Aside from delirium, what other psychiatric complication has been reported in AIDS patients?
   (A) loss of intellectual abilities
   (B) feelings of persecution
   (C) fears such as claustrophobia and agoraphobia

4. What helps AIDS patients who are HIV-positive and asymptomatic and have a depressed CD4+ count?
   (A) injections of antibiotic drugs
   (B) a drug that blocks the growth of HIV
   (C) safe sex

5. CD4+ T cell counts that are below 500 mean that
   (A) red blood cells are very low
   (B) there are low levels of T cell helper lymphocytes
   (C) platelets are severely deficient

6. Metastatic carcinoma means that
   (A) the tumor has spread to a secondary location
   (B) lymph nodes are not usually affected
   (C) tumor is localized

7. Hodgkin's disease
   (A) commonly affects elderly people
   (B) is a type of lymphoma affecting young adults
   (C) is an infectious disease

8. What condition may indicate AIDS virus infection?
   (A) high blood sugar
   (B) oral leukoplakia
   (C) fungal infection of the mouth

IX. Exercises

Remember to check your answers carefully with those given in Section X, Answers to Exercises.

A. *Name the structure or fluid from its meaning below.*

1. stationary lymph tissue along the path of lymph vessels all over the body

   _____

2. large lymph vessel in the chest that drains lymph from the lower part and left side of the body above the

   diaphragm _____

3. organ near the stomach that produces, stores, and eliminates blood cells

   _____

4. masses of lymph tissue in the nasopharynx _____

5. organ in the mediastinum that produces T cell lymphocytes and helps in the immune response

   _____

6. tiniest lymph vessels _____

7. large lymph vessel in the chest that drains lymph from the upper right part of the body

   _____

8. fluid that lies between cells and becomes lymph as it enters lymph capillaries

   _____

B. *Give the locations of the following lymph nodes.*

1. inguinal nodes _____

2. axillary nodes _____

3. cervical nodes _____

4. mediastinal nodes _____

C. Circle the correct answer in each sentence.

1. An immune response in which B cells transform into plasma cells and secrete antibodies is known as (cell-mediated immunity, humoral immunity).

2. Lymphocytes, formed in the thymus gland, that act on antigens are (B cells, T cells, macrophages).

3. An immune reponse in which T cells destroy antigens is called (cell-mediated immunity, humoral immunity).

4. Lymphocytes that transform into plasma cells and secrete antibodies are called (B cells, T cells, macrophages).

D. Match the following cell names with their meanings below.

helper cell   plasma cell   suppressor cell
macrophage   cytotoxic cell

1. cell that originates from a B cell lymphocyte and is capable of secreting antibody

   _____

2. large phagocyte found in lymph nodes and other tissues of the body _____

3. T cell that aids B cells in recognizing antigens; also called a T4 cell _____

4. T cell that directly kills foreign antigens; a killer cell _____

5. T cell that inhibits the activity of B cell lymphocytes _____

E. Match the following terms in column I with their descriptions in column II.

Column I

1. immunoglobulins _____

2. toxins   _____

3. helper cells   _____

4. suppressor cells _____

5. cytotoxic cells   _____

6. plasma cells   _____

7. interferons   _____

Column II

A. antibodies—IgA, IgE, IgG, IgM, IgD
B. T cell lymphocytes—stimulate antibody production—T4 cells
C. poisons (antigens)
D. T cell lymphocytes that inhibit the activity of B cell lymphocytes
E. antiviral proteins secreted by T cells
F. transformed B cells that secrete antibodies
G. T cell lymphocytes—killer cells—T8 cells

F. Build medical terms.

1. removal of the spleen _____

2. enlargement of the spleen _____

3. formation of lymph _____

4. tumor of the thymus gland _____

5. inflammation of lymph glands (nodes) _____

6. deficiency of lymph cells _____

7. pertaining to poison _____

8. disease of lymph glands (nodes) _____

G. Match the following terms with their meanings below.

thymectomy   lymphedema   anaphylaxis
lymphoid organs   hypersplenism   AIDS
allergen   Hodgkin's disease

1. syndrome marked by enlargement of the spleen and associated with anemia, leukopenia, and anemia

   _____

2. an extraordinary hypersensitivity to a foreign protein; marked by hypotension, shock, respiratory

   distress _____

3. an antigen capable of causing allergy (hypersensitivity) _____

4. disorder in which the immune system is suppressed by exposure to HIV

   _____

5. removal of a mediastinal organ _____

6. malignant tumor of lymph nodes and spleen marked by Reed-Sternberg cells identified in lymph nodes

   _____

7. tissue that produces lymphocytes—spleen, thymus, tonsils, and adenoids

   _____

8. swelling of tissues due to interstitial fluid accumulation _____

H. Match the following terms or abbreviations related to AIDS with their meanings below.

opportunistic infections   zidovudine   Kaposi's sarcoma
HIV   ELISA   T4 helper lymphocytes
Western blot   PCP

1. a cancerous condition associated with AIDS (bluish-red skin nodules appear)

   _____

2. human immunodeficiency virus; the retrovirus that causes AIDS _____

3. white blood cells that are destroyed by the AIDS virus _____

4. a pneumonia (*Pneumocystis carinii* pneumonia) that often occurs in AIDS patients

   _____

5. group of infectious diseases associated with AIDS _____

6. test used to screen blood for antibody to AIDS virus _____

7. test used to detect the AIDS virus in the blood _____

8. drug used to treat AIDS by blocking the growth of the AIDS virus _____

I. Give the meanings for the terms or abbreviations below related to the lymphatic and immune systems.

1. lymphangiogram _____

2. CT scan _____

3. CD4+ _____

4. immunoglobulins _____

5. HIV _____

6. KS _____

7. Histo _____

J. Complete the following terms from their definitions. Pay close attention to proper spelling of each term.

1. an inflammatory disease in which small nodules form in lymph nodes and other organs:

   sarc _____

2. an acute infectious disease with enlarged lymph nodes and increased numbers of lymphocytes and

    monocytes in the blood: mono _____

3. a malignant tumor of lymph nodes; histiocytic and lymphocytic are types of this disease:

    non- _____

4. conditions in which the body reacts with an exaggerated immune response:

    hyper _____

5. a substance capable of causing an exaggerated immune response: al _____

6. fluid that lies between cells throughout the body: inter _____ fluid

7. formation of lymphocytes or lymphoid tissue: lympho _____

8. chronic swelling of a part of the body due to collection of fluid between tissues secondary to obstruction

    of lymph vessels and nodes: lymph _____

9. protein with known antibody activity that is made by plasma cells:

    immuno _____

10. an unusual or exaggerated allergic reaction to a foreign protein: ana _____

11. introduction of altered antigens to produce an immune response and protection from disease:

    vac _____

K. Select the correct term to complete each sentence.

1. Mr. Blake had been HIV-positive for 5 years before he developed (PCP, mononucleosis, sarcoidosis) and
    was diagnosed with (Hodgkin's disease, non-Hodgkin's lymphoma, AIDS).

2. Mary developed rhinitis, rhinorrhea, and red eyes every spring when pollen was prevalent. She consulted
    her doctor about her bad (hypersplenism, allergies, lymphadenitis).

3. Paul felt some marble-size lumps in his left groin. His doctor told him that he had an infection in his foot
    and developed secondary (axillary, cervical, inguinal) lymphadenopathy.

4. Mr. Jones was referred to a dermatologist and an oncologist when his primary physician noticed purple
    spots on his arms and legs. Because he had AIDS, his doctor was worried about (Kaposi's sarcoma,
    splenomegaly, thrombocytopenic purpura).

5. Suzy and her friends had been staying up late for weeks cramming for exams. She developed a sore throat,
    began to feel very tired, and had swollen lymph nodes in her neck. Dr. Hershirt did a blood test and
    diagnosed her condition as (lymphedema, anaphylaxis, mononucleosis).

X. Answers to Exercises

A

1. lymph nodes
2. thoracic duct
3. spleen
4. adenoids
5. thymus gland
6. lymph capillaries
7. right lymphatic duct
8. interstitial fluid

B

1. groin region
2. armpit region
3. neck (of the body) region
4. space between the lungs in the chest

C

1. humoral immunity
2. T cells
3. cell-mediated immunity
4. B cells

D

1. plasma cell
2. macrophage
3. helper cell
4. cytotoxic cell
5. suppressor cell

E

1. A
2. C
3. B
4. D
5. G
6. F
7. E

F

1. splenectomy
2. splenomegaly
3. lymphopoiesis
4. thymoma
5. lymphadenitis
6. lymphocytopenia
7. toxic
8. lymphadenopathy

G

1. hypersplenism
2. anaphylaxis
3. allergen
4. AIDS
5. thymectomy
6. Hodgkin's disease
7. lymphoid organs
8. lymphedema

H

1. Kaposi's sarcoma
2. HIV
3. T4 helper lymphocytes
4. PCP
5. opportunistic infections
6. ELISA (enzyme-linked immunosorbent assay)
7. Western blot
8. zidovudine

I

1. x-ray record of lymph vessels after injecting dye into tissue in the feet
2. x-ray images taken in the transverse plane
3. protein on T cell helper lymphocyte
4. antibodies produced by plasma cells; act against antigens
5. human immunodeficiency virus; virus that causes AIDS
6. Kaposi's sarcoma; a malignant condition that occurs in association with AIDS and infection by HIV
7. histoplasmosis; an opportunistic lung infection that occurs in association with AIDS

J

1. sarcoidosis
2. mononucleosis
3. non-Hodgkin's lymphoma
4. hypersensitivity
5. allergen
6. interstitial fluid
7. lymphopoiesis
8. lymphedema
9. immunoglobulin
10. anaphylaxis
11. vaccination

K

1. AIDS
2. allergies
3. inguinal
4. Kaposi's sarcoma
5. mononucleosis

Answers to Practical Applications

1. B
2. A
3. A
4. B
5. B
6. A
7. B
8. C

XI. Pronunciation of Terms

To test your understanding of the terminology in this chapter, write the meaning of each term in the space provided. In addition, you may wish to cover the terms and write them by looking at your definitions. Make sure your spelling is correct. The page number after each term indicates where it is defined or used in the text so you can easily check your responses. (If you are not sure what the pronunciation symbols mean, refer to page 21.)

Term	Pronunciation	Meaning
adenoids (474)	ĂD-ĕ-noydz	
acquired immunity (474)	ă-KWĪ-erd ĭ-MŪ-nĭ-tē	
acquired immunodeficiency syndrome (477)	ă-KWĪ-ĕrd ĭm-ū-nō-dĕ-FĬSH-ĕn-sē SĬN-drōm	
allergen (481)	ĂL-ĕr-jĕn	
allergy (481)	ĂL-ĕr-jē	
anaphylaxis (481)	ăn-ă-fă-LĂK-sĭs	
antibodies (474)	ĂN-tĭ-bŏ-dēz	
axillary nodes (474)	ĂKS-ĭ-lăr-ē nōdz	
cell-mediated immunity (475)	sĕl-MĒ-dē-ā-tĕd ĭ-MŪ-nĭ-tē	
cervical nodes (475)	SĔR-vĭ-k'l nōdz	
cytotoxic cells (475)	sī-tō-TŎK-sĭk sĕlz	
Hodgkin's disease (480)	HŎJ-kĭnz dĭ-ZĒZ	
human immunodeficiency virus (481)	HŪ-măn ĭm-ū-nō-dĕ-FĬSH-ĕn-sē VĪ-rŭs	
humoral immunity (475)	HŪ-mŏr-ăl ĭ-MŪ-nĭ-tē	
hypersensitivity (479)	hī-pĕr-sĕn-sĭ-TĬV-ĭ-tē	
hypersplenism (480)	hī-pĕr-SPLĔN-ĭzm	
immune response (475)	ĭ-MŪN rĕ-SPŎNS	
immunoglobulins (475)	ĭm-ū-nō-GLŎB-ū-lĭnz	
immunology (476)	ĭm-ū-NŎL-ō-jē	
inguinal nodes (475)	ĬNG-gwĭ-năl nōdz	
interferons (475)	ĭn-tĕr-FĔR-ŏnz	

interleukins (475)	ĭn-tĕr-LOO-kĭnz	_____
interstitial fluid (475)	ĭn-tĕr-STĬSH-ăl FLOO-ĭd	_____
Kaposi's sarcoma (481)	KĂ-pō-sēz săr-KŌ-mă	_____
lymph (475)	lĭmf	_____
lymphadenitis (477)	lĭm-FĂH-dĕ-nī-tĭs	_____
lymphadenopathy (477)	lĭm-făd-ĕ-NŎP-ăh-thē	_____
lymphangiogram (477)	lĭm-FĂN-jē-ō-grăm	_____
lymph capillaries (475)	lĭmf KĂP-ĭ-lă-rēz	_____
lymphedema (477)	lĭmf-ĕ-DĒ-mă	_____
lymph nodes (475)	lĭmf nōdz	_____
lymphocytes (474)	LĬM-fō-sītz	_____
lymphocytosis (477)	lĭm-fō-sī-TŌ-sĭs	_____
lymphocytopenia (477)	lĭm-fō-sī-tō-PĒ-nē-ă	_____
lymphoid organs (475)	LĬM-foid ŎR-gănz	_____
lymphoma (480)	lĭm-FŌ-mă	_____
lymphopoiesis (476)	lĭm-fō-poy-Ē-sĭs	_____
lymph vessels (475)	lĭmf VĔS-ĕlz	_____
macrophage (475)	MĂK-rō-făj	_____
mediastinal nodes (476)	mē-dē-ăs-TĪ-năl nōdz	_____
mononucleosis (480)	mŏn-ō-nū-klē-Ō-sĭs	_____
non-Hodgkin's lymphoma (480)	nŏn-HŎJ-kĭnz lĭm-FŌ-mă	_____
opportunistic infections (481)	ŏp-pŏr-tū-NĬS-tĭk ĭn-FĔK-shŭnz	_____
plasma cell (476)	PLĂZ-mă sĕl	_____
retrovirus (481)	rĕ-trō-VĪ-rŭs	_____
right lymphatic duct (476)	rīt lĭm-FĂ-tĭk dŭkt	_____
sarcoidosis (480)	săr-koy-DŌ-sĭs	_____
spleen (476)	splēn	_____

splenectomy (477)   splĕ-NĔK-tō-mē   _____

splenomegaly (477)   splĕ-nō-MĔG-ă-lē   _____

thoracic duct (476)   thō-RĂ-sĭk dŭkt   _____

thymectomy (477)   thī-MĔK-tō-mē   _____

thymoma (480)   thī-MŌ-mă   _____

thymus gland (476)   THĪ-mŭs glănd   _____

tonsils (476)   TŎN-sĭlz   _____

toxic (477)   TŎK-sĭk   _____

toxins (476)   TŎK-sĭnz   _____

vaccination (476)   văk-sĭ-NĀ-shun   _____

XII. Review Sheet

Write the meaning of each word part in the space provided. Check your answers with the information in the chapter or in the Glossary (Medical Terms—English) at the end of the book.

Combining Forms

Combining Form	Meaning	Combining Form	Meaning
axill/o	_____	lymphaden/o	_____
cervic/o	_____	lymphangi/o	_____
immun/o	_____	splen/o	_____
inguin/o	_____	thym/o	_____
lymph/o	_____	tox/o	_____

Suffixes

Suffix	Meaning	Suffix	Meaning
-cytosis	_____	-pathy	_____
-edema	_____	-penia	_____
-globulin	_____	-phylaxis	_____
-megaly	_____	-poiesis	_____
-oid	_____	-stitial	_____

Prefixes

Prefix	Meaning
ana-	_____
inter-	_____
retro-	_____

Musculoskeletal System

In this Chapter you will

■ Define terms relating to the structure and function of bones, joints, and muscles;

■ Describe the process of bone formation and growth;

■ Locate and name the major bones of the body;

■ Analyze the combining forms, prefixes, and suffixes used to describe bones, joints, and muscles;

■ Explain various musculoskeletal disease conditions and terms related to bone fractures; and

■ Identify important laboratory tests, clinical procedures, and abbreviations relating to the musculoskeletal system.

I. Introduction

The musculoskeletal system includes the bones, muscles, and joints. All have important functions in the body. **Bones** provide the framework around which the body is constructed and protect and support internal organs. Bones also assist the body in movement because they are a point of attachment for muscles. The inner core of bones is composed of hematopoietic tissue (red bone marrow manufactures blood cells), whereas other parts of bone are storage areas for minerals necessary for growth, such as calcium and phosphorus.

Joints are the places at which bones come together. Several different types of joints are found within the body. The type of joint found in any specific location is determined by the need for greater or lesser flexibility of movement.

Muscles, whether attached to bones or to internal organs and blood vessels, are responsible for movement. Internal movement involves the contraction and relaxation of muscles that are a part of viscera, and external movement is accomplished by the contraction and relaxation of muscles that are attached to the bones.

Doctors who treat bones and bone diseases are **orthopedists.** Originally, orthopedics was a branch of medicine dealing with correcting deformities in children (**orth/o** means straight, **ped/o** means child). **Rheumatologists** are doctors who treat joint diseases. **Rheumat/o** means watery flow and relates to joint diseases because various forms of arthritis are marked by collection of fluid in the joint spaces.

Osteopaths practice osteopathy, which is a separate school of medicine using diagnostic and therapeutic measures and based on the belief that the body is capable of healing itself when bones are in proper position and adequate nutrition is provided. **Chiropractors (chir/o** means hand) are neither physicians nor osteopaths, and they use physical means to manipulate the spinal column, believing that disease is caused by pressure on nerves.

II. Bones

A. Formation and Structure

Formation

Bones are complete organs, chiefly composed of connective tissue called **osseous** (bony) **tissue** plus a rich supply of blood vessels and nerves. Osseous tissue is a dense connective tissue that consists of **osteocytes** (bone cells) surrounded by a hard, intercellular substance filled with calcium salts.

During fetal development, the bones of the fetus are composed of **cartilage tissue,** which resembles osseous tissue but is more flexible and less dense because of a lack of calcium salts in its intercellular spaces. As the embryo develops, the process of depositing calcium salts in the soft, cartilaginous bones occurs and continues throughout the life of the individual after birth. The gradual replacement of cartilage and its intercellular substance by immature bone cells and calcium deposits is called **ossification** (bone formation).

Osteoblasts are the immature osteocytes that produce the bony tissue that replaces cartilage during ossification. **Osteoclasts** (**-clast** means to break) are large cells that function to reabsorb, or digest, bony tissue. Osteoclasts (also called **bone phagocytes**) digest dead bone tissue from the inner sides of bones and thus enlarge the inner bone cavity so that the bone does not become overly thick and heavy. When a bone breaks, osteoblasts lay down the mineral bone matter (calcium salts), and osteoclasts remove excess bone debris (smooth out the bone).

The formation of bone is dependent to a great extent on a proper supply of **calcium** and **phosphorus** to the bone tissue. These minerals must be taken into the body along with a sufficient amount of vitamin D. Vitamin D helps the passage of calcium through the lining of the small intestine and into the bloodstream. Once calcium and phosphorus are in the bones, osteoblastic activity produces an enzyme that causes the formation of calcium phosphate, a substance giving bone its characteristic hard quality.

Not only are calcium and phosphorus part of the hard structure of bone tissue but calcium is also stored in bones and small quantities are present in the blood. If the proper amount of calcium is lacking in the blood, nerve fibers are unable to transmit impulses effectively to muscles; heart muscle becomes weak, and muscles attached to bones undergo spasms.

The necessary level of calcium in the blood is maintained by the parathyroid gland, which secretes a hormone to release calcium from bone storage. Excess of the hormone (caused by tumor or other pathological process) will raise blood calcium at the expense of the bones, which become weakened by the loss of calcium.

Structure

There are 206 bones of various types in the body. **Long bones** are found in the thigh, lower leg, and upper and lower arm. These bones are very strong, are broad at the ends where they join with other bones, and have large surface areas for muscle attachment.

Short bones are found in the wrist and ankle and have small, irregular shapes. **Flat bones** are found covering soft body parts. These are the shoulder bone, ribs, and pelvic bones. **Sesamoid bones** are small, rounded bones resembling a grain of sesame in shape. They are found near joints; the kneecap is the largest example of this type of bone.

Figure 15–1 shows the anatomical divisions of a long bone such as the thigh bone or upper arm bone. Label the figure as you read the following.

The shaft, or middle region, of a long bone is called the **diaphysis** (1). Each end of a long bone is called an **epiphysis** (2). The **epiphyseal line** or **plate** (3) represents an area of cartilage tissue that is constantly being replaced by new bony tissue as the bone grows. Cartilage cells at the edges of the epiphyseal plate form new bone, and this is responsible for the lengthening of bones during childhood and adolescence. The plate calcifies and disappears when the bone has achieved its full growth.

Figure 15–1

Divisions of a long bone.

Figure 15–2 shows some of the structures that are part of the composition of the epiphysis and diaphysis. The **periosteum** (1) is a strong, fibrous, vascular membrane that covers the surface of a long bone, except at the ends of the epiphyses. Bones other than long bones are completely covered by the periosteum. Beneath the periosteum is the layer of osteoblasts, which deposit calcium phosphate in the bony tissue.

The ends of long bones are covered by a thin layer of cartilage called **articular cartilage** (2). This cartilage layer cushions the bones at the place where they meet with other bones (joints).

Compact (cortical) bone (3) is a layer of hard, dense tissue that lies under the periosteum in all bones and chiefly around the diaphysis of long bones. Within the compact bone is a system of small canals containing blood vessels that bring oxygen and nutrients to the bone and remove waste products such as carbon dioxide. The inset in Figure 15–2 shows these channels, called **haversian canals** (4), in the compact bone. Compact bone is tunneled out in the shaft of the long bones by a central **medullary cavity** (5) that contains **yellow bone marrow** (6). Yellow bone marrow is chiefly composed of fat cells.

Cancellous bone (7), sometimes called **spongy** or **trabecular bone,** is much more porous and less dense than compact bone. The mineral matter in it is laid down in a series of separated bony fibers called a spongy latticework or **trabeculae.** It is found largely in the epiphyses of long bones and in the middle portion of most other bones of the body as well. Spaces in cancellous bone contain **red bone marrow.** This marrow, as opposed to yellow marrow, which is fatty tissue, is richly supplied with blood and consists of immature and mature blood cells in various stages of development.

In an adult, the ribs, pelvic bone, sternum (breastbone), and vertebrae, as well as the epiphyses of long bones, contain red bone marrow within cancellous tissue. The red marrow in the long bones is plentiful in young children but decreases through the years and is replaced by yellow marrow.

B. Processes and Depressions in Bones

Bone processes are enlarged tissues that normally extend out from bones to serve as attachments for muscles and tendons. Label Figure 15–3, which shows the shapes of some of the common bony processes:

1. **Bone head**—rounded end of a bone separated from the body of the bone by a neck.
2. **Tubercle**—small, rounded process on many bones for attachment of tendons or muscles.
3. **Trochanter**—large process on the femur for attachment of muscle.
4. **Tuberosity**—large, rounded process on many bones for attachment of muscles or tendons.
5. **Condyle**—rounded, knuckle-like process at the joint.

Bone depressions are the openings or hollow regions in a bone that help to join one bone to another and serve as passageways for blood vessels and nerves. The names of some common depressions in bone are:

Fossa—shallow cavity in or on a bone.
Foramen—opening for blood vessels and nerves.
Fissure—a narrow, deep, slit-like opening.
Sulcus—a groove or furrow.
Sinus—a hollow cavity within a bone.

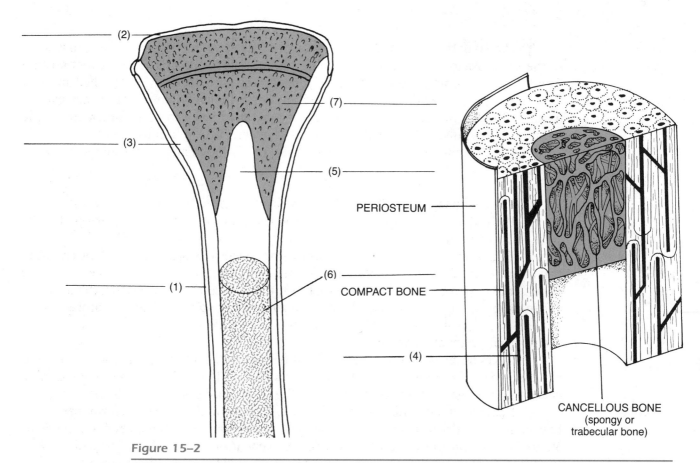

Figure 15–2

Interior bone structure.

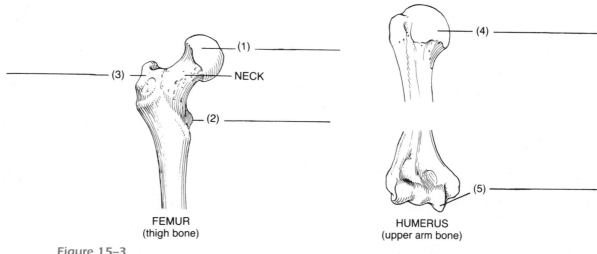

FEMUR
(thigh bone)

HUMERUS
(upper arm bone)

Figure 15–3

Bone processes.

C. Cranial Bones

The bones of the skull, or cranium, protect the brain and structures related to it, such as the sense organs. Muscles for controlling head movements and chewing motions are connected to the cranial bones. The cranial bones join each other at joints called **sutures.**

The cranial bones of a newborn child are not completely joined. There are gaps of unossified tissue in the skull at birth. These are called soft spots, or **fontanelles** (little fountains). The pulse of blood vessels can be felt under the skin in those areas.

Figure 15–4 illustrates the bones of the cranium. Label them as you read the following descriptions:

1. **Frontal bone**—forms the forehead and bony sockets that contain the eyes.

2. **Parietal bone**—there are two parietal bones that form the roof and upper part of the sides of the cranium.

3. **Temporal bone**—two temporal bones form the lower sides and base of the cranium. Each bone encloses an ear and contains a fossa for joining with the mandible (lower jaw bone). The **temporomandibular joint (TMJ)** is the area of connection between the temporal and mandibular bones. The **mastoid process** is a round (**mast/o** means breast) process of the temporal bone behind the ear. The **styloid process** (**styl/o** means pole or stake) projects downward from the temporal bone.

4. **Occipital bone**—forms the back and base of the skull and joins the parietal and temporal bones, forming a suture. The inferior portion of the occipital bone has an opening called the **foramen magnum** through which the spinal cord passes (Fig. 15–5).

5. **Sphenoid bone**—this bat-shaped bone extends behind the eyes and forms part of the base of the skull. Because it joins with the frontal, occipital, and ethmoid bones, it serves as an anchor to hold those skull bones together (**sphen/o** means wedge). The **sella turcica** (meaning Turkish saddle) is a depression in the sphenoid bone in which the pituitary gland is located (Fig. 15–5).

6. **Ethmoid bone**—this thin, delicate bone is composed primarily of spongy, cancellous bone. It supports the nasal cavity and forms part of the orbits of the eyes (**ethm/o** means sieve).

Study Figure 15–5, which shows these cranial bones as viewed looking downward at the floor of the cranial cavity.

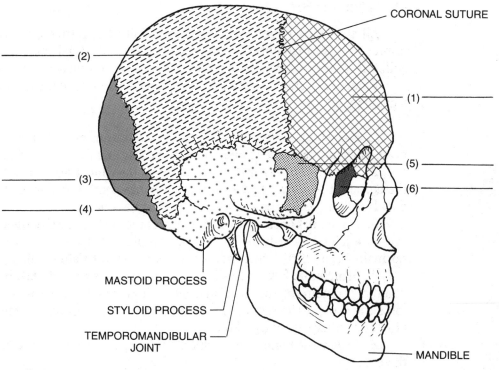

CORONAL SUTURE

(2)

(1)

(5)

(6)

(3)

(4)

MASTOID PROCESS

STYLOID PROCESS

TEMPOROMANDIBULAR
JOINT

MANDIBLE

Figure 15–4

Cranial bones, lateral view.

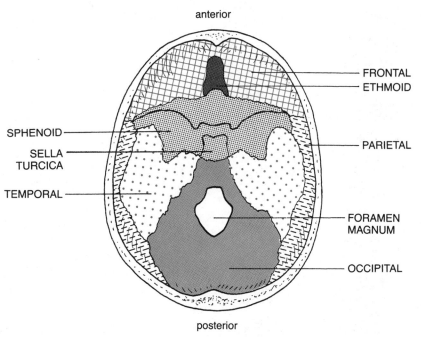

anterior

FRONTAL
ETHMOID

SPHENOID

SELLA
TURCICA

PARIETAL

TEMPORAL

FORAMEN
MAGNUM

OCCIPITAL

posterior

Figure 15–5

Bones of the skull, looking downward at the floor of the cranial cavity.

D. Facial Bones

All the facial bones, except one, are joined together by sutures, so that they are immovable. The mandible (lower jaw bone) is the only facial bone capable of movement. This ability is necessary for activities such as mastication (chewing) and speaking.

Figure 15–6 shows the facial bones; label it as you read the following descriptions of the facial bones:

1. **Nasal bones**—two slender nasal (**nas/o** means nose) bones support the bridge of the nose. They join with the frontal bone superiorly and form part of the nasal septum.

2. **Lacrimal bones**—two paired lacrimal (**lacrim/o** means tear) bones are located one at the corner of each eye. These thin, small bones contain fossae for the lacrimal gland (tear gland) and canals for the passage of the lacrimal duct.

3. **Maxillary bones**—two large bones compose the massive upper jaw bones **(maxillae).** They are joined by a suture in the median plane. If the two bones do not come together normally before birth, the condition known as **cleft palate** results.

4. **Mandibular bone**—this is the lower jaw bone **(mandible).** Both the maxilla and the mandible contain the sockets called alveoli in which the teeth are embedded. The mandible joins the skull at the region of the temporal bone, forming the temporomandibular joint (TMJ) on either side of the skull.

5. **Zygomatic bones**—two bones, one on each side of the face, form the high portion of the cheek.

6. **Vomer**—this thin, single, flat bone forms the lower portion of the nasal septum.

Sinuses, or air cavities, are located in specific places within the cranial and facial bones to lighten the skull and warm and moisten air as it passes through. Figure 15–7 shows the sinuses of the skull.

Figure 15–6

Facial bones.

Figure 15–7

Sinuses of the skull.

E. Vertebral Column and Structure of Vertebrae

The **vertebral**, or **spinal, column** is composed of 26 bone segments, called vertebrae, that are arranged in five divisions from the base of the skull to the tailbone.

Figure 15–8 illustrates these divisions of the vertebral column; label it as you read the following:

The first 7 bones of the vertebral column, forming the neck bone, are the **cervical (C1–C7) vertebrae** (1). These vertebrae do not articulate (join) with the ribs.

The second set of 12 vertebrae are known as the **thoracic (T1–T12 or D1–D12) vertebrae** (2). These vertebrae articulate with the 12 pairs of ribs.

The third set of 5 vertebral bones are the **lumbar (L1–L5) vertebrae** (3). They are the strongest and largest of the back bones.

INTERVERTEBRAL DISKS

Figure 15–8

Vertebral column.

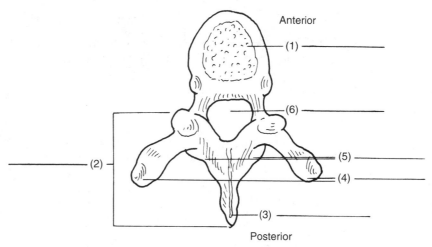

Figure 15–9

General structure of a vertebra, viewed from above.

The **sacrum** (4) is a slightly curved, triangularly shaped bone. At birth it is composed of 5 separate segments (sacral bones); these gradually become fused in the young child.

The **coccyx** (5) is the tailbone, and it, too, is a fused bone, having been formed from 4 small coccygeal bones.

Figure 15–9 illustrates the general structure of a vertebra. Although the individual vertebrae in the separate regions of the spinal column are all slightly different in structure, they do have several parts in common.

A vertebra is composed of an inner, thick, disk-shaped portion called the **vertebral body** (1). Between the body of one vertebra and the bodies of vertebrae lying beneath and above are **cartilaginous disks (discs),** which help to provide flexibility and cushion most shocks to the vertebral column.

The **vertebral arch** (2) is the posterior part of the vertebra, and it consists of a **spinous process** (3), **transverse processes** (4), and **laminae** (5). The **neural canal** (6) is the space between the vertebral body and the vertebral arch through which the spinal cord passes. Figure 15–10 shows a lateral view of several vertebrae. Note the location of the spinal cord running through the neural canal.

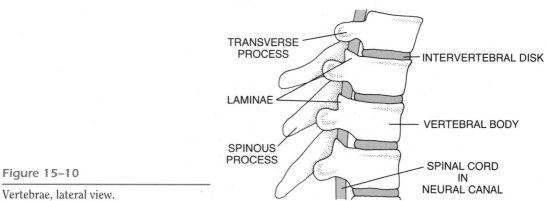

Figure 15–10

Vertebrae, lateral view.

F. Bones of the Thorax, Pelvis, and Extremities

Label Figure 15–11 as you read the following descriptions of the bones of the thorax (chest cavity), pelvis (hip bone), and extremities (arms and legs):

Figure 15–11

Bones of the thorax, pelvis, and extremities.

Bones of the Thorax

1. **Clavicle**—collar bone; a slender bone, one on each side of the body, connecting the breastbone to each shoulder bone.

2. **Scapula**—shoulder bone; two flat, triangular bones, one on each dorsal side of the thorax. The extension of the scapula that joins with the clavicle to form the joint of the shoulder is called the **acromion** (**acr/o** means extremity, **om/o** means shoulder). Figure 15–12 shows a posterior view of the scapula.

3. **Sternum**—breastbone; a flat bone extending down the midline of the chest. The uppermost part of the sternum articulates on the sides with the clavicle and ribs, and the lower, narrower portion is attached to the diaphragm and abdominal muscles. The lower portion of the sternum is called the **xiphoid process** (**xiph/o** means sword).

4. **Ribs**—there are 12 pairs of ribs. The first 7 pairs join the sternum anteriorly through cartilaginous attachments called **costal cartilages.** Ribs 1-7 are called **true ribs.** They join with the sternum anteriorly and with the vertebral column in the back. Ribs 8–10 are called **false ribs.** They join with the vertebral column in the back but join the 7th rib anteriorly instead of attaching to the sternum. Ribs 11 and 12 are the **floating ribs** because they are completely free at their anterior extremity. Figure 15–12 shows a posterior view of the rib cage.

Bones of the Arm and Hand

These are described as if the patient is in the anatomical position—palms forward.

5. **Humerus**—upper arm bone; the large head of the humerus is rounded and joins with the scapula and clavicle.

6. **Ulna**—medial lower arm bone; the proximal bony process of the ulna at the elbow is called the **olecranon** (elbow bone).

7. **Radius**—lateral lower arm bone (on line with the thumb).

8. **Carpals**—wrist bones; there are two rows of 4 bones each in the wrist.

9. **Metacarpals**—these are 5 radiating bones to the fingers.

10. **Phalanges** (singular: **phalanx**)—finger bones; each finger (except the thumb) has 3 phalanges: a proximal, middle, and distal phalanx. The thumb has only 2 phalanges.

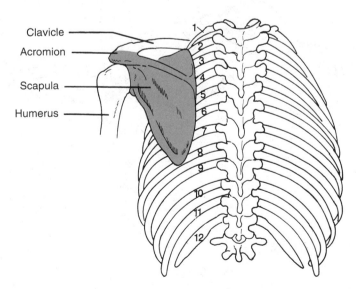

Figure 15–12

Posterior view of the scapula and rib cage.

Bones of the Pelvis

11. **Pelvic girdle**—hip bone; this large bone supports the trunk of the body and articulates with the thigh bone and sacrum. The adult pelvic bone is composed of 3 pairs of fused bones: the ilium, ischium, and pubis.

The **ilium** is the uppermost and largest portion. Dorsally, the two parts of the ilium do not meet. Rather, they join the sacrum on either side. The connection between the iliac bones and the sacrum is so firm that they are commonly spoken of as one bone: the sacroiliac. The superior part of the ilium is known as the iliac crest. It is filled with red bone marrow and serves as an attachment for abdominal wall muscles.

The **ischium** (**isch/o** means back) is the posterior part of the pelvis. The ischium and the muscles attached to it are what you sit on.

The **pubis** is the anterior part and contains suture marks where the two pubes join by way of a cartilaginous disk (disc). This area of fusion is called the **pubic symphysis.**

The region within the ring of bone formed by the pelvic girdle is called the **pelvic cavity.** The rectum, sigmoid colon, bladder, and female reproductive organs lie within the pelvic cavity.

Bones of the Leg and Foot

12. **Femur**—thigh bone; this is the longest bone in the body. At its proximal end it has a rounded head that fits into a depression, or socket, in the hip bone. This socket is called the **acetabulum.** The acetabulum was named because of its resemblance to a rounded cup the Romans used for vinegar *(acetum).*

Figure 15–13

Bones of the foot, lateral view *(left),* and right foot, viewed from above *(right).*

13. **Patella**—kneecap; this is a small, flat bone that lies in front of the articulation between the femur and one of the lower leg bones called the tibia. It is surrounded by protective tendons and held in place by muscle attachments.

14. **Tibia**—largest of 2 bones of the lower leg; the tibia (meaning flute) runs under the skin in the front part of the leg. It joins with the femur at the patella, and at its distal end (ankle) forms a swelling that is the bony prominence (medial **malleolus**) at the inside of the ankle. The tibia is commonly called the **shin bone.**

15. **Fibula**—smaller of 2 lower leg bones; this thin bone, well hidden under the leg muscles, joins at its proximal end with the tibia laterally and joins at its distal end with the tibia and ankle bones to form the bony prominence (lateral **malleolus**) on the outside of the ankle.

16. **Tarsals**—ankle bones; these are 7 short bones that resemble the carpal bones of the wrist but are larger. The **calcaneus** is the largest of these bones and is also called the **heel bone** (Fig. 15–13).

17. **Metatarsals**—there are 5 metatarsal bones—each leads to the phalanges of the toes.

18. **Phalanges of the toes**—there are 2 phalanges in the big toe and 3 in each of the other four toes.

Figure 15–13 illustrates the bones of the foot.

G. Vocabulary

This list will help you review many of the new terms introduced in the text. Short definitions will reinforce your understanding of the terms. See Section IX of this chapter for help in pronouncing the more difficult terms.

acetabulum	Rounded depression, or socket, in the pelvic bone where the thigh bone joins with the pelvis.
acromion	Outward extension of the shoulder bone forming the point of the shoulder.
articular cartilage	Thin layer of cartilage at the ends of long bones.
calcium	One of the mineral constituents of bone.
cancellous bone	Spongy, porous, trabecular bone tissue.
cartilage tissue	Flexible, rubbery connective tissue found on joint surfaces and in the embryonic skeleton.
compact bone	Hard, dense bone tissue.
condyle	Knuckle-like process at the end of a bone near the joint.
cranial bones	Skull bones: ethmoid, frontal, occipital, parietal, sphenoid, and temporal.
diaphysis	Shaft, or midportion, of a long bone.
disk (disc)	Flat, round, plate-like structure. An intervertebral disk is a fibrocartilaginous substance between the vertebrae.

epiphyseal plate	Cartilaginous area at the ends of long bones where lengthwise growth takes place.
epiphysis	Each end of a long bone.
facial bones	Bones of the face: lacrimal, mandible, maxillae, nasal, vomer, and zygomatic.
false ribs	Ribs 8–10.
fissure	Narrow, slit-like opening between bones.
floating ribs	Ribs 11 and 12.
fontanelle	Soft spot (incomplete bone formation) between the skull bones of an infant.
foramen	Opening or passage in bones where blood vessels and nerves enter and leave. The **foramen magnum** is the opening of the occipital bone through which the spinal cord passes.
fossa	Shallow cavity in a bone.
haversian canals	Minute spaces filled with blood vessels, found in compact bone.
malleolus	Round process on both sides of the ankle joint.
mastoid process	Round projection on the temporal bone behind the ear.
medullary cavity	Central, hollowed-out area in the shaft of a long bone.
olecranon	Large process forming the elbow.
osseous tissue	Bone tissue.
ossification	Process of bone formation.
osteoblast	Bone cell that helps form bone tissue.
osteoclast	Bone cell that absorbs and removes unwanted bone tissue.
periosteum	Membrane surrounding bones.
phosphorus	Mineral substance found in bones in combination with calcium.
pubic symphysis	Area of fusion of the two pubic bones. They are joined (sym- means together, -physis means to grow) by a piece of fibrocartilage.
red bone marrow	Found in cancellous bone; site of hemopoiesis.
sinus	Cavity within a bone.
styloid process	Pole-like process on the temporal bone.

sulcus	Groove-like depression.
trabeculae	Supporting bundles of bony fibers in cancellous (spongy) bone.
trochanter	Large process below the neck of the femur.
tubercle	Small, rounded process on a bone.
tuberosity	Large, rounded process on a bone.
vertebra	Back bone, composed of: vertebral body, vertebral arch, spinous process, transverse processes, lamina, and neural canal.
xiphoid process	Lower, narrow portion of the sternum.
yellow bone marrow	Fatty tissue found in the diaphyses of long bones.

H. Combining Forms and Suffixes

These are divided into two groups: general terms and terms related to specific bones. Write the meaning of the medical term in the space provided.

GENERAL TERMS
Combining Forms

Combining Form	Meaning	Terminology	Meaning
calc/o	calcium	hyper<u>calc</u>emia _____	
calci/o		de<u>calci</u>fication _____	
		de- means less or lack of; -fication is the process of making.	
kyph/o	humpback (posterior curvature in the thoracic region)	<u>kyph</u>osis _____	
		The term (from the Greek) means hill or mountain, indicating a hump on the back. A person's height is reduced, and kyphosis may lead to pressure on the spinal cord or peripheral nerves. See page 518, Figure 15–16 in Section II(I), Pathological Conditions and Fractures, under osteoporosis.	
lamin/o	lamina (part of the vertebral arch)	<u>lamin</u>ectomy _____	
		An operation often performed to relieve the symptoms of a ruptured intervertebral disk (disc).	
lord/o	curve, swayback (anterior curvature in the lumbar region)	<u>lord</u>osis _____	
		This term is used to describe the normal anterior curvature of the spinal column in the lumbar region and an excessive, abnormal	

anterior curvature, or swayback, condition. The word is derived from the Greek, describing a person leaning backward in a lordly fashion.

lumb/o	loins, lower back	lumbar _____
		lumbosacral _____
		lumbodynia _____
		Also called lumbago.

myel/o	bone marrow	myelopoiesis _____

orth/o	straight	orthopedic _____
		Ped/o means child.

oste/o	bone	osteitis _____
		osteodystrophy _____
		osteogenesis _____

Osteogenesis imperfecta is an inherited congenital anomaly marked by brittle bones and multiple fractures; also called brittle bone disease.

scoli/o	crooked, bent (lateral curvature)	scoliosis _____

The spinal column is bent from side to side (Fig. 15–14).

spondyl/o (used to make words about conditions of the structure)	vertebra	spondylitis _____
		spondylosis _____

This term indicates degeneration of the intervertebral disks (discs) in the cervical, thoracic, and lumbar regions. Symptoms include pain and restriction of movement.

vertebr/o (used to describe the structure)	vertebra	vertebral _____

Figure 15–14

Scoliosis (lateral curvature of the spine). (From Dorland's Illustrated Medical Dictionary, 27th ed. Philadelphia, WB Saunders, 1988, p 1497.)

Suffixes

Suffix	Meaning	Terminology	Meaning
-blast	embryonic or immature cell	osteoblast _____	
-clast	to break	osteoclast _____	
		This cell breaks down bone to remove bone tissue.	
-listhesis	slipping	spondylolisthesis _____	
		(spŏn-dĭ-lō-lĭs-THĒ-sĭs) Forward slipping (subluxation) of a vertebra over a lower vertebra.	
-malacia	softening	osteomalacia _____	
		A condition in which vitamin D deficiency leads to decalcification of bones; known as rickets in children.	
-physis	to grow	epiphysis _____	
		pubic symphysis _____	
-porosis	pore, passage	osteoporosis _____	
		Loss of bony tissue and decreased mass of bone. See page 517, Section II(I), Pathological Conditions and Fractures.	
-tome	instrument to cut	osteotome _____	
		This surgical chisel is designed to cut bone.	

TERMS RELATED TO SPECIFIC BONES
Combining Forms

Combining Form	Meaning	Terminology	Meaning
acetabul/o	acetabulum (hip socket)	acetabular _____	
calcane/o	calcaneus (heel bone)	calcaneal _____	
		The calcaneus is one of the tarsal (foot) bones.	
carp/o	carpals (wrist bones)	carpal _____	
clavicul/o	clavicle (collar bone)	supraclavicular _____	
		supra- means above.	

cost/o	ribs (true ribs, false ribs, and floating ribs)	sub<u>costal</u> _____
		chondro<u>costal</u> _____
		Cartilage that is attached to the ribs.
crani/o	cranium (skull bones)	<u>crani</u>otomy _____
		<u>crani</u>otome _____
femor/o	femur (thigh bone)	<u>femor</u>al _____
fibul/o	fibula (smaller lower leg bone)	<u>fibul</u>ar _____
		See perone/o.
humer/o	humerus (upper arm bone)	<u>humer</u>al _____
ili/o	ilium (upper part of the pelvic bone)	<u>ili</u>ac _____
isch/o	ischium (posterior part of the pelvic bone)	<u>isch</u>ial _____
malleol/o	malleolus (process on each side of the ankle)	<u>malleol</u>ar _____
		The medial malleolus is at the lower end of the tibia, and the lateral malleolus is at the lower end of the fibula.
mandibul/o	mandible (lower jaw bone)	<u>mandibul</u>ar _____
maxill/o	maxilla (upper jaw bone)	<u>maxill</u>ary _____
metacarp/o	metacarpals (hand bones)	<u>metacarp</u>ectomy _____
metatars/o	metatarsals (foot bones)	<u>metatars</u>algia _____
olecran/o	olecranon (elbow)	<u>olecran</u>al _____
patell/a **patell/o**	patella (kneecap)	<u>patell</u>apexy _____
		sub<u>patell</u>ar _____

pelv/i	pelvis (hip bone)	pelvimetry _____
perone/o	fibula	peroneal _____
phalang/o	phalanges (finger bones)	phalangeal _____
pub/o	pubis (anterior part of the pelvic bone)	pubic _____
radi/o	radius (lower arm bone— thumb side)	radial _____
scapul/o	scapula (shoulder bone)	scapular _____
stern/o	sternum (breast bone)	sternal _____
tars/o	tarsals (ankle bones)	tarsectomy _____
tibi/o	tibia (shin bone)	tibial _____
uln/o	ulna (lower arm bone—little finger side)	ulnar _____

I. Pathological Conditions and Fractures

Ewing's sarcoma

Malignant bone tumor.

Pain and swelling are common, with the tumor sometimes involving the entire shaft (medullary cavity) of a long bone. This tumor usually occurs at an early age (5–15 years old), and radiotherapy with chemotherapy represents the best chance for cure (60–70 per cent of patients are cured before metastases occur).

exostosis

Bony growth arising from the surface of bone (ex- means out, -ostosis means condition of bone).

Osteochondromas (composed of cartilage and bone) are **exostoses** and are usually found on the diaphysis of long bones near the epiphyseal plate.

A **bunion** is a swelling of the metatarsophalangeal joint near the base of the big toe and is accompanied by build up of soft tissue and underlying bone.

fracture   Sudden breaking of a bone.

A **simple** (closed) **fracture** means that a bone is broken but there is no open wound in the skin, whereas a **compound** (open) **fracture** means a bone is broken with an open wound in the skin. A **pathological fracture** is caused by disease of the bone or change in the tissue surrounding the bone, making it weak. **Crepitus** is the crackling sound produced when ends of bone rub each other or against roughened cartilage.

Some examples of fractures (Fig. 15–15) are:

Colles' fracture—occurs in the wrist at the lower end of the radius.
comminuted fracture—bone is splintered or crushed.
compression fracture—bone is compressed; often occurs in vertebrae.
greenstick fracture—bone is partially broken and partially bent on the opposite side, as when a green stick breaks.
impacted fracture—fracture in which one fragment is driven firmly into the other.

Treatment of fractures involves **reduction,** which is the restoration of the bone to its normal position. A **closed reduction** is manipulative reduction without an

Compound   Comminuted   Colles'

Impacted   Greenstick

Figure 15–15

Types of fractures. (Colles' fracture from Dorland's Illustrated Medical Dictionary, 28th ed. Philadelphia, WB Saunders, 1994, p 661.)

incision; in an **open reduction,** an incision is made into the fracture site. A **cast** (solid mold of the bone) is applied to fractures to immobilize the injured bone.

osteogenic sarcoma

Malignant tumor arising from bone **(osteosarcoma).**

This is the most common type of malignant bone tumor. Osteoblasts multiply without control and form large tumors, especially at the ends of long bones (half the lesions are located just below or just above the knee). Metastasis is through the bloodstream and often occurs in the lungs. Surgical resection with chemotherapy improves the survival rate.

osteomalacia

Softening of bone with inadequate amounts of mineral (calcium) in the bone.

Osteomalacia primarily occurs as a disease of infancy and childhood and is then known as **rickets.** Bones fail to receive adequate amounts of calcium and phosphorus, and they become soft, bend easily, and become deformed.

Vitamin D is usually deficient in the diet, and this prevents calcium and phosphorus from being absorbed into the bloodstream from the intestines. Vitamin D is formed by the action of sunlight on certain compounds (such as cholesterol) in the skin; thus rickets is more common in large, smoky cities during the winter months.

Treatment consists of administration of large daily doses of vitamin D and an increase in dietary intake of calcium and phosphorus.

osteomyelitis

Inflammation of the bone and bone marrow.

Bacteria enter the body through a wound and spread from an infection near the bone or come from a skin or throat infection. Children are most often affected, and the infection usually occurs in the long bones of the legs and arms.

The lesion begins as an **abscess** (inflammation with pus collection). Pus tends to spread down the medullary cavity and outward to the periosteum. Antibiotic therapy corrects the condition, so that abscess can be prevented.

osteoporosis

Decrease in bone density (mass); thinning and weakening of bone.

This condition is also called **osteopenia,** because the interior of bones is diminished in structure, as if the steel skeleton of a building had been rusted and worn down. Osteoporosis commonly occurs in older women as a consequence of estrogen deficiency with menopause. Lack of estrogen promotes excessive bone resorption (osteoclast activity) and less bone deposition. Weakened bones are subject to fractures (as in the hip); loss of height and kyphosis occur as vertebrae collapse (Fig. 15–16).

Estrogen replacement therapy and increased intake of calcium may be helpful for some patients. A weight-bearing daily exercise program is also important.

Osteoporosis can occur with atrophy of disuse as in a limb that is in a cast, or in the legs of a paraplegic, or in a bedridden patient. It may also occur in men as part of the aging process and in patients who have been given corticosteroid (hormones made by the adrenal gland and used to treat inflammatory conditions) therapy.

talipes

Clubfoot.

This congenital deformity of the bones of the foot means that the patient cannot stand with the sole of the foot flat on the ground. The defect can be corrected by orthopedic splinting in the early months of infancy (Fig. 15–17).

Age   40   60   70

Figure 15–16

Loss of bone mass due to osteoporosis produces posterior curvature of the spine in the thoracic region (kyphosis). A normal spine is shown at age 40 years, and osteoporotic changes are illustrated at 60 and 70 years of age. (From O'Toole M [ed]: Miller-Keane Encyclopedia and Dictionary of Medicine, Nursing, and Allied Health, 5th ed. Philadelphia, WB Saunders, 1992, p 1079.)

Talipes equinus	Talipes calcaneus	Talipes cavus
Talipes varus	Talipes equinovarus	Talipes calcaneovarus
Talipes valgus	Talipes calcaneovalgus	Talipes equinovalgus

Figure 15–17

Types of talipes. Equinus means horse; calcaneus refers to the heel; cavus means hollow; varus means bent inward; valgus means bent outward. (From O'Toole M [ed]: Miller-Keane Encyclopedia and Dictionary of Medicine, Nursing, and Allied Health, 5th ed. Philadelphia, WB Saunders, 1992, p 1458.)

Figure 15–18

Synovial joint.

III. Joints

A. Types of Joints

A joint (articulation) is a coming together of two or more bones. Some joints are immovable, such as the **suture joints** between the skull bones. Other joints, such as those between the vertebrae, are partially movable. Most joints, however, allow considerable movement. These freely movable joints are called **synovial joints.** Examples of synovial joints are the ball-and-socket type (hip joint; the head of the femur fits into the acetabular fossa of the ilium) and hinge type (elbow, knee, and ankle joints). Label the structures in Figure 15–18 as you read the following description of a synovial joint:

The bones in a synovial joint are separated by a **joint capsule** (1) composed of fibrous cartilage tissue. **Ligaments** (fibrous bands, or sheets, of connective tissue) often anchor the bones together around the joint capsule to strengthen it. The surface of the bones at the joint is covered with a smooth cartilage surface called the **articular cartilage** (2). The **synovial membrane** (3) lies under the joint capsule and lines the **synovial cavity** (4) between the bones. The synovial cavity is filled with a special lubricating fluid produced by the synovial membrane. This **synovial fluid** contains water and nutrients that nourish as well as lubricate the joints, so that friction on the articular cartilage is minimal.

B. Bursae

Bursae (singular: **bursa**) are closed sacs of synovial fluid lined with a synovial membrane and are located near a joint. They are formed in the spaces between **tendons** (connective tissue binding muscles to bones), **ligaments** (connective tissue binding bones to bones), and bones. Bursae lubricate these areas where friction would normally develop close to the joint capsule.

Some common bursae locations are at the elbow joint (olecranon bursa), knee joint (patellar bursa), and shoulder joint (subacromial bursa). Figure 15–19 shows a lateral view of the knee joint with bursae.

Figure 15–19

Knee joint (lateral view) with bursae expanded for clarity. (From Jacob S, Francone A: Elements of Anatomy and Physiology, 2nd ed. Philadelphia, WB Saunders, 1989, p 68.)

C. Vocabulary

This list will help you review many of the new terms introduced in this text. Short definitions will reinforce your understanding of the terms. See Section IX of this chapter for help in pronouncing the more difficult terms.

articulation	Joint.
bursa (plural: **bursae**)	Sac of fluid near a joint.
ligament	Connective tissue binding bones to other bones; supports and strengthens the joint.
suture joint	Type of joint in which apposed surfaces are closely united.
synovial cavity	Space between bones at a synovial joint.
synovial fluid	Viscous (sticky) fluid within the synovial cavity. Synovial fluid is similar in viscosity to egg white; this accounts for the origin of the term (syn- means like, ov/o means egg).
synovial joint	A freely movable joint.
synovial membrane	Membrane lining the synovial cavity.
tendon	Connective tissue that binds muscles to bones.

D. Combining Forms and Suffixes

Write the meaning of the medical term in the space provided.

Combining Forms

Combining Form	Meaning	Terminology	Meaning
ankyl/o	crooked, bent, stiff	ankylosis _____	
		*This term indicates a fusion of the bones across a joint space by either bony tissue (**bony ankylosis**) or growth of fibrous tissue (**fibrous ankylosis**). This immobility and stiffening of the joint most often occurs in rheumatoid arthritis.*	
arthr/o	joint	arthroplasty _____	
		Replacement arthroplasty is the replacement of one or both bone ends by a prosthesis (artificial part) of metal or plastic.	

arthrotomy _____

hemarthrosis _____

hydrarthrosis _____

Synovial fluid collects abnormally in the joint.

periarthritis _____

articul/o joint articular cartilage _____

burs/o bursa bursitis _____

Etiology may be related to stress placed on the bursa or diseases such as gout or rheumatoid arthritis. Movement becomes limited and painful. Intrabursal injection of corticosteroids as well as rest and splinting of the limb is helpful in treatment.

chondr/o cartilage achondroplasia _____

This is an inherited condition in which the bones of the arms and legs fail to grow to normal size owing to a defect in cartilage and bone formation. Dwarfism occurs, with short limbs and a normal-sized head and body.

chondroma _____

chondromalacia _____

Chondromalacia patellae *is a roughening of the inner surface of the kneecap, resulting in pain, a grating sensation, and instability of movement.*

ligament/o ligament ligamentous _____

rheumat/o watery flow rheumatologist _____

Various forms of arthritis are marked by collection of fluid in joint spaces.

synov/o synovial membrane synovitis _____

ten/o tendon tenorrhaphy _____

tenosynovitis _____

synov/o here refers to the sheath (covering) around the tendon.

tendin/o tendon tendinitis _____

Suffixes			
Suffix	Meaning	Terminology	Meaning

-desis	to bind, tie together	arthro<u>desis</u> _____	
		Bones are fused across the joint space by surgery (artificial ankylosis). This operation is performed when a joint is very painful, unstable, or chronically infected.	
-stenosis	narrowing	spinal <u>stenosis</u>	
		Narrowing of the neural canal or nerve root canals in the lumbar spine. Symptoms (pain, paresthesias, urinary retention, or incontinence) come from compression of the cauda equina (nerves that spread out from the lower end of the spinal cord like a horse's tail).	

E. Pathological Conditions

arthritis

Inflammation of joints.

Some of the more common forms are:

ankylosing spondylitis

Chronic, progressive arthritis with stiffening of joints, primarily of the spine.

Bilateral sclerosis (hardening) of the sacroiliac joints is a diagnostic sign. Joint changes are similar to those seen in rheumatoid arthritis, and the condition responds to corticosteroids and anti-inflammatory drugs.

gouty arthritis

Inflammation of joints caused by excessive uric acid in the body.

A defect in metabolism of uric acid causes too much of it to accumulate in blood **(hyperuricemia),** joints, and soft tissues near joints. The uric acid crystals (salts) destroy the articular cartilage and damage the synovial membrane. A joint chiefly affected is the big toe; hence, the condition is often called **podagra** (pod/o means foot, -agra means excessive pain). Treatment consists of drugs to lower uric acid production (allopurinol) and to prevent inflammation (colchicine), and a special diet that avoids foods that are rich in uric acid, such as red meats.

osteoarthritis

Progressive, degenerative joint disease characterized by loss of articular cartilage and hypertrophy of bone at articular surfaces.

This condition, also known as **degenerative joint disease,** occurs mainly in the hips and knees of older individuals and is marked by a narrowing of the joint space (due to loss of cartilage). Treatment consists of aspirin and other analgesics to reduce inflammation and pain and physical therapy to loosen impaired joints. Figure 15–20 compares a normal joint with those that have changes characteristic of osteoarthritis and rheumatoid arthritis.

rheumatoid arthritis

A chronic disease in which joints become inflamed and painful. It is believed to be caused by an immune (autoimmune) reaction against joint tissues.

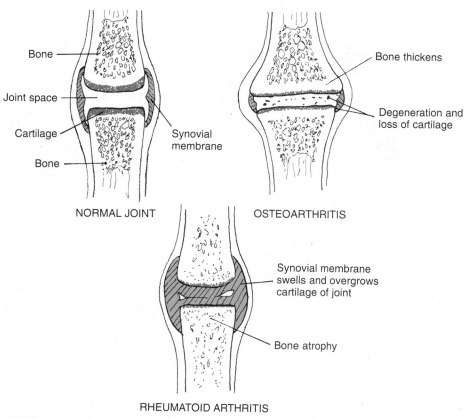

Bone

Joint space

Cartilage

Synovial membrane

Bone

NORMAL JOINT

Bone thickens

Degeneration and loss of cartilage

OSTEOARTHRITIS

Synovial membrane swells and overgrows cartilage of joint

Bone atrophy

RHEUMATOID ARTHRITIS

Figure 15–20

Changes in a joint with osteoarthritis and rheumatoid arthritis.

The small joints of the hands and feet are affected first and larger joints later. Women are more commonly afflicted than men. Synovial membranes become inflamed and thickened, damaging the articular cartilage and preventing easy movement (Fig. 15–20). Sometimes fibrous tissue forms and calcifies, creating a bony **ankylosis** (union) at the joint and preventing any movement at all. Swollen, painful joints accompanied by **pyrexia** (fever) are symptoms.

Diagnosis is by a blood test that shows the presence of the rheumatoid factor (an antibody) and x-rays revealing changes around the affected joints. Treatment consists of heat applications and drugs (aspirin, gold compounds, and corticosteroids) to reduce inflammation and pain.

bunion

Abnormal swelling of the joint between the big toe and the first metatarsal bone.

A bursa often develops over the site, and chronic irritation from ill-fitting shoes can cause a build-up of soft tissue and underlying bone. Bunionectomy may be indicated if other measures (changing shoes and use of anti-inflammatory agents) fail.

carpal tunnel syndrome (CTS)

Compression (by a wrist ligament) of the median nerve as it passes between the ligament and the bones and tendons of the wrist (the carpal tunnel) (Fig. 15–21).

This condition most often affects middle-aged women, and pain and burning sensations occur in the fingers and hand, sometimes extending to the elbow.

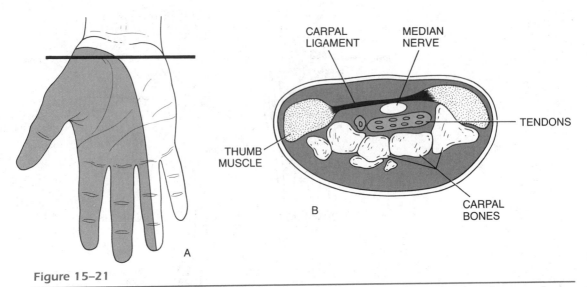

Figure 15–21

Carpal tunnel syndrome. *(A)* The median nerve's sensory distribution in the thumb, first three fingers, and palm. (The palm is facing forward.) *(B)* Cross section of a right hand at the level indicated in *A*. Note the position of the median nerve between the carpal ligament and the tendons and carpal bones.

Figure 15–22

Ganglion.

Figure 15–23

Protrusion of an intervertebral disk (disc) (looking down on a vertebra). Note how the inner portion (nucleus pulposus) of the disk (disc) herniates and presses on the spinal nerve.

Excessive wrist movement, arthritis, hypertrophy of bone, and swelling of the wrist can produce CTS.

Treatment is splinting the wrist to immobilize it, and sometimes surgical resection of the carpal ligament is helpful.

dislocation	Displacement of a bone from its joint.

Dislocations must be **reduced** (restored to normal position) and the joint then immobilized for healing of torn ligaments and tendons.

A **subluxation** is a partial or incomplete dislocation.

ganglion	A cystic mass arising from a tendon in the wrist (Fig. 15–22).

herniation of an intervertebral disk (disc)	Abnormal protrusion of a cartilaginous intervertebral pad into the neural canal or spinal nerves.

This condition is commonly referred to as **slipped disk (disc).** Pain is experienced as the protruded disk (disc) (Fig. 15–23) presses on spinal nerves or cord. Low-back pain, cervical pain, and **sciatica** (pain radiating down the leg) are symptoms, depending on the location of the disk. Bed rest, physical therapy, and drugs for pain help in initial treatment. In patients with chronic or recurrent disk herniation, **laminectomy** (surgical removal of a portion of the vertebral arch to allow more room for the protruded disk) may be advised. Spinal fusion of the two vertebrae with removal of the damaged, herniated disk may be necessary as well. **Aspiration percutaneous diskectomy** is a new technique of removing the disk by inserting a tube through the skin and aspirating the disk through the tube. Chemonucleolysis is injection of a disk-dissolving enzyme (such as chymopapain) into the center of a herniated disk.

Lyme disease	A recurrent disorder marked by severe arthritis, myalgia, malaise, neurologic and cardiac symptoms.

Also known as **Lyme arthritis,** the etiology of the condition is a spirochete (bacterium) that is carried by a tick. It was first reported in Old Lyme, Connecticut, and is now found occurring throughout the eastern coast of the United States. It is treated with antibiotics.

sprain	Trauma to a joint with pain, swelling, and injury to ligaments.

Sprains may also involve damage to blood vessels, muscles, tendons, and nerves. A **strain** is a less serious injury with overstretching of muscle. Application of ice and elevation of the joint are immediate measures to relieve pain and prevent swelling due to sprains.

systemic lupus erythematosus (SLE)	A chronic inflammatory disease involving joints, skin, kidneys, nervous system, heart, and lungs.

This condition affects connective tissue (specifically a protein component called **collagen**) such as in tendons, ligaments, bones, and cartilage all over the body. Typically, there is a red scaly rash on the face over the nose and cheeks, so that the patient resembles a wolf (lupus means wolf). Patients, usually women, experience joint pain (polyarthralgia), pyrexia, and malaise. SLE is believed to be an autoimmune disease that can be diagnosed by the presence of abnormal antibodies in the bloodstream and characteristic white blood cells called LE cells. Treatment is with corticosteroids, which are hormones made by the adrenal gland and used to treat inflammatory conditions.

IV. Muscles

A. Types of Muscles

There are three types of muscles in the body. Label Figure 15–24 as you read the following descriptions of the various types of muscles:

Striated muscles (1), also called **voluntary** or **skeletal muscles,** are the muscle fibers that move all bones as well as the face and eyes. Through the central and peripheral nervous system, we have conscious control over these muscles. Striated muscle fibers (cells) have a pattern of dark and light bands, or fibrils, in their cytoplasm. Fibrous tissue that envelops and separates muscles is called **fascia,** which contains the muscle's blood, lymph, and nerve supply.

Smooth muscles (2), also called **involuntary** or **visceral muscles,** are those muscle fibers that move internal organs such as the digestive tract, blood vessels, and secretory ducts leading from glands. These muscles are controlled by the autonomic nervous system. They are called smooth because they have no dark and light fibrils in their cytoplasm. Skeletal muscle fibers are arranged in bundles, while smooth muscle forms sheets of fibers as it wraps around tubes and vessels.

Cardiac muscle (3) is striated in appearance but like smooth muscle in its action. Its movement cannot be consciously controlled. The fibers of cardiac muscle are branching fibers and are found in the heart.

B. Actions of Skeletal Muscles

Skeletal (striated) muscles (over 400 in the human body) are the muscles that move bones. Figure 15–25 shows some skeletal muscles of the head, neck, and torso and muscles

(1) _____

(2) _____

(3) _____

Figure 15–24

Types of muscles. (From O'Toole M [ed]: Miller-Keane Encyclopedia and Dictionary of Medicine, Nursing, and Allied Health, 5th ed. Philadelphia, WB Saunders, 1992, p 945.)

Figure 15–25

(A) Selected muscles of the head, neck, and torso and their functions. (B) Selected muscles of the buttock and thigh and their functions.

of the leg. When a muscle contracts, one of the bones to which it is joined remains virtually stationary as a result of other muscles that hold it in place. The point of attachment of the muscle to the stationary bone is called the **origin (beginning)** of that muscle. However, when the muscle contracts, another bone to which it is attached does move. The point of junction of the muscle to the bone that moves is called the **insertion** of the muscle.

Figure 15–26 shows the biceps and triceps muscles in the upper arm. One origin of the biceps is at the scapula, and its insertion is at the radius. Tendons are the connective tissue bands that connect muscles to the bones that they move.

Figure 15–26

Origin and insertion of the biceps in the upper arm. (From O'Toole M [ed]: Miller-Keane Encyclopedia and Dictionary of Medicine, Nursing, and Allied Health, 5th ed. Philadelphia, WB Saunders, 1992, p 945.)

Muscles can perform a variety of actions. Some of the terms used to describe those actions are listed here with a short description of the specific type of movement performed (Fig. 15–27):

Action	Meaning
flexion	Decreasing the angle between two bones; bending a limb.
extension	Increasing the angle between two bones; straightening out a limb.
abduction	Movement away from the midline of the body.
adduction	Movement toward the midline of the body.
rotation	Circular movement around an axis.
dorsiflexion	Decreasing the angle of the ankle joint so that the foot bends backward (upward).
plantar flexion	The motion that extends the foot downward toward the ground as when pointing the toes. Plant/o means sole of the foot.
supination	As applied to the hand, the act of turning the palm forward.
pronation	As applied to the hand, the act of turning the palm backward.

Your medical dictionary will have a complete list of the muscles of the body, with a description of their origin, insertion, and various actions.

C. Vocabulary

This list will help you review many of the new terms introduced in the text. Short definitions will reinforce your understanding of the terms. See Section IX of this chapter for help in pronouncing the more difficult terms.

abduction	Movement away from the midline of the body.
adduction	Movement toward the midline of the body.
dorsiflexion	Backward (upward) bending of the foot.
extension	Straightening of a flexed limb.

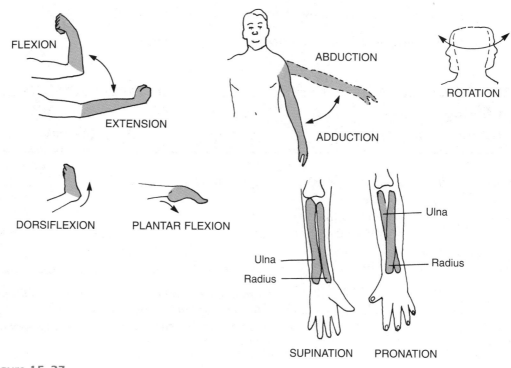

Figure 15–27

Types of muscular actions.

fascia	Fibrous membrane separating and enveloping muscles.
flexion	Bending.
insertion of a muscle	Connection of the muscle to the bone that moves.
origin of a muscle	Connection of the muscle to a stationary bone.
plantar flexion	Bending the sole of the foot downward toward the ground.
pronation	Turning the palm backward.
rotation	Circular movement around a central point.
skeletal muscle	Muscle connected to bones; voluntary or striated muscle.
smooth muscle	Muscle connected to internal organs; involuntary or visceral muscle.
striated muscle	Skeletal muscle.
supination	Turning the palm forward.
visceral muscle	Smooth muscle.

D. Combining Forms, Suffixes, and Prefixes

Write the meaning of the medical term in the space provided.

Combining Forms

Combining Form	Meaning	Terminology	Meaning
fasci/o	fascia (forms sheaths enveloping muscles)	fasciectomy _____	
fibr/o	fibrous connective tissue	fibromyalgia _____	

*Chronic pain and stiffness in muscles and fibrous tissue especially of the back, shoulders, neck, hips, and knees. Fatigue is a common complaint. The condition has previously been called **fibrositis** or **rheumatism**.*

Combining Form	Meaning	Terminology	Meaning
leiomy/o	smooth (visceral) muscle that lines the walls of internal organs	leiomyoma _____	
		leiomyosarcoma _____	
my/o	muscle	myalgia _____	
		electromyography _____	
		myopathy _____	
myocardi/o	heart muscle	myocardial _____	
myos/o	muscle	myositis _____	
plant/o	sole of the foot	plantar flexion _____	
rhabdomy/o	skeletal (striated) muscle connected to bones	rhabdomyoma _____	
		rhabdomyosarcoma _____	

| Suffixes | | | |
Suffix	Meaning	Terminology	Meaning
-asthenia	lack of strength	my<u>asthenia</u> gravis _____	
		Muscles lose strength because of a failure in transmission of the nervous impulse from the nerve to the muscle cell.	
-trophy	development, nourishment	a<u>trophy</u> _____	
		Decrease in size of an organ or tissue.	
		hyper<u>trophy</u> _____	
		Increase in size of an organ or tissue.	
		amyo<u>trophic</u> _____	
		*In **amyotrophic lateral sclerosis** (Lou Gehrig's disease), muscles are affected (paralysis occurs) by degeneration of nerves in the spinal cord and lower region of the brain.*	

| Prefixes | | | |
Prefix	Meaning	Terminology	Meaning
ab-	away from	<u>ab</u>duction _____	
		duct/o means to lead.	
ad-	toward	<u>ad</u>duction _____	
dorsi-	back	<u>dorsi</u>flexion _____	
poly-	many, much	<u>poly</u>myalgia _____	

E. Pathological Conditions

muscular dystrophy A group of inherited diseases characterized by progressive weakness and degeneration of muscle fibers without involvement of the nervous system.

Duchenne's dystrophy is the most common form. Muscles enlarge **(pseudohypertrophy)** as fat replaces functional muscle cells that have degenerated and atrophied. Onset of muscle weakness occurs soon after birth, and diagnosis can be made by muscle biopsy and electromyography.

polymyositis Chronic inflammatory myopathy.

This condition is marked by symmetrical muscle weakness and pain, often accompanied by a rash around the eyes, face, and limbs. Evidence that polymyositis is an autoimmune disorder is growing stronger, and some patients recover completely with immunosuppressive therapy.

V. Laboratory Tests, Clinical Procedures, and Abbreviations

Laboratory Tests

antinuclear antibody test (ANA)	A sample of plasma is tested for the presence of antibodies that are found in patients with systemic lupus erythematosus.
erythrocyte sedimentation rate (ESR)	This test measures the rate at which erythrocytes fall to the bottom of a test tube. Elevated sedimentation rates are associated with inflammatory disorders such as rheumatoid arthritis.
rheumatoid factor test	A sample of blood is tested for the presence of the rheumatoid factor (antibody found in the serum of patients with rheumatoid arthritis).
serum calcium (Ca)	Measurement of the amount of calcium in blood (serum).
serum creatine phosphokinase (CPK)	Creatine phosphokinase is an enzyme normally present in skeletal and cardiac muscle. Elevated serum CPK levels are found in muscular dystrophy, myocardial infarction, and skeletal muscle disorders.
serum phosphorus (P)	Measurement of the amount of phosphorus in a sample of serum.

Figure 15–28

Radiographs of hip joint degeneration and hip prosthesis (arthroplasty). *A,* This radiograph shows degeneration of the hip joint. *B,* this radiograph shows the same hip after a Charnley total hip arthroplasty. (*A* and *B,* From Petty W: Total Joint Replacement. Philadelphia, WB Saunders, 1991.)

Figure 15–29

Arthroscopy. An arthroscope is used in the diagnosis of pathological changes. (From Kelley WN, Harris ED Jr, Ruddy S, Sledge CB: Textbook of Rheumatology, 4th ed. Philadelphia, WB Saunders, 1993, p 640.)

uric acid test

This test measures the amount of uric acid in a sample of blood. High values are associated with gouty arthritis.

Clinical Procedures

arthrocentesis

Surgical puncture of the joint space with a needle. Synovial fluid is removed for analysis.

arthrography

Process of taking x-ray pictures of a joint after injection of opaque contrast material.

arthroplasty

Surgical repair of a joint. Total hip arthroplasty is replacement of the femoral head and acetabulum with prostheses that are cemented into the bone (see Fig. 15–28).

arthroscopy

Visual examination of the inside of a joint with an endoscope. Surgical instruments can be passed through the arthroscope to remove tissue and repair the joint. Arthroscopy is primarily used to visualize the knee, ankle, and shoulder (Fig. 15–29).

bone scan

A radioactive phosphate substance is injected intravenously, and uptake of the substance in bone is measured by a special scanning device. Areas that take up excessive amounts of radioactive substance may contain tumors, infection, inflammation, or other destructive changes.

electromyography

The process of recording the strength of muscle contraction as a result of electrical stimulation.

muscle biopsy

Removal of muscle tissue for microscopic examination.

photon absorptiometry

Rays (resembling x-rays) are passed through bones, and a machine measures how well the rays can penetrate the bone. This is a test of bone density, and it is used to detect osteoporosis.

ABBREVIATIONS

ANA	Antinuclear antibody	LE cell	Lupus erythematosus cell
C1–C7	Cervical vertebrae	Ortho.	Orthopedics, orthopaedics
Ca	Calcium	P	Phosphorus
CPK	Creatine phosphokinase	RA	Rheumatoid arthritis
CTS	Carpal tunnel syndrome	RF	Rheumatoid factor
DTR	Deep tendon reflexes	ROM	Range of motion
EMG	Electromyography	SLE	Systemic lupus erythematosus
ESR	Erythrocyte sedimentation rate	T1–T12	Thoracic vertebrae
IM	Intramuscular	TMJ	Temporomandibular joint
L1–L5	Lumbar vertebrae		

VI. Practical Applications

This section contains an actual medical report using terms that you have studied in this and previous chapters. Explanations of more difficult terms are added in brackets.

Skeletal Memorial Hospital—Department of Radiology

PA [posteroanterior] and lateral chest: The heart is enlarged in its transverse diameter. The lungs are fully expanded and free of active disease.

The thoracic spine shows a scoliosis of the upper thoracic spine convex to the left. There is 50 per cent wedge compression fracture of T6 and slight wedge compression fracture of T5. There is also anterior wedge compression fracture of T12.

Lumbar spine shows 90 per cent compression fractures of L1 and L3 with 30 per cent compression fractures L2 and L5. All bones are markedly osteoporotic. There is calcification within the aortic arch. There are gallstones in the right upper quadrant. The findings in the spine are most compatible with osteoporotic compression fractures. During the procedure, the patient had a sickable* episode and fell, striking her head. A skull series, done at no cost to the patient, shows no evidence of bony fracture. The pineal gland is calcified and has a midline location. The sella turcica is normal.

---

* This word was incorrectly transcribed. The correct term is syncopal.

Operating Schedule—Skeletal Memorial Hospital

Match the operation in column I with an accompanying diagnosis or reason for surgery in column II.

Answers can be found at the end of Answers to Exercises section, page 548.

COLUMN I—*Operations*	COLUMN II — *Diagnoses*
1. Excision, osteochondroma, R calcaneus _____	A. fracture of the ankle bone
2. TMJ arthroscopy with probable arthrotomy _____	B. patellar ligament injury
3. L4–5 laminectomy and diskectomy _____	C. neoplastic lesion in brain
4. Arthroscopy, left knee _____	D. exostosis on heel bone
5. Open reduction, malleolar fracture _____	E. pelvic fracture
6. R occipital craniotomy with tumor resection _____	F. pain and malocclusion of jaw bones
7. Excision, distal end right clavicle, with prob. acromioplasty _____	G. lower back pain radiating down one leg
8. Acetabuloplasty with open reduction hip _____	H. pain in shoulder joint with bone tumor evident on x-ray

VII. Exercises

Remember to check your answers carefully with those given in Section VIII, Answers to Exercises.

A. *Complete the following sentences.*

1. Bones are composed of bony connective tissue called _____ tissue.

2. Bone cells are called _____ .

3. The bones of a fetus are mainly composed of _____ tissue.

4. During bone development, immature bone cells called _____ produce bony tissue.

5. Large bone cells called _____ digest bone tissue to shape the bone and smooth it out.

6. Two mineral substances necessary for proper development of bones are _____

   and _____ .

7. A round, small bone resembling a sesame seed in shape and covering the knee joint is called a (an)

    _____ bone.

8. The shaft of a long bone is called the _____ .

9. The ends of a long bone are called the _____ .

10. The cartilaginous area at the end of long bones where growth takes place is called the

    _____ .

11. Red bone marrow is found in spongy or _____ bone.

12. Yellow bone marrow is composed of _____ tissue.

13. The strong membrane surrounding the surface of a bone is the _____ .

14. Hard, dense bone tissue lying under the periosteum is _____ .

15. A series of canals containing blood vessels lie within the outer dense tissue of bone and are called

    the _____ canals.

16. A thin layer of cartilage surrounding the ends of bones at the joint is called

    _____ .

17. The _____ is a central, hollowed-out area in the shaft of long bones.

18. A physician who treats bones and bone diseases is called a (an) _____ .

19. A person who uses his or her hands to manipulate the spinal column (in the belief that diseases are caused

    by pressure on spinal nerves) is a (an) _____ .

20. A doctor who treats patients based on the belief that the body can be healed when bones are in proper

    position and adequate nutrition is provided is a (an) _____ .

B. Identify each of the following as a bone process or depression and give a short description of each.

1. sulcus _____

2. sinus _____

3. tubercle _____

4. condyle _____

5. fossa _____

6. tuberosity _____

7. trochanter _____

8. foramen _____

9. fissure _____

10. bone head _____

C. *Match the following cranial and facial bones with their meanings below.*

mandible	nasal bone	maxilla	vomer
ethmoid bone	temporal bone	parietal bone	lacrimal bone
zygomatic bone	occipital bone	sphenoid bone	frontal bone

1. forms the roof and upper side parts of the skull _____

2. delicate bone, composed of spongy, cancellous tissue; supports the nasal cavity and orbits of the eye

_____

3. forms the back and base of the skull _____

4. forms the forehead _____

5. bat-shaped bone that extends behind the eyes to form the base of the skull

_____

6. bone near the ear and connecting to the lower jaw _____

7. cheek bone _____

8. bone that supports the bridge of the nose _____

9. thin, flat bone forming the lower portion of the nasal septum _____

10. lower jaw bone _____

11. upper jaw bone _____

12. two paired bones located one at the corner of each eye _____

D. *Name the five divisions of the spinal column.*

1. _____   4. _____

2. _____   5. _____

3. _____

E. Identify the following parts associated with a vertebra.

1. space through which the spinal cord passes _____

2. piece of cartilage between each vertebra _____

3. posterior part of a vertebra _____

4. anterior part of a vertebra _____

F. Give the medical names for the following bones.

1. shoulder bone _____

2. upper arm bone _____

3. breastbone _____

4. thigh bone _____

5. finger bones _____

6. hand bones _____

7. medial lower arm bone

_____

8. lateral lower arm bone

_____

9. collar bone _____

10. wrist bones _____

11. backbone _____

12. kneecap _____

13. shin bone (larger of two lower leg bones)

_____

14. smaller of two lower leg bones

_____

15. three parts of the hip bone are:

_____ , _____ ,

and _____

16. foot bones _____

G. Give the meanings for the following terms associated with bones.

1. foramen magnum _____

2. calcaneus _____

3. acromion _____

4. xiphoid process _____

5. lamina _____

6. malleolus _____

7. acetabulum _____

8. pubic symphysis _____

9. olecranon _____

10. fontanelle _____

11. mastoid process _____

12. styloid process _____

H. Give the meanings for the following terms.

1. osteogenesis _____

2. hypercalcemia _____

3. spondylosis _____

4. epiphyseal _____

5. decalcification _____

6. ossification _____

7. osteitis _____

8. costoclavicular _____

I. Build medical terms.

1. pertaining to the shoulder bone _____

2. instrument to cut the skull _____

3. pertaining to the upper arm bone _____

4. fixation of the kneecap _____

5. softening of cartilage _____

6. pertaining to a toe bone _____

7. removal of hand bones _____

8. pertaining to the shin bone _____

9. pertaining to the heel bone _____

10. poor bone development _____

11. removal of the lamina of the vertebral arch _____

12. pertaining to the sacrum and ilium _____

J. Give medical terms for the following.

1. formation of bone marrow _____

2. clubfoot _____

3. humpback _____

4. high levels of calcium in the blood _____

5. benign tumors arising from the bone surface _____

6. brittle bone disease _____

7. lateral curvature of the spine _____

8. abnormal anterior curvature of the spine _____

9. forward slipping (subluxation) of a vertebra over a lower vertebra _____

10. pain in the lumbar spine; lumbago _____

K. Match the term in column I with its description in column II. Write the letter of the description in the space provided.

Column I

1. greenstick fracture _____

2. simple fracture _____

3. comminuted fracture _____

4. compound fracture _____

5. Colles' fracture _____

6. cast _____

7. open reduction _____

8. closed reduction _____

9. impacted fracture _____

10. compression fracture _____

Column II

A. fracture of the lower end of the radius at the wrist
B. break in bone with wound in the skin
C. one side of the bone is fractured; the other side is bent
D. bone is put in proper place without incision of skin
E. mold of the bone applied to fractures to immobilize the injured bone
F. bone is broken by pressure from another bone; often in vertebrae
G. bone is splintered or crushed
H. bone is put in proper place after incision through the skin
I. bone is broken and one end is wedged into the interior of the adjoining bone
J. break in the bone without an open skin wound

L. Give the meanings for the following terms.

1. osteoporosis _____

2. osteomyelitis _____

3. osteogenic sarcoma _____

4. crepitus _____

5. osteomalacia _____

6. abscess _____

7. osteopenia _____

8. Ewing's sarcoma _____

M. Complete the following sentences.

1. A joint in which apposed bones are closely united as in the skull bones is called a (an)

_____ .

2. Connective tissue that binds muscles to bones is a (an) _____ .

3. Another term for a joint is a (an) _____ .

4. Connective tissue that binds bones to other bones is a (an) _____ .

5. Fluid found within a joint is called _____ .

6. The membrane that lines the joint cavity is the _____ .

7. A sac of fluid near a joint is a (an) _____ .

8. Smooth cartilage that surrounds the surface of bones at joints is _____ .

9. Surgical repair of a joint is called _____ .

10. Inflammation surrounding a joint is known as _____ .

N. Complete the following terms from their definition.

1. inflammation of a tendon: _____ itis

2. tumor (benign) of cartilage: _____ oma

3. tumor (malignant) of cartilage: _____ oma

4. incision of a joint: arthr _____

5. softening of cartilage: chondro _____

6. abnormal condition of blood in the joint: _____ osis

7. inflammation of a sac of fluid near the joint: _____ itis

8. a doctor who specializes in treatment of joint disorders: _____ logist

9. abnormal condition of a crooked, stiffened, immobile joint: _____ osis

10. suture of a tendon: ten _____

O. Select from the following terms to name the abnormal conditions below.

systemic lupus erythematosus	achondroplasia	ankylosing spondylitis
gouty arthritis	rheumatoid arthritis	bunion
tenosynovitis	osteoarthritis	carpal tunnel syndrome
dislocation	ganglion	Lyme disease

1. an inherited condition in which the bones of the arms and the legs fail to grow normally because of a

   defect in cartilage and bone formation; type of dwarfism _____

2. degenerative joint disease; chronic inflammation of bones and joints

   _____

3. inflammation of joints caused by excessive uric acid in the body (hyperuricemia)

   _____

4. chronic joint disease; inflamed and painful joints owing to autoimmune reaction against normal joint

   tissue, and synovial membranes become swollen and thickened _____

5. tick-borne bacterium causes this condition marked by arthritis, myalgia, malaise, and neurological and

   cardiac symptoms _____

6. abnormal swelling of a metatarsophalangeal joint _____

7. cystic mass arising from a tendon in the wrist _____

8. chronic, progressive arthritis with stiffening of joints, especially of the spine (vertebrae)

   _____

9. chronic inflammatory disease affecting not only the joints but also the skin (red rash on the face),

   kidneys, heart, and lungs _____

10. inflammation of a tendon sheath _____

11. compression of the median nerve in the wrist as it passes through an area between a ligament and

    tendons, bones, and connective tissue _____

12. displacement of a bone from its joint _____

P. Give the meanings for the following terms.

1. subluxation _____

2. arthrodesis _____

3. pyrexia _____

4. podagra _____

5. sciatica _____

6. herniation of an intervertebral disk (disc) _____

7. laminectomy _____

8. sprain _____

9. strain _____

10. hyperuricemia _____

Q. Select the term that best fits the definition given.

1. fibrous membrane separating and enveloping muscles: (fascia, flexion)

2. movement away from the midline of the body: (abduction, adduction)

3. connection of the muscle to a stationary bone: (insertion, origin) of the muscle

4. connection of the muscle to the bone that moves: (insertion, origin) of the muscle

5. muscle that is connected to internal organs; involuntary muscle: (skeletal, visceral) muscle

6. muscle that is connected to bones; voluntary muscle: (skeletal, visceral) muscle

7. pain of many muscles: (myositis, polymyalgia)

8. pertaining to heart muscle: (myocardial, myasthenia)

9. process of recording electricity within muscles: (muscle biopsy, electromyography)

10. increase in development (size) of an organ or tissue: (hypertrophy, atrophy)

R. Match the term for muscle action with its meaning. Write the letter of the meaning in the space provided.

Column I

1. extension _____

2. rotation _____

3. flexion _____

4. adduction _____

5. supination _____

6. abduction _____

7. pronation _____

8. dorsiflexion _____

9. plantar flexion _____

Column II

A. movement away from the midline
B. turning the palm backward
C. turning the palm forward
D. straightening out a limb
E. bending the sole of the foot downward
F. circular movement around an axis
G. bending a limb
H. movement toward the midline
I. backward (upward) bending of the foot

S. Give the meanings for the following abnormal conditions affecting muscles.

1. leiomyosarcoma _____

2. rhabdomyoma _____

3. polymyositis _____

4. fibromyalgia _____

5. muscular dystrophy _____

6. myasthenia gravis _____

7. amyotrophic lateral sclerosis _____

T. Match the term in column I with its meaning in column II. Write the letter of the answer in the space provided.

Column I   *Column II*

  1. antinuclear antibody test   _____   A. radioactive substance is injected and traced in tissue
                                            B. chemical found in myoneural space

  2. serum creatine phosphokinase   _____   C. test for presence of an antibody found in the serum of patients with rheumatoid arthritis

  3. uric acid test   _____   D. substance necessary for proper bone development
                                            E. visual examination of a joint

  4. rheumatoid factor test   _____   F. test tells if patient has gouty arthritis
                                            G. test tells if patient has systemic lupus erythematosus

  5. bone scan   _____   H. removal of tissue for microscopic examination
                                            I. process of taking x-ray pictures of a joint

  6. muscle biopsy   _____   J. elevated levels of this enzyme are found in muscular disorders

  7. arthroscopy   _____

  8. acetylcholine   _____

  9. phosphorus   _____

10. arthrography   _____

U. Select the term that best completes the meaning of the sentence.

1. Selma, a 40-year-old secretary, had been complaining of wrist pain with tingling sensations in her fingers for months. Dr. Ayres diagnosed her condition as (osteomyelitis, rheumatoid arthritis, carpal tunnel syndrome).

2. Daisy tripped while playing tennis and landed on her hand. She had excruciating pain and a (Ewing's, Colles', pathological) fracture that required casting.

3. In her 50s, Estee started hunching over more and more. Her doctor realized that she was developing (gouty arthritis, osteoarthritis, osteoporosis) and prescribed calcium pills and exercise.

4. Paul had a skiing accident and tore ligaments in his knee. Dr. Miller recommended (electromyography, hypertrophy, arthroscopic surgery) to repair the ligaments.

5. For several months after her first pregnancy Else noticed a red rash on her face and cheeks. Her joints were giving her pain and she had a slight fever. Her ANA was elevated and her doctor suspected that she had (SLE, polymyositis, muscular dystrophy).

V. Give the meanings for the following abbreviations.

  1. Ca _____

  2. P _____

  3. SLE _____

4. EMG _____

5. IM _____

6. Ortho. _____

7. ESR _____

8. T1–T12 _____

9. C1–C5 _____

10. CPK _____

VIII. Answers to Exercises

A

1. osseous
2. osteocytes
3. cartilage
4. osteoblasts
5. osteoclasts
6. calcium and phosphorus
7. sesamoid
8. diaphysis
9. epiphyses
10. epiphyseal plate
11. cancellous or trabecular
12. fat
13. periosteum
14. compact bone
15. haversian
16. articular cartilage
17. medullary cavity
18. orthopedist
19. chiropractor
20. osteopath

B

1. depression—a groove or furrow
2. depression—a hollow cavity within the bone
3. process—small, rounded process for attachment of tendons or muscles
4. process—rounded, knuckle-like process at the joint
5. depression—shallow cavity in or on a bone
6. process—large, rounded process for attachment of muscles or tendons
7. process—large process on the femur for attachment of muscles
8. depression—opening in a bone for blood vessels and nerves
9. depression—narrow, deep, slit-like opening
10. process—rounded end of a bone separated from the rest of the bone by a neck

C

1. parietal bone
2. ethmoid bone
3. occipital bone
4. frontal bone
5. sphenoid bone
6. temporal bone
7. zygomatic bone
8. nasal bone
9. vomer
10. mandible
11. maxilla
12. lacrimal bones

D

1. cervical
2. thoracic
3. lumbar
4. sacral
5. coccygeal

E

1. neural canal
2. intervertebral disk (disc)
3. vertebral arch
4. vertebral body

F

1. scapula
2. humerus
3. sternum
4. femur
5. phalanges
6. metacarpals
7. ulna
8. radius
9. clavicle
10. carpals
11. vertebral column
12. patella
13. tibia
14. fibula
15. ilium, ischium, pubis
16. metatarsals

G

1. opening of the occipital bone through which the spinal cord passes
2. heel bone; largest of the tarsal (ankle) bones
3. extension of the scapula
4. lower portion of the sternum
5. portion of the vertebral arch
6. the bulge on either side of the ankle joint; the lower end of the fibula is the lateral malleolus, and the lower end of the tibia is the medial malleolus

G

7. depression in the hip bone into which the femur fits
8. area of fusion of the two pubis bones, at the midline

9. bony process at the proximal end of the ulna; elbow joint
10. soft spot between the bones of the skull in an infant

11. round process on the temporal bone behind the ear
12. pole-like process projecting downward from the temporal bone

H

1. formation of bone; osteogenesis imperfecta is known as brittle bone disease
2. excessive calcium in the blood
3. abnormal condition of the vertebrae; degenerative changes in the spine

4. pertaining to the epiphysis
5. removal of calcium from bones
6. formation of bone
7. inflammation of bone; osteitis deformans

or Paget's disease causes deformed bones, such as bowed legs
8. pertaining to the ribs and clavicle

I

1. scapular
2. craniotome
3. humeral
4. patellapexy

5. chondromalacia
6. phalangeal
7. metacarpectomy
8. tibial

9. calcaneal
10. osteodystrophy
11. laminectomy
12. sacroiliac

J

1. myelopoiesis
2. talipes
3. kyphosis
4. hypercalcemia

5. exostoses
6. osteogenesis imperfecta
7. scoliosis

8. lordosis
9. spondylolisthesis
10. lumbodynia

K

1. C
2. J
3. G
4. B

5. A
6. E
7. H

8. D
9. I
10. F

L

1. increased porosity in bone; decrease in bone density
2. inflammation of bone and bone marrow
3. cancerous tumor of bone; osteoblasts multiply at the ends of long bones

4. crackling sensation as broken bones move against each other
5. softening of bones; rickets in children due to loss of calcium in bones

6. collection of pus
7. deficiency of bone; occurs in osteoporosis
8. malignant tumor of bone, often involving the entire shaft of a long bone

M

1. suture joint; a synovial joint is a freely movable joint
2. tendon
3. articulation

4. ligament
5. synovial fluid
6. synovial membrane
7. bursa

8. articular cartilage
9. arthroplasty
10. periarthritis

N

1. tendinitis
2. chondroma
3. chondrosarcoma
4. arthrotomy

5. chondromalacia
6. hemarthrosis
7. bursitis

8. rheumatologist
9. ankylosis
10. tenorrhaphy

O

1. achondroplasia
2. osteoarthritis
3. gouty arthritis
4. rheumatoid arthritis

5. Lyme disease
6. bunion
7. ganglion
8. ankylosing spondylitis

9. systemic lupus erythematosus
10. tenosynovitis
11. carpal tunnel syndrome
12. dislocation

P

1. partial or incomplete displacement of a bone from the joint
2. surgical fixation of a joint (binding it together by fusing the joint surfaces)
3. fever; increase in body temperature
4. pain in the big toe from gouty arthritis
5. pain radiating from the back to the leg

(along the sciatic nerve); most commonly caused by a protruding intervertebral disk
6. protrusion (prolapse) of a disk (piece of cartilage between the vertebrae) into the neural canal or the spinal nerves
7. removal of a portion of the vertebral arch

(laminae) to relieve pressure from a protruding intervertebral disk
8. trauma to a joint with pain, swelling, and injury to ligaments
9. overstretching of a muscle
10. high levels of uric acid in the bloodstream; a symptom of gouty arthritis

Q

1. fascia
2. abduction
3. origin of the muscle
4. insertion of the muscle

5. visceral muscle
6. skeletal muscle
7. polymyalgia

8. myocardial
9. electromyography
10. hypertrophy

R

1. D	4. H	7. B
2. F	5. C	8. I
3. G	6. A	9. E

S

1. malignant tumor of smooth (involuntary, visceral) muscle
2. benign tumor of striated (voluntary, skeletal) muscle
3. inflammation of many muscles; polymyositis rheumatica is a chronic inflammatory condition causing muscle weakness and pain
4. pain of muscle and fibrous tissue (especially of the back); also called fibrositis or rheumatism
5. group of inherited muscular diseases marked by progressive weakness and degeneration of muscles without nerve involvement
6. loss of strength of muscles (often with paralysis) owing to a defect at the space between the nerve and the muscle cell
7. muscles degenerate (paralysis occurs) owing to degeneration of nerves in the spinal cord and lower region of the brain; Lou Gehrig's disease

T

1. G	5. A	8. B
2. J	6. H	9. D
3. F	7. E	10. I
4. C		

U

1. carpal tunnel syndrome
2. Colles'
3. osteoporosis
4. arthroscopic surgery
5. SLE

V

1. calcium
2. phosphorus
3. systemic lupus erythematosus
4. electromyography
5. intramuscular
6. orthopedics (orthopaedics)
7. erythrocyte sedimentation rate
8. first through twelve thoracic vertebrae
9. first through five cervical vertebrae
10. creatine phosphokinase

Answers to Practical Applications

1. D	4. B	7. H
2. F	5. A	8. E
3. G	6. C	

IX. Pronunciation of Terms

To test your understanding of the terminology in this chapter, write the meaning of each term in the space provided. In addition, you may wish to cover the terms and write them by looking at your definitions. Make sure your spelling is correct. The page number after each term indicates where it is defined or used in the text so you can easily check your responses. (If you are not sure what the pronunciation symbols mean, refer to page 21.)

Terms Related to Bones

Term	Pronunciation	Meaning
acetabulum (509)	ăs-ĕ-TĂB-ū-lŭm	_____
acromion (509)	ă-KRŌ-mē-ŏn	_____
articular cartilage (509)	ăr-TĬK-ū-lăr KĂR-tĭ-lăj	_____
calcaneal (513)	kăl-KĀ-nē-ăl	_____
calcaneus (513)	kăl-KĀ-nē-ŭs	_____

calcium (509)	KĂL-sē-ŭm	
cancellous bone (509)	KĂN-sĕ-lŭs bōn	
carpals (513)	KĂR-pălz	
cartilage (509)	KĂR-tĭ-lĭj	
cervical vertebrae (504)	SĔR-vĭ-kăl VĔR-tĕ-brā	
chondrocostal (514)	kŏn-drō-KŎS-tăl	
clavicle (513)	KLĂV-ĭ-k'l	
coccyx (505)	KŎK-sĭks	
Colles' fracture (516)	KŎL-ēz FRĂK-shŭr	
comminuted fracture (516)	KŎM-ĭ-nūt-ĕd FRĂK-shŭr	
compact bone (498)	KŎM-păkt bōn	
condyle (498)	KŎN-dīl	
cranial bones (509)	KRĀ-nē-ăl bōnz	
craniotome (514)	KRĀ-nē-ō-tōm	
craniotomy (514)	krā-nē-ŎT-ō-mē	
crepitus (516)	KRĔP-ĭ-tŭs	
decalcification (511)	dē-kăl-sĭ-fĭ-KĀ-shŭn	
diaphysis (509)	dī-ĂF-ĭ-sĭs	
epiphyseal plate (510)	ĕp-ĭ-FĬZ-ē-ăl plāt	
epiphysis (510)	ĕ-PĬF-ĭ-sĭs	
ethmoid bone (500)	ĔTH-moyd bōn	
Ewing's sarcoma (515)	Ū-ĭngz săr-kō-mă	
exostosis (515)	ĕk-sŏs-TŌ-sĭs	
facial bones (510)	FĀ-shăl bōnz	
femoral (514)	FĔM-ŏr-ăl	
femur (514)	FĒ-mŭr	
fibula (514)	FĬB-ū-lă	
fibular (514)	FĬB-ū-lăr	

fissure (510)	FĬSH-ŭr	_____
fontanelle (510)	fŏn-tă-NĔL	_____
foramen (510)	fō-RĀ-měn	_____
fossa (510)	FŎS-ă	_____
frontal bone (500)	FRŎN-tăl bōn	_____
haversian canals (510)	hă-VĔR-shăn kă-NĂLZ	_____
humeral (514)	HŪ-měr-ăl	_____
humerus (514)	HŪ-měr-ŭs	_____
hypercalcemia (511)	hī-pěr-kăl-SĒ-mē-ă	_____
iliac (514)	ĬL-ē-ăk	_____
ilium (514)	ĬL-ē-ŭm	_____
impacted fracture (516)	ĭm-PĂK-těd FRĂK-shŭr	_____
ischial (514)	ĬSH-ē-ăl	_____
ischium (514)	ĬSH-ē-ŭm	_____
kyphosis (511)	kī-FŌ-sĭs	_____
lacrimal bones (502)	LĂ-krĭ-măl bōnz	_____
lamina (505)	LĂM-ĭ-nă	_____
laminectomy (511)	lăm-ĭ-NĔK-tō-mē	_____
lordosis (511)	lŏr-DŌ-sĭs	_____
lumbar vertebrae (504)	LŬM-băr VĔR-tě-brā	_____
lumbodynia (512)	lŭm-bō-DĬN-ē-ă	_____
lumbosacral (512)	lŭm-bō-SĀ-krăl	_____
malleolar (514)	mă-LĒ-ō-lăr	_____
malleolus (510)	măl-LĒ-ō-lŭs	_____
mandible (514)	MĂN-dĭ-b'l	_____
mandibular (514)	măn-DĬB-ū-lăr	_____
mastoid process (510)	MĂs-toyd PRŌ-sěs	_____
medullary cavity (510)	MĔD-ū-lăr-ē KĂ-vĭ-tē	_____

metacarpals (514)	mĕt-ă-KĂR-pălz	
metacarpectomy (514)	mĕt-ă-kăr-PĔK-tō-mē	
metatarsalgia (514)	mĕt-ă-tăr-SĂL-jă	
metatarsals (514)	mĕt-ă-TĂR-sălz	
myelopoiesis (512)	mī-ĕ-lō-poy-Ē-sĭs	
nasal bones (502)	NĀ-zăl bōnz	
occipital bone (500)	ŏk-SĬP-ĭ-tăl bōn	
olecranal (514)	ō-LĔK-ră-năl	
olecranon (510)	ō-LĔK-ră-nŏn	
orthopedic (512)	ŏr-thō-PĒ-dĭk	
osseous tissue (510)	ŎS-ē-ŭs TĬSH-ū	
ossification (510)	ŏs-ĭ-fĭ-KĀ-shŭn	
osteitis (512)	ŏs-tē-Ī-tĭs	
osteoblast (510)	ŎS-tē-ō-blăst	
osteochondroma (515)	ŏs-tē-ō-kŏn-DRŌ-mă	
osteoclast (510)	ŎS-tē-ō-klăst	
osteodystrophy (512)	ŏs-tē-ō-DĬS-trō-fē	
osteogenesis imperfecta (512)	ŏs-tē-ō-JĔN-ĕ-sĭs ĭm-pĕr-FĔK-tă	
osteogenic sarcoma (517)	ŏs-tē-ō-JĔN-ĭk săr-KŌ-mă	
osteomalacia (513)	ŏs-tē-ō-mă-LĀ-shă	
osteomyelitis (517)	ŏs-tē-ō-mī-ĕ-LĪ-tĭs	
osteoporosis (517)	ŏs-tē-ō-pŏr-Ō-sĭs	
osteotome (513)	ŎS-tē-ō-tōm	
parietal bones (500)	pă-RĪ-ĭ-tăl bōnz	
patella (514)	pă-TĔL-ă	
patellapexy (514)	pă-TĔL-ă-pĕk-sē	
pelvimetry (515)	pĕl-VĬM-ĕ-trē	
peroneal (515)	pĕr-ō-NĒ-ăl	

phalangeal (515)	fă-lăn-JĒ-ăl	
phalanges (515)	fă-LĂN-jēz	
phosphorous (510)	FŎS-fō-rŭs	
pubic symphysis (510)	PŪ-bĭk SĬM-fĭ-sĭs	
pubis (515)	PŪ-bĭs	
radial (515)	RĀ-dē-ăl	
radius (515)	RĀ-dē-ŭs	
reduction (516)	rĕ-DŬK-shŭn	
sacral vertebrae (505)	SĀ-krăl Vĕr-tĕ-brā	
scapula (515)	SKĂP-ū-lăr	
scapular (515)	SKĂP-ū-lă	
scoliosis (512)	skō-lē-Ō-sĭs	
sinus (510)	SĪ-nŭs	
sphenoid bone (500)	SFĔ-noyd bōn	
spondylitis (512)	spŏn-dĭ-LĪ-tĭs	
spondylolisthesis (513)	spŏn-dĭ-lō-LĬS-thē-sĭs	
spondylosis (512)	spŏn-dĭ-LŌ-sĭs	
sternum (515)	STĔR-nŭm	
styloid process (510)	STĪ-loyd PRŌ-sĕs	
subcostal (514)	sŭb-KŎS-tăl	
subpatellar (514)	sŭb-pă-TĔL-lăr	
supraclavicular (513)	sŭ-pră-klă-VĬK-ū-lăr	
talipes (517)	TĂL-ĭ-pĕz	
tarsals (515)	TĂR-sălz	
tarsectomy (515)	tăr-SĔK-tō-mē	
temporal bones (500)	TĔM-pōr-ăl bōnz	
thoracic vertebrae (504)	thō-RĂS-ĭk VĔR-tĕ-brā	
tibia (515)	TĬB-ē-ă	

tibial (515)	TĬB-ē-ăl
trabeculae (511)	tră-BĔK-ū-lē
trochanter (511)	trō-KĂN-tĕr
tubercle (511)	TŪ-bĕr-k'l
tuberosity (511)	tū-bĕ-RŎS-ĭ-tē
ulna (515)	ŬL-nă
ulnar (515)	ŬL-năr
vomer (502)	VŌ-mĕr
xiphoid process (511)	ZĬF-oyd PRŌ-sĕs
zygomatic bones (502)	zī-gō-MĂ-tĭk bōnz

Terms Related to Joints and Muscles

Term	Pronunciation	Meaning
abduction (528)	ăb-DŬK-shŭn	
achondroplasia (521)	ā-kŏn-drō-PLĀ-zē-ă	
adduction (528)	ă-DŬK-shŭn	
amyotrophic lateral sclerosis (531)	ā-mī-ō-TRŌ-fĭk LĂT-ĕr-ăl sklĕ-RŌ-sĭs	
ankylosing spondylitis (522)	ăng-kĭ-LŌ-sĭng spŏn-dĭ-LĪ-tĭs	
ankylosis (520)	ăng-kĭ-LŌ-sĭs	
arthrocentesis (533)	ăr-thrō-sĕn-TĒ-sĭs	
arthrodesis (522)	ăr-thrō-DĒ-sĭs	
arthrography (533)	ăr-THRŎG-ră-fē	
arthroplasty (533)	ĂR-thrō-plăs-tē	
arthroscopy (533)	ăr-THRŎS-kō-pē	
arthrotomy (521)	ăr-THRŌT-ō-mē	
articular cartilage (521)	ăr-TĬK-ū-lăr KĂR-tĭ-lĭj	
articulation (520)	ăr-tĭk-ū-LĀ-shŭn	
atrophy (531)	ĂT-rō-fē	

bunion (523)	BŬN-yŭn	_____
bursa (plural: bursae) (520)	BĔR-să (BĔR-sē)	_____
bursitis (521)	bŭr-SĪ-tis	_____
carpal tunnel syndrome (523)	KĂR-păl TŬN-nĕl SĬN-drōm	_____
chondroma (521)	kŏn-DRŌ-mă	_____
chondromalacia (521)	kŏn-drō-mă-LĀ-shă	_____
dislocation (525)	dĭs-lō-KĀ-shŭn	_____
dorsiflexion (528)	dŏr-sē-FLĔK-shŭn	_____
electromyography (533)	ē-lĕk-trō-mī-ŎG-ră-fē	_____
extension (528)	ĕk-STĔN-shŭn	_____
fascia (529)	FĂSH-ē-ă	_____
fasciectomy (530)	făsh-ē-ĔK-tō-mē	_____
fibromyalgia (530)	fē-brō-mī-ĂL-jă	_____
flexion (529)	FLĔK-shŭn	_____
ganglion (525)	GĂNG-lē-ŏn	_____
gouty arthritis (522)	GŎW-tē ăr-THRĪ-tĭs	_____
hemarthrosis (521)	hĕm-ăr-THRŌ-sĭs	_____
hydrarthrosis (521)	hī-drăr-THRŌ-sĭs	_____
hypertrophy (531)	hī-PĔR-trō-fē	_____
hyperuricemia (522)	hī-pĕr-ŭr-ĭ-SĒ-mē-ă	_____
leiomyoma (530)	lī-ō-mī-Ō-mă	_____
leiomyosarcoma (530)	lī-ō-mī-ō-săr-KŌ-mă	_____
ligament (520)	LĬG-ă-mĕnt	_____
ligamentous (521)	lĭg-ă-MĔN-tŭs	_____
Lyme disease (525)	līm dĭ-ZĒZ	_____
muscular dystrophy (531)	MŬS-kū-lăr DĬs-trō-fē	_____
myalgia (530)	mī-ĂL-jă	_____
myopathy (530)	mī-ŎP-ă-thē	_____

myositis (530)	mī-ō-SĪ-tĭs	_____
osteoarthritis (522)	ŏs-tē-ō-ăr-THRĪ-tĭs	_____
podagra (522)	pō-DĂG-ră	_____
polymyalgia (531)	pŏl-ē-mĭ-ĂL-jă	_____
polymyositis (531)	pŏl-ē-mī-ō-SĪ-tĭs	_____
pronation (529)	prō-NĀ-shŭn	_____
pyrexia (523)	pī-RĔK-sē-ă	_____
rhabdomyoma (530)	răb-dō-mī-Ō-mă	_____
rhabdomyosarcoma (530)	răb-dō-mī-ō-săr-KŌ-mă	_____
rheumatoid arthritis (522)	ROO-mă-toyd ăr-THRĪ-tĭs	_____
rheumatologist (521)	roo-mă-TŎL-ō-jĭst	_____
rotation (529)	rō-TĀ-shŭn	_____
sprain (525)	sprān	_____
strain (525)	strān	_____
striated muscle (529)	STRĪ-ā-tĕd MŬS-el	_____
subluxation (525)	sŭb-lŭk-SĀ-shŭn	_____
supination (529)	sū-pĭ-NĀ-shŭn	_____
suture joint (520)	SŪ-chŭr joint	_____
synovial fluid (520)	sĭ-NŌ-vē-ăl FLŌO-ĭd	_____
synovial joint (520)	sĭ-NŌ-vē-ăl joint	_____
synovial membrane (520)	sĭ-NŌ-vē-ăl MĔM-brān	_____
synovitis (521)	sĭ-nō-VĪ-tĭs	_____
systemic lupus erythematosus (525)	sĭs-TĔM-ĭk LŪ-pŭs ĕ-rĭ-thē-mă-TŌ-sŭs	_____
tendinitis (521)	tĕn-dĭ-NĪ-tĭs	_____
tendon (520)	TĔN-dŭn	_____
tenorrhaphy (521)	tĕn-ŎR-ă-fē	_____
tenosynovitis (521)	tĕn-ō-sĭ-nō-VĪ-tĭs	_____
visceral muscle (529)	VĬS-ĕr-ăl MŬS-ĕl	_____

X. Review Sheet

Write the meaning of each word part in the space provided. Check your answers with the information in the chapter or in the Glossary (Medical Terms—English) at the end of the book.

Combining Forms

Combining Form	Meaning	Combining Form	Meaning
acetabul/o	_____	crani/o	_____
ankyl/o	_____	fasci/o	_____
arthr/o	_____	femor/o	_____
articul/o	_____	fibr/o	_____
burs/o	_____	fibul/o	_____
calcane/o	_____	humer/o	_____
calc/o	_____	ili/o	_____
calci/o	_____	isch/o	_____
carp/o	_____	kyph/o	_____
cervic/o	_____	lamin/o	_____
chondr/o	_____	leiomy/o	_____
clavicul/o	_____	ligament/o	_____
coccyg/o	_____	lord/o	_____
cost/o	_____	lumb/o	_____

malleol/o	_____	pub/o	_____
mandibul/o	_____	radi/o	_____
maxill/o	_____	rhabdomy/o	_____
metacarp/o	_____	rheumat/o	_____
metatars/o	_____	sacr/o	_____
my/o	_____	sarc/o	_____
myel/o	_____	scapul/o	_____
myocardi/o	_____	scoli/o	_____
myos/o	_____	spondyl/o	_____
olecran/o	_____	stern/o	_____
orth/o	_____	synov/o	_____
oste/o	_____	tars/o	_____
patell/a	_____	ten/o	_____
patell/o	_____	tendin/o	_____
ped/o	_____	thorac/o	_____
pelv/i	_____	tibi/o	_____
perone/o	_____	uln/o	_____
phalang/o	_____	vertebr/o	_____
plant/o	_____		

Continued on following page

Suffixes

Suffix	Meaning	Suffix	Meaning
-algia	_____	-penia	_____
-asthenia	_____	-physis	_____
-blast	_____	-plasty	_____
-clast	_____	-porosis	_____
-desis	_____	-stenosis	_____
-emia	_____	-tome	_____
-listhesis	_____	-trophy	_____
-malacia	_____		

Prefixes

Prefix	Meaning	Prefix	Meaning
a-, an-	_____	peri-	_____
ad-	_____	poly-	_____
ab-	_____	sub-	_____
dorsi-	_____	supra-	_____
exo-	_____	sym-	_____
hyper-	_____		

Skin

This Chapter is divided into the following sections

In this Chapter you will

- Identify the layers of the skin and the accessory structures associated with the skin;
- Build medical words using the combining forms that are related to the specialty of dermatology;
- Describe lesions, symptoms, and pathological conditions that relate to the skin; and
- Identify laboratory tests, clinical procedures, and abbreviations that pertain to the skin.

I. Introduction

The skin and its accessory organs (hair, nails, and glands) are known as the **integumentary system** of the body. Integument means covering, and the skin (weighing 8–10 pounds over an area of 22 square feet in an average adult) is the outer covering for the body. It is, however, more than a simple body covering. The skin, as a complex system of specialized tissues, contains glands that secrete several types of fluids, nerves that carry impulses, and blood vessels that aid in the regulation of the body temperature. The following paragraphs review the many important functions of the skin.

First, as a protective membrane over the entire body, the skin guards the deeper tissues of the body against excessive loss of water, salts, and heat and against invasion of pathogens and their toxins. Secretions from the skin are slightly acid in nature, and this contributes to the skin's ability to prevent bacterial invasion.

Second, the skin contains two types of glands that produce important secretions. These glands under the skin are the **sebaceous** and **sweat glands.** The sebaceous glands produce an oily secretion called **sebum,** and the sweat glands produce a watery secretion called **sweat.** Sebum and sweat are carried to the outer edges of the skin by ducts and excreted from the skin through openings, or pores. Sebum helps to lubricate the surface of the skin, and sweat helps to cool the body as it evaporates from the skin surface.

Third, nerve fibers located under the skin act as receptors for sensations such as pain, temperature, pressure, and touch. Thus, the adjustment of an individual to her or his environment is dependent on the sensory messages relayed to the brain and spinal cord by the sensitive nerve endings in the skin.

Fourth, several different tissues in the skin aid in maintaining the body temperature (thermoregulation). Nerve fibers coordinate thermoregulation by carrying messages to the skin from heat centers in the brain that are sensitive to increases and decreases in body temperature. Impulses from these fibers cause blood vessels to dilate to bring blood to the surface and cause sweat glands to produce the watery secretion that carries heat away.

II. Structure of the Skin

Figure 16–1*A* shows the three layers of the skin. Label these layers from the outer surface inward:

1. **Epidermis**—a thin, cellular membrane layer.
2. **Corium** or **dermis**—dense, fibrous, connective tissue layer.
3. **Subcutaneous tissue**—thick, fat-containing tissue.

Epidermis

The epidermis is the outermost, totally cellular layer of the skin. It is composed of **squamous epithelium.** Epithelium is the covering of both the internal and the external surfaces of the body. Squamous epithelial cells are flat and scale-like. In the outer layer of the skin, these cells are arranged in several layers **(strata)** and are therefore called **stratified squamous epithelium.**

The epidermis lacks blood vessels, lymphatic vessels, and connective tissue (elastic fibers, cartilage, fat) and is therefore dependent on the deeper corium layer and its rich network of capillaries for nourishment. In fact, oxygen and nutrients seep out of the capillaries in the corium, pass through tissue fluid, and supply nourishment to the deeper layers of the epidermis.

Figure 16–1*B* illustrates the multilayered cells of the epidermis. The deepest layer is called the **basal layer** (4). The cells in the basal layer are constantly growing and multiplying and give rise to all the other cells in the epidermis. As the basal layer cells divide, they are pushed upward and away from the blood supply of the dermal layer by a steady stream of younger cells. In their movement toward the most superficial layer of the epidermis, called the **stratum corneum** (5), the cells flatten, shrink, lose their nuclei, and die, becoming filled with a protein called **keratin.** The cells are then called **horny cells,** reflecting their composition of keratin, which is a hard, protein material. Finally, within 3–4 weeks after beginning as a basal cell in the deepest part of the epidermis, the horny, keratinized cell is sloughed off from the surface of the skin. The epidermis is thus constantly renewing itself, cells dying at the same rate at which they are replaced.

The basal layer of the epidermis contains special cells called **melanocytes** (6). Melanocytes form and contain a black pigment called **melanin** that is transferred to other epidermal cells and gives color to the skin. The number of melanocytes in all races is the same but the amount of melanin accounts for the color differences among the races. Individuals with darker skin possess more melanin within the melanocytes, not a greater number of melanocytes. The presence of melanin in the epidermis is vital for protection against the harmful effects of ultraviolet radiation, which can manifest themselves as skin cancer. Individuals who, through a flaw in their chemical makeup, are incapable of forming melanin at all are called **albino** (meaning white). Skin and hair are white. Their eyes are red because in the absence of pigment, the tiny blood vessels are visible in the iris (normally pigmented portion) of the eye.

Melanin production increases with exposure to strong ultraviolet light, and this creates a suntan, which is a protective response. When the melanin cannot absorb all the ultraviolet rays, the skin becomes sunburned and inflamed (redness, swelling, and pain). Over a period of years, excessive exposure to sun can tend to cause wrinkles and cancer of the skin. Since

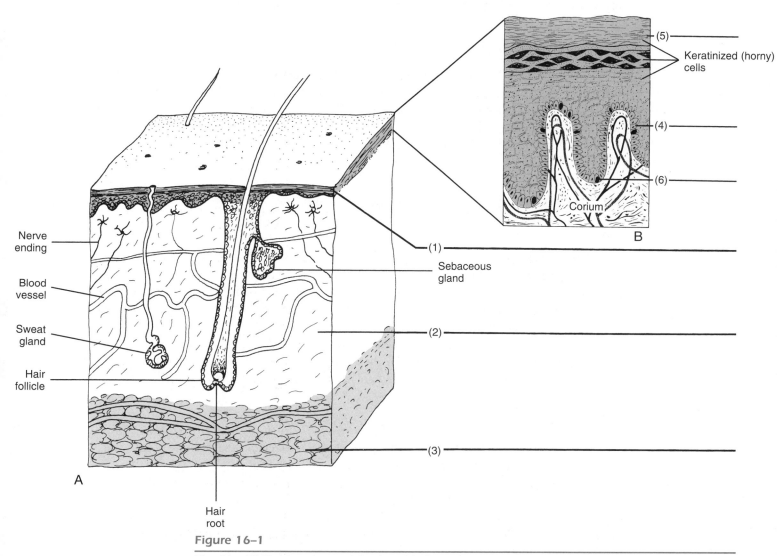

Figure 16–1

The skin. *(A)* The three layers of the skin. *(B)* The epidermis.

dark-skinned people have more melanin, they have fewer wrinkles and they are less likely to develop skin cancer.

Corium (Dermis)

The corium layer, directly below the epidermis, is also called the **dermis.** It is composed of blood and lymph vessels and nerve fibers, as well as the accessory organs of the skin, which are the hair follicles, sweat glands, and sebaceous glands. To support the elaborate system of nerves, vessels, and glands, the corium contains connective tissue cells and fibers that account for the extensibility and elasticity of the skin.

The corium is composed of interwoven elastic and **collagen** fibers. Collagen (**colla** means glue) is a fibrous protein material found in bone, cartilage, tendons, and ligaments, as well as in the skin. It is tough and resistant but also flexible. In the infant, collagen is loose and delicate, and it becomes harder as the body ages. During pregnancy, overstretching of a woman's skin may break the elastic collagen fibers and stretch the collagen resulting in linear markings called striae or stretch marks. Collagen fibers support and protect the blood and nerve networks that pass through the corium. Collagen diseases affect connective tissues of the body. Examples of these connective tissue collagen disorders are systemic lupus erythematosus and scleroderma (see Section VI, under Abnormal Conditions).

Subcutaneous Layer

The subcutaneous layer of the skin is another connective tissue layer; it specializes in the formation of fat. **Lipocytes** (fat cells) are predominant in the subcutaneous layer, and they manufacture and store large quantities of fat. Obviously, areas of the body and individuals vary as far as fat deposition is concerned. Functionally, this layer of the skin is important in protection of the deeper tissues of the body and as a heat insulator.

III. Accessory Organs of the Skin

Hair

A hair fiber is composed of a tightly fused meshwork of horny cells filled with the hard protein called **keratin.** Hair growth is similar to the growth of the epidermal layer of the skin. Deep-lying cells in the hair root (see Fig. 16–1) produce horny cells that move upward through the **hair follicles** (shafts or sacs that hold the hair fibers). Melanocytes are located at the root of the hair follicle, and they support the melanin pigment for the horny cells of the hair fiber. Hair turns gray when the melanocytes stop producing melanin.

Of the 5 million hairs on the body, about 100,000 are on the head. They grow about ½ inch (1.3 cm) a month, and cutting the hair has no effect on its rate of growth.

Nails

Nails are hard, keratin plates covering the dorsal surface of the last bone of each toe and finger. They are composed of horny cells that are cemented together tightly and can extend indefinitely unless cut or broken. A nail grows in thickness and length as a result of division of cells in the region of the nail root, which is at the base (proximal portion) of the nail plate.

Most nails grow about 1 mm a week, which means that fingernails may regrow in 3–5 months. Toenails grow more slowly than fingernails; it takes 12–18 months for toenails to be replaced completely.

Figure 16–2

Parts of the nail.

The **lunula** is a semilunar (half-moon), white region at the base of the nail plate, and it is generally found in the thumbnail of most people and in varying degrees in other fingers. Air mixed in with keratin and cells rich in nuclei give the lunula its whitish color. The **cuticle,** a narrow band of epidermis (layer of keratin), is at the base and sides of the nail plate. Figure 16–2 illustrates the parts of a nail.

Nail growth and appearance are frequently altered during systemic disease. For example, grooves in nails may occur with high fevers and serious illness, and spoon nails (flattening of the nail plate) occurs in iron deficiency anemia.

Glands

Sebaceous Glands

Sebaceous glands are located in the corium layer of the skin over the entire body, with the exception of the palms (hands) and soles (feet). They secrete an oily substance called **sebum.** Sebum, containing lipids, lubricates the skin and minimizes water loss. Sebaceous glands are closely associated with hair follicles, and their ducts open into the hair follicle through which the sebum is released. Figure 16–1 shows the relationship of the sebaceous gland to the hair follicle. The sebaceous glands are influenced by sex hormones, which cause them to hypertrophy at puberty and atrophy in old age. Overproduction of sebum during puberty contributes to blackhead (comedo) formation and acne in some individuals.

Sweat Glands

Sweat glands are tiny, coiled glands found on almost all body surfaces (about 2 million in the body). They are most numerous in the palm of the hand (3000 glands per sq in) and on the sole of the foot. Figure 16–1 illustrates how the coiled sweat gland originates deep in the corium and straightens out to extend up through the epidermis. The tiny opening on the surface is called a **pore.**

Sweat, or perspiration, is almost pure water, with dissolved materials such as salt making up less than 1 per cent of the total composition. It is colorless and odorless. The odor produced when sweat accumulates on the skin is due to the action of bacteria on the sweat.

Sweat cools the body as it evaporates into the air. Perspiration is controlled by the sympathetic nervous system, whose nerve fibers are activated by the heart regulatory center in the hypothalamic region of the brain, which stimulates sweating.

A special variety of sweat gland, active only from puberty onward and larger than the ordinary kind, is concentrated in a few areas of the body near the reproductive organs and in the armpits. These glands secrete an odorless sweat, but it contains certain substances that are easily broken down by bacteria on the skin. The breakdown products are responsible for the characteristic human body odor. The milk-producing mammary gland is another type of modified sweat gland; it secretes milk only after the birth of a child.

IV. Vocabulary

This list will help you review many of the new terms introduced in the text. Short definitions will reinforce your understanding of the terms. See Section XI of this chapter for help in pronouncing the more difficult terms.

albino	A person with skin deficient in pigment.
basal layer	The deepest region of the epidermis; it gives rise to all the epidermal cells.
collagen	Structural protein found in the skin and connective tissue.
corium	The middle layer of the skin; dermis.
cuticle	Band of epidermis at the base and side of the nail plate.
dermis	The corium.
epidermis	The outermost layer of the skin.
epithelium	The layer of skin cells forming the outer and inner surfaces of the body.
hair follicle	The sac or tube within which each hair grows.
horny cell	A keratin-filled cell in the epidermis.
integumentary system	The skin and its accessory structures such as hair and nails.
keratin	A hard, protein material found in the epidermis, hair, and nails. Keratin means horn and is commonly found in the horns of animals.
lipocyte	A fat cell.
lunula	The half-moon–shaped, white area at the base of a nail.
melanin	A black pigment formed by melanocytes in the epidermis.
sebaceous gland	An oil-secreting gland in the corium that is associated with hair follicles.
sebum	An oily substance secreted by sebaceous glands.
squamous epithelium	Flat, scale-like cells composing the epidermis.
stratified	Arranged in layers.
stratum (plural: **strata**)	A layer (of cells).
stratum corneum	The outermost layer of the epidermis, which consists of flattened, keratinized (horny) cells.
subcutaneous tissue	Innermost layer of the skin, containing fat tissue.

V. Combining Forms and Suffixes

Write the meaning of the medical term in the space provided.

Combining Forms

Combining Form	Meaning	Terminology	Meaning
adip/o	fat (see **lip/o** and **steat/o**)	adipose _____	
albin/o	white	albinism _____	

Table 16–1 lists combining forms for colors and examples of terms using those combining forms.

Combining Form	Meaning	Terminology	Meaning
caus/o	burn, burning	causalgia _____	

Intensely unpleasant burning sensation in skin and muscles when there is damage to nerves.

Combining Form	Meaning	Terminology	Meaning
cutane/o	skin (see **derm/o**)	subcutaneous _____	
derm/o **dermat/o**	skin	epidermis _____	
		dermatitis _____	
		dermatoplasty _____	
		dermatologist _____	
		epidermolysis _____	

Loosening of the epidermis with the development of large blisters; occurs after injury.

Combining Form	Meaning	Terminology	Meaning
diaphor/o	profuse sweating (see **hidr/o**)	diaphoresis _____	

Table 16–1 COLORS

Combining Form	Meaning	Terminology
albin/o	white	*albin*ism
anthrac/o	black (as coal)	*anthrac*osis
chlor/o	green	*chlor*ophyll
cirrh/o	tawny yellow	*cirrh*osis
cyan/o	blue	*cyan*osis
eosin/o	rosy	*eosin*ophil
erythr/o	red	*erythr*ocyte
jaund/o	yellow	*jaund*ice
leuk/o	white	*leuk*oderma
lute/o	yellow	corpus *lute*um
melan/o	black	*melan*ocyte
poli/o	gray	*poli*omyelitis
xanth/o	yellow	*xanth*oma

erythem/o	redness	erythema _____
erythemat/o		*Flushing; widespread redness of the skin.*
		erythematous _____
hidr/o	sweat	anhidrosis _____
		Do not confuse hidr/o with hydr/o (water)!
ichthy/o	scaly, dry (fish-like)	ichthyosis _____
		A hereditary condition in which the skin is dry, rough, and scaly because of a defect in keratinization. Ichthyosis can also be acquired, appearing with malignancies such as lymphomas and multiple myeloma.
kerat/o	hard, horny tissue	keratosis _____
		See page 572, Section VI, under Skin Neoplasms.
leuk/o	white	leukoplakia _____
		-plakia means plaques.
lip/o	fat	lipoma _____
melan/o	black	melanocyte _____
		melanoma _____
		This is a malignant skin tumor. See page 573, Section VI, under Skin Neoplasms.
myc/o	fungus (fungi include yeasts, molds, and mushrooms)	dermatomycosis _____
		An example is ringworm (athlete's foot).
onych/o	nail (see **ungu/o**)	onycholysis _____
		Separation of the nail plate from the nail bed in fungal infections or after trauma.
		onychomycosis _____
		The nails become white, opaque, thickened, and brittle.
		paronychia _____
		par- means near or bedside. Paronychia is inflammation and swelling of the soft tissue around the nail and is associated with torn cuticles or ingrown nails.

phyt/o	plant	dermatophytosis _____	

Examples are fungal infections of the hands and feet.

pil/o	hair (see **trich/o**), hair follicle	pilosebaceous _____

sebace/o means a gland that secretes sebum.

seb/o	sebum (oily secretion from sebaceous glands)	seborrhea _____

*Excessive secretion from sebaceous glands. **Seborrheic dermatitis** is commonly known as **dandruff.***

squam/o	scale-like	squamous epithelium _____

Cells are flat and scale-like.

steat/o	fat	steatoma _____

***Sebaceous cyst;** this is a cystic collection of sebum (fatty material) that forms in a sebaceous gland and can become infected.*

trich/o	hair	trichomycosis _____
ungu/o	nail	subungual _____
xanth/o	yellow	xanthoma _____

Nodules develop under the skin owing to excess lipid deposits. Usually associated with a high cholesterol level. Plaques that appear on the eyelids of elderly people are called xanthelasmas (-elasma means a flat plate).

xer/o	dry	xeroderma _____

-derma means skin. This is a mild form of ichthyosis.

Suffixes

Suffix	Meaning	Terminology	Meaning
-derma	skin	pyoderma _____	
		leukoderma _____	

VI. Lesions, Symptoms, Abnormal Conditions, and Skin Neoplasms

Cutaneous Lesions

A **lesion** is an area of damaged tissue, caused by disease or trauma. The following terms describe common skin lesions, which are illustrated in Figure 16–3.

cyst	A thick-walled, closed sac or pouch containing fluid or semisolid material.
	Examples of cysts are: **pilonidal cyst,** which is found over the sacral area of the back in the midline and contains hairs (**pil/o** means hair, **nid/o** means nest); and **sebaceous cyst,** which is a collection of yellowish, cheesy sebum commonly found on the scalp, vulva, and scrotum.
fissure	A groove or crack-like sore.
	An anal fissure is a break in the skin lining and anal canal.
macule	A discolored (often reddened) flat lesion.
	Freckles, tattoo marks, and flat moles are examples.
papule	A small (less than 1 cm in diameter), solid elevation of the skin.
	Pimples are examples of papules. A larger, solid elevation is called a **nodule.**
polyp	A mushroom-like growth extending on a stalk from the surface of mucous membrane.

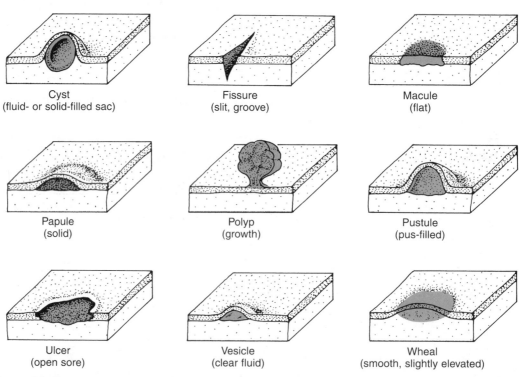

Cyst
(fluid- or solid-filled sac)

Fissure
(slit, groove)

Macule
(flat)

Papule
(solid)

Polyp
(growth)

Pustule
(pus-filled)

Ulcer
(open sore)

Vesicle
(clear fluid)

Wheal
(smooth, slightly elevated)

Figure 16–3

Cutaneous lesions.

Polyps are commonly found in the nose and sinuses, urinary bladder, and uterus.

pustule

A small elevation of the skin containing pus.

A pustule is a small **abscess** on the skin.

ulcer

An open sore or erosion of the skin or mucous membrane.

Decubitus ulcers (bedsores) are due to pressure from lying in one position (**decubitus** means lying down). Ulcers usually involve loss of tissue substance and pus formation.

vesicle

A small collection of clear fluid (serum); **blister.**

Vesicles are found in burns, allergies, and dermatitis. **Bullae** (singular: **bulla**) are large vesicles or blisters.

wheal

A smooth, slightly elevated, edematous (swollen) area that is redder or paler than the surrounding skin; **hives.**

Wheals may be circumscribed, as in a mosquito bite, or involve a wide area, as in allergic reactions. Wheals (hives) are often accompanied by itching.

Symptoms

alopecia

Absence of hair from areas where it normally grows.

Alopecia or baldness may be hereditary (usual progressive loss of scalp hair in men); or it may be due to disease, injury, or treatment (chemotherapy) or occur in old age. **Alopecia areata** is an idiopathic condition in which hair falls out in patches.

ecchymosis (plural: **ecchymoses**

Bluish-black mark (macule) on the skin; **black-and-blue mark.**

Ecchymoses (**ec-** means out, **chym/o** means to pour) are caused by hemorrhages into the skin from injury or spontaneous leaking of blood from vessels.

petechia (plural: **petechiae**)

Small, pinpoint hemorrhage.

Petechiae are smaller versions of ecchymoses.

pruritus

Itching.

Pruritus is associated with most forms of dermatitis and with other conditions as well. It arises as a result of stimulation of nerves in the skin by enzymes released in allergic reactions or by irritation caused by substances from the blood or from foreign bodies.

purpura

Merging ecchymoses and petechiae over any part of the body.

urticaria (hives)

An acute allergic reaction in which red, round wheals develop on the skin.

Pruritus may be intense, and etiology is commonly allergy to foods (such as shellfish or strawberries). Localized edema (swelling) occurs as well.

vitiligo

Loss of pigment (depigmentation) in areas of the skin (milk-white patches).

Also known as **leukoderma.** There is an increased association of vitiligo with

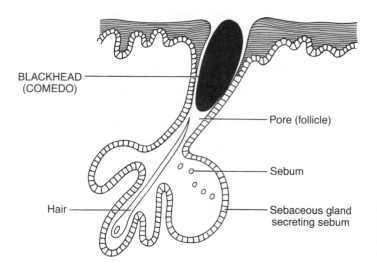

BLACKHEAD
(COMEDO)

Pore (follicle)

Sebum

Hair

Sebaceous gland
secreting sebum

Figure 16–4

Formation of a blackhead (comedo) in a dilated pore filled with sebum, bacteria, and pigment.

certain autoimmune conditions such as thyroiditis, hyperthyroidism, and diabetes mellitus.

Abnormal Conditions

acne

Papular and pustular eruption of the skin.

Acne vulgaris (**vulgaris** means ordinary) is caused by the buildup of sebum and keratin in the pores of the skin. A **blackhead** or **comedo** (plural: **comedones**) is a sebum plug partially blocking the pore (Fig. 16–4). If the pore becomes completely blocked, a **whitehead** forms. Bacteria in the skin break down the sebum, producing inflammation in the surrounding tissue. Papules, pustules, and cysts can thus form. Treatment consists of long-term antibiotic use and medications to dry the skin. Benzoyl peroxide and tretinoin (Retin-A) are medications to prevent comedo formation; isotretinoin (Accutane) is used in severe cystic acne.

burns

Injury to tissues caused by heat contact.

Examples are dry heat (fire), moist heat (steam or liquid), chemicals, lightning, electricity, or radiation. Burns are classified into three types:

Figure 16–5

Burns. *(A)* A second-degree burn injury. *(B)* A third-degree burn injury. (*A* and *B,* From Ignatavicius DD, Bayne MV: Medical-Surgical Nursing: A Nursing Process Approach. Philadelphia, WB Saunders, 1991, pp 364, 366.)

first-degree burns—superficial epidermal lesions, erythema, hyperesthesia and no blisters. Sunburn is an example.
second-degree burns—epidermal and dermal lesions, erythema, blisters, and hyperesthesia (Fig. 16–5).
third-degree burns—epidermis and dermis are destroyed (necrosis of skin), and subcutaneous layer is damaged leaving charred, white tissue (Fig. 16–5).

eczema   Inflammatory skin disease with erythematous, papulovesicular lesions.

This chronic or acute dermatitis is often accompanied by pruritus and may occur without any obvious cause. It is a common allergic reaction in children and also occurs in adults. Allergy may be to foods, dust, or pollens. Treatment depends on the cause but usually includes the use of corticosteroids.

exanthematous viral diseases   Rash **(exanthem)** of the skin due to a viral infection.

Examples are **rubella** (German measles), **rubeola** (measles), and **varicella** (chickenpox).

gangrene   Death of tissue associated with loss of blood supply.

In this condition, ischemia resulting from injury, inflammation, frostbite, diseases such as diabetes, or arteriosclerosis can lead to necrosis of tissue followed by bacterial invasion and putrefaction (proteins are decomposed by bacteria).

impetigo   Bacterial inflammatory skin disease characterized by vesicles, pustules, and crusted-over lesions.

This is a contagious **pyoderma** (**py/o** means pus) and is usually caused by staphylococci or streptococci. Systemic use of antibiotics and proper cleansing of lesions are effective treatments.

psoriasis   Chronic, recurrent dermatosis marked by itchy, scaly, red patches covered by silvery gray scales.

Psoriasis commonly forms on the forearms, knees, legs, and scalp. It is neither infectious nor contagious, but it is caused by an increased rate of growth of the basal layer of the epidermis. Etiology is unknown, but the condition runs in families and may be brought on by anxiety. Treatment is palliative (relieving but not curing) with topical lubricants, keratolytics, and steroids. PUVA (psoralen–ultraviolet A) light therapy is also used.

scabies   A contagious, parasitic infection of the skin with intense pruritus.

Scabies (from *scabere,* meaning to scratch) is often spread through sexual contact, and commonly affected areas are the penis, groin, nipples, and skin between the fingers. Treatment is topical medicated cream to destroy the scabies mites (tiny parasites).

scleroderma   A chronic progressive disease of the skin with hardening and shrinking of connective tissue.

Fibrous scar tissue infiltrates the skin and the heart, lungs, kidney, and esophagus may be affected as well. Skin is thickened, hard, and rigid, and pigmented patches may occur. Etiology is not known; palliative treatment consists of drugs, such as immunosuppressives and anti-inflammatory agents, and physical therapy.

systemic lupus erythematosus (SLE)

Chronic inflammatory disease of collagen in the skin, of joints, and of internal organs.

Lupus (meaning wolf-like; physicians thought the shape and color of the skin lesions resembled the bite of a wolf) produces a characteristic "butterfly" pattern of redness over the cheeks and nose. In more severe cases, the extent of erythema increases and all exposed areas of the skin may be involved. Primarily a disease of females, lupus is an autoimmune condition. High levels of antibodies are found in the patient's blood. Corticosteroids and immunosuppressive drugs are used to control symptoms.

SLE should be differentiated from chronic **discoid lupus erythematosus (DLE),** which is a milder, scaling, plaque-like, superficial eruption of the skin confined to the face, scalp, ears, chest, arms, and back. The reddish patches heal and leave scars.

tinea

Infection of the skin caused by a fungus.

Tinea or **ringworm,** because the infection is in a ring-like pattern, is highly contagious and causes severe pruritus. Examples are **tinea pedis** (athlete's foot), which affects the skin between the toes, **tinea capitis** (ringworm of the scalp), and **tinea barbae** (ringworm of the skin under a beard). Treatment is with antifungal agents.

Skin Neoplasms

Benign Neoplasms

callus

Increased growth of cells in the horny layer of the epidermis due to pressure or friction.

The feet and the hands are common sites. A **corn** is a type of callus that develops a hard core (a whitish, corn-like central kernel).

keloid

Hypertrophied, thickened scar after trauma or surgical incision.

Keloids occur from excessive collagen formation in the corium during connective tissue repair. The term comes from the Greek *kelis* meaning a blemish.

keratosis

Thickened area of the epidermis.

Some keratoses are red and are due to excessive exposure to light **(actinic keratosis). Seborrheic keratoses** are yellow or brown and are also called **senile warts.** Both types occur in middle age and old age.

leukoplakia

White, thickened patches on mucous membrane tissue of the tongue or cheek.

This is a precancerous lesion. It is common in smokers and may be caused by chronic inflammation.

nevus (plural: nevi)

Pigmented lesion of the skin.

Nevi include dilated blood vessels (telangiectasis) radiating out from a point (vascular spiders), hemangiomas, and moles. Many are present at birth, but some are acquired.

Dysplastic nevi are moles that do not form properly and may progress to form a type of skin cancer called melanoma (see **malignant melanoma).**

wart (verruca)	Epidermal growth caused by a virus.

Plantar warts (verrucae) occur on the soles of the feet, juvenile warts occur on the hands and face of children, and venereal warts occur on the genitals and around the anus. Warts may be removed by use of acids, electrocautery, or freezing with liquid nitrogen (cryosurgery). If the virus remains in the skin, the wart can regrow.

Cancerous Lesions

basal cell carcinoma	Malignant tumor of the basal cell layer of the epidermis.

This is the most frequent type of skin cancer. It is a slow-growing tumor that usually occurs on the upper half of the face, near the nose. It almost never metastasizes (Fig. 16–6).

Kaposi's sarcoma	Malignant, vascular, neoplastic growth characterized by cutaneous nodules usually on the lower extremities. Nodules range in color from deep pink to dark blue and purple. The condition is associated with acquired immuno-deficiency syndrome (AIDS).

malignant melanoma	Cancerous growth composed of melanocytes.

This malignancy is attributed to the intense exposure to sunlight that many people experience. Melanoma usually begins as a mottled, light brown to black, flat

Figure 16–6

Basal cell carcinoma. (From Wyngaarden JB, Smith LH Jr, Bennett JC [eds]: Cecil Textbook of Medicine, 19th ed. Philadelphia, WB Saunders, 1992, p 2315.)

Figure 16–7

Melanoma. (From Wyngaarden JB, Smith LH Jr, Bennett JC [eds]: Cecil Textbook of Medicine, 19th ed. Philadelphia, WB Saunders, 1992, p 2317.)

macule with irregular borders (Fig. 16–7). The lesions may turn shades of red, blue, and white and may crust on the surface and bleed. Melanomas often arise in preexisting moles (dysplastic nevi) and frequently appear on the upper back, lower legs, head, and neck.

Biopsy is required to diagnose melanoma, and prognosis following excision is determined by the depth of invasion through the skin layers. On this basis melanomas have been classified levels I to V. Level I indicates that the growth is confined to the epidermis, and levels IV and V represent penetration to the lower levels of the dermis and subcutaneous layer (Fig. 16–8).

Melanomas often metastasize to the lung, liver, and brain. Treatment includes excision of the tumor, regional lymphadenectomy, chemotherapy/immunotherapy, or radiotherapy to prevent metastasis.

squamous cell carcinoma Malignant tumor of the squamous epithelial cells of the epidermis.

This tumor may grow in places other than the skin, wherever squamous epithelium is found (mouth, larynx, bladder, esophagus, and so forth). It may arise from actinic (sun-related) keratoses and metastasize to lymph nodes. Treatment is surgical excision or radiotherapy.

Figure 16–8

Staging of melanoma by depth of invasion. A progressively worse prognosis is associated with increasing invasion of the dermis and subcutaneous layers of skin.

VII. Laboratory Tests, Clinical Procedures, and Abbreviations

Laboratory Tests

bacterial analyses	Samples of **purulent** (pus-filled) material or **exudate** (fluid that accumulates in a space or passes out of tissues) are sent to the laboratory for examination to determine what type of bacteria are present.
fungal tests	Scrapings from skin lesions are placed on a growth medium for several weeks and then examined microscopically for evidence of fungal growth.

Clinical Procedures

cryosurgery	Tissue is destroyed by the application of intensely cold liquid nitrogen.
Mohs' surgery	Thin layers of a malignant growth are removed, and each is examined under the microscope; also called **microscopically controlled surgery.**
skin biopsy	Skin lesions, such as pigmented nevi, chronic dermatoses, or any lesion in which there is the possibility of present or future malignant change, are removed and sent to the pathology laboratory for examination. A **punch biopsy** (used to obtain tissue in cases in which complete excision is not feasible) involves use of a surgical instrument that removes a core of tissue by rotation of its sharp, circular edge. In a **shave biopsy,** tissue is excised using a cut parallel to the surface of the surrounding skin.
skin testing for allergy or disease	The **patch test** is performed by applying to the skin a small piece of gauze or filter paper on which has been placed a suspected allergy-causing substance. If the area becomes reddened or swollen, the result is considered positive. The **scratch test** involves making several scratches in the skin and inserting a very minute amount of test material in the scratches. The test is considered negative if no reaction occurs. **Intradermal tests** are performed by injection of a reactive substance between layers of the skin and observation of the skin for a subsequent reaction. This test is used for the detection of sensitivity to infectious agents such as tuberculosis **(Mantoux tests, PPD test)** or diphtheria **(Schick test).** Strong reactions indicate ongoing infection.

ABBREVIATIONS

bx	Biopsy	**PUVA**	Psoralen–ultraviolet A light therapy
Derm.	Dermatology	**SLE**	Systemic lupus erythematosus
DLE	Discoid lupus erythematosus	**subq**	Subcutaneous
PPD	Purified protein derivative		

VIII. Practical Applications

This section contains actual medical reports using terms that you have studied in this and previous chapters. Explanations of more difficult terms are added in brackets.

Disease Descriptions

1. **Candidiasis** [*Candida* is a yeast-like fungus]: This fungus is normally found on mucous membranes, skin, and vaginal mucosa. Under certain circumstances (excessive warmth; administration of birth control pills, antibiotics and corticosteroids; debilitated states; infancy), it can change to a pathogen and cause localized or generalized mucocutaneous disease. Examples are paronychial lesions, lesions in areas of the body where rubbing opposed surfaces is common (groin, perianal, axillary, inframammary, and interdigital), thrush (white plaques attached to oral or vaginal mucous membranes), and vulvovaginitis.

2. **Cellulitis:** This is a common nonsuppurative infection of connective tissue with severe inflammation of the dermal and subcutaneous layers of the skin. Cellulitis appears on an extremity as a reddish-brown area of edematous skin. A surgical wound, puncture, skin ulcer, or patch of dermatitis is the usual means of entry for bacteria (most cases are caused by streptococci). Therapy entails rest, elevation, hot wet packs, and penicillin. Any cellulitis on the face should be given special attention because the infection may extend directly to the brain.

3. **Mycosis fungoides:** This is a rare, chronic skin condition caused by the infiltration of malignant lymphocytes. It is characterized by generalized erythroderma and large, reddish raised tumors that spread and ulcerate. In some cases, the malignant cells may involve lymph nodes and other organs. Treatment with topical nitrogen mustard and radiation can be effective in controlling the disease.

Write Up: Physical Examination of the Skin

A wide variety of lesions are seen on the face, shoulders, and back. The predominant lesions are pustules on an inflammatory base. Many pustules are confluent [running together] over the chin and forehead. Comedones are present on the face, especially along the nasolabial folds. Inflammatory papules are present on the lower cheeks and chin. Large abscesses and ulcerated cysts are present over the upper shoulder area. Numerous scars are present over the face and upper back.

IX. Exercises

Remember to check your answers carefully with those given in Section X, Answers to Exercises.

A. Select from the following terms to complete the sentences below.

corium	sebum	cuticle
melanin	basal layer	stratum corneum
keratin	lunula	lipocyte
collagen		

1. A fat cell is a (an) _____ .

2. The half-moon–shaped white area at the base of a nail is the _____ .

3. A structural protein found in skin and connective tissue is _____ .

4. A black pigment found in the epidermis is _____ .

5. The deepest region of the epidermis is the _____ .

6. The outermost layer of the epidermis, which consists of flattened, keratinized cells, is the

   _____ .

7. An oily substance secreted by sebaceous glands is _____ .

8. The middle layer of the skin is the dermis or _____ .

9. A hard, protein material found in epidermis, hair, and nails is _____ .

10. A band of epidermis at the base and side of the nail plate is the _____ .

B. Complete the following terms from their meanings given below.

1. The outermost layer of skin: epi _____

2. Profuse sweating: dia _____

3. Excessive secretion from sebaceous glands: sebo _____

4. Inflammation and swelling of soft tissue around a nail: par _____

5. Fungal infections of hands and feet: dermato _____

6. Burning sensation (pain) in skin: caus _____

C. *Match the term in column I with a related term in column II. Write the letter of the answer in the space provided.*

Column I

1. squamous epithelium _____

2. sebaceous gland _____

3. albino _____

4. horny cell _____

5. subcutaneous tissue _____

6. collagen _____

7. corium _____

8. melanocyte _____

9. erythema _____

Column II

A. keratin-filled
B. dermis
C. flat, scale-like cells
D. connective tissue protein
E. pigment deficiency
F. melanin
G. widespread redness of skin
H. lipocytes
I. oil-producing

D. *Build medical terms from the definitions and word parts given.*

1. surgical repair of the skin: dermato _____

2. pertaining to under the skin: sub _____

3. abnormal condition of lack of sweat: an _____

4. abnormal condition of proliferation of horny, keratinized cells: kerat _____

5. abnormal condition of dry, scaly skin: _____ osis

6. loosening of the epidermis: epidermo _____

7. yellow tumor (nodule undeer the skin): _____oma

8. under the nail: sub _____

9. abnormal condition of fungus in the hair: _____ mycosis

10. abnormal condition of nail fungus: onycho _____

E. Give the meanings for the following combining forms.

1. melan/o _____

2. adip/o _____

3. squam/o _____

4. xanth/o _____

5. myc/o _____

6. onych/o _____

7. pil/o _____

8. xer/o _____

9. steat/o _____

10. trich/o _____

11. erythem/o _____

12. albin/o _____

13. ichthy/o _____

14. hist/o _____

15. ungu/o _____

F. Match the cutaneous lesion with its meaning below.

polyp	wheal	macule
papule	ulcer	cyst
vesicle	fissure	nodule
pustule		

1. circumscribed collection of clear fluid (blister) _____

2. smooth, slightly elevated edematous area (hive) _____

3. discolored, flat lesion (freckle) _____

4. a groove or crack-like sore _____

5. a mushroom-like growth extending from the surface of a mucous membrane _____

6. circumscribed collection of pus (small abscess) _____

7. a closed sac containing fluid or semisolid material _____

8. open sore or erosion of the skin _____

9. solid elevation of the skin (pimple) _____

10. larger than 1 cm solid elevation of the skin _____

G. Give the medical terms for the following.

1. baldness _____

2. purplish, macular patch caused by hemorrhages into the skin _____

3. itching _____

4. acute allergic reaction in which red, round wheals develop on the skin _____

5. loss of pigment in areas of the skin _____

6. merging ecchymoses over the body _____

7. blackhead _____

8. small, pinpoint hemorrhages _____

H. Match the pathological skin condition with its description below.

impetigo   tinea   squamous cell carcinoma
psoriasis   scleroderma   acne
gangrene   malignant melanoma decubitus ulcer
eczema   basal cell carcinoma systemic lupus erythematosus

1. malignant neoplasm originating in scale-like cells of the epidermis _____

2. build up of sebum and keratin in pores of the skin leading to papular and pustular eruptions

_____

3. fungal skin infection _____

4. chronic disease marked by hardening and shrinking of connective tissue in the skin

_____

5. bedsore _____

6. necrosis of skin tissue resulting from ischemia _____

7. chronic or acute inflammatory skin disease with erythematous, pustular, or papular lesions

_____

8. widespread inflammatory disease of the joints and collagen of the skin with "butterfly" rash on the face

_____

9. cancerous tumor composed of melanocytes _____

10. chronic, recurrent dermatosis marked by silvery gray scales covering red patches on the skin

_____

11. malignant neoplasm originating from the basal layer of the epidermis _____

12. contagious, infectious pyoderma _____

I. Select the term that best fits the definition given.

1. contagious parasitic infection with intense pruritus: (scleroderma, scabies)

2. measles: (rubella, rubeola)

3. chickenpox: (varicella, eczema)

4. thickened scar: (tinea, keloid)

5. white patches on mucous membrane of tongue or cheek: (leukoplakia, albinism)

6. characterized by a rash: (gangrene, exanthematous)

7. thickening of epidermis related to sunlight exposure: (actinic keratosis, callus)

8. small, pinpoint hemorrhages: (psoriasis, petechiae)

9. large blisters: (bullae, purpura)

10. colored pigmentation of skin (mole): (nevus, verruca)

11. sac of fluid and hair over sacral region: (ecchymosis, pilonidal cyst)

12. acute allergic reaction in which hives develop: (vitiligo, urticaria)

J. Describe the following types of burns.

1. second-degree burn _____

2. first-degree burn _____

3. third-degree burn _____

K. Match the following medical terms with their more common meanings below.

pruritus   seborrheic dermatitis   alopecia
decubitus ulcer   comedones   vesicles
nevi   verrucae   tinea pedis
ecchymosis   wheals   exanthem

1. blackheads _____

2. moles _____

3. baldness _____

4. itching _____

5. hives _____

6. bedsore _____

7. warts _____

8. athlete's foot _____

9. black-and-blue mark _____

10. dandruff _____

11. blisters _____

12. rash _____

L. What is wrong with the skin?

1. pyoderma _____

2. xeroderma _____

3. leukoderma _____

4. erythema _____

5. dermatomycosis _____

6. callus _____

7. keloid _____

8. purpura _____

9. telangiectasis _____

10. gangrene _____

M. Give short answers for the following.

1. Two skin tests for allergy are _____ and _____.

2. The _____ test is an intradermal test for diphtheria.

3. The _____ test or _____ test is a test for tuberculosis.

4. Purulent means _____.

5. A surgical procedure to core out a disk of skin for microscopic analysis is a (an)

   _____.

6. The procedure in which thin layers of a malignant growth are removed, and each is examined under the

   microscope is called _____.

7. A type of skin cancer associated with AIDS and marked by dark blue-purple lesions over the skin is

   called _____.

8. Moles that do not form properly and may progress to form melanomas are called

   _____.

9. Removal of skin tissue using a cut parallel to the surface of the surrounding skin is called

   _____.

10. Destruction of tissue by use of intensely cold temperatures is called _____.

N. Circle the term that best completes the meaning of the sentence.

1. Since he was a teenager, Mike had red, scaly patches on his elbows and backs of his knees. Dr. Horm diagnosed Mike's dermatologic condition as (vitiligo, impetigo, psoriasis) and prescribed a special cream.

2. Clarissa noticed a rash across the bridge of her face and aching in her joints. She saw a rheumatologist who did some blood work and diagnosed her condition as (rheumatoid arthritis, systemic lupus erythematosus, scleroderma).

3. Bea had large, red patches all over her trunk and neck after eating shrimp. The doctor prescribed hydrocortisone cream to relieve her itching (seborrhea, acne, urticaria).

4. The poison ivy caused incredible (pruritus, calluses, keratosis) and Maggie was scratching her arms raw.

5. Kelly was fair-skinned with red hair. She had many benign nevi on her arms and legs, but Dr. Keefe was especially worried about one lesion with an irregular, raised border that he biopsied and found to be malignant (melanoma, Kaposi's sarcoma, pyoderma).

X. Answers to Exercises

A

1. lipocyte
2. lunula
3. collagen
4. melanin
5. basal layer
6. stratum corneum
7. sebum
8. corium
9. keratin
10. cuticle

B

1. epidermis
2. diaphoresis
3. seborrhea
4. paronychia
5. dermatophytosis
6. causalgia

C

1. C
2. I
3. E
4. A
5. H
6. D
7. B
8. F
9. G

D

1. dermatoplasty
2. subcutaneous
3. anhidrosis
4. keratosis
5. ichthyosis
6. epidermolysis
7. xanthoma
8. subungual
9. trichomycosis
10. onychomycosis

E

1. black
2. fat
3. scale-like
4. yellow
5. fungus
6. nail
7. hair
8. dry
9. fat, sebum
10. hair
11. redness
12. white
13. scaly, dry
14. tissue
15. nail

F

1. vesicle
2. wheal
3. macule
4. fissure
5. polyp
6. pustule
7. cyst
8. ulcer
9. papule
10. nodule

G

1. alopecia
2. ecchymosis
3. pruritus
4. urticaria
5. vitiligo
6. purpura
7. comedo
8. petechiae

H

1. squamous cell carcinoma
2. acne
3. tinea
4. scleroderma
5. decubitus ulcer
6. gangrene
7. eczema
8. systemic lupus erythematosus
9. malignant melanoma
10. psoriasis
11. basal cell carcinoma
12. impetigo

I

1. scabies
2. rubeola
3. varicella
4. keloid
5. leukoplakia
6. exanthematous
7. actinic keratosis
8. petechiae
9. bullae
10. nevus
11. pilonidal cyst
12. urticaria

J

1. damage to the epidermis and corium with blisters, erythema, and hyperesthesia
2. damage to the epidermis with erythema and hyperesthesia; no blisters
3. destruction of both epidermis and corium and damage to subcutaneous layer

K

1. comedones
2. nevi
3. alopecia
4. pruritus
5. wheals
6. decubitus ulcer
7. verrucae
8. tinea pedis
9. ecchymosis
10. seborrheic dermatitis
11. vesicles
12. exanthem

L

1. collections of pus in the skin
2. dry skin
3. white patches of skin (vitiligo)
4. redness of skin
5. abnormal condition of fungal infection in the skin
6. increased growth of epidermal horny layer cells due to excess pressure or friction
7. thickened, hypertrophied scar tissue
8. merging ecchymoses (purple patches) under the skin
9. abnormal dilation (-ectasis) of tiny blood vessels (angi/o) under the skin (tel- means complete)
10. necrosis (death) of skin tissue

M

1. scratch; patch
2. Schick
3. Mantoux; PPD
4. pus-filled

5. punch biopsy
6. Mohs' surgery
7. Kaposi's sarcoma

8. dysplastic nevi
9. shave biopsy
10. cryosurgery

N

1. psoriasis
2. systemic lupus erythematosus
3. urticaria

4. pruritus
5. melanoma

XI. Pronunciation of Terms

To test your understanding of the terminology in this chapter, write the meaning of each term in the space provided. In addition, you may wish to cover the terms and write them by looking at your definitions. Make sure your spelling is correct. The page number after each term indicates where it is defined or used in the text so you can easily check your responses. (If you are not sure what the pronunciation symbols mean, refer to page 21.)

Vocabulary, Combining Forms, and Suffixes

Term	Pronunciation	Meaning
adipose (565)	ĂD-ĭ-pōs	
albinism (565)	ĂL-bĭ-nĭzm	
albino (564)	ăl-BĪ-nō	
alopecia (569)	ăl-ō-PĒ-shē-ă	
anhidrosis (566)	ăn-hī-DRŌ-sĭs	
basal layer (564)	BĀ-săl LĀ-ĕr	
causalgia (565)	kăw-ZĂL-jă	
collagen (564)	KŎL-ă-jĕn	
corium (564)	KŌ-rē-ŭm	
cuticle (564)	KŪ-tĭ-k'l	
dermatologist (565)	dĕr-mă-TŎL-ō-jĭst	
dermatomycosis (566)	dĕr-mă-tō-mī-KŌ-sĭs	
dermatophytosis (567)	dĕr-mă-tō-fī-TŌ-sĭs	
dermatoplasty (565)	DĔR-mă-tō-plăs-tē	
dermis (564)	DĔR-mĭs	
diaphoresis (565)	dī-ă-fŏr-RĒ-sĭs	

epidermis (564)	ĕp-ĭ-DĔR-mĭs	_____
epidermolysis (565)	ĕp-ĭ-dĕr-MŎL-ĭ-sĭs	_____
epithelium (564)	ĕp-ĭ-THĒL-ē-ŭm	_____
erythema (566)	ĕr-ĭ-THĒ-mă	_____
erythematous (566)	ĕr-ĭ-THĒ-mă-tŭs	_____
hair follicle (564)	hār FŎL-ĭ-k'l	_____
ichthyosis (566)	ĭk-thē-Ō-sĭs	_____
integumentary system (564)	ĭn-tĕg-ū-MĔN-tăr-ē SĬS-tĕm	_____
keratin (564)	KĔR-ă-tĭn	_____
keratosis (566)	kĕr-ă-TŌ-sĭs	_____
leukoderma (567)	lū-kō-DĔR-mă	_____
leukoplakia (566)	lū-kō-PLĀ-kē-ă	_____
lipocyte (564)	LĬP-ō-sīt	_____
lipoma (566)	lī-PŌ-mă or lĭ-PŌ-mă	_____
lunula (564)	LŪ-nū-lă	_____
melanin (564)	MĔL-ă-nĭn	_____
melanocyte (566)	mĕ-LĂN-ō-sīt	_____
melanoma (566)	mĕl-ă-NŌ-mă	_____
onycholysis (566)	ŏn-ĭ-kē-ŎL-ĭ-sĭs	_____
onychomycosis (566)	ŏn-ĭ-kō-mī-KŌ-sĭs	_____
paronychia (566)	păr-ō-NĬK-ē-ă	_____
pilosebaceous (567)	pī-lō-sĕ-BĀ-shŭs	_____
pyoderma (567)	pī-ō-DĔR-mă	_____
sebaceous gland (564)	sĕ-BĀ-shŭs glănd	_____
seborrhea (567)	sĕb-ō-RĒ-ă	_____
seborrheic dermatitis (567)	sĕb-ō-RĒ-ĭk dĕr-mă-TĪ-tĭs	_____
sebum (564)	SĒ-bŭm	_____
squamous epithelium (564)	SKWĀ-mŭs ĕp-ĭ-THĒ-lē-ŭm	_____

steatoma (567)	stē-ă-TŌ-mă	_____
stratified (564)	STRĂT-ĭ-fīd	_____
stratum (plural: strata) (564)	STRĂ-tŭm (STRă-tă)	_____
subcutaneous (564)	sŭb-kū-TĀ-nē-ŭs	_____
subungual (567)	sŭb-ŬNG-wăl	_____
trichomycosis (567)	trĭk-ō-mī-KŌ-sĭs	_____
xanthoma (567)	zăn-THŌ-mă	_____
xeroderma (567)	zē-rō-DĔR-mă	_____

Lesions, Symptoms, Abnormal Conditions, and Neoplasms; Laboratory Tests and Clinical Procedures

Term	Pronunciation	Meaning
acne (570)	ĂK-nē	_____
basal cell carcinoma (572)	BĀ-săl sĕl kăr-sĭ-NŌ-mă	_____
bulla (plural: bullae) (569)	BŬL-ă (BŬL-ē)	_____
callus (572)	KĂL-ŭs	_____
comedo (plural: comedones) (570)	KŎM-ĕ-dō (kŏm-ĕ-DŌNZ)	_____
cyst (568)	sĭst	_____
decubitus ulcer (569)	dē-KŪ-bĭ-tŭs ŬL-sĕr	_____
ecchymosis (plural: ecchymoses) (569)	ĕk-ĭ-MŌ-sĭs (ĕk-ĭ-MŌ-sēz)	_____
eczema (571)	ĔK-zĕ-mă	_____
exanthematous viral disease (571)	ĕg-zăn-THĔM-ă-tŭs VĪ-răl dĭ-ZĒZ	_____
fissure (568)	FĬSH-ŭr	_____
fungal tests (575)	FŬNG-ăl tĕsts	_____
gangrene (571)	găng-GRĒN	_____
impetigo (571)	ĭm-pĕ-TĪ-gō	_____
Kaposi's sarcoma (573)	KĂH-pō-sēz săr-KŌ-mă	_____
keloid (572)	KĒ-lŏyd	_____

macule (568)	MĂK-ūl	_____
Moh's surgery (575)	mōz SŬR-jĕ-rē	_____
nevus (plural: nevi) (572)	NĒ-vŭs (NĒ-vī)	_____
papule (568)	PĂP-ūl	_____
petechia (plural: petechiae) (569)	pĕ-TĒ-kē-ă (pĕ-TĒ-kē-ī)	_____
pilonidal cyst (568)	pī-lō-NĪ-dăl sĭst	_____
polyp (568)	PŎL-ĭp	_____
pruritus (569)	proo-RĪ-tŭs	_____
psoriasis (571)	sō-RĪ-ă-sĭs	_____
purpura (569)	PĔR-pĕr-ă	_____
purulent (575)	PŪ-roo-lĕnt	_____
pustule (569)	PŬS-tūl	_____
rubella (571)	roo-BĔL-ă	_____
rubeola (571)	roo-bē-Ō-lă	_____
scabies (571)	SKĀ-bēz	_____
scleroderma (571)	sklĕr-ō-DĔR-mă	_____
squamous cell carcinoma (574)	SKWĀ-mŭs sĕl kăr-sĭ-NŌ-mă	_____
systemic lupus erythematosus (572)	sĭs-TĔM-ĭk LOO-pŭs ĕr-ĭ-thē-mă-TŌ-sĭs	_____
tinea (572)	TĬN-ē-ă	_____
ulcer (569)	ŬL-sĕr	_____
urticaria (569)	ŭr-tĭ-KĀ-rē-ă	_____
varicella (571)	văr-ĭ-SĔL-ă	_____
verruca (plural: verrucae) (573)	vĕ-ROO-kă (vĕ-ROO-kē)	_____
vesicle (569)	VĔS-ĭ-k'l	_____
vitiligo (569)	vĭt-ĭ-LĪ-gō	_____
wheal (569)	wēl	_____

XII. Review Sheet

Write the meanings of each word part in the space provided and test yourself. Check your answers with the information in the chapter or in the Glossary (Medical Terms—English) at the end of the book.

Combining Forms

Combining Form	Meaning	Combining Form	Meaning
adip/o		lip/o	
albin/o		melan/o	
caus/o		myc/o	
cauter/o		onych/o	
cutane/o		phyt/o	
derm/o		pil/o	
dermat/o		py/o	
diaphor/o		seb/o	
erythem/o		sebace/o	
erythemat/o		squam/o	
hidr/o		steat/o	
hydr/o		trich/o	
ichthy/o		ungu/o	
kerat/o		xanth/o	
leuk/o		xer/o	

Continued on following page

Suffixes

Suffix	Meaning	Suffix	Meaning
-algia	_____	-osis	_____
-derma	_____	-ous	_____
-esis	_____	-plakia	_____
-lysis	_____	-plasty	_____
-ose	_____	-rrhea	_____

Give combining forms for the following (first letters are given).

fat	a _____	yellow	x _____
	l _____	dry	x _____
	s _____	scaly, dry	i _____
white	a _____	redness	e _____
	l _____		e _____
skin	c _____	hard, horny	k _____
	d _____	burn, burning	c _____
nail	o _____	black	m _____
	u _____	fungus	m _____
hair	p _____	plant	p _____
	t _____		_____
sweat	d _____		_____
	h _____		_____

Sense Organs:
The Eye and the Ear

In this Chapter you will
- Identify the location and function of the major parts of the eye and the ear;
- Name the combining forms, prefixes, and suffixes most commonly used to describe these organs and their parts;
- Describe the pathological conditions that may affect the eye and ear; and
- Identify clinical procedures that pertain to ophthalmology and otology.

I. Introduction

In the previous chapter, we learned that the sensitive nerve endings in the corium layer of the skin receive impulses from various stimuli applied to the external surfaces of the body. These nerve endings transmit electrical messages, initiated by the stimuli, to regions of the brain (cerebrum and thalamus) so that we can recognize sensations such as temperature, touch, pain, and pressure. In Chapter 10 (Nervous System), we learned that nerve cells that carry impulses from a sense organ or sensory receptor area, such as the skin, taste buds, and **olfactory** regions (centers of smell in the nose), to the brain are called **afferent sensory neurons.**

The **eye** and the **ear** are sense organs, like the skin, taste buds, and olfactory regions. As such, they are receptors whose sensitive cells may be activated by a particular form of energy or stimulus in the external or internal environment. The sensitive cells in the eye and ear respond to the stimulus by initiating a series of nerve impulses along afferent sensory neurons that lead to the brain.

No matter what kind of stimulus is applied to a particular receptor, the sensation felt is determined by the regions in the brain that are connected to that receptor. Thus, mechanical injury that might stimulate receptor cells in the eye and the ear would produce sensations of vision (flashes of light) and sound (ringing in the ears). Similarly, if one could make a nerve connection between the sensitive receptor cells of the ear and the area in the brain associated with sight, it would be possible to perceive, or "see," sounds.

Figure 17–1 recapitulates the general pattern of events when such stimuli as light and sound are applied to sense organs such as the eye and ear.

II. The Eye

A. Anatomy and Physiology

Label Figure 17–2 as you read the following:

Light rays enter the dark center of the eye, the **pupil** (1). The **conjunctiva** (2) is a mucous membrane that lines the eyelids and coats the anterior portion of the eyeball over the white of the eye. The conjunctiva is clear and colorless except when blood vessels are dilated. Dust or smoke may cause the blood vessels to dilate and give the conjunctiva a reddish appearance, commonly known as bloodshot eyes.

The **cornea** (3) is a fibrous, transparent tissue that extends over the pupil and colored portion of the eye. The function of the cornea is to bend, or **refract,** the rays of light, so that they are focused properly on the sensitive receptor cells in the posterior region of the eye. The cornea is avascular (has no blood vessels) but receives its nourishment from blood vessels near its junction with the white of the eye, the **sclera** (4). Corneal transplants for people with scarred or opaque corneas are successful because the cornea has no blood supply and antibodies responsible for rejection of foreign tissue do not reach it. The sclera is a tough, fibrous, supportive, connective tissue that extends from the cornea on the anterior surface of the eyeball to the optic nerve in the back of the eye.

The **choroid** (5) is a dark brown membrane inside the sclera. It contains many blood vessels that supply nutrients to the eye. The choroid is continuous with the pigment-containing **iris** (6) and the **ciliary body** (7) on the anterior surface of the eye.

The iris is the colored (it can appear blue, green, hazel, gray, or brown) portion of the eye that surrounds the pupil. Muscles of the iris constrict the pupil in bright light and dilate the pupil in dim light, thereby regulating the amount of light entering the eye. The inset in Figure 17–2 shows the iris and its relationship to the pupil.

The ciliary body, on each side of the **lens** (8), contains muscles that can adjust the shape and thickness of the lens. These changes in the shape of the lens aid in the **refraction** of light

STIMULUS $\xrightarrow[\text{to}]{\text{applied}}$ RECEPTOR CELLS IN EAR AND EYE $\xrightarrow[\text{excite}]{\text{which}}$ AFFERENT NERVE FIBERS $\xrightarrow[\text{impulse to}]{\text{which carry}}$ BRAIN $\Big\}$ where nerve impulses are translated into sound sensations and visual images

Figure 17–1

Pattern of events in stimulation of a sense organ.

rays. The lens is thinned or flattened (for distant vision) and thickened (for close vision) by the muscles of the ciliary body. This refractive power of the lens is called **accommodation.**

Besides regulating the shape of the lens, the ciliary body also secretes a fluid called **aqueous humor,** which flows through the **posterior chamber** (9) and **anterior chamber** (10) of the eye. The fluid is constantly produced and leaves the eye through a canal that carries it into the bloodstream. Another cavity of the eye is called the **vitreous chamber** (11), which is a large region behind the lens filled with a soft, jelly-like material, the **vitreous humor.** Vitreous humor maintains the shape of the eyeball and is not constantly reformed. Its escape from the eye can cause blindness. Both the aqueous and the vitreous humors function to further refract light rays.

The **retina** (12) is the thin, delicate, and sensitive nerve layer of the eye. As light energy, in the form of waves, travels through the eye, it is refracted (by the cornea, lens, and fluids), so that it focuses on sensitive receptor cells of the retina called the **rods** and **cones.** There are approximately 6.5 million cones and 120 million rods in the retina. The cones function in bright levels of light and are responsible for color and central vision. There are three types of cones, each type stimulated by one of the primary colors in light (red, green, or violet). Most cases of color blindness affect either the green or red receptors, so that the two colors cannot be distinguished from each other. Rods function at reduced levels of light and are responsible for peripheral vision.

RETINAL ARTERIES AND VEINS

EYELID

SCLERA

INSET

PUPIL

IRIS

Figure 17–2

The eye.

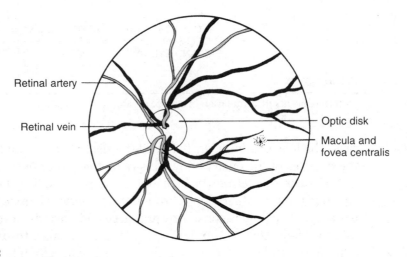

Figure 17–3

The posterior, inner part (fundus) of the eye, showing the retina as seen through an ophthalmoscope.

Figure 17–4

Visual pathway.

Light energy, when focused on the retina, causes a chemical change in the rods and cones, initiating nerve impulses that then travel from the eye to the brain via the **optic nerve** (13). The region in the eye where the optic nerve meets the retina is called the **optic disk** (14). The optic disk is known as the blind spot of the eye. The **macula** (15) is a small, oval, yellowish area to the side of the optic disk. It contains a central depression called the **fovea centralis** (16) composed largely of cones, and is the location of sharpest vision in the eye. If a portion of the fovea or macula is damaged, vision is reduced and central vision blindness occurs. Figure 17–3 shows the retina of a normal eye as seen through an ophthalmoscope. The **fundus** of the eye is this posterior, inner part that is visualized through the ophthalmoscope.

Figure 17–4 illustrates the pathway of the light-stimulated nervous impulse from the sensitive cells of the retina to the visual region of the cerebral cortex in the brain. The rods and cones in the **retina** synapse (meet) with neurons that lead to the **optic nerve fibers.** As the optic nerve fibers travel into the brain, the fibers located more medially cross in an area called the **optic chiasm.** Nerve fibers from the right half of each retina now form an **optic tract,** synapsing in the **thalamus** of the brain and ending in the right visual region of the **cerebral cortex.** Similarly, fibers from the left half of each retina merge to form the optic tract and pass from the thalamus to the left region of the **cerebral cortex.** In the visual area of the cerebral cortex, the images (one from each eye) are fused, and a single visual sensation with a three-dimensional effect is experienced. This is called **binocular vision.**

Damage to nerve cells in the **right cerebral cortex** (such as due to a stroke) causes loss of vision in the left visual field. Similarly, damage in the **left cerebral cortex** causes loss of vision in the right visual field. This loss of vision in the contralateral (opposite side) visual field is called **hemianopsia** (**hemi-** means half, **an-** means without, **-opsia** means vision).

Study Figure 17–5, which summarizes the pathway of light rays from the conjunctival membrane to the inner visual region in the cerebral cortex of the brain.

B. Vocabulary

This list will help you review many of the new items introduced in the text. Short definitions will reinforce your understanding of the terms. See Section VII of this chapter to help in pronouncing the more difficult terms.

accommodation	The normal adjustment of the eye for seeing objects at various distances. The lens is made thinner or fatter by the ciliary body to bring an object into focus on the retina.
anterior chamber	The area behind the cornea and in front of the lens and iris. It contains aqueous humor.
aqueous humor	Fluid produced by the ciliary body and found in the anterior and posterior chambers.
biconvex	Having two sides that are rounded, elevated, and curved evenly, like part of a sphere. The lens of the eye is a biconvex body.
choroid layer	The middle, vascular layer of the eye, between the retina and the sclera.
ciliary body	Structure on each side of the lens that connects the choroid and the iris. It contains ciliary muscles, which control the shape of the lens, and secretes aqueous humor.

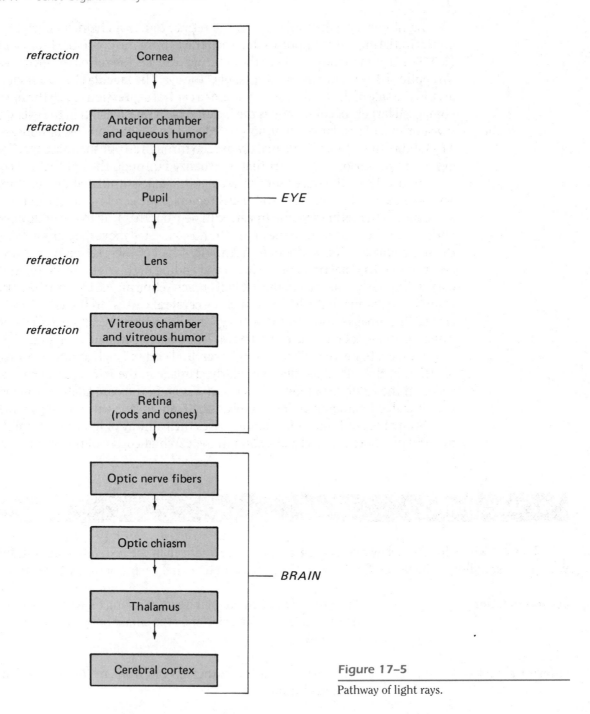

Figure 17–5

Pathway of light rays.

cones	Photosensitive receptor cells in the retina that transform light energy into a nerve impulse. Cones are responsible for color and central vision.
conjunctiva	A delicate membrane lining the eyelids and covering the anterior eyeball.
cornea	Fibrous transparent layer of clear tissue that extends over the anterior portion of the eyeball.
fovea centralis	The tiny pit or depression in the retina that is the region of clearest vision.
fundus of the eye	The posterior, inner part of the eye.
iris	The colored portion of the eye.
lens	A transparent, biconvex body behind the pupil of the eye. It bends light rays to bring them into focus on the retina.
macula	A yellowish region on the retina lateral to and slightly below the optic disk; contains the fovea centralis.
optic chiasm	The point at which the fibers of the optic nerve cross in the brain (**chiasm** means crossing).
optic disk	The region at the back of the eye where the optic nerve meets the retina. It is the blind spot of the eye because it contains only nerve fibers and no rods or cones and is thus insensitive to light.
optic nerve	The cranial nerve that carries impulses from the retina to the brain (cerebral cortex).
posterior chamber	The area behind the iris; contains aqueous humor.
pupil	The dark opening of the eye, surrounded by the iris, through which light rays pass.
refraction	Bending of light rays by the cornea, lens, and fluids of the eye to bring the rays into focus on the retina. **Refract** means to break (-fract) back (re-).
retina	The light-sensitive nerve cell layer of the eye that contains receptor cells called rods and cones.
rods	Photosensitive receptor cells of the retina that are essential for vision in dim light and for peripheral vision.
sclera	The tough, white, outer coat of the eyeball.
vitreous chamber	Area behind the lens of the eye. It contains vitreous humor.
vitreous humor	Soft, jelly-like material behind the lens; helps to maintain the shape of the eyeball.

C. Combining Forms, Suffixes, and Terminology: Structures and Fluids; Conditions

Write the meaning of the medical term in the space provided.

STRUCTURES AND FLUIDS
Combining Forms

Combining Form	Meaning	Terminology	Meaning
aque/o	water	aqueous humor	
blephar/o	eyelid (see also **palpebr/o**)	blepharitis	
		blepharoptosis	
		blef-ă-rŏp-TŌ-sis. Also called ptosis (Fig. 17–6).	
conjunctiv/o	conjunctiva	conjunctivitis	
		Commonly called pinkeye.	
cor/o	pupil (see also **pupill/o**)	anisocoria	
		anis/o means unequal. Anisocoria may be an indication of neurological injury or disease.	
corne/o	cornea (see also **kerat/o**)	corneal ulcer	
		From the Latin corneus meaning horny. Perhaps, as it protrudes outward, the cornea was thought to resemble the bud of a growing horn.	
cycl/o	ciliary body or muscle of the eye	cycloplegic	
dacry/o	tears, tear duct (see also **lacrim/o**)	dacryoadenitis	
		See Figure 17–7 for a picture of tear (lacrimal) glands.	
ir/o irid/o	iris (colored portion of the eye around the pupil)	iritis	
		iridic	

Figure 17–6

Ptosis (prolapse) of the right eyelid.

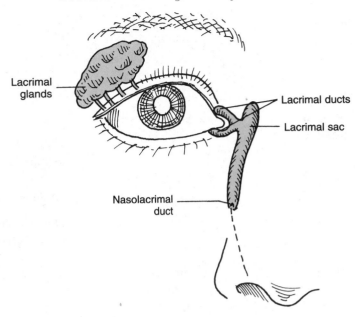

Figure 17–7

Lacrimal glands, lacrimal sac, nasolacrimal duct, and lacrimal ducts.

		<u>irid</u>ectomy _____
kerat/o	cornea	<u>kerat</u>itis _____
		<u>kerat</u>otomy _____

In radial keratotomy slit-like cuts are made in the cornea to flatten it for a correction of myopia (near-sightedness).

lacrim/o	tears	<u>lacrim</u>al _____
		<u>lacrim</u>ation _____
ocul/o	eye	intra<u>ocul</u>ar _____
ophthalm/o	eye	<u>ophthalm</u>ologist _____

A medical doctor who specializes in treating disorders of the eye.

		<u>ophthalm</u>ic _____
		<u>ophthalm</u>oplegia _____
opt/o **optic/o**	eye, vision	<u>opt</u>ic _____
		<u>opt</u>ometrist _____

A nonmedical person who can examine eyes to determine vision problems and prescribe lenses.

		optician _____

A nonmedical person who grinds lenses and fits glasses but cannot prescribe lenses.

palpebr/o	eyelid	<u>palpebr</u>al _____

papill/o	optic disk; nipple-like	papilledema _____

-edema means swelling. This condition is associated with increased intracranial pressure and hyperemia (increased blood flow) in the region of the optic disk.

phac/o **phak/o**	lens of the eye	phacoemulsification _____

This is a technique of cataract extraction using ultrasonic vibrations to fragment (emulsify) the lens and aspirate it out of the eye.

aphakia _____

This may be congenital, but most often it is the result of extraction of a cataract (clouded lens).

pupill/o	pupil	pupillary _____
retin/o	retina	retinitis _____

diabetic <u>retin</u>opathy _____

See Section II(E), Pathological Conditions.

scler/o	sclera (white of the eye)	corneo<u>scler</u>al _____

scleritis _____

uve/o	uvea; vascular layer of the eye (iris, ciliary body, and choroid)	<u>uve</u>itis _____
vitre/o	glassy	<u>vitre</u>ous humor _____

CONDITIONS
Combining Forms

Combining Form	Meaning	Terminology	Meaning
ambly/o	dull, dim	amblyopia _____	

-opia means vision. Amblyopia is a partial loss of sight and is also known as lazy eye. This is because it is associated with failure of the eyes to work together to focus on the same point.

dipl/o	double	diplopia _____	
glauc/o	gray	glaucoma _____	

-oma here means mass or collection of fluid (aqueous humor). The term comes from the dull gray-green gleam of the affected eye in advanced cases. See page 604, Section II(E), Pathological Conditions.

mi/o	smaller, less	miosis _____	

Contraction of the pupil. A **miotic** *is a drug (such as pilocarpine) that causes the pupil to contract.*

mydr/o	widen, enlarge	mydriasis _____

Enlargement of pupils. Atropine and cocaine cause dilation or enlargement of pupils.

nyct/o	night	nyctalopia _____

-opia means vision; al comes from ala meaning blindness. Night blindness is poor vision at night, but good vision on bright days. Deficiency of vitamin A leads to nyctalopia.

phot/o	light	photophobia _____

Sensitivity to light.

presby/o	old age	presbyopia _____

See page 604, Section II(D), Errors of Refraction.

scot/o	darkness	scotoma _____

An area of depressed vision surrounded by an area of normal vision; a blind spot. This can result from damage to the retina or the optic nerve.

xer/o	dry	xerophthalmia _____

Suffixes

Suffix	Meaning	Terminology	Meaning
-opia	vision	hyperopia _____	

Hypermetropia (farsightedness). See Section II(D), Errors of Refraction.

-opsia	vision	hemianopsia _____

Absence of vision in half of the visual field (space of vision of each eye). Stroke victims frequently have damage to the brain on one side of the visual cortex and experience hemianopsia (the visual loss is in the right or left visual field of both eyes).

-tropia	to turn	esotropia _____

Inward (eso-) turning of an eye. **Exotropia** *is an outward turning of an eye. These are examples of* **strabismus** *(defect in eye muscles so that both eyes cannot be focused on the same point at the same time).*

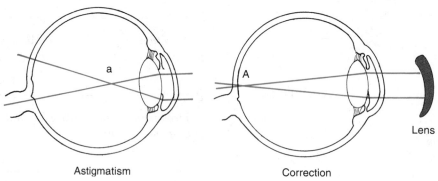

Astigmatism   Correction

Figure 17–8

Astigmatism and its correction. Point a is improper focus of light due to abnormal curvature of the lens or cornea. Point A is the point of focus after a proper lens has corrected the refractive error.

D. Errors of Refraction

astigmatism   Defective curvature of the cornea or lens of the eye.

This problem results from one or more abnormal curvatures of the cornea or lens. This causes light rays to be unevenly and not sharply focused on the retina, so

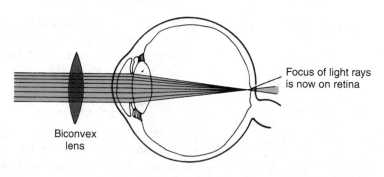

Figure 17–9

Hyperopia and its correction.

that the image is distorted. A cylindrical lens placed in the proper position in front of the eye can correct this problem (Fig. 17–8).

hyperopia (hypermetropia)   Farsightedness.

As Figure 17–9 illustrates, the eyeball in this condition is too short or the refractive power of the lens is too weak. Parallel rays of light tend to focus behind the retina, and this results in a blurred image. A convex lens (thicker in the middle than at the sides) bends the rays inward before they reach the cornea, and thus the rays can be focused properly on the retina.

myopia   Nearsightedness.

In myopia (**my-** comes from Greek *myein* meaning to shut, referring to the observation that myopic persons usually peer through half-closed eyelids), the eyeball is too long or the refractive power of the lens so strong that light rays do not properly focus on the retina. The image perceived is blurred because the light rays are focused in front of the retina. Concave glasses (thicker at the periphery than in the middle) correct this condition because the lenses spread the rays out before they reach the cornea, and thus they can be properly focused directly on the retina (Fig. 17–10).

MYOPIC EYE

CORRECTION FOR MYOPIA

Figure 17–10

Myopia and its correction.

presbyopia

Impairment of vision due to old age.

With increasing age, loss of elasticity of the ciliary body impairs its ability to adjust the lens for accommodation to near vision. The lens of the eye cannot become fat to bend the rays coming from near objects (less than 20 feet). The light rays focus behind the retina, as in hyperopia. Therefore, a convex lens is needed to refract the rays coming from objects closer than 20 feet.

E. Pathological Conditions

cataract

Clouding of the lens, causing decreased vision.

A cataract is a type of degenerative eye disease and is linked to the process of aging (senile cataracts). Some cataracts, however, may be present at birth, and others may occur with diabetes mellitus, ocular trauma, and prolonged high-dose corticosteroid administration. Vision appears blurred as the lens clouds over and becomes opaque. Lens cloudiness can be seen with an ophthalmoscope or the naked eye. Surgical removal of the lens and implantation of an artificial lens behind the iris are treatments for cataracts. If an intraocular lens cannot be inserted, the patient may wear eyeglasses or contact lenses to help refraction.

chalazion

Small, hard, cystic mass on the eyelid; formed from chronic inflammation of a sebaceous gland (meibomian gland).

Chalazions (kă-LĀ-zē-ŏnz) often require incision and drainage.

diabetic retinopathy

Retinal effects of diabetes mellitus include microaneurysms, hemorrhages, dilation of retinal veins, and neovascularization (new blood vessels forming near the optic disk).

Edema (macular edema) occurs as fluid leaks from blood vessels into the retina and vision is blurred. Fatty **exudates** (fluid leaking from the blood) appear in the retina as yellow-white spots. Laser photocoagulation and vitrectomy (see page 609, Section II[F], Clinical Procedures) are helpful to patients in whom hemorrhaging has been severe.

glaucoma

Increased intraocular pressure results in damage to the retina and optic nerve.

Intraocular pressure in the anterior and posterior chambers is elevated because of the inability of aqueous humor to drain from the eye and enter the bloodstream. Aqueous humor, which is normally formed by the ciliary body, flows into the posterior chamber and then into the anterior chamber, leaving the eye at the angle where the cornea and iris meet (Fig. 17–11).

Glaucoma is diagnosed by means of **tonometry** (see page 606, Section II[F], Clinical Procedures), with an instrument applied externally to the eye after administration of local anesthetic.

Administration of drugs (miotics) to lower intraocular pressure may prove effective in controlling the condition. Sometimes, laser therapy is used to tighten fibers in the ciliary body or to create a hole in the periphery of the iris, which allows aqueous humor to flow from the posterior to the anterior chamber and thus reduce intraocular pressure.

hordeolum (stye)

A localized, purulent, inflammatory staphylococcal infection of a sebaceous gland in the eyelid.

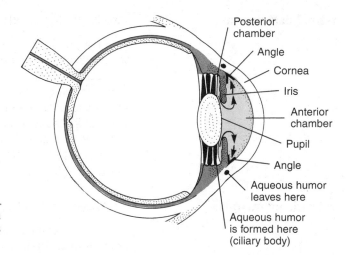

Figure 17–11

Circulation of aqueous humor. Circulation is impaired in glaucoma, so that fluid builds up in the anterior chamber.

Hot compresses may help localize the infection and promote drainage. In some cases, surgical incision may be necessary. **Hordeolum** (hŏr-DĒ-ō-lŭm) means barley corn.

macular degeneration   Deterioration of the macula of the retina.

This condition may be inherited, drug-induced, or age-related, and it leads to a severe loss of central vision (Fig. 17–12). Peripheral vision (using the part of the retina that is outside the macular region) is retained.

There is no known medical treatment, although certain forms of the condition may be treated with laser photocoagulation to destroy blood vessels that grow beneath the macula (the vessels leak fluid and blood and cause injury to macular nerve cells).

Figure 17–12

(A) Normal vision. *(B)* The same scene as it would appear to someone with macular degeneration. (*A* and *B*, Reprinted from *Seeing It Their Way,* published by the National Association for Visually Handicapped, New York.)

retinal detachment Two layers of the retina separate from each other.

Trauma to the eyeball, head injuries, bleeding, scarring from infection, or shrinkage of the vitreous humor can produce holes or tears in the retina leading to separation of layers. Patients often see flashes of light and then later notice cloudy vision or loss of central vision. Photocoagulation (making pinpoint burns to form scar tissue and seal holes) and cryotherapy (creating a "freezer burn" that forms a scar and knits a tear together) are used to repair retinal tears. A **scleral buckle** (see page 609, Section II[F], Clinical Procedures) made of silicone may be sutured to the sclera directly over the detached portion of the retina to push the two retinal layers together.

retinitis pigmentosa Progressive retinal sclerosis, pigmentation, and atrophy.

The major characteristic of this condition is the deposition of a pigmented scar on the retina. This is an inherited disease associated with decreased vision, especially **nyctalopia** (night blindness).

strabismus Abnormal deviation of the eye.

A failure of the eyes to look in the same direction because of weakness of a muscle controlling the position of one eye. Different forms of strabismus include **esotropia** (one eye turns inward; cross-eyed) **exotropia** (one eye turns outward; wall-eyed) and **hypertropia** (upward deviation of one eye). Treatment includes corrective lenses, eye exercises and patching of the normal eye, or surgery to restore muscle balance.

In children, strabismus may lead to **diplopia** and possibly **amblyopia** (partial loss of vision or lazy eye). Amblyopia is reversible until the retina is fully developed at about 7 years of age.

F. Clinical Procedures

Diagnostic

fluorescein angiography Fluorescein (a dye) is injected intravenously, and movement of blood is then observed by ophthalmoscopy to detect diabetic or hypertensive retinopathy and lesions in the macular area of the retina.

ophthalmoscopy This is a visual examination of the interior of the eye. The pupil is dilated so that the physician can see lesions of the cornea, lens, and retina (Fig. 17–13).

slit lamp ocular examination The slit lamp (Fig. 17–14) is an instrument that permits examination of anterior ocular structures under microscopic magnification.

tonometry This is measurement of the tension (**ton/o** means tension) or pressure within the eye and is useful in detecting glaucoma (Fig. 17–15).

Figure 17–13

Ophthalmoscopy. (From Swartz MH: Textbook of Physical Diagnosis: History and Examination. Philadelphia, WB Saunders, 1989, p 1005.)

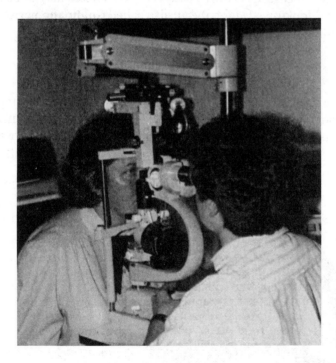

Figure 17–14

Slit lamp ocular examination. (From Ignatavicius DD, Bayne MV: Medical-Surgical Nursing: A Nursing Process Approach. Philadelphia, WB Saunders, 1991, p 1007.)

Figure 17–15

Measurement of intraocular pressure by tonometry. (From Ignatavicius DD, Bayne MV: Medical-Surgical Nursing: A Nursing Process Approach. Philadelphia, WB Saunders, 1991, p 1008.)

visual acuity (clearness) test

A test of clarity of vision. The patient reads a chart (standard is the Snellen eye chart) that contains black letters of gradually decreasing size. The chart is placed at a distance of 20 feet. Visual acuity is expressed as a ratio, such as 20/20. The first number is the distance at which the patient reads the chart. The second number is the distance at which a person with normal vision can read the same line of the chart. If the best a person can see is the 20/200 line, this means that at 20 feet the patient can see what a person with normal vision can see at 200 feet.

visual field examination

This test measures the area within which objects may be seen when the eye is fixed, looking straight ahead; also called **Goldmann perimeter visual field examination.**

Treatment

cataract surgery

There are two general methods of removing a cataract: intracapsular and extracapsular. **Intracapsular extraction** is removal of the entire lens, including its capsule. **Extracapsular extraction** involves removal of most lens tissue, but the back part of the lens capsule is left in place. This can be

Figure 17–16

Appearance of the eye with sutures in place after keratoplasty (corneal transplant). (From Ignatavicius DD, Bayne MV: Medical-Surgical Nursing: A Nursing Process Approach. Philadelphia, WB Saunders, 1991, p 1033.)

performed by **aspiration-irrigation** (a hollow needle withdraws the lens material, and the anterior chamber of the eye is washed out) and **phacoemulsification** (ultrasonic vibration is used to break up portions of the lens, so that it can be aspirated through the ultrasonic probe). Some patients develop clouding of the back part of the lens capsule after extracapsular extraction and may need further treatment with an ophthalmic laser (neodymium-YAG or "cold" laser).

In most patients, an intraocular lens (IOL) is implanted at the same time the defective lens is removed.

keratoplasty	This procedure, also called **corneal transplant,** involves replacement of a section of a scarred or opaque cornea with normal, transparent cornea in an effort to restore vision (Fig. 17–16).
laser photocoagulation	Argon laser (high-energy light) beams are used to stimulate coagulation of tissue (blood vessels) in the interior of the eye. Photocoagulation is useful to treat diabetic retinopathy and age-related macular degeneration (blood vessels are sealed to prevent leakage, or abnormal growth of blood vessels is prevented). Laser is an acronym for <u>l</u>ight <u>a</u>mplification by <u>s</u>timulated <u>e</u>mission of <u>r</u>adiation.
scleral buckle	Suture of a silicone band to the sclera directly over a detached portion of the retina. The band pushes the two parts of the retina against each other to bring together the two layers of a detached retina.
vitrectomy	Removal of the vitreous humor and its replacement with a clear solution. This is necessary when blood and scar tissue accumulate in the vitreous humor (a complication of diabetic retinopathy).

G. Abbreviations

IOL	Intraocular lens	**OU**	Each eye (Latin, *oculus uterque*)
IOP	Intraocular pressure	**PERRLA**	Pupils equal, round, reactive to light and accommodation
OD	Right eye (Latin, *oculus dexter*)	**VA**	Visual acuity
OS	Left eye (Latin, *oculus sinister*)	**VF**	Visual field

III. The Ear

A. Anatomy and Physiology

Sound waves are received by the outer ear, conducted to special receptor cells within the ear, and transmitted by those cells to nerve fibers that lead to the auditory region of the brain in the cerebral cortex. It is within the nerve fibers of the cerebral cortex that the sensations of sound are perceived.

Figure 17–17

The ear.

Label Figure 17–17 as you read the following paragraphs describing the anatomy and physiology of the ear.

The ear can be divided into three separate regions—outer ear, middle ear, and inner ear. The outer and middle ears function in the conduction of sound waves through the ear, and the inner ear contains structures that receive the auditory waves and relay them to the brain.

Outer Ear

Sound waves enter the ear through the **pinna,** also called the **auricle** (1), which is the projecting part, or flap, of the ear. The **external auditory meatus (auditory canal)** (2) leads from the pinna and is lined with numerous glands that secrete a yellowish-brown, waxy substance called **cerumen.** Cerumen lubricates and protects the ear.

Middle Ear

Sound waves travel through the auditory canal and strike a membrane between the outer and the middle ear. This is the **tympanic membrane, or eardrum** (3). As the eardrum vibrates, it moves three small bones, or **ossicles,** that conduct the sound waves through the middle ear. These bones, in the order of their vibration, are the **malleus** (4), the **incus** (5), and the **stapes** (6). As the stapes moves, it touches a membrane called the **oval window** (7), which separates the middle from the inner ear.

Before proceeding with the pathway of sound conduction and reception into the inner ear, an additional structure that affects the middle ear should be mentioned. The **auditory** or **eustachian tube** (8) is a canal leading from the middle ear to the pharynx. It is normally closed but opens upon swallowing. In an efficient way, this tube can prevent damage to the eardrum and shock to the middle and inner ears. Normally the pressure of air in the middle ear is equal to the pressure of air in the external environment. However, if you ascend in the atmosphere, as in flying an airplane, climbing a high mountain, or riding a fast elevator, the atmospheric pressure, and that in the outer ear, will drop, while the pressure in the middle ear remains the same—greater than that in the outer ear. This inequality of air pressure on the inside and outside of the eardrum forces the eardrum to bulge outward and eventually to burst. Swallowing will open the eustachian tube, so that air can leave the middle ear and enter the throat until the atmospheric and middle ear pressures are balanced. The eardrum then relaxes, and the danger of its bursting is averted.

Inner Ear

Sound vibrations, having been transmitted by the movement of the eardrum to the bones of the middle ear, reach the inner ear via the fluctuations of the oval window that separates the middle and inner ears. The inner ear is also called the **labyrinth** because of its circular, maze-like structure. The part of the labyrinth that leads from the oval window is a bony, snail-shaped structure called the **cochlea** (9). The cochlea contains special auditory liquids called **perilymph** and **endolymph** through which the vibrations travel. Also present in the cochlea is a sensitive auditory receptor area called the **organ of Corti.** In the organ of Corti, tiny hair cells receive vibrations from the auditory liquids and relay the sound waves to **auditory nerve fibers** (10), which end in the auditory center of the cerebral cortex, where these impulses are interpreted and "heard."

Study Figure 17–18, which is a schematic representation of the pathway of sound vibrations from the outer ear to the brain.

The ear is an important organ of equilibrium (balance), as well as an organ for hearing. Within the inner ear are three organs responsible for equilibrium. Refer back to Figure 17–17 and label these three organs: **semicircular canals** (11), **saccule** (12), and **utricle** (13). These organs contain the fluid called endolymph, as well as sensitive hair cells. In an intricate manner, the fluid and hair cells fluctuate in response to the movement of the head. This sets up impulses in nerve fibers that lead to the brain. Messages are then sent to muscles in all parts of the body to assure that equilibrium is maintained.

B. Vocabulary

This list will help you review many of the new terms introduced in the text. Short definitions will reinforce your understanding of the terms. See Section VII of this chapter for help in pronouncing the more difficult terms.

auditory canal	The channel that leads from the pinna to the eardrum.
auditory meatus	Auditory canal.
auditory nerve fibers	These nerves carry nerve impulses from the inner ear to the brain (cerebral cortex).
auditory tube	Channel between the middle ear and the nasopharynx; eustachian tube.
auricle	The flap of the ear; protruding part of the external ear or **pinna.**
cerumen	A waxy substance secreted by the external ear; also called **ear wax.**
cochlea	A snail-shaped, spirally wound tube in the inner ear; contains hearing-sensitive receptor cells.

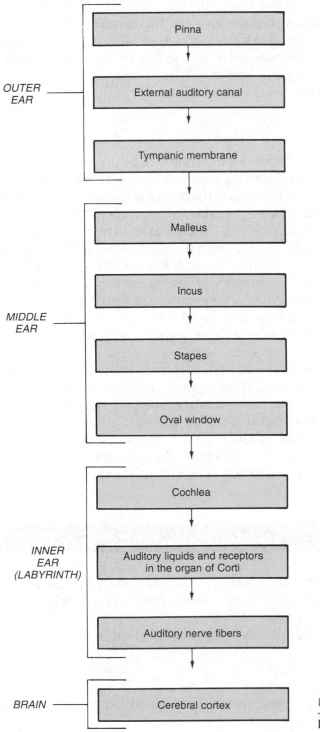

Figure 17–18

Pathway of sound vibrations.

endolymph	Fluid within the labyrinth of the inner ear.
eustachian tube	Auditory tube.
incus	The second ossicle (bone) of the middle ear; also called the **anvil.**
labyrinth	The maze-like series of canals in the inner ear. This includes the cochlea, semicircular canals, saccule, and utricle.
malleus	The first ossicle of the middle ear; also called the **hammer.**
organ of Corti	A sensitive auditory receptor area found in the cochlea of the inner ear.
ossicle	Small bone.
oval window	A membrane between the middle and the inner ears.
perilymph	Fluid contained in the labyrinth of the inner ear.
pinna	The auricle; flap of the ear.
saccule	An organ in the inner ear that is associated with maintaining equilibrium; saccule means little bag.
semicircular canals	Passages in the inner ear that are associated with maintaining equilibrium.
stapes	The third ossicle of the middle ear. **Stapes** means stirrup.
tympanic membrane	A membrane between the outer and the middle ear; also called the **eardrum.**
utricle	A tiny, sac-like structure in the inner ear that, along with the saccule and semicircular canals, is associated with maintaining equilibrium.

C. Combining Forms, Suffixes, and Terminology

Write the meaning of the medical term in the space provided.

Combining Forms			
Combining Form	Meaning	Terminology	Meaning
acous/o	hearing	acoustic _____	
audi/o	hearing, the sense of hearing	audiometer _____	
		audiogram _____	

audit/o	hearing	auditory _____
aur/o **auricul/o**	ear (see also ot/o)	aural _____
		postauricular _____
cochle/o	cochlea	cochlear _____
mastoid/o	mastoid process	mastoiditis _____

The mastoid process is the posterior portion of the temporal bone that extends downward behind the external auditory meatus. Mastoiditis is usually caused by bacterial infection that spreads from the middle ear.

myring/o	eardrum, tympanic membrane (see also tympan/o)	myringotomy _____
		myringitis _____
ossicul/o	ossicle	ossiculoplasty _____
ot/o	ear	otic _____
		otomycosis _____
		otopyorrhea _____
		otolaryngologist _____
salping/o	eustachian tube, auditory tube	salpingopharyngeal _____

In the context of female anatomy, salping/o means the fallopian tubes.

staped/o	stapes (third bone of the middle ear)	stapedectomy _____

After stapedectomy a prosthetic device is used to connect the incus and the oval window (Fig. 17–19).

tympan/o	eardrum, middle ear	tympanoplasty _____

Surgical reconstruction of the bones of the middle ear with reconnection of the eardrum to the oval window.

Suffixes			
Suffix	Meaning	Terminology	Meaning
-cusis	hearing	presbycusis _____	

This type of nerve deafness occurs with the process of aging.

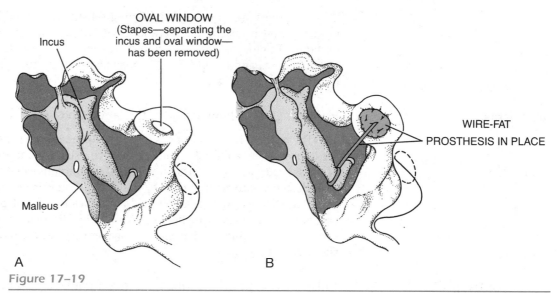

Figure 17–19

(A) Stapedectomy and *(B)* prosthesis to correct otosclerosis. (*A* and *B*, Modified from O'Toole M [ed]: Miller-Keane Encyclopedia and Dictionary of Medicine, Nursing, and Allied Health, 5th ed. Philadelphia, WB Saunders, 1992, p 1408.)

-otia	ear condition	macr<u>otia</u> _____
		Abnormally large ears; congenital anomaly.
		micr<u>otia</u> _____
		Abnormally small ears; congenital anomaly.

D. Abnormal and Pathological Conditions

Deafness is usually divided into two types: nerve deafness and conduction deafness. Nerve deafness is caused by impairment of the cochlea or auditory (acoustic) nerve. Conduction deafness is caused by impairment of the middle ear ossicles and membranes that transmit sound waves into the cochlea.

acoustic neuroma

Benign tumor arising from the acoustic nerve (eighth cranial nerve) in the brain.

This tumor causes tinnitus (ringing in the ears), vertigo (dizziness), and decreased hearing as its initial symptoms. Small tumors may be resected by surgical techniques, or ablated (removed) by radiosurgery (using radiation rather than a surgical incision).

cholesteatoma

Collection of skin cells and cholesterol in a sac within the middle ear.

These cyst-like masses are most often the result of chronic otitis media and associated with perforations of the tympanic membrane.

Ménière's disease

Disorder of the labyrinth of the inner ear marked by elevated endolymph pressure within the cochlea.

Symptoms are tinnitus, heightening sensitivity to loud sounds, progressive loss of hearing, headache, nausea, and vertigo. Attacks may last minutes or continue for hours. Etiology is unknown, and treatment is bed rest, sedation, and drugs to combat nausea and vertigo. Surgery may be necessary to relieve accumulation of fluid from the inner ear.

otosclerosis

Hardening of the bony tissue of the labyrinth of the ear.

The result of this condition is that bone forms around the oval window and can cause fixation or **ankylosis** (stiffening) of the stapes bone (ossicle). Conduction deafness occurs as the ossicles cannot pass on vibrations when sound enters the ear. Stapedectomy with replacement by tissue **graft** (substitute for the damaged part) using fatty tissue from the ear lobe and a **prosthesis** (artificial part) of stainless steel wire is effective in restoring hearing (see Fig. 17–19). In order to do this operation, the oval window must be **fenestrated** (opened) so that the otosclerotic area of the stapes can be removed.

serous otitis media

Inflammation (noninfectious) of the middle ear with accumulation of serum.

Treatment may include myringotomy to aspirate fluid and tympanostomy tubes placed in the eardrum to allow ventilation of the middle ear.

suppurative otitis media

Inflammation of the middle ear caused by bacterial infection and with pus formation.

Staphylococcus, streptococcus, or pneumococcus may be the infecting organism. Antibiotics are an excellent treatment. Myringotomy (surgical evacuation of the purulent material through the tympanic membrane) will prevent hearing loss and mastoiditis.

tinnitus

Noise (ringing, buzzing, roaring) sound in the ears.

This is a disease symptom and causes include presbycusis, Ménière's disease, otosclerosis, chronic otitis, labyrinthitis, and other disorders. Tinnitus can be persistent and severe and can interfere with a patient's daily life. Treatment may include biofeedback to help the patient relax and exert control over stress and anxiety if these are contributing factors.
Tinnitus, a Latin-derived term, means tinkling.

vertigo

Sensation of irregular or whirling motion either of oneself or of external objects.

Vertigo may result from disease in the labyrinth of the inner ear or the nerve that carries messages from the semicircular canals, utricle, and saccule to the brain. Equilibrium and balance are affected, and nausea may occur as well.

E. Clinical Procedures

audiometry

An instrument (audiometer) delivers acoustic stimuli of specific frequencies to determine the patient's hearing for each frequency. Test results are plotted on a graph called an **audiogram.**

cochlear implant

A device allowing deaf people to understand spoken words. It consists of a microphone, speech processor, external transmitter, and implanted receiver. The receiver is implanted under the skin near the mastoid process

LENS AND
VIEWING PIECE

SPECULUM

LIGHT

BATTERY
AND
HANDLE

Figure 17–20

Otoscope.

above and behind the ear. It sends electrical signals to electrodes planted within the cochlea, which stimulate auditory nerves leading to the brain.

otoscopy Visual examination of the ear with an otoscope (Fig. 17–20).

pneumatic otoscopy Visual examination of the external ear and tympanic membrane using air to change pressure in the external auditory canal. By increasing and decreasing the pressure in the external canal, the normal tympanic membrane should move in and out, respectively.

tuning fork tests A vibration source (tuning fork) is placed on the mastoid process and then in front of the external auditory meatus to test bone and air conduction **(Rinne test).** The **Weber test** compares bone conduction in the two ears (a vibrating tuning fork is placed on the center of the forehead).

F. Abbreviations

AD	Right ear (Latin, *auris dextra*)	**EENT**	Eyes, ears, nose, and throat
AS	Left ear (Latin, *auris sinistra*)	**ENT**	Ears, nose, and throat
AU	Both ears (Latin, *auris uterque*)	**PE tube**	Polyethylene ventilating tube (placed in the eardrum)

IV. Practical Applications

This section contains two listings of services and diagnoses and a medical report using terms that you have studied in this and previous chapters. Explanations of more difficult terms are added in brackets.

Operating Schedule and Diagnoses: Eye and Ear Hospital

Match the operation in column I with a diagnosis in column II. Answers are found at the end of Answers to Exercises section, page 629.

Operation—Column I

1. extracapsular cataract extraction with IOL; O.S. _____

2. blepharoplasty _____

3. scleral buckle _____

4. vitrectomy _____

5. radical mastoidectomy _____

6. keratoplasty _____

7. cochlear implant _____

8. argon laser photocoagulation of the macula _____

9. incision and drainage of hordeolum _____

Diagnosis—Column II

A. scarred and torn cornea
B. ptosis of eyelid skin
C. retinal detachment
D. diabetic retinopathy
E. macular degeneration
F. chronic stye
G. chronic infection of a bone behind the ear
H. deafness
I. senile cataract; left eye

Operative Report

Preoperative Diagnosis. Bilateral chronic serous otitis media adenotonsillitis.

Operation. Bilateral myringotomies and ventilation tube insertion adenotonsillectomy.

Procedure. With the patient in the supine position and under general endotracheal anesthesia, inspection of AD was made under the operating microscope. The external canal was clear, tympanic membrane was divided. A purulent discharge appeared to be present. This drainage was suctioned out and the ear thoroughly lavaged [washed out]. A ventilating tube was put in place and otic drops were administered. Same procedure for AS.

The patient was placed in the Rose position [supine with the head over the table edge in full extension] and the adenoids removed with adenoid curettes and adenoid biopsy forceps. A nasopharyngeal sponge was put in place. The right tonsil was then grasped with tonsil forceps, dissected free, and removed with snare. Bleeding was controlled with suction cautery. The nasopharyngeal sponge was removed and no further bleeding noted. The patient tolerated the procedure well and left the OR in good condition.

V. Exercises

Remember to check your answers carefully with those given in Section VI, Answers to Exercises.

A. *Match the structure of the eye with its description below. Write the letter of the description in the space provided.*

Column I

1. pupil _____

2. conjunctiva _____

3. cornea _____

4. sclera _____

5. choroid _____

6. iris _____

7. ciliary body _____

8. lens _____

9. retina _____

10. vitreous humor _____

Column II

A. contains sensitive cells called rods and cones that transform light energy into a nerve impulse

B. contains muscles that control the shape of the lens and secretes aqueous humor

C. transparent structure behind the iris and in front of the vitreous humor; it refracts light rays onto the retina

D. jelly-like material behind the lens that helps to maintain the shape of the eyeball

E. dark center of the eye through which light rays enter

F. vascular layer of the eyeball that is continuous with the iris

G. delicate membrane lining the eyelids and covering the anterior eyeball

H. fibrous layer of clear tissue that extends over the anterior portion of the eyeball

I. colored portion of the eye; surrounds the pupil

J. tough, white, outer coat of the eye

B. **Supply the term to complete the following sentences.**

1. The region at the back of the eye where the optic nerve meets the retina is the

   _____ .

2. The normal adjustment of the lens (becoming fatter or thinner) to bring an object into focus on the

   retina is called _____ .

3. A yellowish region on the retina lateral to the optic disk is the

   _____ .

4. The tiny pit or depression in the retina that is the region of clearest vision is the

   _____ .

5. The bending of light rays by the cornea, lens, and fluids of the eye is called

   _____ .

6. The point at which the fibers of the optic nerve cross in the brain is the

_____ .

7. The photosensitive receptor cells in the retina that make the perception of color possible are the

_____ .

8. The photosensitive receptor cells in the retina that make vision in dim light possible are the

_____ .

9. The _____ is the area behind the cornea and in front of the lens and iris. It contains aqueous humor.

10. The _____ is an area behind the iris, and it contains aqueous humor.

C. Give the meanings for the following terms.

1. optic nerve _____

2. biconvex _____

3. anisocoria _____

4. cycloplegic _____

5. palpebral _____

6. mydriasis _____

7. miosis _____

8. papilledema _____

9. photophobia _____

10. scotoma _____

D. Complete the medical term from its meaning and word parts given.

1. inflammation of an eyelid: _____ itis

2. inflammation of the conjunctiva: _____ itis

3. inflammation of a tear gland: _____ itis

4. inflammation of the iris: _____ itis

5. inflammation of the cornea: _____ itis

6. inflammation of the white of the eye: _____ itis

7. inflammation of the retina: _____ itis

8. prolapse of the eyelid: blephar _____

9. pertaining to tears: _____ al

10. pertaining to within the eye: intra _____

E. Match the following terms with their meanings below.

optician	xerophthalmia	corneal ulcer
ophthalmologist	uveitis	esotropia
optometrist	retinitis	exotropia
aphakia	hemianopsia	hypertropia

1. the fibrous layer of clear tissue over the front of the eyeball has a defect resulting from trauma or

   infection _____

2. inflammation of the vascular layer of the eye (iris, ciliary body, and choroid)

   _____

3. condition of dry eyes _____

4. absence of vision in half of the visual field _____

5. the eye abnormally turns outward _____

6. a medical doctor who treats diseases of the eyes _____

7. a nonmedical person who can examine eyes and prescribe glasses _____

8. a nonmedical person who grinds lenses and fits glasses _____

9. absence of the lens of the eye _____

10. the eye abnormally turns inward _____

F. Describe the following visual conditions.

1. amblyopia _____

2. hyperopia _____

3. presbyopia _____

4. myopia _____

5. nyctalopia _____

6. diplopia _____

7. astigmatism _____

G. *Complete the following sentences.*

1. In the myopic eye, light rays do not focus properly on the _____. Either the eyeball

   is too _____ or the refractive power of the lens is too

   _____ , so that the image is blurred and comes to a focus in

   _____ of the retina. The type of lens used to correct this refractive error is

   called a _____ lens.

2. In the hyperopic eye, the eyeball is too _____ or the refractive power of the lens

   too _____ , so that the image is blurred and focused in

   _____ of the retina. The type of lens used to correct this refractive error is called

   a _____ lens.

3. A miotic is a drug that _____ the pupil of the eye.

4. A mydriatic is a drug that _____ the pupil of the eye.

H. *Match the following abnormal conditions of the eye with their meanings below.*

glaucoma	diabetic retinopathy	retinitis pigmentosa
cataract	strabismus	retinal detachment
chalazion	hordeolum (stye)	macular degeneration

1. retinal microaneurysms, hemorrhages, dilation of retinal veins, and neovascularization occur secondary

   to an abnormal endocrine condition _____

2. two layers of the retina separate from each other _____

3. abnormal deviations of the eye occur (esotropia and exotropia) _____

4. clouding of the lens causes decreased vision _____

5. loss of central vision caused by deterioration of the macula of the retina _____

6. a localized, purulent infection of a sebaceous gland in the eyelid _____

7. a small, hard, cystic mass on the eyelid; formed from chronic inflammation of a sebaceous gland

_____

8. increased intraocular pressure results in retinal and optic nerve damage _____

9. progressive retinal sclerosis, pigmentation, and atrophy; inherited condition leading to nyctalopia

_____

I. The picture below shows how a patient with one of the following conditions would view the scene. What is the patient's condition?

1. glaucoma
2. cataract
3. stroke (hemianopsia)
4. macular degeneration

(Reprinted from *Seeing It Their Way,* published by the National Association for Visually Handicapped, New York.)

J. Give the meanings for the following combining forms.

1. lacrim/o _____

2. dacry/o _____

3. kerat/o _____

4. corne/o _____

5. blephar/o _____

6. palpebr/o _____

7. cor/o _____

8. pupill/o _____

9. phac/o _____

10. phak/o _____

11. ocul/o _____

12. ophthalm/o _____

13. opt/o _____

14. scot/o _____

K. Match the following clinical procedures with their meanings below.

tonometry   ophthalmoscopy   radial keratotomy
fluorescein angiography   visual acuity test   keratoplasty
visual field examination   slit lamp ocular examination   phacoemulsification
laser photocoagulation   vitrectomy   scleral buckle

1. ultrasonic vibrations break up the lens, and it is aspirated from the eye _____

2. test of clearness of vision _____

3. measurement of tension or pressure within the eye; glaucoma test _____

4. high-energy light radiation beams are used to stop retinal hemorrhaging

   _____

5. slit-like incisions are made in the cornea to change its shape and correct myopia

   _____

6. intravenous injection of dye followed by examination of the eyes and blood vessels

   _____

7. suture of a silicone band to the sclera to correct retinal detachment _____

8. test to measure the area within which objects are seen when the eyes are looking straight ahead

   _____

9. removal (and replacement) of diseased fluid in the chamber behind the lens of the eye

   _____

10. visual examination of the interior of the eye after dilation of the pupil _____

11. use of an instrument for microscopic examination of parts of the eye _____

12. corneal transplant surgery _____

L. Give the meaning of the following abbreviations.

1. OU _____

2. VA _____

3. OD _____

4. OS _____

5. VF _____

6. IOL _____

7. IOP _____

8. PERRLA _____

M. *Arrange the following terms in the correct order to indicate their sequence in the transmission of sound waves to the brain from the outer ear.*

incus, tympanic membrane, pinna, cochlea, malleus, oval window,

external auditory canal, auditory liquids and receptors, stapes,

auditory nerve fibers, cerebral cortex

1. _____   7. _____

2. _____   8. _____

3. _____   9. _____

4. _____   10. _____

5. _____   11. _____

6. _____

N. *Give the meanings for the following medical terms.*

1. labyrinth _____

2. semicircular canals _____

3. auditory (eustachian) tube _____

4. stapes _____

5. organ of Corti _____

6. perilymph and endolymph _____

7. cerumen _____

8. utricle _____

9. oval window _____

10. tympanic membrane _____

O. Complete the following terms from their definitions.

1. instrument to examine the ear: _____ scope

2. removal of the third bone of the middle ear: _____ ectomy

3. pertaining to the auditory tube and throat: _____ pharyngeal

4. flow of pus from the ear: oto _____

5. instrument to measure hearing: _____ meter

6. incision of the eardrum: _____ tomy

7. surgical repair of the eardrum: _____ plasty

8. deafness due to old age: _____ cusis

9. small ear: micr _____

10. inflammation of the middle ear: ot _____ _____

P. Give the meanings for the following medical terms.

1. vertigo _____

2. Ménière's syndrome _____

3. otosclerosis _____

4. tinnitus _____

5. labyrinthitis _____

6. cholesteatoma _____

7. suppurative otitis media _____

8. acoustic neuroma _____

9. mastoiditis _____

10. myringitis _____

Q. Give the meanings for the following abbreviations relating to otology.

1. AU _____

2. AS _____

3. AD _____

4. EENT _____

5. ENT _____

6. PE tube _____

R. Select the correct term to complete each sentence.

1. Dr. Jones specializes in pediatric ophthalmology. His examination of children with poor vision often leads to the diagnosis of (cataract, amblyopia, glaucoma) or lazy eye.

2. Stella's vision became progressively worse as she aged. Her physician told her that she had a common condition called (presbyopia, detached retina, anisocoria), which many elderly patients develop.

3. Matthew rubbed his itchy eyes constantly and thus spread his "pink eye" or (conjunctivitis, blepharitis, myringitis) from one eye to the other. Dr. Chang prescribed antibiotics for this common condition.

4. As David's (mastoiditis, otitis media, tinnitus) became progressively worse, his doctor worried that this ringing in his ears might be caused by a benign brain tumor, a(an) (cholesteatoma, acoustic neuroma, glaucoma).

5. Baby Sally had so many episodes of (vertigo, otosclerosis, suppurative otitis media) that Dr. Sills recommended the placement of PE tubes.

VI. Answers to Exercises

A

1. E	5. F	8. C
2. G	6. I	9. A
3. H	7. B	10. D
4. J		

B

1. optic disk	5. refraction	8. rods
2. accommodation	6. optic chiasm	9. anterior chamber
3. macula	7. cones	10. posterior chamber
4. fovea centralis		

C

1. cranial nerve that carries impulses from the retina to the brain	4. pertaining to paralysis of the ciliary muscles	8. swelling in the region of the optic disk
2. having two sides that are rounded, elevated, and curved evenly	5. pertaining to the eyelid	9. condition of sensitivity ("fear") to light
3. condition of pupils of unequal (anis/o) size	6. condition of enlargement of the pupil	10. blind spot; area of darkened (diminished vision) surrounded by clear vision
	7. condition of narrowing of the pupil	

D

1. blepharitis	5. keratitis	8. blepharoptosis
2. conjunctivitis	6. scleritis	9. lacrimal
3. dacryoadenitis	7. retinitis	10. intraocular
4. iritis		

E

1. corneal ulcer
2. uveitis
3. xerophthalmia
4. hemianopsia

5. exotropia
6. ophthalmologist
7. optometrist

8. optician
9. aphakia
10. esotropia

F

1. dimness of vision; lazy eye (resulting from strabismus and diplopia)
2. farsightedness
3. decreased vision resulting from old age
4. nearsightedness

5. night blindness; decreased vision at night
6. double vision
7. defective curvature of the lens and cornea leading to blurred vision

G

1. retina; long; strong; front; concave
2. short; weak; back; convex
3. constricts
4. dilates

H

1. diabetic retinopathy
2. retinal detachment
3. strabismus

4. cataract
5. macular degeneration
6. hordeolum (stye)

7. chalazion
8. glaucoma
9. retinitis pigmentosa

I

1. C is the correct answer—loss of half of the visual field caused by a stroke occurring in the left visual cortex. Glaucoma would cause loss of peripheral vision (darkness around the edges of the picture). A cataract would cause blurred vision. Macular degeneration would produce loss of central vision.

J

1. tears
2. tears
3. cornea
4. cornea
5. eyelid

6. eyelid
7. pupil
8. pupil
9. lens
10. lens

11. eye
12. eye
13. eye
14. darkness

K

1. phacoemulsification
2. visual acuity test
3. tonometry
4. laser photocoagulation

5. radial keratotomy
6. fluorescein angiography
7. scleral buckle
8. visual field examination

9. vitrectomy
10. ophthalmoscopy
11. slit lamp ocular examination
12. keratoplasty

L

1. each eye
2. visual acuity
3. right eye

4. left eye
5. visual field
6. intraocular lens

7. intraocular pressure
8. pupils equal, round, reactive to light and accommodation

M

1. pinna (auricle)
2. external auditory canal
3. tympanic membrane
4. malleus

5. incus
6. stapes
7. oval window
8. cochlea

9. auditory liquids and receptors
10. auditory nerve fibers
11. cerebral cortex

N

1. cochlea and organs of equilibrium (semicircular canals, saccule, and utricle)
2. organ of equilibrium in the inner ear
3. passageway between the middle ear and the throat
4. third ossicle (little bone) of the middle ear

5. region in the cochlea that contains auditory receptors
6. auditory fluids circulating within the inner ear
7. wax in the external auditory meatus
8. tiny sac in the inner ear associated with

the semicircular canals and important in maintaining equilibrium and balance
9. delicate membrane between the middle and the inner ears
10. eardrum

O

1. otoscope
2. stapedectomy
3. salpingopharyngeal
4. otopyorrhea
5. audiometer
6. myringotomy (tympanotomy)
7. tympanoplasty (myringoplasty)
8. presbycusis
9. microtia
10. otitis media

P

1. sensation of irregular or whirling motion either of oneself or of external objects
2. disorder of the labyrinth marked by elevation of ear fluids and pressure within the cochlea (tinnitus, vertigo, and nausea result)
3. hardening of the bony tissue of the labyrinth of the inner ear
4. noise (ringing, buzzing) in the ears
5. inflammation of the labyrinth of the inner ear
6. collection of skin cells and cholesterol in a sac within the middle ear
7. inflammation of the middle ear with bacterial infection and pus collection
8. benign tumor arising from the acoustic nerve in the brain
9. inflammation of the mastoid process (behind the ear)
10. inflammation of the eardrum

Q

1. both ears
2. left ear
3. right ear
4. eyes, ears, nose, and throat
5. ears, nose, and throat
6. ventilating tube placed in the eardrum

R

1. amblyopia
2. presbyopia
3. conjunctivitis
4. tinnitus; acoustic neuroma
5. suppurative otitis media

Answers to Practical Applications

1. I
2. B
3. C
4. D
5. G
6. A
7. H
8. E
9. F

VII. Pronunciation of Terms

To test your understanding of the terminology in this chapter, write the meaning of each term in the space provided. In addition, you may wish to cover the terms and write them by looking at your definitions. Make sure your spelling is correct. The page number after each term indicates where it is defined or used in the text so you can easily check your responses. (If you are not sure what the pronunciation symbols mean, refer to page 21.)

Eye

Term	Pronunciation	Meaning
accommodation (595)	ă-kŏm-ō-DĀ-shŭn	_____
ambylopia (600)	ăm-blē-Ō-pē-ă	_____
anisocoria (598)	ăn-ī-sō-KŌ-rē-ă	_____
anterior chamber (595)	ăn-TĒ-rē-ŏr CHĀM-bĕr	_____
aphakia (600)	ă-FĀ-kē-ă	_____

aqueous humor (595)	ĂK-wē-ŭs or Ā-kwē-ŭs HŪ-měr	_____
astigmatism (602)	ă-STĬG-mă-tĭsm	_____
biconvex (595)	bī-KŌN-věks	_____
blepharitis (598)	blěf-ă-RĪ-tĭs	_____
blepharoptosis (598)	blěf-ă-rŏp-TŌ-sĭs	_____
cataract (604)	KĂT-ă-răkt	_____
chalazion (604)	kă-LĀ-zē-ŏn	_____
choroid layer (595)	KŎR-oyd LĀ-ěr	_____
ciliary body (595)	SĬL-ē-ăr-ē BŎD-ē	_____
cones (597)	kōnz	_____
conjunctiva (597)	kŏn-jŭnk-TĪ-vă	_____
conjunctivitis (598)	kŏn-jŭnk-tĭ-VĪ-tĭs	_____
cornea (597)	KŎR-nē-ă	_____
corneal ulcer (598)	KŎR-nē-ăl ŬL-sěr	_____
corneoscleral (600)	kŏr-nē-ō-SKLĚ-răl	_____
cycloplegic (598)	sī-klō-PLĒ-jĭk	_____
dacryoadenitis (598)	dăk-rē-ō-ăd-ĕ-NĪ-tĭs	_____
diabetic retinopathy (604)	dī-ă-BĚT-ĭk rě-tĭn-NŎP-ă-thē	_____
diplopia (600)	dĭp-LŌ-pē-ă	_____
esotropia (601)	ěs-ō-TRŌP-pē-ă	_____
exotropia (601)	ěk-sō-TRŌ-pē-ă	_____
fluorescein angiography (606)	floo-ō-RĚS-ē-ĭn ăn-jē-ŎG-ră-fē	_____
fovea centralis (597)	FŌ-vē-ă sěn-TRĂ-lĭs	_____
fundus (597)	FŬN-dŭs	_____
glaucoma (604)	glăw-KŌ-mă	_____
hemianopsia (601)	hě-mē-ă-NŎP-sē-ă	_____
hordeolum (604)	hŏr-DĒ-ō-lŭm	_____

hyperopia (603)	hī-pĕr-Ō-pē-ă	
hypertropia (606)	hī-pĕr-TRŌ-pē-ă	
intraocular (599)	ĭn-tră-ŎK-ū-lăr	
iridectomy (599)	ĭr-ĭ-DĔK-tō-mē	
iridic (598)	ĭ-RĬD-ĭk	
iris (597)	Ī-rĭs	
iritis (598)	ī-RĪ-tĭs	
keratitis (599)	kĕr-ă-TĪ-tĭs	
keratoplasty (609)	kĕr-ă-tō-PLĂS-tē	
keratotomy (599)	kĕ-ră-TŎT-ō-mē	
lacrimal (599)	LĂK-rĭ-măl	
lacrimation (599)	lă-krĭ-MĀ-shŭn	
laser photocoagulation (609)	LĀ-zĕr fō-tō-kō-ăg-ū-LĀ-shŭn	
lens (597)	lĕnz	
macula (597)	MĂK-ū-lă	
macular degeneration (605)	MĂK-ū-lăr dē-jĕn-ĕ-RĀ-shŭn	
miosis (601)	mī-Ō-sĭs	
miotic (601)	mī-ŎT-ĭk	
mydriasis (601)	mĭ-DRĪ-ă-sĭs	
myopia (603)	mī-Ō-pē-ă	
nyctalopia (601)	nĭk-tă-LŌ-pē-ă	
ophthalmic (599)	ŏf-THĂL-mĭk	
ophthalmologist (599)	ŏf-thăl-MŎL-ō-jĭst	
ophthalmoplegia (599)	ŏf-thăl-mō-PLĒ-jă	
ophthalmoscopy (606)	ŏf-thăl-MŎS-kō-pē	
optic chiasm (597)	ŎP-tĭk KĪ-azm	
optic disk (597)	ŎP-tĭk dĭsk	
optician (599)	ŏp-TĬSH-ăn	

optic nerve (597)	ŎP-tĭk nĕrv	_____
optometrist (599)	ŏp-TŎM-ĕ-trĭst	_____
palpebral (599)	PĂL-pĕ-brăl	_____
papilledema (600)	păp-ĕ-lĕ-DĒ-mă	_____
phacoemulsification (600)	făk-ō-ĕ-mŭl-sĭ-fĭ-KĀ-shŭn	_____
photophobia (601)	fō-tō-FŌ-bē-ă	_____
presbyopia (604)	prĕz-bē-Ō-pē-ă	_____
pupil (597)	PŪ-pĭl	_____
pupillary (600)	PŪ-pĭ-lăr-ē	_____
refraction (597)	rē-FRĂK-shŭn	_____
retina (597)	RĔT-ĭ-nă	_____
retinal detachment (606)	RĔ-tĭ-năl dē-TĂCH-mĕnt	_____
retinitis pigmentosa (606)	rĕt-ĭ-NĪ-tĭs pĭg-mĕn-TŌ-să	_____
sclera (597)	SKLĔ-ră	_____
scleral buckle (609)	SKLĔ-răl BŬK'l	_____
scleritis (600)	sklĕ-RĪ-tĭs	_____
scotoma (601)	skō-TŌ-mă	_____
slit lamp ocular examination (606)	slĭt lămp ŏk-ū-lăr ĕk-zăm-ĭ-NĀ-shŭn	_____
strabismus (606)	stră-BĬZ-mŭs	_____
tonometry (606)	tō-NŎM-ĕ-trē	_____
uveitis (600)	ū-vē-Ī-tĭs	_____
visual acuity (608)	VĬZ-ū-ăl ă-KŪ-ĭ-tē	_____
visual field examination (608)	VĬZ-ū-ăl fēld ĕk-zăm-ĭ-NĀ-shŭn	_____
vitrectomy (609)	vĭ-TRĔK-tō-mē	_____
vitreous humor (597)	VĬT-rē-ŭs Ū-mĕr	_____
xerophthalmia (601)	zĕr-ŏf-THĂL-mē-ă	_____

Ear

Term	Pronunciation	Meaning
acoustic (613)	ă-KŌŌS-tĭk	_____
acoustic neuroma (615)	ă-KŌŌS-tĭk nū-RŌ-mă	_____
audiogram (613)	ĂW-dē-ō-grăm	_____
audiometer (613)	ăw-dē-ŎM-ĕ-tĕr	_____
audiometry (616)	ăw-dē-ŎM-ĕ-trē	_____
auditory canal (611)	ăw-dĭ-TŌ-rē kă-NĂL	_____
auditory meatus (611)	ăw-dĭ-TŌ-rē mē-Ā-tŭs	_____
auditory tube (611)	ăw-dĭ-TŌ-rē tōōb	_____
aural (613)	ĂW-răl	_____
auricle (611)	ĂW-rĭ-k'l	_____
cerumen (611)	sĕ-RŌŌ-mĕn	_____
cholesteatoma (615)	kō-lē-stē-ă-TŌ-mă	_____
cochlea (611)	KŎK-lē-ă	_____
cochlear (614)	KŎK-lē-ăr	_____
endolymph (613)	ĔN-dō-lĭmf	_____
eustachian tube (613)	ū-STĀ-shŭn or ū-STĀ-kē-ăn	_____
incus (613)	ĬNG-kŭs	_____
labyrinth (613)	LĂB-ĭ-rĭnth	_____
macrotia (615)	măk-RŌ-shē-ă	_____
malleus (613)	MĂL-ē-ŭs	_____
mastoiditis (614)	măs-toy-DĪ-tĭs	_____
Ménière's disease (615)	mĕn-ē-ĀRZ dĭ-ZĒZ	_____
microtia (615)	mī-KRŌ-shē-ă	_____
myringitis (614)	mĭr-ĭn-JĪ-tĭs	_____
myringotomy (614)	mĭr-ĭn-GŎT-ō-mē	_____

ossicle (613)	ŎS-ĭ-k'l	_____
ossiculoplasty (614)	ŏs-ĭ-kū-lō-PLĂS-tē	_____
otic (614)	Ō-tĭk	_____
otolaryngologist (614)	ō-tō-lă-rĭn-GŎL-ō-jĭst	_____
otomycosis (614)	ō-tō-mī-KŌ-sĭs	_____
otopyorrhea (614)	ō-tō-pī-ō-RĒ-ă	_____
otosclerosis (616)	ō-tō-sklĕ-RŌ-sĭs	_____
otoscopy (617)	ō-TŎS-kō-pē	_____
oval window (613)	Ō-văl WĬN-dō	_____
perilymph (613)	PĔR-ĭ-lĭmf	_____
pinna (613)	PĬN-ă	_____
pneumatic otoscopy (617)	nū-MĂ-tĭk ō-TŎS-kō-pē	_____
postauricular (614)	pōst-ăw-RĬK-ū-lăr	_____
presbycusis (614)	prĕz-bē-KŪ-sĭs	_____
saccule (613)	SĂK-ūl	_____
salpingopharyngeal (614)	săl-pĭng-gō-fă-RĬN-gē-ăl	_____
semicircular canals (613)	sĕ-mē-SĔR-kū-lăr kă-NĂLZ	_____
serous otitis media (616)	SĔR-ŭs ō-TĪ-tĭs MĒ-dē-ă	_____
stapedectomy (614)	stā-pĕ-DĔK-tō-mē	_____
stapes (613)	STĀ-pēz	_____
suppurative otitis media (616)	SŪ-pĕr-ă-tĭv ō-TĪ-tĭs MĒ-dē-ă	_____
tinnitus (616)	tĭ-NĪ-tĭs	_____
tuning fork tests (617)	TOO-nēng fork tests	_____
tympanic membrane (613)	tĭm-PĂN-ĭk MĔM-brān	_____
tympanoplasty (614)	tĭm-pă-nō-PLĂS-tē	_____
utricle (613)	Ū-trĭ-k'l	_____
vertigo (616)	VĔR-tĭ-gō	_____

VIII. Review Sheet

Write the meaning of each word part in the space provided and test yourself. Check your answers with the information in the chapter or in the Glossary (Medical Terms—English) at the end of the book.

Combining Forms

Combining Form	Meaning	Combining Form	Meaning
acous/o		lacrim/o	
ambly/o		mastoid/o	
anis/o		mi/o	
aque/o		myc/o	
audi/o		mydr/o	
audit/o		myring/o	
aur/o		nyct/o	
auricul/o		ocul/o	
blephar/o		ophthalm/o	
conjunctiv/o		opt/o	
cor/o		optic/o	
corne/o		ossicul/o	
cycl/o		ot/o	
dacry/o		palpebr/o	
dipl/o		papill/o	
glauc/o		phac/o	
ir/o		phak/o	
irid/o		phot/o	
kerat/o		presby/o	

pupill/o _____   staped/o _____

retin/o _____   tympan/o _____

salping/o _____   uve/o _____

scler/o _____   vitre/o _____

scot/o _____   xer/o _____

Suffixes

Suffix	Meaning	Suffix	Meaning
-cusis	_____	-phobia	_____
-opia	_____	-plegic	_____
-opsia	_____	-tropia	_____
-otia	_____		

Endocrine System

This Chapter is divided into the following sections

In this Chapter you will

- Identify the endocrine glands and their hormones;
- Gain an understanding of the functions of these hormones in the body;
- Analyze medical terms related to the endocrine glands and their hormones;
- Describe the abnormal conditions resulting from excessive and deficient secretions of the endocrine glands; and
- Identify laboratory tests, clinical procedures, and abbreviations related to endocrinology.

I. Introduction

The endocrine system is composed of **glands** located in many different regions of the body, all of which release specific chemical substances directly into the bloodstream. These chemical substances, called **hormones** (from the Greek work *hormōn,* meaning urging on), can regulate the many and varied functions of an organism. For example, one hormone stimulates the growth of bones, another causes the maturation of sex organs and reproductive cells, and another controls the metabolic rate (metabolism) within all the individual cells of the body. In addition, one powerful endocrine gland near the brain secretes a wide variety of different hormones that travel through the bloodstream and regulate the activities of other endocrine glands.

Hormones produce their effects by binding to **receptors,** which are recognition sites in the various **target** tissues on which the hormones act. The receptors initiate specific biological effects when the hormones bind to them. Each hormone has its own receptor, and binding of a receptor by a hormone is much like the interaction of a key and a lock.

All the **endocrine glands,** no matter which hormones they produce, secrete their hormones directly into the bloodstream rather than into ducts leading to the exterior of the body. Those glands that send their chemical substances into ducts and out of the body are called **exocrine glands.** Examples of exocrine glands are sweat, mammary, mucous, salivary, and lacrimal (tear) glands.

The ductless, internally secreting **endocrine glands** are listed below. Locate these glands on Figure 18–1.

(1) thyroid gland
(2) parathyroid glands (four glands)
(3) adrenal glands (one pair)
(4) pancreas (islets of Langerhans)
(5) pituitary gland
(6) ovaries in female (one pair)
(7) testes in male (one pair)
(8) pineal gland
(9) thymus gland

The last two glands on this list, the pineal and the thymus glands, are included as endocrine glands because they are ductless, although little is known about their endocrine function in the human body. The **pineal gland,** located in the central portion of the brain, is believed to secrete a substance called **melatonin.** Melatonin contributes to the process of skin pigmentation in lower animals, such as frogs and fishes. In mammals, melatonin is believed to affect the brain and influence the rate of gonad (ovary and testis) maturation. Calcification of the pineal gland can occur and can be an important radiological landmark when x-rays of the brain are examined.

The **thymus gland,** located behind the sternum in the mediastinum, resembles a lymph gland in structure. It contains lymphatic tissue and antibody-producing lymphocytes. The gland produces a hormone, **thymosin,** and is important in the development of immune responses in newborns (it is large in children but shrinks in adults). Its endocrine function is not well understood. Removal of the thymus gland is helpful in treating a muscular-neurological disorder called myasthenia gravis.

Some hormones are produced by organs other than the endocrine glands already mentioned. For example, the kidney secretes a hormone called **erythropoietin,** which stimulates the production of red blood cells by the bone marrow. The gastrointestinal tract secretes three hormones, **gastrin, secretin,** and **cholecystokinin.** These hormones stimulate the secretion of gastric acid and enzymes (gastrin), the secretion of pancreatic enzymes (secretin), and the contraction of the gallbladder (cholecystokinin). The skin produces **vitamin D,** which is also considered a hormone. Vitamin D stimulates the absorption of calcium from the gastrointestinal tract and is necessary for the maintenance of proper amounts of calcium in the bones and in the bloodstream.

Figure 18–1

The endocrine system.

Table 18–1. ENDOCRINE TISSUE (APART FROM MAJOR GLANDS): LOCATION, SECRETION, AND ACTION

Location	Secretion	Action
Body cells	Prostaglandins	Contract uterus Lower blood pressure Clump platelets Lower acid secretion in stomach
Gastrointestinal tract	Cholecystokinin Gastrin Secretin	Contracts gallbladder Stimulates gastric secretion Stimulates pancreatic enzymes
Kidney	Erythropoietin	Stimulates erythrocyte production
Pineal gland	Melatonin	Affects brain and releases hormones (gonadotropins)
Skin	Vitamin D	Affects absorption of calcium
Thymus gland	Thymosin	Affects immune response

Prostaglandins are hormone-like substances that affect the body in many ways. First found in semen (produced by the prostate gland) but now recognized in cells throughout the body, prostaglandins stimulate the contraction of the uterus; regulate body temperature, platelet aggregation, and acid secretion in the stomach; and have the ability to lower blood pressure.

Endocrine tissue (apart from the major glands) is reviewed in Table 18–1. Use it as a reference.

II. Thyroid Gland

A. Location and Structure

Label Figure 18–2.

The **thyroid gland** is composed of a **right** and a **left lobe** (1) on either side of the **trachea** (2), just below a large piece of cartilage called the **thyroid cartilage** (3). The thyroid cartilage covers the larynx and produces the prominence on the neck known as the Adam's apple. The **isthmus** (4) of the thyroid gland is a narrow strip of glandular tissue that connects the two lobes on the ventral surface of the trachea.

B. Function

Two of the hormones secreted by the thyroid gland are **thyroxine** or **tetraiodothyronine (T_4) and triiodothyronine (T_3). These hormones are synthesized in the thyroid gland from iodine,** which is picked up from the blood circulating through the gland, and from an amino acid called tyrosine. T_4 (containing four atoms of iodine) is much more concentrated in the blood, whereas T_3 (containing three atoms of iodine) is far more potent in affecting the metabolism of cells. Most thyroid hormone is bound to protein molecules as it travels in the bloodstream.

T_4 and T_3 are necessary in the body to maintain a normal level of metabolism in all body cells. Cells need oxygen to carry on metabolic processes, one aspect of which is the burning of food to release the energy stored within the food. Thyroid hormone aids cells in their

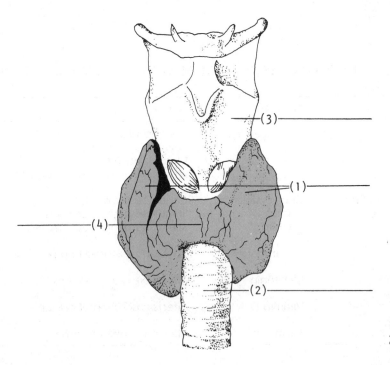

Figure 18–2

Thyroid gland, ventral view.

Figure 18–3

The thyroid gland, its hormones and actions.

uptake of oxygen and thus supports the metabolic rate in the body. Injections of thyroid hormone will raise the metabolic rate, whereas removal of the thyroid gland, diminishing thyroid hormone content in the body, will result in a lower metabolic rate, heat loss, and poor physical and mental development.

A more recently discovered hormone produced by the thyroid gland is called **calcitonin (thyrocalcitonin).** Calcitonin is secreted when calcium levels in the blood are high. It stimulates calcium to leave the blood and enter the bones, thus lowering blood calcium back to normal. Figure 18–3 summarizes the hormones secreted by the thyroid glands.

III. Parathyroid Glands

A. Location and Structure

Label Figure 18–4.

The **parathyroid glands** are four small oval bodies (1) located on the dorsal aspect of the **thyroid gland** (2).

B. Function

Parathyroid hormone (PTH) is secreted by the parathyroid glands. This hormone (also known as **parathormone**) mobilizes **calcium** (a mineral substance) from bones into the

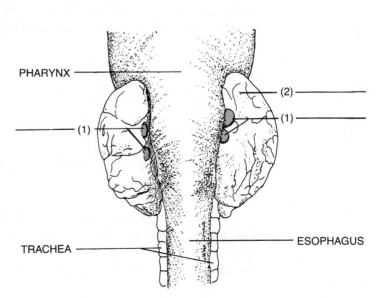

Figure 18–4

Parathyroid glands, dorsal view.

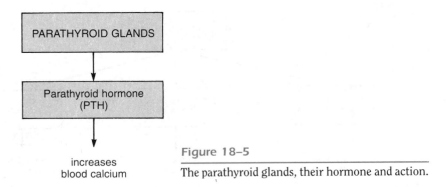

Figure 18–5

The parathyroid glands, their hormone and action.

bloodstream, where calcium is necessary for the proper functioning of body tissues, especially muscles. Normally, calcium in the food we eat is absorbed from the intestine and carried, by the blood, to the bones, where it is stored. The adjustment of the level of calcium in the blood is a good example of the way hormones in general control the **homeostasis** (equilibrium or constancy in the internal environment) of the body. If there is a decrease in blood calcium (as in pregnancy or rickets, a vitamin D–deficiency disease), parathyroid hormone is secreted in larger amounts to cause calcium to leave the bones and enter the bloodstream. Thus, blood calcium levels are brought back to normal (Fig. 18–5). Conversely, any situation of increase in calcium in the bloodstream, such as excess quantity of calcium or vitamin D in the diet, will lead to decreased parathyroid hormone secretion (calcium then leaves the blood to enter bones), decreasing blood calcium, so that homeostasis is again achieved.

IV. Adrenal Glands

A. Location and Structure

Label Figure 18–6.

The **adrenal glands,** also called the **suprarenal glands,** are two small glands situated one on top of each **kidney** (1). Each gland consists of two parts, an outer portion called the **adrenal cortex** (2) and an inner portion called the **adrenal medulla** (3). The cortex and medulla are two glands in one, each secreting its own different endocrine hormones. The cortex secretes hormones called **corticosteroids** (complex chemicals derived from cholesterol), and the medulla secretes hormones called **catecholamines** (chemicals derived from amino acids).

B. Function

The **adrenal cortex** secretes three types of steroid hormones known as **corticosteroids.**

1. **Mineralocorticoids**—These hormones are essential to life because they regulate the amounts of mineral salts (also called **electrolytes**) that are retained in the body. A proper balance of water and salts in the blood and tissues is essential to the normal functioning of the body.

The most important mineralocorticoid hormone is called **aldosterone.** The secretion of aldosterone by the adrenal cortex increases the reabsorption into the bloodstream of **sodium** (a mineral electrolyte commonly found in salts) by the kidney tubules. At the same time, aldosterone stimulates the excretion of another electrolyte called **potassium.**

The secretion of aldosterone increases manyfold in the face of a severe sodium-restricted diet, thereby enabling the body to hold needed salt in the bloodstream.

2. **Glucocorticoids**—These steroid hormones have an important influence on the metabolism of sugars, fats, and proteins within all body cells and have a powerful anti-inflammatory effect.

Cortisol (also called **hydrocortisone**) is the most important glucocorticoid hormone. Cortisol increases the ability of cells to make new sugars out of fats and proteins (gluconeogenesis) and regulates the quantity of sugars, fats, and proteins in the blood and cells.

Cortisone is a hormone very similar to cortisol and can be prepared synthetically. Cortisone is useful in treating inflammatory conditions such as rheumatoid arthritis.

3. **Androgens, Estrogens, and Progestins**—These are male and female hormones that maintain the secondary sex characteristics, such as beard and breast development, and are necessary for reproduction. These hormones are also produced in the ovaries and testes. Excess adrenal androgen secretion in females leads to **virilism** (development of male characteristics), and excess adrenal estrogen and progestin secretion in males produces **feminization** (development of feminine characteristics).

The adrenal medulla secretes two types of **catecholamine** hormones:

1. **Epinephrine (adrenaline)**—This hormone increases cardiac rate, dilates bronchial tubes, and stimulates the production of glucose from a storage substance called glycogen when glucose is needed by the body.
2. **Norepinephrine (noradrenaline)**—This hormone constricts vessels and raises blood pressure.

Both epinephrine and norepinephrine are called **sympathomimetic** agents because they mimic, or copy, the actions of the sympathetic nervous system. During times of stress, these

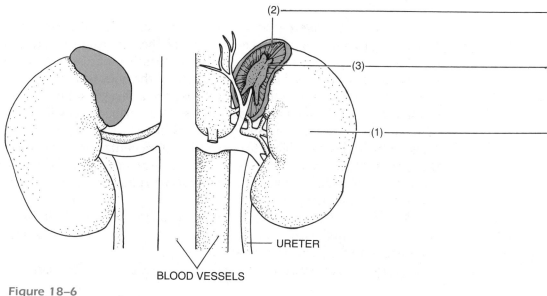

(2) —

(3) —

(1) —

URETER

BLOOD VESSELS

Figure 18–6

The adrenal glands.

Figure 18–7

The adrenal cortex, adrenal medulla, their hormones and actions.

hormones are secreted by the adrenal medulla in response to nervous stimulation. They help the body respond to crisis situations by raising blood pressure, increasing heartbeat and respiration, and bringing sugar out of storage in the cells.

Figure 18–7 summarizes the hormones that are secreted by the adrenal glands, and their actions.

V. Pancreas

A. Location and Structure

Label Figure 18–8.

The **pancreas** (1) is located behind the **stomach** (2) in the region of the first and second lumbar vertebrae. The specialized cells in the pancreas that produce hormones are called the **islets of Langerhans** (islet cells of the pancreas).

B. Function

The islets of Langerhans produce two hormones, **insulin** (produced by beta cells) and **glucagon** (produced by alpha cells). Both of these hormones play a role in the proper metabolism of sugars and starches in the body. Insulin is necessary in the bloodstream so that sugars can pass from the blood into the cells of the body where they are burned to release energy. When blood sugar **(glucose)** is above normal level, insulin is released by the islet cells of the pancreas. The insulin causes glucose to enter body cells to be used for energy and stimulates the conversion of **glucose** to **glycogen** (a starch-storage form of sugar) in the liver. Thus, sugar can leave the blood to be stored (as glycogen) or used to release energy. Glucagon, the opposite "twin" of insulin, is released into the blood when sugar levels are below normal. It causes the breakdown of stored liver **glycogen** to **glucose,** so that there is a rise in the sugar content of blood leaving the liver.

The islets of Langerhans carry on the endocrine functions of the pancreas, and other cells within the organ carry on its exocrine functions. These cells secrete digestive enzymes and juices into the gastrointestinal tract (see Chapter 5).

Figure 18–9 reviews the secretions from the islet cells of the pancreas and their actions.

Figure 18–8

The pancreas.

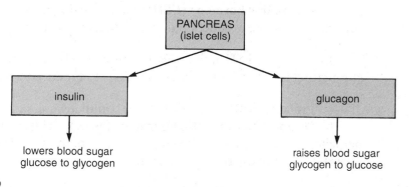

Figure 18–9

The pancreas (islets of Langerhans), its hormones and actions.

VI. Pituitary Gland

A. Location and Structure

Label Figure 18–10.

The **pituitary gland,** also called the **hypophysis,** is a small, pea-sized gland located at the base of the brain in a small, pocket-like depression of the skull called the **sella turcica.** It is a well-protected gland with the entire mass of the brain above it and the nasal cavity below. The ancient Greeks imagined that its function was to produce *pituita* or nasal secretion.

The pituitary consists of two distinct parts: an **anterior lobe** called the **adenohypophysis** (1), which is formed by an upgrowth from the pharynx and is glandular in nature; and a **posterior lobe** called the **neurohypophysis** (2), which is derived from a downgrowth from the base of the brain and is composed of nervous tissue. The **hypothalamus** (3) is a region of the brain that is in close proximity to the pituitary gland. Signals transmitted from the hypothalamus control the secretions by the pituitary gland. Secretion from the neurohypophysis is controlled by nerve fibers originating in the hypothalamus and ending in the neurohypophysis. Secretion by the adenohypophysis is controlled by special hormones called **releasing** and **inhibiting factors.** These hormones are secreted by the hypothalamus and pass to the adenohypophysis by way of special capillaries.

B. Function

The hormones of the **anterior pituitary gland** are

1. **Growth hormone (GH; also called somatotropin)**—This hormone acts on bone tissue to accelerate its growth in the body.
2. **Thyroid-stimulating hormone (TSH; also called thyrotropin)**—This hormone stimulates the growth of the thyroid gland and its secretion of thyroxine.
3. **Adrenocorticotropic hormone (ACTH)**—This hormone stimulates the growth of the adrenal cortex and increases its secretion of steroid hormones (primarily cortisol).
4. **Gonadotropic hormones**—There are several gonadotropic hormones that influence the growth and hormone secretion of the ovaries in females and testes in males. In the female, **follicle-stimulating hormone (FSH)** and **luteinizing hormone (LH)** stimulate the growth of eggs in the ovaries, production of hormones, and ovulation.

In the male, FSH influences the production of sperm and LH (as interstitial cell–stimulating hormone) stimulates the testes to produce testosterone.

5. **Prolactin (PRL)**—This hormone stimulates and sustains milk production after birth.
6. **Melanocyte-stimulating hormone (MSH)**—This hormone influences the formation of melanin and causes increased pigmentation of the skin. This effect is observed only when hypersecretion of the hormone occurs.

The **posterior pituitary gland** secretes two important hormones. These hormones are formed in the hypothalamus but secreted through the posterior pituitary gland:

1. **Antidiuretic hormone (ADH)**—This hormone, also known as **vasopressin,** stimulates the reabsorption of water by the kidney tubules. In addition, ADH can also increase blood pressure by constricting arterioles.
2. **Oxytocin**—This hormone stimulates the uterus to contract during childbirth and maintains labor during childbirth. Oxytocin is also secreted during suckling and causes the production of milk from the mammary glands.

Figure 18–11 reviews the hormones secreted by the pituitary gland and their functions.

Figure 18–10

Pituitary gland.

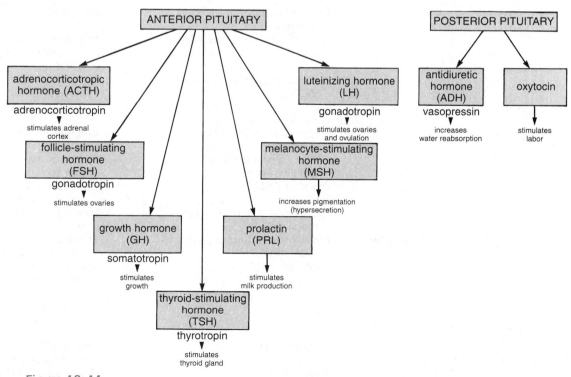

Figure 18–11

The pituitary gland, its hormones and actions.

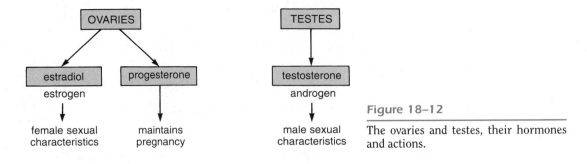

Figure 18–12

The ovaries and testes, their hormones and actions.

Table 18–2. MAJOR ENDOCRINE GLANDS, THE HORMONES THEY PRODUCE, AND THEIR ACTIONS

Endocrine Gland	Hormone	Action
Thyroid	Thyroxin, triiodothyronine	Increases metabolism in body cells
	Calcitonin	Lowers blood calcium
Parathyroids	Parathyroid hormone	Increases blood calcium
Adrenals		
Cortex	Aldosterone (mineralocorticoid)	Increases reabsorption of sodium
	Cortisol (glucocorticoid)	Increases blood sugar
	Androgens, estrogens, and progestins	Maintain secondary sex characteristics
Medulla	Epinephrine (adrenaline)	Sympathomimetic
	Norepinephrine (noradrenaline)	Sympathomimetic
Pancreas		
Islet cells	Insulin	Decreases blood sugar (glucose to glycogen)
	Glucagon	Increases blood sugar (glycogen to glucose)
Pituitary		
Anterior lobe	Growth hormone (GH; somatotropin)	Increases bone and tissue growth
	Thyroid-stimulating hormone (TSH)	Stimulates production of thyroxine and growth of the thyroid gland
	Adrenocorticotropic hormone (ACTH)	Stimulates secretion of hormones from the adrenal cortex, especially cortisol
	Gonadotropins Follicle-stimulating hormone (FSH)	Oogenesis and spermatogenesis
	Luteinizing hormone (LH); or ICSH in a male	Promotes ovulation; testosterone secretion
	Prolactin (PRL)	Promotes growth of breast tissue and milk secretion
	Melanocyte-stimulating hormone (MSH)	Increases pigmentation of the skin
Posterior lobe	Antidiuretic hormone (ADH; vasopressin)	Stimulates reabsorption of water by kidney tubules
	Oxytocin	Stimulates contraction of the uterus during labor and childbirth
Ovaries	Estradiol	Develops and maintains secondary sex characteristics in the female
	Progesterone	Prepares and maintains the uterus in pregnancy
Testes	Testosterone	Promotes growth and maintenance of secondary sex characteristics in the male

VII. Ovaries

A. Location and Structure

The **ovaries** are two small glands located in the lower abdominal region of the female. The ovaries produce the female gamete, the ovum, as well as hormones that are responsible for female sex characteristics and regulation of the menstrual cycle.

B. Function

The ovarian hormones are **estradiol** (an estrogen) and **progesterone.** Estradiol is responsible for the development and maintenance of secondary sex characteristics, such as hair and breast development. Progesterone is responsible for the preparation and maintenance of the uterus in pregnancy.

VIII. Testes

A. Location and Structure

The **testes** are two small, ovoid glands suspended from the inguinal region of the male by the spermatic cord and surrounded by the scrotal sac. The testes produce the male gametes, spermatozoa, as well as the male hormone called **testosterone.**

B. Function

Testosterone is an **androgen** (male steroid hormone) that stimulates and promotes the growth of secondary sex characteristics in the male (development of beard and pubic hair, deepening of voice, and distribution of fat).

Figure 18–12 reviews the hormones secreted by the ovaries and testes.

Table 18–2 lists the major endocrine glands, their hormones, and the actions they produce.

IX. Vocabulary

This list will help you review many of the new terms introduced in the text. Short definitions will reinforce your understanding of the terms. See Section XVIII of this chapter for help in pronouncing the more difficult terms.

Major Glands

adrenal cortex   The outer section of each adrenal gland.

adrenal medulla   The inner section of each adrenal gland.

ovaries   Two endocrine glands in a female's lower abdomen; responsible for egg production and estrogen and progesterone secretion.

pancreas   Endocrine gland behind the stomach. Islet cells (islets of Langerhans) secrete hormones from the pancreas.

parathyroid glands	Four small endocrine glands on the posterior side of the thyroid gland.
pituitary gland (hypophysis)	Endocrine gland at the base of the brain; composed of an anterior **(adeno-hypophysis)** and a posterior **(neurohypophysis)** lobe.
testes	Two endocrine glands enclosed in the scrotal sac of a male; responsible for sperm production and testosterone secretion.
thyroid gland	Endocrine gland in the neck.

Hormones

adrenaline	Produced by the adrenal medulla; also called **epinephrine.** Adrenaline increases heart rate and blood pressure.
adrenocorticotropic hormone (ACTH)	Produced by the anterior lobe of the pituitary gland (adenohypophysis); also called **adrenocorticotropin.** ACTH stimulates the adrenal cortex.
aldosterone	Produced by the adrenal cortex; increases salt (sodium) reabsorption.
androgen	Male hormone produced by the testes and to a lesser extent by the adrenal cortex; testosterone is an example.
antidiuretic hormone (ADH)	Secreted by the posterior lobe of the pituitary gland (neurohypophysis). ADH increases reabsorption of water by the kidney and is also known as **vaso-pressin.**
calcitonin	Produced by the thyroid gland. Calcitonin lowers blood calcium. Also called **thyrocalcitonin.**
cortisol	Produced by the adrenal cortex; increases blood sugar.
epinephrine	Produced by the adrenal medulla; also called **adrenaline.** Epinephrine (a sympathomimetic) increases heart rate and blood pressure, and dilates airways.
estradiol	An estrogen (female hormone) produced by the ovaries.
estrogen	Female hormone produced by the ovaries and to a lesser extent by the adrenal cortex.
follicle-stimulating hormone (FSH)	Hormone produced by the anterior lobe of the pituitary gland (adenohypophysis). FSH stimulates hormone secretion and egg production by the ovaries and sperm production by the testes.
glucagon	Hormone produced by the islet cells of the pancreas; increases blood sugar by conversion of glycogen (starch) to glucose.
growth hormone (GH)	Produced by the anterior lobe of the pituitary gland (adenohypophysis); also called **somatotropin.** GH stimulates the growth of bones and tissues.

insulin	Produced by the islet cells (**insula** means island) of the pancreas. Insulin lowers blood sugar by transport and conversion of glucose to glycogen (starch).
luteinizing hormone (LH)	Produced by the anterior lobe of the pituitary gland (adenohypophysis). LH stimulates ovulation in females and (as ICSH) stimulates testosterone secretion in males.
melanocyte-stimulating hormone (MSH)	Produced by the anterior lobe of the pituitary gland (adenohypophysis). High levels of MSH increase pigmentation of the skin.
norepinephrine	Produced by the adrenal medulla; also called **noradrenaline.** Norepinephrine (a sympathomimetic) increases heart rate and blood pressure. Nor- in chemistry means a parent compound from which another is derived.
oxytocin	Secreted by the posterior lobe of the pituitary gland (neurohypophysis). Oxytocin stimulates contraction of the uterus during labor and childbirth.
parathormone (PTH)	Produced by the parathyroid gland; also called **parathyroid hormone.** PTH increases blood calcium.
progesterone	Produced by the ovaries. Progesterone prepares the uterus for pregnancy.
prolactin (PRL)	Produced by the anterior lobe of the pituitary gland (adenohypophysis). PRL promotes milk secretion.
somatotropin	Produced by the anterior lobe of the pituitary gland (adenohypophysis); also called **growth hormone.**
testosterone	Male hormone produced by the testes.
thyroid-stimulating hormone (TSH)	Produced by the anterior lobe of the pituitary gland (adenohypophysis). TSH acts on the thyroid gland to promote its functioning; also called **thyrotropin.**
thyroxine (T_4)	Produced by the thyroid gland; also called **tetraiodothyronine.** T_4 increases metabolism in cells.
triiodothyronine (T_3)	Produced by the thyroid gland; T_3 increases metabolism in cells.
vasopressin	Secreted by the posterior lobe of the pituitary gland (neurohypophysis); also called **antidiuretic hormone.**

Related Terms

catecholamines	Hormones derived from an amino acid and secreted by the adrenal medulla. Epinephrine is a catecholamine.
corticosteroids	Hormones (steroid) produced by the adrenal cortex. Glucocorticoids and mineralocorticoids are examples.

electrolyte	A mineral salt found in the blood and tissues and necessary for proper functioning of cells; potassium, sodium, and calcium are examples.
glucocorticoid	Hormone secreted by the adrenal cortex; necessary for use of sugars, fats, and proteins by the body and for the body's normal response to stress. Cortisol is an example.
homeostasis	The tendency in an organism to maintain a constant internal environment.
hormone	A substance that is produced by an endocrine gland and that travels through the blood to a distant organ or gland where it acts to modify the structure or function of that organ or gland.
hypothalamus	A region of the brain that lies below the thalamus and above the pituitary gland. It produces releasing factors that stimulate the pituitary gland to release hormones.
mineralocorticoid	Steroid hormone produced by the adrenal cortex to regulate the mineral salts (electrolytes) and water balance in the body. Aldosterone is an example.
sella turcica	The cavity in the skull that contains the pituitary gland.
steroid	Complex substance related to fats (derived from a sterol, such as cholesterol) and of which many hormones are made. Examples of steroids are estrogens, androgens, glucocorticoids and mineralocorticoids. **Ster/o** means solid, **-ol** means oil.
sympathomimetic	Pertaining to mimicking or copying the effect of the sympathetic nervous system. Adrenaline is a sympathomimetic hormone (raises blood pressure and heart rate and dilates airways).

X. Combining Forms, Suffixes, Prefixes, and Terminology: Glands and Related Terms

Write the meaning of the medical term in the space provided.

Glands

Combining Forms			
Combining Form	Meaning	Terminology	Meaning
aden/o	gland	adenectomy _____
adren/o	adrenal glands	adrenopathy _____
adrenal/o	adrenal glands	adrenalectomy _____

gonad/o	sex glands (ovaries and testes)	gonadotropin _____

-tropin means to act upon, to turn. A gonadotropin acts on (stimulates) the gonads. Examples are FSH and LH.

hypogonadism _____

Deficiency of gonadotropins can produce hypogonadism.

pancreat/o	pancreas	pancreatectomy _____
parathyroid/o	parathyroid gland	parathyroidectomy _____
pituitar/o	pituitary gland	hypopituitarism _____

Pituitary dwarfism (see page 662, Section XI, Abnormal Conditions) is caused by hypopituitarism.

thyr/o	thyroid gland	thyrotropin hormone _____

Thyroid-stimulating hormone (TSH).

thyroid/o	thyroid gland	thyroiditis _____

Related Terms

Combining Forms

Combining Form	Meaning	Terminology	Meaning
andr/o	male	androgen _____	

Androgens are produced by the testes in males and by the adrenal cortex in males and females.

calc/o	calcium	hypercalcemia _____	
		hypocalcemia _____	
cortic/o	cortex, outer region	corticosteroid _____	

Cortisol is an example of a corticosteroid.

crin/o	secrete	endocrinologist _____	
dips/o	thirst	polydipsia _____	

Symptom associated with both diabetes mellitus and diabetes insipidus (see page 660, Section XI, Abnormal Conditions).

estr/o	female	estrogenic _____
gluc/o	sugar	glucagon _____

-agon means to assemble or gather together. Glucagon raises blood sugar by stimulating its release from glycogen into the bloodstream.

glyc/o	sugar	hyperglycemia _____
		glycogen _____

Glycogen is animal starch that can be broken down to glucose by the hormone glucagon.

home/o	sameness	homeostasis _____

-stasis means to control.

hormon/o	hormone	hormonal _____
insulin/o	insulin	hypoinsulinism _____
kal/i	potassium (an electrolyte)	hypokalemia _____

This condition can occur in dehydration and with excessive vomiting and diarrhea. The heart is particularly sensitive to potassium loss.

lact/o	milk	prolactin _____

-in means a substance.

myx/o	mucus	myxedema _____

Mucus-like material accumulates under the skin. See page 656, Section XI, Abnormal Conditions, under hypothyroidism.

natr/o	sodium (an electrolyte)	hyponatremia _____

Occurs with hyposecretion of the adrenal cortex as salts and water leave the body.

phys/o	growing	hypophysectomy _____

The hypophysis is the pituitary gland, which is so named because it grows from the undersurface of the brain.

somat/o	body	somatotropin _____

Also called growth hormone.

ster/o	solid structure	steroid _____

This complex, solid, ring-shaped molecule resembles a sterol (such as cholesterol); many hormones (androgens, estrogens, glucocorticoids, and mineralocorticoids) are steroids.

toc/o	childbirth	oxy<u>toc</u>in _____
		oxy- means swift, rapid.
toxic/o	poison	thyro<u>toxic</u>osis _____
		This condition is caused by excessive thyroid gland activity and oversecretion of thyroid hormone. Symptoms are sweating, weight loss, tachycardia, and nervousness.
ur/o	urine	antidi<u>ur</u>etic hormone _____
		This posterior pituitary hormone affects the kidneys and reduces water loss.

Suffixes

Suffix	Meaning	Terminology	Meaning
-agon	assemble, gather together	gluc<u>agon</u> _____	
-in, ine	a substance	epinephr<u>ine</u> _____	
-tropin	stimulating the function of (to turn or act upon)	adrenocortico<u>tropin</u> _____	
		-tropic is the adjective form (adrenocorticotropic hormone).	
-uria	urine condition	glycos<u>uria</u> _____	
		A symptom of diabetes mellitus.	

Prefixes

Prefix	Meaning	Terminology	Meaning
eu-	good, normal	<u>eu</u>thyroid _____	
oxy-	rapid, sharp, acid	<u>oxy</u>tocin _____	
pan-	all	<u>pan</u>hypopituitarism _____	
tetra-	four	<u>tetra</u>iodothyronine _____	
		iod/o means iodine.	
tri-	three	<u>tri</u>iodothyronine _____	

XI. Abnormal Conditions

Thyroid Gland

Enlargement of the thyroid gland is known as **goiter.** Goiter may be a symptom of many different conditions. **Endemic (en-** means in; **dem/o** means people) **goiter** occurs in certain regions and peoples as a result of deficiency of **iodine** in the diet. A glue-like or gelatinous material called **colloid** collects in the thyroid, and the gland enlarges as it works harder to compensate for the scarcity of iodine. Treatment of this type of goiter is to increase the supply of iodine in the diet.

Another type of goiter is **nodular** or **adenomatous goiter,** in which hyperplasia occurs as well as nodules and adenomas. Some patients develop hyperthyroidism with symptoms such as rapid pulse, tremors, nervousness, and excessive sweating. Treatment consists of use of thyroid hormone to suppress the normal thyroid functioning (by reducing TSH production).

Hypersecretion

hyperthyroidism

Overactivity of the thyroid gland.

The most common form of this condition is known as **thyrotoxicosis** or **Graves' disease.** Hyperplasia of the thyroid parenchyma (glandular cells) occurs, so that excessive hormone is produced. The metabolic rate in cells is increased, leading to thyrotoxic symptoms as in nodular or adenomatous goiter. In addition, **exophthalmia** (protrusion of the eyeballs) occurs as a result of swelling of tissue behind the eyeball. The etiology is unclear, although it is currently thought to be an immunological disorder. Treatment may include thyroidectomy, management with antithyroid drugs that reduce the amount of thyroid hormone produced from the gland, or administration of radioactive iodine, which destroys the overactive glandular tissue. Figure 18–13 shows a patient with exophthalmia and Graves' disease.

Hyposecretion

hypothyroidism

Underactivity of the thyroid gland.

Any one of several conditions can produce hypothyroidism (thyroidectomy, endemic goiter, destruction of the gland by irradiation), but all have similar physiological effects. These include fatigue, muscular and mental sluggishness, and constipation. Two examples of hypothyroidism are

Myxedema—This is advanced hypothyroidism in adulthood. Atrophy of the thyroid gland occurs, and practically no hormone is produced. The skin becomes dry and puffy (edema) because of collection of mucus-like **(myx/o** means mucus) material under the skin. Many patients also develop atherosclerosis because lack of thyroid hormone increases the quantity of blood lipids (fats). Recovery may be complete if thyroid hormone is given soon after symptoms appear. Figure 18–14 shows a patient with myxedema.

Cretinism—Extreme hypothyroidism during infancy and childhood leads to a lack of normal physical and mental growth. Skeletal growth is more inhibited than soft tissue growth, so the **cretin** has the appearance of an obese, short, and stocky child (Fig. 18–15). Treatment consists of administration of thyroid hormone, which may be able to reverse some of the hypothyroid effects.

Figure 18–13

Exophthalmia in Graves' disease. (From Jacob SW, Francone CA, Lossow WJ: Structure and Function in Man, 5th ed. Philadelphia, WB Saunders, 1982, p 555.)

Figure 18–14

Myxedema. (From Jacob SW, Francone CA, Lossow WJ: Structure and Function in Man, 5th ed. Philadelphia, WB Saunders, 1982, p 555.)

Figure 18–15

Cretinism. (From Sheldon H: Boyd's Introduction to the Study of Disease, 10th ed. Philadelphia, Lea & Febiger, 1988, p 562.)

Neoplasms

thyroid carcinoma

Cancer of the thyroid gland.

Some tumors are very slow growing, and others may metastasize widely. Adenomas (benign growths) can be distinguished from carcinomas (malignant growths) by radioactive iodine tracer scans. "Hot" tumor areas (those collecting more radioactivity than surrounding tissues) usually indicate hyperthyroidism and benign growth; "cold," nonfunctional nodules can be either benign or malignant. Ultimately, fine-needle aspiration, surgical biopsy, or excision is often required to make the diagnosis.

Parathyroid Glands

Hypersecretion

hyperparathyroidism

Excessive production of parathormone.

Hypercalcemia occurs as calcium leaves the bones and enters the bloodstream. Bones are decalcified and susceptible to fractures and cysts, as in **osteitis fibrosa cystica.** Kidney stones can occur from hypercalcemia. Etiology is often a parathyroid tumor, which is resected as treatment for the condition.

Hyposecretion

hypoparathyroidism

Deficient production of parathyroid hormone.

Hypocalcemia results as calcium remains in bones and is unable to enter the bloodstream. This leads to muscle and nerve weakness with spasms of muscles, a condition called **tetany** (constant muscle contraction). Administration of calcium plus large quantities of vitamin D (to promote absorption of calcium) can control the calcium level in the bloodstream.

Adrenal Cortex

Hypersecretion

adrenal virilism

Excessive output of adrenal androgens.

Adrenal hyperplasia or tumor can cause this condition in adult women. Symptoms include amenorrhea, **hirsutism** (excessive hair on the face and body), acne, and deepening of the voice. Drug therapy to suppress androgen production and adrenalectomy are possible treatments.

Cushing's syndrome

A group of symptoms produced by excess of cortisol from the adrenal cortex.

Obesity, moon-like fullness of the face, excess deposition of fat in the thoracic region of the back (so-called buffalo hump), hyperglycemia, hypernatremia, hypokalemia, osteoporosis, and hypertension occur with excess cortisol secretion. Etiology may be excess ACTH secretion (called Cushing's disease) or tumor of the adrenal cortex. Figure 18–16 shows a woman with Cushing's syndrome.

Hyposecretion

Addison's disease

Hypofunctioning of the adrenal cortex.

Mineralocorticoids and glucocorticoids are produced in deficent amounts. Hypoglycemia (from deficient glucocorticoids), hyponatremia (excretion of large amounts of water and salts from deficient mineralocorticoids), weakness, weight loss, and darker pigmentation of the skin (because of increased blood levels of MSH) are symptoms of the condition. Treatment consists of daily cortisone administration and intake of salts.

Figure 18–16

(A) A patient with Cushing's syndrome. *(B)* Signs and symptoms disappeared after adrenalectomy and therapy. (*A* and *B*, From Forsham PH: The adrenal cortex. *In* Williams RH [ed]: Textbook of Endocrinology, 4th ed. Philadelphia, WB Saunders, 1968, p 352.)

Adrenal Medulla

Hypersecretion

pheochromocytoma

Tumor of the adrenal medulla (tumor cells stain a dark or dusky **[phe/o]** color **[chrom/o]**).

The tumor cells produce excess secretion of epinephrine and norepinephrine. Symptoms are hypertension, palpitations, severe headaches, sweating, flushing of the face, and muscle spasms. Surgery to remove the tumor and administration of antihypertensive drugs are possible treatments.

Pancreas

Hypersecretion

hyperinsulinism

Excess secretion of insulin causing hypoglycemia.

Etiology may be a tumor of the pancreas (benign adenoma or carcinoma) or overdose of insulin. Hypoglycemia occurs as insulin draws sugar out of the bloodstream. Fainting spells, convulsions, and loss of consciousness are common because a minimal level of blood sugar is necessary for proper mental functioning.

Hyposecretion

diabetes mellitus

Lack of insulin secretion or resistance of insulin to promote sugar, starch, and fat metabolism in cells.

In diabetes mellitus, insulin insufficiency or ineffectiveness prevents sugar from leaving the blood (hyperglycemia occurs) and entering the body cells, where it is normally used to produce energy. There are two major types of diabetes mellitus.

Type I diabetes, also called **insulin-dependent diabetes mellitus (IDDM),** with onset usually in childhood, involves destruction of the beta islet cells of the pancreas with complete deficiency of insulin in the body. Patients are usually thin and require frequent injections of insulin to maintain a normal level of glucose in the blood.

Type II diabetes, also called **non–insulin-dependent diabetes mellitus (NIDDM)** is a separate disease from type I, with a different inheritance pattern. Patients are usually older, and obesity is very common. The islet cells are not destroyed, and there is a relative deficiency of insulin secretion with a resistance by target tissues to the action of insulin. Treatment is with diet, weight reduction, exercise, and if necessary, insulin or oral hypoglycemic agents. The oral hypoglycemic agents can stimulate the release of insulin from the pancreas and improve the body's sensitivity to insulin.

Diabetes is associated with both primary and secondary complications. **Primary complications** include **ketoacidosis** (fats are improperly burned, leading to an accumulation of ketones in the body) and **coma** when blood sugar concentration gets too high or the patient receives an insufficient amount of insulin. **Hypoglycemia** can occur when too much insulin is taken by the patient.

Secondary (long-term) **complications** occur over many years after the patient develops diabetes. These include destruction of the blood vessels of the retina **(diabetic retinopathy),** causing visual loss and blindness; destruction of the kidneys **(diabetic nephropathy),** causing renal insufficiency and often requiring hemodialysis or renal transplantation; destruction of blood vessels, with **atherosclerosis;** and destruction of nerves **(diabetic neuropathy)** involving pain or loss of sensation, most commonly in the extremities.

Pituitary Gland (Anterior Lobe)

Hypersecretion

acromegaly

Enlargement of the extremities (**acr/o** means extremities) caused by hypersecretion of the anterior pituitary *after puberty*.

An excess of growth hormone is produced by adenomas of the pituitary gland that occur during adulthood. This causes the bones in the hands, feet, face, and jaw to grow abnormally large in size, producing a characteristic Frankenstein-type facial appearance. The pituitary adenoma can be irradiated or surgically removed. Figure 18–17 shows a woman with acromegaly.

Figure 18–17

Progression of acromegaly: *(A)* patient at age 9; *(B)* age 16, with possible early features of acromegaly; *(C)* age 33, well established acromegaly; *(D)* age 52, end-stage acromegaly. *(A–D,* From Clinical Pathological Conference. Am J Med 20:133, 1956.)

gigantism

Hyperfunctioning of the pituitary gland *before puberty,* leading to abnormal overgrowth of the body.

Benign adenomas of the pituitary gland that occur before a child reaches puberty produce an excess of growth hormone. Gigantism can be corrected by early diagnosis in childhood, followed by resection of the tumor or irradiation of the pituitary.

Hyposecretion

dwarfism

Congenital hyposecretion of growth hormone; hypopituitary dwarfism.

The children affected are normal mentally, but their bones remain small and underdeveloped. Treatment consists of administration of growth hormone. Achondroplastic dwarfs differ from hypopituitary dwarfs in that they suffer from a genetic defect in cartilage formation that adversely affects the growth of bones.

panhypopituitarism

All pituitary hormones are deficient.

Tumors of the sella turcica as well as arterial aneurysms may be etiological factors. Functions of target glands (adrenals, thyroid, ovaries, and testes) are also adversely affected.

Pituitary Gland (Posterior Lobe)

Hypersecretion

syndrome of inappropriate ADH (SIADH)

Excessive secretion of antidiuretic hormone.

Hypersecretion of ADH produces excess water retention in the body. Treatment consists of dietary water restriction. Tumor, drug reactions, and head injury are some of the possible etiological factors.

Table 18–3. ABNORMAL CONDITIONS OF ENDOCRINE GLANDS

Endocrine Gland	Hypersecretion	Hyposecretion
Adrenal cortex	Adrenal virilism Cushing's syndrome	Addison's disease
Adrenal medulla	Pheochromocytoma	
Pancreas	Hyperinsulinism	Diabetes mellitus
Parathyroid glands	Hyperparathyroidism (osteitis fibrosa cystica)	Hypoparathyroidism (tetany, hypocalcemia)
Pituitary (anterior lobe)	Acromegaly Gigantism	Dwarfism Panhypopituitarism
Pituitary (posterior lobe)	Syndrome of inappropriate antidiuretic hormone	Diabetes insipidus
Thyroid gland	Exophthalmic goiter (Graves' disease, thyrotoxicosis) Nodular (adenomatous) goiter	Cretinism (children) Endemic goiter Myxedema (adults)

Hyposecretion

diabetes insipidus	Insufficient secretion of antidiuretic hormone (vasopressin).

Deficient antidiuretic hormone causes the kidney tubules to fail to hold back (reabsorb) needed water and salts. Clinical symptoms include polyuria and polydipsia. Synthetic preparations of ADH are administered with nasal sprays or intramuscularly as treatment. **Insipidus** means tasteless, reflecting the condition of dilute urine.

Table 18–3 reviews the abnormal conditions associated with hypersecretions and hyposecretions of the endocrine glands.

XII. Laboratory Tests

serum and urine tests	These tests measure hormones and other substances (electrolytes and glucose) in blood and urine as indicators of endocrine function.
glucose tolerance test (GTT)	This test measures the glucose levels in a blood sample from a fasting patient **(fasting blood sugar)** and in specimens taken 30 minutes, 1 hour, 2 hours, and 3 hours after ingestion of 100 gm of glucose. Delayed return of blood glucose to normal level indicates diabetes mellitus.
radioimmunoassay (RIA)	This test measures hormone levels in plasma. The test is based on the ability of antibodies to bind specifically to radioactively labeled hormone molecules and to nonradioactively labeled molecules.
thyroid function tests	These tests measure the levels of T_4, T_3, and TSH in the bloodstream.

XIII. Clinical Procedures

exophthalmometry	This test measures the extent of eyeball protrusion as evidenced in Graves' disease.
CT scans (computed tomography)	These transverse views of the pituitary gland and other endocrine organs are useful in diagnosis of pathological conditions.
thyroid scan	A radioactive compound is administered and localizes in the thyroid gland. The gland is then visualized with a scanner device to detect tumors or nodules.
radioactive iodine uptake	Radioactive iodine is administered orally, and its uptake into the thyroid gland is measured as evidence of thyroid function.
skull x-ray and tomography of the sella turcica	The fossa in the base of the cranium that houses the pituitary gland is x-rayed, and pictures are taken in sections to show the area in depth.

XIV. ABBREVIATIONS

ACTH	Adrenocorticotropic hormone	LH	Luteinizing hormone
ADH	Antidiuretic hormone (vasopressin)	MSH	Melanocyte-stimulating hormone
BMR	Basal metabolic rate (an indicator of thyroid function, but not in current use)	Na	Sodium
		NIDDM	Non-insulin-dependent diabetes mellitus
DI	Diabetes insipidus		
DM	Diabetes mellitus	17-OH	17-hydroxycorticosteroids
FBS	Fasting blood sugar	PRL	Prolactin
FSH	Follicle-stimulating hormone	PTH	Parathyroid hormone (parathormone)
GH	Growth hormone	RIA	Radioimmunoassay; measures hormone levels in plasma
GTT	Glucose tolerance test		
hGH	Human growth hormone	SIADH	Syndrome of inappropriate ADH
ICSH	Interstitial cell-stimulating hormone	T_3	Triiodothyronine
IDDM	Insulin-dependent diabetes mellitus	T_4	Thyroxine
K	Potassium	TFT	Thyroid function test
		TSH	Thyroid-stimulating hormone

XV. Practical Applications

Answers to the questions in each case report are on page 673 at the end of Answers to Exercises section.

Case Report 1

A 24-year-old college student, known diabetic, was admitted for treatment of ketoacidosis. He had a several-year history of diabetes and had been taking insulin in the morning and in the evening. After the history was pieced together from the patient and his friends, it appeared that he had been getting progressively ill over several days following a flu-like episode and may well not have taken his insulin on the day of admission. He was found, slightly drowsy and confused, by classmates. His respirations were rapid, his pulse was 126, and he offered no sensible answers to questions. Blood sugar level was elevated at 728 mg/dL [100 mg/dL is normal], and blood ketones were positive. The patient was treated with insulin intravenously, and over the course of the next 24 hours the ketoacidosis cleared.

Questions

1. Ketoacidosis is a complication of
   (A) Diabetes insipidus
   (B) Diabetes mellitus
   (C) Both A and B
2. A symptom of ketoacidosis is
   (A) Tachypnea
   (B) Bradycardia

(C) Hypoglycemia

3. Ketoacidosis occurs when
    (A) Insulin blood levels are high
    (B) Sugar is not transported to cells and fats are burned improperly
    (C) Insulin is given intravenously

Case Report 2

A 42-year-old woman presented with a 6-month history of progressive weakness. She had facial and central obesity with muscle wasting in the extremities. As an initial screening test, a 24-hour urine collection for cortisol determination revealed high levels. Her ACTH level was low. On CT scan a 3-cm mass was found in the left adrenal. When the mass was resected, it proved to be a 3-cm, smooth, yellow adrenocortical adenoma that secreted cortisol. The patient's condition (Cushing's syndrome) normalized after surgery.

Questions

1. Symptoms of Cushing's syndrome are
    (A) Hirsutism and hypergonadism
    (B) Palpitations
    (C) Moon-like fullness of the face and deposition of fat

2. What factors pointed to a diagnosis of Cushing's syndrome?
    (A) Pituitary gland tumor on CT scan
    (B) Hypersecretion of ACTH
    (C) Hypersecretion of cortisol and adrenal mass on CT scan

3. Surgery performed to correct this condition was
    (A) Adrenocortical adenoma resection
    (B) Hypophysectomy
    (C) Both A and B

Case Report 3

Graves' disease, as characterized by exophthalmia and stare, was diagnosed in a 51-year-old man. Examination revealed a history of nervousness, palpitation, weight loss, diarrhea, dyspnea on exertion, insomnia, heat intolerance, and fatigue. An ECG showed atrial fibrillation with a ventricular rate of about 180 beats per minute, which was treated with digoxin and propranolol. A chest x-ray film disclosed cardiomegaly. Thyroid function tests showed T_4 and T_3 levels to be elevated, and a thyroid scan showed diffuse enlargement of the gland. The patient was treated with radioactive iodine and is now euthyroid. The exophthalmia has not resolved, however.

Questions

1. Symptoms of Graves' disease are
    (A) bulging eyeballs
    (B) difficult breathing on exertion
    (C) A and B

2. Atrial fibrillation means that
   (A) the heart is enlarged
   (B) the heart rate is less than 180 beats per minute
   (C) the heart rate is rapid and irregular
3. Blood tests revealed that
   (A) the thyroid gland was hypersecreting
   (B) the thyroid gland was hyposecreting
   (C) goiter was present
4. The patient was treated and
   (A) exophthalmia has regressed
   (B) is still having palpitations
   (C) his thyroid gland is functioning normally

XVI. Exercises

Remember to check your answers carefully with those given in Section XVII, Answers to Exercises.

A. Name the endocrine organs (including appropriate lobe or region) that produce the following hormones.

1. follicle-stimulating hormone _____

2. vasopressin _____

3. aldosterone _____

4. insulin _____

5. thyroxine _____

6. cortisol _____

7. gonadotropic hormones _____

8. epinephrine _____

9. oxytocin _____

10. prolactin _____

11. growth hormone _____

12. glucagon _____

13. adrenocorticotropic hormone _____

14. estradiol _____

15. progesterone _____

16. testosterone _____

17. melanocyte-stimulating hormone _____

B. *Give the meaning of the following abbreviations for hormones.*

1. ADH _____

2. ACTH _____

3. LH _____

4. FSH _____

5. TSH _____

6. PTH _____

7. GH _____

8. PRL _____

9. T_4 _____

10. T_3 _____

C. *Match the following hormones with their actions.*

insulin   ADH   thyroxine   ACTH
parathyroid hormone   aldosterone   estradiol   cortisol
testosterone   epinephrine

1. sympathomimetic; raises heart rate and blood pressure _____

2. promotes growth and maintenance of male sex characteristics _____

3. stimulates water reabsorption by kidney tubules; decreases urine output _____

4. increases metabolism in body cells _____

5. raises blood calcium _____

6. increases reabsorption of sodium by kidney tubules _____

7. stimulates secretion of hormones from the adrenal cortex _____

8. increases blood sugar _____

9. helps transport glucose to cells and decreases blood sugar _____

10. develops and maintains female sex characteristics _____

D. *Indicate whether the following conditions are related to hypersecretion or hyposecretion. Also, select from the following the endocrine gland and hormone involved in each disease.*

Glands

thyroid	neurohypophysis
adrenal cortex	adenohypophysis
pancreas	parathyroid gland
testes	ovaries
adrenal medulla	

Hormones

GH	ADH
parathyroid hormone	insulin
cortisol	aldosterone
thyroxine	epinephrine

Disease	*Hypo or Hyper*	*Gland and Hormone*
1. Cushing's syndrome	_____	_____
2. tetany	_____	_____
3. Graves' disease	_____	_____
4. diabetes insipidus	_____	_____
5. acromegaly	_____	_____
6. myxedema	_____	_____
7. osteitis fibrosa cystica	_____	_____
8. diabetes mellitus	_____	_____
9. Addison's disease	_____	_____
10. gigantism	_____	_____
11. endemic goiter	_____	_____
12. cretinism	_____	_____
13. pheochromocytoma	_____	_____

E. Build medical terms from their definitions and word parts given.

1. abnormal condition (poison) of the thyroid gland: thyro _____

2. removal of the pancreas: _____ ectomy

3. condition of deficiency or underdevelopment of the sex organs: hypo _____

4. pertaining to producing female (characteristics): _____ genic

5. removal of the pituitary gland: _____ ectomy

6. deficiency of calcium in the blood: hypo _____

7. excessive sugar in the blood: _____ emia

8. inflammation of the thyroid gland: _____ itis

9. specialist in the study of hormone disorders: _____ ist

10. disease condition of the adrenal glands: adren _____

F. Give the meanings for the following conditions.

1. hyponatremia _____

2. polydipsia _____

3. hyperkalemia _____

4. hypercalcemia _____

5. hypoglycemia _____

6. glycosuria _____

7. euthyroid _____

8. hyperthyroidism _____

9. tetany _____

10. ketoacidosis _____

G. The following hormones are all produced by the anterior lobe of the pituitary gland (note that they all have the same suffix, -tropin). Name the target tissue they act on or stimulate in the body.

1. gonadotropins _____

2. somatotropin _____

3. thyrotropin _____

4. adrenocorticotropin _____

H. Give the meanings for the following medical terms.

1. steroids _____

2. catecholamines _____

3. adenohypophysis _____

4. tetany _____

5. exophthalmia _____

6. mineralocorticoids _____

7. homeostasis _____

8. sympathomimetic _____

9. glucocorticoids _____

10. epinephrine _____

11. glycogen _____

12. androgen _____

13. corticosteroid _____

14. oxytocin _____

15. tetraiodothyronine _____

16. adrenal virilism _____

17. thyroid carcinoma _____

18. hirsutism _____

19. acromegaly _____

20. estradiol _____

I. Give the meanings for the following terms or abbreviations related to diabetes mellitus.

1. IDDM _____

2. diabetic neuropathy _____

3. ketoacidosis _____

4. hypoglycemia _____

5. NIDDM _____

6. diabetic retinopathy _____

7. diabetic coma _____

8. diabetic nephropathy _____

9. atherosclerosis _____

10. hyperglycemia _____

J. Explain the following laboratory tests or clinical procedures related to the endocrine system.

1. thyroid scan _____

2. glucose tolerance test _____

3. RIA _____

4. exophthalmometry _____

5. skull x-ray and tomography of the sella turcica _____

K. Circle the term that best fits the meaning of the sentence.

1. Phyllis was diagnosed with Graves' disease when her husband noticed her (panhypopituitarism, hirsutism, exophthalmia). Her eyes seemed to be bulging out of their sockets.

2. Helen had a primary brain tumor called a (pituitary, thyroid, adrenal) adenoma. Her entire endocrine system was disrupted and her physician recommended surgery and radiation to help relieve her symptoms.

3. Bessie's facial features gradually became "rough" in her late thirties and forties. By the time she was fifty, her children noticed her very large hands and recommended that she see an endocrinologist, who diagnosed her chronically progressive condition as (hyperinsulism, gigantism, acromegaly).

4. Bobby was brought in the emergency room because he was found passed out in the kitchen. He had forgotten his insulin and had now developed (Cushing's disease, hyperparathyroidism, diabetic ketoacidosis).

5. Because her 1-hour test of blood sugar was slightly abnormal, Selma's obstetrician ordered a (glucose tolerance test, thyroid function test, Pap smear) to rule out gestational (hyperthyroidism, chlamydial infection, diabetes).

XVII. Answers to Exercises

A

1. anterior lobe of the pituitary gland (adenohypophysis)
2. posterior lobe of the pituitary gland (neurohypophysis)
3. adrenal cortex
4. islet cells of the pancreas
5. thyroid gland
6. adrenal cortex
7. anterior lobe of the pituitary gland; these hormones are FSH and LH
8. adrenal medulla
9. posterior lobe of the pituitary gland
10. anterior lobe of the pituitary gland
11. anterior lobe of the pituitary gland
12. islet cells of the pancreas
13. anterior lobe of the pituitary gland
14. ovaries
15. ovaries
16. testes
17. anterior lobe of the pituitary gland

B

1. antidiuretic hormone
2. adrenocorticotropin
3. luteinizing hormone
4. follicle-stimulating hormone
5. thyroid-stimulating hormone
6. parathyroid hormone
7. growth hormone
8. prolactin
9. thyroxine
10. triiodothyronine

C

1. epinephrine
2. testosterone
3. ADH
4. thyroxine
5. parathyroid hormone
6. aldosterone
7. ACTH
8. cortisol
9. insulin
10. estradiol

D

1. hypersecretion; adrenal cortex; cortisol
2. hyposecretion; parathyroid gland; parathyroid hormone
3. hypersecretion; thyroid gland; thyroxine
4. hyposecretion; neurohypophysis; ADH
5. hypersecretion; adenohypophysis; GH
6. hyposecretion; thyroid gland; thyroxine
7. hypersecretion; parathyroid gland; parathyroid hormone
8. hyposecretion; pancreas; insulin
9. hyposecretion; adrenal cortex; aldosterone and cortisol
10. hypersecretion; adenohypophysis; GH
11. hyposecretion; thyroid gland; thyroxine
12. hyposecretion; thyroid gland; thyroxine
13. hypersecretion; adrenal medulla; epinephrine

E

1. thyrotoxicosis
2. pancreatectomy
3. hypogonadism
4. estrogenic
5. hypophysectomy
6. hypocalcemia
7. hyperglycemia
8. thyroiditis
9. endocrinologist
10. adrenopathy

F

1. deficient sodium in the blood
2. condition of excessive thirst
3. excessive potassium in the blood
4. excessive calcium in the blood
5. deficient sugar in the blood
6. condition of sugar in the urine
7. normal thyroid function
8. condition of increased secretion from the thyroid gland
9. constant muscle contraction (result of hypoparathyroidism)
10. condition of excessive ketones (acids) in the blood as a result of diabetes mellitus

G

1. the male and female sex organs (ovaries and testes); examples of gonadotropins are FSH and LH
2. bones; another name for somatotropin is growth hormone
3. thyroid gland; another name for thyrotropin is thyroid-stimulating hormone
4. adrenal cortex; another name for adrenocorticotropin is adrenocorticotropic hormone (ACTH)

H

1. Complex substances derived from cholesterol; hormones from the adrenal cortex and sex hormones are steroids.
2. Complex substances derived from an amino acid; epinephrine (adrenaline) and norepinephrine (noradrenaline) are examples.
3. Anterior lobe of the pituitary gland.
4. Continuous contractions of muscles associated with low levels of parathyroid hormone.
5. Eyeballs that bulge outward (exophthalmia); associated with hyperthyroidism.
6. Steroid hormones from the adrenal cortex (outer region of the adrenal gland) that influence salt (minerals such as sodium and potassium) metabolism.
7. A state of equilibrium in the body with respect to function, fluids, and times.
8. A substance that mimics the action of the sympathetic nerves; epinephrine (adrenaline) is an example.
9. Steroid hormones from the adrenal cortex that influence sugar metabolism in the body.
10. Catecholamine hormone from the adrenal medulla; adrenaline.
11. Animal starch; storage form of glucose.
12. Male hormone; testosterone is an example.
13. Hormone secreted by the adrenal cortex; cortisol is an example.
14. Hormone from the posterior lobe of the pituitary that stimulates contraction of the uterus during labor.
15. Major hormone from the thyroid gland; thyroxine (contains four iodine atoms).
16. Abnormal secretion of androgens from the adrenal cortex produces masculine characteristics in a female.
17. Cancerous tumor of the thyroid gland.
18. Excessive hair on the body (result of excessive secretion of androgens).
19. Enlargement of extremities (excessive secretion of growth hormone after puberty).
20. Female hormone; an estrogen.

I

1. Insulin-dependent diabetes mellitus; characterized by destruction of the islets of Langerhans.
2. Destruction of nerves as a secondary complication of diabetes mellitus.
3. Abnormal condition of high levels of ketones (acids) in the blood as a result of improper burning of fats. Fats are burned because the cells do not have sugar available because of lack of insulin or inability of insulin to act.
4. Too little sugar in the blood. This can occur if too much insulin is taken by a diabetic patient.
5. Non–insulin-dependent diabetes mellitus; characterized by insulin deficiency and resistance by target tissue to the action of insulin.
6. Destruction of blood vessels in the retina as a secondary complication of diabetes mellitus.
7. Unconsciousness due to high levels of sugar in the blood. Water leaves cells to balance the large amounts of sugar in the blood, leading to cellular dehydration.
8. Destruction of the kidneys as a secondary complication of diabetes mellitus.
9. Collection of fatty plaque in arteries.
10. High level of sugar in the blood; insulin is unavailable or unable to transport sugar from the blood into cells.

J

1. A radioactive compound is given, and the thyroid gland is pictured with a scanner device.
2. Measurement of blood sugar levels in a fasting patient, and after intervals of 30 minutes, and 1, 2, and 3 hours following ingestion of glucose.

3. Radioimmunoassay; hormone concentrations are measured by using antibodies, nonradioactively labeled hormone, and radioactively labeled hormone.

4. Measurement of eyeball protrusion (symptoms of Graves' disease).
5. X-ray of the cranium and cavity in the skull that houses the pituitary gland; serial x-rays show the gland in depth.

K

1. exophthalmia
2. pituitary
3. acromegaly

4. diabetic ketoacidosis
5. glucose tolerance test; diabetes

Answers to Practical Applications

Case Report 1—1. B, 2. A, 3. B
Case Report 2—1. C, 2. C, 3. A
Case Report 3—1. C, 2. C, 3. A, 4. C

XVIII. Pronunciation of Terms

To test your understanding of the terminology in this chapter, write the meaning of each term in the space provided. In addition, you may wish to cover the terms and write them by looking at your definitions. Make sure your spelling is correct. The page number after each term indicates where it is defined or used in the text so you can easily check your responses. (If you are not sure what the pronunciation symbols mean, refer to page 21.)

Vocabulary and Terminology

Term	Pronunciation	Meaning
adenectomy (652)	ăd-ĕ-NĔK-tō-mē	_____
adenohypophysis (650)	ăd-ĕ-nō-hī-PŎF-ĭ-sĭs	_____
adrenal cortex (649)	ă-DRĒ-năl KŎR-tĕks	_____
adrenalectomy (652)	ă-drē-năl-ĔK-tō-mē	_____
adrenaline (650)	ă-DRĔN-ă-lĭn	_____
adrenal medulla (649)	ă-DRĒ-năl mĕ-DŪ-lă	_____
adrenocorticotropic hormone (650)	ă-drē-nō-kŏr-tĭ-kō-TRŌP-ĭk HŎR-mōn	_____
adrenocorticotropin (650)	ă-drē-nō-kŏr-tĭ-kō-TRŌ-pĭn	_____
adrenopathy (652)	ă-drē-NŎP-ă-thē	_____
aldosterone (650)	ăl-DŎS-tĕ-rōn or ăl-dō-STĔR-ŏn	_____
androgen (650)	ĂN-drō-jĕn	_____

antidiuretic hormone (650)	ăn-tĭ-dī-ū-RĔT-ĭk HŎR-mōn	_____
calcitonin (650)	kăl-sĭ-TŌ-nĭn	_____
catecholamines (651)	kăt-ĕ-KŌL-ă-mēnz	_____
corticosteroid (651)	kŏr-tĭ-kō-STĔ-royd	_____
cortisol (650)	KŎR-tĭ-sōl	_____
electrolyte (652)	ĕ-LĔK-trō-līt	_____
endocrinologist (653)	ĕn-dō-krĭ-NŎL-ō-jĭst	_____
epinephrine (650)	ĕp-ĭ-NĔF-rĭn	_____
estradiol (650)	ĕs-tră-DĪ-ŏl	_____
estrogen (650)	ĔS-trō-jĕn	_____
estrogenic (654)	ĕs-trō-JĔN-ĭk	_____
euthyroid (655)	ū-THĪ-royd	_____
follicle-stimulating hormone (650)	FŎL-ĭ-k'l STĬM-ū-lā-tĭng HŎR-mōn	_____
glucagon (650)	GLOO-kă-gŏn	_____
glucocorticoid (652)	gloo-kō-KŎR-tĭ-koyd	_____
glycogen (654)	GLĪ-kō-jĕn	_____
glycosuria (655)	glī-kōs-Ū-rē-ă	_____
gonadotropin (653)	gō-năd-ō-TRŌ-pĭn	_____
growth hormone (650)	GRŌ-TH HŎR-mōn	_____
homeostasis (652)	hō-mē-ō-STĀ-sĭs	_____
hormonal (654)	hŏr-MŌ-năl	_____
hormone (652)	HŎR-mōn	_____
hypercalcemia (653)	hī-pĕr-kăl-SĒ-mē-ă	_____
hyperglycemia (654)	hī-pĕr-glī-SĒ-mē-ă	_____
hypocalcemia (653)	hī-pō-kăl-SĒ-mē-ă	_____
hypogonadism (653)	hī-pō-GŌ-năd-ĭzm	_____
hypoinsulinism (654)	hī-pō-ĬN-sū-lĭn-ĭzm	_____
hypokalemia (654)	hī-pō-kā-LĒ-mē-ă	_____

hyponatremia (654)	hī-pō-nā-TRĒ-mē-ă	
hypophysectomy (654)	hī-pō-fĭ-SĔK-tō-mē	
hypophysis (650)	hī-PŎF-ĭ-sĭs	
hypopituitarism (653)	hī-pō-pĭ-TOO-ĭ-tă-rĭzm	
hypothalamus (652)	hī-pō-THĂL-ă-mŭs	
insulin (651)	ĬN-sū-lĭn	
luteinizing hormone (651)	LŪ-tē-ĭn-īz-ĭng HŎR-mōn	
mineralocorticoid (652)	mĭn-ĕr-ăl-ō-KŎR-tĭ-koyd	
neurohypophysis (650)	nū-rō-hī-PŎF-ĭ-sĭs	
norepinephrine (651)	nŏr-ĕp-ĭ-NĔF-rĭn	
oxytocin (651)	ŏk-sĕ-TŌ-sĭn	
pancreas (649)	PĂN-krē-ăs	
pancreatectomy (653)	păn-krē-ă-TĔK-tō-mē	
parathormone (651)	păr-ă-THŎR-mōn	
parathyroidectomy (653)	păr-ă-thī-roy-DĔK-tō-mē	
parathyroid glands (650)	păr-ă-THĪ-royd glănz	
pineal gland (638)	pī-NĒ-ăl glănd	
pituitary gland (650)	pĭ-TOO-ĭ-tĕr-ē glănd	
polydipsia (653)	pŏl-ē-DĬP-sē-ă	
progesterone (651)	prō-JĔS-tĕ-rōn	
prolactin (654)	prō-LĂK-tĭn	
sella turcica (652)	SĔL-ă TŬR-sĭ-kă	
somatotropin (651)	sō-mă-tō-TRŌ-pĭn	
steroid (652)	STĔR-oyd	
sympathomimetic (652)	sĭm-pă-thō-mĭ-MĔT-ĭk	
testosterone (651)	tĕs-TŎS-tĕ-rōn	
tetraiodothyronine (651)	tĕ-tră-ī-ō-dō-THĪ-rō-nēn	
thyroid gland (650)	THĪ-royd glănd	

thyroiditis (653)	thī-royd-Ī-tĭs	_____
thyrotropin (651)	thī-rō-TRŌ-pĭn	_____
thyroxine (651)	thī-RŎK-sĭn	_____
triiodothyronine (651)	trī-ī-ō-dō-THĪ-rō-nēn	_____
vasopressin (651)	văz-ō-PRĔS-ĭn	_____

Abnormal Conditions, Laboratory Tests, and Clinical Procedures

Term	Pronunciation	Meaning
acromegaly (661)	ăk-rō-MĔG-ă-lē	_____
Addison's disease (659)	ĂD-ĭ-sŏnz dĭ-ZĒZ	_____
adrenal virilism (659)	ă-DRĒ-năl VĬR-ĭ-lĭzm	_____
cretinism (656)	KRĒ-tĭn-ĭzm	_____
Cushing's disease (659)	KŬSH-ĭngz dĭ-ZĒZ	_____
diabetes insipidus (663)	dī-ă-BĒ-tēz ĭn-SĬP-ĭ-dŭs	_____
diabetes mellitus (660)	dī-ă-BĒ-tēz MĔL-ĭ-tŭs or mĕ-LĪ-tŭs	_____
dwarfism (662)	DWARF-izm	_____
endemic goiter (656)	ĕn-DĔM-ĭk GOY-tĕr	_____
exophthalmia (656)	ĕk-sŏf-THĂL-mē-ă	_____
exophthalmometry (663)	ĕk-sŏf-thăl-MŎM-ĕ-trē	_____
gigantism (662)	JĪ-găn-tĭzm	_____
glucose tolerance test (663)	GLŪ-kōs TŎL-ĕr-ăns test	_____
goiter (656)	GOY-tĕr	_____
Graves' disease (656)	GRĀVZ dĭ-ZĒZ	_____
hirsutism (659)	HĔR-so͞ot-ĭzm	_____
hyperinsulinism (660)	hī-pĕr-ĬN-sū-lĭn-ĭzm	_____
hyperparathyroidism (658)	hī-pĕr-pă-ră-THĪ-royd-ĭzm	_____
hypoparathyroidism (658)	hī-pō-pă-ră-THĪ-royd-ĭzm	_____

hypothyroidism (656)	hī-pō-THĪ-royd-ĭzm	_____
ketoacidosis (660)	kē-tō-ă-sĭ-DŌ-sĭs	_____
myxedema (656)	mĭk-sĕ-DĒ-mă	_____
nodular goiter (656)	NŎD-ū-lăr GOY-tĕr	_____
panhypopituitarism (662)	păn-hī-pō-pĭ-TŪ-ĭ-tăr-ĭzm	_____
pheochromocytoma (660)	fē-ō-krō-mō-sī-TŌ-mă	_____
radioactive iodine uptake (663)	rā-dē-ō-ĂK-tĭv Ī-ō-dīn ŬP-tāk	_____
radioimmunoassay (663)	rā-dē-ō-ĭm-ū-nō-ĂS-ā	_____
tetany (658)	TĔT-ă-nē	_____
thyroid carcinoma (658)	THĪ-royd kăr-sĭ-NŌ-mă	_____
thyroid function tests (663)	THĪ-royd FŬNK-shŭn tests	_____
thyroid scan (663)	THĪ-royd skăn	_____
thyrotoxicosis (655)	thī-rō-tŏk-sĭ-KŌ-sĭs	_____

XIX. Review Sheet

Write the meaning of each word part in the space provided and test yourself. Check your answers with the information in the chapter or in the Glossary (Medical Terms—English) at the end of the book.

Combining Forms

Combining Form	Meaning	Combining Form	Meaning
aden/o	_____	home/o	_____
adren/o	_____	kal/i	_____
adrenal/o	_____	lact/o	_____
andr/o	_____	myx/o	_____
calc/o	_____	natr/o	_____
cortic/o	_____	pancreat/o	_____
crin/o	_____	parathyroid/o	_____
dips/o	_____	phys/o	_____
estr/o	_____	pituitar/o	_____
gluc/o	_____	somat/o	_____
glyc/o	_____	ster/o	_____
gonad/o	_____	thyr/o	_____

thyroid/o   _____   toxic/o   _____

toc/o   _____   ur/o   _____

Suffixes

Suffix	Meaning	Suffix	Meaning
-agon		-osis	
-ectomy		-physis	
-emia		-stasis	
-genic		-tocin	
-in, -ine		-tropin	
-megaly		-uria	
-oid			

Prefixes

Prefix	Meaning	Prefix	Meaning
eu-		pan-	
hyper-		tetra-	
hypo-		tri-	
oxy-			

19

Cancer Medicine (Oncology)

This Chapter is divided into the following sections

In this Chapter you will

- Describe medical terms related to the pathological appearance and the growth and spread of tumors;
- Recognize how tumors are classified and named;
- Become familiar with terms related to the causes, diagnosis, and treatment of cancer;
- Understand the methods used by physicians for determining the extent of tumor spread (staging); and
- Recognize combining forms, procedures, tests, and abbreviations that pertain to cancer medicine.

I. Introduction

Cancer is a disease characterized by unrestrained and excessive multiplication of body cells. It may occur in any body tissue and at any age, although cancer is found most frequently in older people. Cancerous cells accumulate as growths called **malignant tumors,** which penetrate, compress, and ultimately destroy the surrounding normal tissue. In addition to their local growth, cancerous cells also have the ability to spread throughout the body by way of the bloodstream or lymphatic vessels. In most patients, the spread of cancers from their site of origin to distant organs is responsible for causing death.

Although half of all patients who develop cancer will be cured of their disease, it is currently the cause of about one-fifth of all deaths in the United States. Lung, breast, and colorectal cancers rank highest in percentage of deaths for women, whereas lung, colorectal, and prostate cancers are highest in percentage of deaths for men. This chapter will explore the terminology related to this common, and often fatal, disease process.

II. Characteristics of Tumors

Tumors (also called **neoplasms**) are masses, or growths, that arise from normal tissue. They may be either **malignant** (progressive and life-threatening) or **benign** (nonprogressive and not life-threatening). There are several differences between benign and malignant tumors. Some of these differences are

1. Benign tumors grow slowly, and malignant tumor cells multiply rapidly.
2. Benign tumors are often **encapsulated** (contained within a fibrous capsule or cover), so that the tumor cells do not invade the surrounding tissue. Malignant tumor growth is characteristically **invasive** and **infiltrative,** extending beyond the tissue or origin into adjacent organs.
3. Benign tumors are composed of highly organized and specialized **(differentiated)** cells, which closely resemble normal, mature tissue. Malignant tumors are composed of cancerous cells that resemble primitive, or embryonic, cells that do not have the capacity for mature cellular functions. This characteristic of malignant tumors is called **anaplasia.** Anaplasia means that the cancerous cells are **dedifferentiated** (reverting to a less developed state) in contrast to the normal, differentiated tissue of their origin. Anaplastic cells lack an orderly arrangement. Instead, the tumor cells are found piled one on top of the other in a disorganized fashion. Figure 19–1 compares normal fibroblast cells (connective tissue–forming cells) with cancerous anaplastic fibroblasts (both grown in culture).
4. Cells from benign tumors do not spread to form secondary tumor masses in other places in the body. Malignant tumors, however, can detach themselves from the primary (original) tumor site, travel through the bloodstream and lymphatic system, and establish a new tumor site at a distant region within the body. This secondary growth is called a **metastasis.** Figure 19–2 shows a liver filled with metastatic cancer.

III. Carcinogenesis

The transformation of a normal cell to a cancerous one is only partially understood at the present time. The key to understanding the process of malignant transformation lies in the operation of the genetic material, or **DNA (deoxyribonucleic acid),** of the cell. Strands

Figure 19-1

(A) Normal fibroblast cells (connective tissue–forming cells). *(B)* Cancerous anaplastic fibroblasts. (*A* and *B*, Courtesy of Dr. Tom Wright, Brigham and Women's Hospital and Harvard Medical School, Boston, MA.)

of DNA in the cell nucleus form chromosomes, which are easily seen at times during the growth cycle of the cell.

DNA controls not only the production of new cells but also the cell's ability to grow. It contains codes or programs called genes that direct the production of new proteins **(protein synthesis).** When a cell divides, the DNA material copies itself, so that exactly the same DNA is passed to two new cells that are formed. This process is called **mitosis** or **self-replication** (Fig. 19–3).

Figure 19-2

A liver studded with metastatic cancer. (From Robbins SL, Kumar V: Basic Pathology, 4th ed. Philadelphia, WB Saunders, 1987, p 194.)

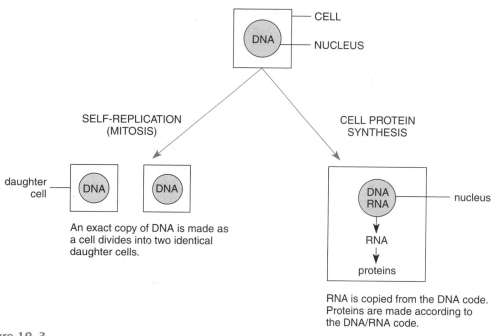

Figure 19–3

The two functions of DNA.

Between cycles of replication, DNA serves as the computer program that directs the cell's life functions. DNA sends a molecular message to the cytoplasm of the cell so that proteins (such as hormones and enzymes) can be made for cellular growth. This program is transmitted in the following way. In the nucleus, a coded message is copied from DNA onto another molecule called **RNA (ribonucleic acid).** RNA travels from nucleus to cytoplasm carrying the message that directs the formation of specific proteins in the cell. Figure 19–3 illustrates these two important functions of DNA.

When a cell becomes malignant, however, the process of mitosis is disturbed (cancer cells reproduce almost continuously). They also become anaplastic; that is, their DNA stops making the codes that allow cells to carry on normal function and instead makes new signals that lead to movement of cells, invasion of adjacent tissue, and metastasis. All these changes are characteristic of malignant cells and occur as the result of changes in DNA.

The changes in DNA that result in malignancy occur as the result of environmental factors, such as toxic chemicals, sunlight, a host of other sources of injury, and rarely, by certain viral and bacterial infections. Once these changes are established in a cell, they are passed on to its daughter cells. Such an inheritable change in a cell is called a **mutation.** Cellular mutations thus lead to malignant growths.

Although most DNA changes, or mutations, lead to higher than normal rates of growth, some mutations found in cancer cells prevent the cells from dying. In recent years, scientists have recognized that some types of cancers have lost the normal blueprints that direct aging or damaged cells to die. Normal cells undergo spontaneous disintegration by a process known as **apoptosis,** or programmed cell death. Cancer cells have lost this program and thus can live forever.

Environmental Agents

Agents from the environment—such as chemicals and drugs, radiation, and viruses—can cause changes in DNA and thus produce cancer. These environmental agents are called **carcinogens.**

Chemical carcinogens are found in a variety of products and drugs including **hydrocarbons** (in cigarette, cigar, and pipe smoke and automobile exhaust), insecticides, dyes, industrial chemicals, insulation, and hormones. For example, the hormone diethylstilbestrol (DES) causes a malignant tumor, carcinoma of the vagina in females.

Radiation, whatever its source—sunlight, x-rays, radioactive substances, nuclear fission—is a wave of energy. When it interacts with DNA it causes breaks or mutations that lead to cancer. Thus, leukemia is an occupational hazard of radiologists, who are routinely exposed to x-rays. There is also a high incidence of leukemia and other cancers among survivors of atomic bomb explosions, as at Hiroshima and Nagasaki. **Ultraviolet radiation** given off by the sun can cause skin cancer (basal cell carcinoma, squamous cell carcinoma, and melanoma), especially in persons with lightly pigmented, or fair, skin.

Some **viruses** have been proved to be carcinogenic in a variety of animals. For example, the human T cell leukemia virus (HTLV) causes a form of leukemia in adults. A related virus, HIV (human immunodeficiency virus), causes AIDS (acquired immunodeficiency syndrome). Other viruses have been implicated as the cause of cervical cancer (papilloma virus) and Burkitt's lymphoma (Epstein-Barr virus). **Oncogenic (onc/o** means tumor) viruses fall into two categories: RNA viruses (composed of RNA and known as retroviruses) and DNA viruses (composed of DNA). In addition to transmission of cancer by whole viruses, pieces of viral DNA (called **viral oncogenes**) or similar broken or dislocated pieces of human DNA (called **cellular oncogenes**) can cause normal cells to become malignant if they are activated by mutations. An **oncogene** is a piece of DNA whose activation is associated with the conversion of normal cells into cancer cells.

Heredity

Causes of cancer not only come from the environment but may also originate within the body. Susceptibility to some forms of cancer is transmitted from parents to offspring through defects in the DNA of the egg and sperm cells. Examples of known inherited cancers are retinoblastoma (tumor of the retina of the eye), xeroderma pigmentosum (tumors on skin exposed to sunlight), certain types of malignant melanoma, and polyposis coli syndrome (polyps that grow in the colon and rectum). Each of these diseases is believed to be caused by specific breaks or rearrangements of the DNA code. These changes can be seen in special studies of the DNA molecule.

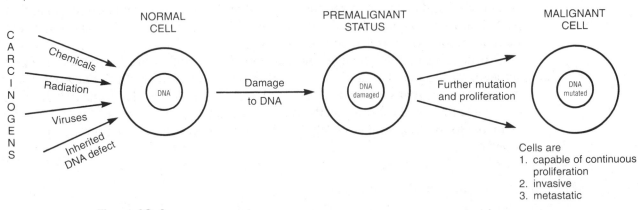

Figure 19–4

The role of carcinogens and heredity in carcinogenesis.

In many cases it is believed that these tumors arise because of inherited or acquired abnormalities in so-called suppressor genes. In normal individuals, these suppressor genes control growth and differentiation. Loss of a normal suppressor gene in effect takes the brake off the reproductive process, leading to cancer.

Figure 19–4 summarizes the role of environmental agents and heredity in carcinogenesis.

IV. Classification of Cancerous Tumors

About half of all cancer deaths are caused by malignancies that originate in lung, breast, or colon. However, in all there are more than 100 distinct types of cancer, each having a unique set of symptoms and requiring a specific type of therapy. It is possible to divide these specific types of cancer into three broad groups on the basis of histogenesis—that is, by identifying the particular tissue (**hist/o**) from which the tumor cells arise (**-genesis**). These major groups are called **carcinomas, sarcomas,** and **mixed-tissue tumors.**

Carcinomas

Carcinomas, the largest group, are **solid tumors** that are derived from epithelial tissue that lines external and internal body surfaces, including skin, glands, and digestive, urinary, and reproductive organs. Approximately 90 per cent of all malignant neoplasms are carcinomas.

Table 19–1 gives examples of specific carcinomas and the epithelial tissue from which they derive. Benign tumors of epithelial origin are usually designated by adding the suffix **-oma** to the type of tissue in which the tumor occurs. For example, a **gastric adenoma** is a benign tumor of the glandular (aden/o) epithelial cells lining the stomach. Malignant tumors of epithelial origin are named by using **carcinoma** added to the type of tissue in which the tumor occurs. Thus, a **gastric adenocarcinoma** is a cancerous tumor arising from glandular cells lining the stomach.

Sarcomas

Sarcomas are less common than carcinomas and are derived from supportive and connective tissue, such as bone, fat, muscle, cartilage, and bone marrow, and from cells of the immune (lymph) system. Sarcomas account for approximately 5 per cent of all malignant neoplasms.

Table 19–2 gives examples of specific types of sarcomas and the connective tissue from which they derive. Benign tumors of connective tissue origin are named by adding the suffix **-oma** to the type of tissue in which the tumor occurs. For example, a benign tumor of bone is called an **osteoma.** Malignant tumors of connective tissue origin are often named by using **sarcoma** (sarc/o means flesh) added to the type of tissue in which the tumor occurs. For example, an **osteosarcoma** is a malignant tumor of bone.

Mixed-tissue Tumors

Mixed-tissue tumors are derived from tissue that is capable of differentiating into both epithelial and connective tissue. These uncommon tumors are thus composed of several different types of cells. Examples of mixed-tissue tumors (Table 19–3) can be found in the kidney, ovaries, and testes.

Table 19–1. CARCINOMAS AND THE EPITHELIAL TISSUES FROM WHICH THEY DERIVE

Type of Epithelial Tissue	Malignant Tumor
GASTROINTESTINAL TRACT	
Stomach	Gastric adenocarcinoma
Esophagus	Esophageal carcinoma
Colon	Adenocarcinoma of the colon
Liver	Hepatocellular carcinoma, also called hepatoma
GLANDULAR TISSUE	
Thyroid	Carcinoma of the thyroid
Adrenal glands	Carcinoma of the adrenals
Pancreas	Carcinoma of the pancreas (pancreatic adenocarcinoma)
Breast	Carcinoma of the breast
Prostate	Carcinoma of the prostate
SKIN	
Squamous cell layer	Squamous cell carcinoma
Basal cell layer	Basal cell carcinoma
Melanocyte	Malignant melanoma
LUNG	Adenocarcinoma of the lung
	Small cell carcinoma
	Epidermoid carcinoma
KIDNEY AND BLADDER	Renal cell carcinoma (hypernephroma)
	Transitional cell carcinoma of the bladder
REPRODUCTIVE ORGANS	Cystadenocarcinoma of the ovaries
	Adenocarcinoma of the uterus
	Squamous cell (epidermoid) carcinoma of the vagina or cervix
	Carcinoma of the penis
	Seminoma and embryonal cell carcinoma (testes)
	Choriocarcinoma of the uterus or testes

Table 19–2. SARCOMAS AND THE CONNECTIVE TISSUES FROM WHICH THEY DERIVE

Type of Connective Tissue	Malignant Tumor
BONE	Osteosarcoma (osteogenic sarcoma)
	Ewing's sarcoma
MUSCLE	
Smooth (visceral) muscle	Leiomyosarcoma
Striated (skeletal) muscle	Rhabdomyosarcoma
CARTILAGE	Chondrosarcoma
FAT	Liposarcoma
FIBROUS TISSUE	Fibrosarcoma
BLOOD VESSEL TISSUE	Angiosarcoma
BLOOD-FORMING TISSUE	
Leukocytes	Leukemia
Lymphocytes	Hodgkin's disease
	Non–Hodgkin's lymphomas
	Burkitt's lymphoma
Plasma cells	Multiple myeloma
NERVE TISSUE	
Embryonic nerve tissue	Neuroblastoma
Neuroglial tissue	Astrocytoma (tumor of neuroglial cells called astrocytes)

Table 19–3. MIXED-TISSUE TUMORS

Type of Tissue	Malignant Tissue
Kidney	Wilms' tumor (embryonal adenosarcoma)
Ovaries and testes	Teratoma (tumor composed of bone, muscle, skin, gland cells, cartilage, etc.)

V. Pathological Descriptions

The following terms are used to describe the appearance of a malignant tumor, either on gross (visual) or on microscopic examination.

Gross Descriptions

cystic
Forming large open spaces filled with fluid. **Mucinous** tumors are filled with mucus (thick, sticky fluid), and **serous** tumors are filled with a thin, watery fluid resembling serum. The most common site of cystic tumors is in ovaries.

fungating
Mushrooming pattern of growth in which tumor cells pile one on top of another and project from a tissue surface. Tumors found in the colon are of this type.

inflammatory
Having the features of inflammation; that is, redness, swelling, and heat. These tumors characteristically occur in the breast.

medullary
Pertaining to large, soft, fleshy tumors. Thyroid and breast tumors may be medullary.

necrotic
Containing dead tissue. Any type of tumor can outgrow its blood supply and undergo necrosis.

polypoid
Growths that are like projections extending outward from a base. **Sessile** polypoid tumors extend from a broad base, and **pedunculated** polypoid tumors extend from a stem or stalk. Both benign and malignant tumors of the colon may grow as polyps.

ulcerating
Characterized by an open, exposed surface resulting from death of overlying tissue. Ulcerating tumors are often found in the stomach, breast, colon, and skin.

verrucous
Resembling a wart-like growth. Tumors of the gingiva (cheek) are frequently verrucous.

Microscopic Descriptions

alveolar
Tumor cells form patterns resembling small, microscopic sacs; commonly found in tumors of muscle, bone, fat, and cartilage.

carcinoma in situ
Referring to localized tumor cells that have not invaded adjacent structures. Cancer of the cervix may begin as carcinoma in situ.

diffuse
Spreading evenly throughout the affected tissue. Malignant lymphomas may display diffuse involvement of lymph nodes.

dysplastic
Pertaining to abnormal formation of cells. These tumors display a highly abnormal but not clearly cancerous appearance. Dysplastic nevi (moles on skin) are an example.

epidermoid
Resembling squamous epithelial cells (thin, plate-like), often occurring in the respiratory tract.

follicular	Forming small, microscopic, gland-type sacs. Thyroid gland cancer is an example.
nodular	Forming multiple areas of tightly packed clusters of cells with lightly populated areas in between. Malignant lymphomas may display a nodular pattern of lymph node involvement.
papillary	Forming small, finger-like or nipple-like projections of cells. Bladder cancer may be described as papillary.
pleomorphic	Composed of a variety of types of cells. Mixed-cell tumors are examples.
scirrhous	Densely packed (scirrhous means hard) tumors, overgrown with fibrous tissue; commonly found in breast or stomach cancers.
undifferentiated	Lacking microscopic structures typical of normal mature cells.

VI. Grading and Staging Systems

Tumors are classified on the basis of their location, microscopic appearance, and extent of spread. Of particular importance are the tumor's **grade** (its degree of maturity or differentiation under the microscope) and its **stage** (its extent of spread within the body). These two properties influence the prognosis (the chances of successful treatment and survival) and determine the specific treatment to be used.

When grading a tumor, the pathologist is concerned with the microscopic appearance of the tumor cells, specifically with their degree of maturation or differentiation. Often, four grades are used. **Grade I** tumors are very well differentiated, so that they closely resemble the normal parent tissue of their origin. **Grade IV** tumors are so undifferentiated or anaplastic that even recognition of the tumor's tissue of origin may be difficult. **Grades II** and **III** are intermediate in appearance, moderately or poorly differentiated, as opposed to well differentiated (grade I) and dedifferentiated (grade IV).

Grading is often of value in the prognosis of certain types of cancers, such as cancer of the urinary bladder and ovary and brain tumors (astrocytomas). Patients with grade I tumors have a high survival rate, and patients with grades II, III, and IV tumors have a poorer survival rate. Grading is also used in evaluating cells obtained from body fluids in preventive screening tests, such as **Papanicolaou's (Pap) smears** of the uterine cervix, tracheal secretions, or stomach secretions.

The staging of cancerous tumors is based on the extent of spread of the tumor rather than on its microscopic appearance. An example of a staging system is the **TNM staging system.** It has been applied to malignancies such as lung cancer, as well as many other tumors. **T** refers to the size and degree of local extension of the **tumor; N** refers to the number of regional lymph **nodes** that have been invaded by tumor; and **M** refers to the presence or absence of **metastases** (spreads to distant sites) of the tumor cells. Subscripts are used to denote size and degree of involvement: For example, 0 indicates undetectable, and 1, 2, 3, and 4 a progressive increase in size or involvement. A tumor may be described as $T_1 N_2 M_0$ (a small tumor with spread to regional nodes, but no distant metastases). Table 19–4 presents the notations in the TNM staging system.

Other staging systems use letters such as A, B, C, and D or I, II, III, and IV to indicate the extent of spread of tumor in the body.

Table 19–4. A TNM STAGING SYSTEM

Tumor	
T_0	No evidence of primary tumor
T_{IS}	Carcinoma in situ
T_1 T_2 T_3 T_4	Progressive increase in tumor size and involvement
T_x	Tumor cannot be assessed
Nodes	
N_0	Regional lymph nodes not demonstrably abnormal
N_1 N_2 N_3 N_4	Increasing numbers or increasingly distant location of spread to regional lymph nodes
N_x	Regional lymph nodes cannot be assessed clinically
Metastasis	
M_0	No evidence of distant metastasis
M_1 M_2 M_3	Ascending degrees of distant metastasis

VII. Cancer Treatment

Four major approaches to cancer treatment are **surgery, radiation therapy, chemotherapy,** and **biological therapy.** Each method **(modality)** may be used alone, but often they are coordinated in combined modality programs to improve the overall treatment result.

Surgery

In many patients with cancer, the tumor is discovered before it has spread, and it may be cured by surgical excision. Some common cancers in which surgery may be curative are those of the stomach, breast, and uterus (endometrium).

The following is a list of terms that describe surgical procedures used in treating cancer.

cryosurgery	Malignant tissue is frozen and thus destroyed. This procedure is often used to treat brain and bladder tumors.
electrocauterization	Malignant tissue is destroyed by burning. Electrocauterization is often used in treating tumors of the rectum and colon.
en bloc resection	Tumor is removed along with a large area of surrounding tissue containing lymph nodes. Modified radical mastectomy, colectomy, and gastrectomy are examples.
excisional biopsy	Removal of tumor and a margin of normal tissue. This procedure provides a specimen for diagnosis and may be curative for small tumors.
exenteration	A wide resection involving removal of the tumor, its organ of origin, and all surrounding tissue in the body space, such as in the pelvis.
fulguration	Destruction of tissue by electric sparks generated by a high-frequency current.
incisional biopsy	A piece of tumor is removed for examination to establish a diagnosis. Other forms of treatment, such as chemotherapy or x-ray, may then be used to treat the bulk of the tumor.

Radiation

The goal of radiation therapy is to deliver a maximal dose of ionizing radiation to the tumor tissue and a minimal dose to surrounding normal tissue. In reality, this goal is difficult to achieve, and usually one accepts a degree of residual normal cell damage **(morbidity)** as a side effect of the destruction of the tumor. High-dose radiation produces damage to DNA.

Some terms used in the field of radiation therapy for cancer are listed below:

electron beams	Low-energy beams for treatment of skin or surface tumors.
fractionation	A method of giving radiation in small, repeated doses rather than a few large doses. Fractionation allows larger total doses to be given with less damage to normal tissue.
linear accelerator	A large electronic device that produces high-energy x-ray beams for treatment of deep-seated tumors.
radiocurable tumor	Tumor that can be completely eradicated by radiation therapy. These are usually localized tumors with no evidence of metastasis. Lymphomas and Hodgkin's disease are examples.
radioresistant tumor	Tumor that requires large doses of radiation to produce death of cells. The high doses of radiation may have a damaging effect on surrounding normal tissues. Connective tissue tumors are the most radioresistant.
radiosensitive tumor	Tumor in which irradiation can cause death of cells without serious damage to surrounding normal tissue. Tumors of hematopoietic and lymphatic origins are radiosensitive.
radiosensitizers	Drugs that increase the sensitivity of tumors to x-rays.

Cancer Chemotherapy and Biological Therapy

Chemotherapy

Cancer chemotherapy is the treatment of cancer using drugs. It is the standard treatment for many types of cancer, and it produces cures of most patients who have choriocarcinoma, testicular cancer, acute lymphocytic leukemia, or Hodgkin's disease. Chemotherapy may be used alone or in combination with surgery and irradiation.

The field of **pharmacokinetics** (-kinetic means pertaining to movement) is concerned with the study of the distribution and disappearance of drugs in the body. Obviously, the ideal is to develop drugs that kill large numbers of tumor cells without harming normal cells. Because some normal tissue cells, such as bone marrow and gastrointestinal lining cells, have a rapidly dividing cell population, they suffer considerable damage from antitumor drugs. Scientists working in the field of pharmacokinetics study the appearance and disappearance of drugs in various body fluids, such as blood plasma and urine, and use the information to design drug dosages and schedules of administration to achieve the greatest tumor kill with the least toxicity to normal cells.

Combination chemotherapy refers to the use of two or more antitumor drugs together to kill a specific type of malignant growth. In chemotherapy, drugs are given according to a written **protocol,** or plan, that details exactly how the drugs will be given. Usually drug therapy is continued until the patient achieves a complete **remission,** which is the absence of all signs of disease. At times, chemotherapy is given as an **adjuvant** (an aid) to surgery. This means that the drugs are used to kill possible hidden disease in patients who, after surgery, are otherwise free of any evidence of malignancy.

The following are categories of cancer chemotherapeutic agents:

1. **Alkylating agents**—These are synthetic compounds containing two or more chemical groups called alkyl groups. The drugs interfere with the process of DNA synthesis by attaching to DNA molecules. Toxic side effects include nausea and vomiting, diarrhea, bone marrow depression (myelosuppression), and alopecia (hair loss). These are common side effects because the cells in the gastrointestinal tract, bone marrow, and scalp are rapidly dividing cells (high growth fraction) that, along with tumor cells, are susceptible to the lethal effects of chemotherapeutic drugs. The side effects disappear after treatment is suspended.

2. **Antibiotics**—These drugs are produced by bacteria or fungi. Many of these drugs act by binding to DNA and RNA in the cell, thus preventing normal replication. Toxic effects from their use include alopecia, stomatitis, myelosuppression, and gastrointestinal disturbances.

3. **Antimetabolites**—These drugs inhibit the synthesis of substances that are the necessary components of DNA or may directly block the replication or copying of DNA. Side effects are myelosuppression, with leukopenia, thrombocytopenia, and bleeding; and oral and digestive tract toxicity, including stomatitis (sore mouth), nausea, and vomiting.

4. **Plant derivatives**—These drugs are chemicals derived from plants. They are used frequently in combination with other chemotherapeutic agents. Side effects include myelosuppression, alopecia, and nerve damage.

5. **Steroids**—These are a class of chemicals made by glands in the body, and they have important effects on reproduction, energy production, and aging. Examples are **estrogens** and **androgens.** These hormones exert their action by attaching to receptor proteins in target tissues. The growth of some tumors (breast and prostate) is often dependent on steroid hormones. Some breast cancers have **estrogen receptors (ER)** and will respond to the removal of estrogen by oophorectomy or the use of antiestrogen drugs, such as **tamoxifen,** that block estrogenic effects. Fluid retention, masculinization or feminization, nausea, and vomiting are some possible side effects of various steroids.

Biological Therapy

A more recent approach to cancer treatment is the use of the body's own defense mechanisms to fight tumor cells. Investigators explore how the elements of the immune system can be restored, enhanced, mimicked, and manipulated to destroy cancerous cells. Substances produced by normal cells that either directly block tumor growth or stimulate the immune system and other body defenses are called **biological response modifiers.** Examples of these substances are **interferon** (made by lymphocytes), **monoclonal antibodies** (made by mouse cells and capable of binding to human tumors), **colony-stimulating factors (CSFs)** that stimulate blood-forming cells and reverse the effects of chemotherapy, and **interleukins** that stimulate the immune system to destroy tumors.

Table 19–5 summarizes the categories of chemotherapeutic and biological agents and gives specific examples.

Table 19–5. CANCER CHEMOTHERAPEUTIC AND BIOLOGICAL AGENTS

Chemotherapeutic Agents

ALKYLATING AGENTS
  Carmustine (BCNU)
  Cisplatin, carboplatin
  Cyclophosphamide (Cytoxan)
  Melphalan (Alkeran)
  Nitrogen mustard
  Chlorambucil
ANTIBIOTICS
  Actinomycin D
  Bleomycin sulfate
  Daunorubicin hydrochloride
  Doxorubicin hydrochloride (Adriamycin)
  Idarubicin
  Mitomycin C
ANTIMETABOLITES
  Cytosine arabinoside (ara-C)
  5-fluorouracil (5-FU)
  Methotrexate (MTX)
  6-thioguanine (6-TG)
  Fludarabine
  Pentostatin

Biological Agents

  Colony-stimulating factors (CSFs)
  Interferon
  Interleukins (IL-1, IL-2, IL-3)
  Monoclonal antibodies
PLANT DERIVATIVES
  Vinblastine sulfate (Velban)
  Vincristine sulfate (Oncovin)
  VP-16 (etoposide)
  VM-26 (teniposide)
  Taxol
STEROIDS
  Dexamethasone (Decadron)
  Diethylstilbestrol (DES)
  Flutamide
  Leuprolide
  Prednisone
  Tamoxifen citrate
  Testosterone
MISCELLANEOUS DRUGS
  Dacarbazine
  L-asparaginase
  Lomustine
  Procarbazine hydrochloride

VIII. Vocabulary

This list will help you review many of the new terms introduced in the text. Short definitions will reinforce your understanding of the terms. See Section XVI of this chapter for help in pronouncing the more difficult terms.

adjuvant therapy — Assisting primary treatment. Drugs are given early in the course of treatment, along with surgery or radiation to attack cancer cells that may be too small to be detected by diagnostic techniques.

alkylating agents — Synthetic chemicals containing alkyl groups that interfere with DNA synthesis.

anaplasia — Loss of differentiation of cells; reversion to a more primitive cell type.

antibiotics — Chemical substances, produced by bacteria, that inhibit the growth of cells; used in cancer chemotherapy.

antimetabolites — Chemicals that prevent cell division by inhibiting the formation of substances necessary to make DNA; used in cancer chemotherapy.

apoptosis — Programmed cell death. Apo- means off, away, and -ptosis means to fall. Normal cells undergo apoptosis when they are damaged or aging. Some cancer cells have lost the ability to undergo apoptosis and live forever.

benign — Noncancerous.

biological response modifiers	Substances produced by normal cells that either directly block tumor growth or stimulate the immune system.
biological therapy	Use of the body's own defense mechanisms to fight tumor cells.
carcinogens	Agents that cause cancer; chemicals and drugs, radiation, and viruses.
carcinoma	Cancerous tumor made up of cells of epithelial origin.
cellular oncogenes	Pieces of DNA that, when broken or dislocated, can cause a normal cell to become malignant.
chemotherapy	Treatment with drugs.
combination chemotherapy	Use of several chemotherapeutic agents together in the treatment of tumors.
dedifferentiation	Loss of differentiation of cells; reversion to a more primitive, embryonic cell type; anaplasia.
deoxyribonucleic acid (DNA)	Genetic material within the nucleus of a cell; controls cell division and protein synthesis.
differentiation	Specialization of cells.
electron beams	Low-energy beams of radiation for treatment of skin or surface tumors.
encapsulated	Surrounded by a capsule; benign tumors are encapsulated.
fractionation	Giving radiation in small, repeated doses.
grading of tumors	Evaluating the degree of maturity of tumor cells.
gross description of tumors	Visual appearance of tumors: cystic, fungating, inflammatory, medullary, necrotic, polypoid, ulcerating, and verrucous.
infiltrative	Extending beyond normal tissue boundaries.
invasive	Having the ability to enter and destroy surrounding tissue.
linear accelerator	Device that produces high-energy x-ray beams for treatment of deep-seated tumors.
malignant	Tending to become worse and result in death; tumors having the characteristics of invasiveness, anaplasia, and metastasis.
metastasis	Spread of a malignant tumor to a secondary site; literally, beyond (meta-) control (-stasis).
microscopic description (of tumors)	The appearance of tumors as seen under the microscope: alveolar, carcinoma in situ, diffuse, dysplastic, epidermoid, follicular, nodular, papillary, pleomorphic, scirrhous, undifferentiated.

mitosis	Replication of cells; a stage in the cell life cycle involving the production of two identical cells from a parent cell.
mixed-tissue tumors	Tumors composed of different types of tissue (epithelial as well as connective tissue).
modality	Method of treatment, such as surgery, chemotherapy, or radiation.
morbidity	The condition of being diseased.
mucinous	Containing mucus.
mutation	Change in the genetic material (DNA) of a cell; may be caused by chemicals, radiation, or viruses or may occur spontaneously.
neoplasm	New growth; benign or malignant tumors.
oncogene	A region of DNA (genetic material) found in tumor cells (cellular oncogene) or in viruses that cause cancer (viral oncogene). Oncogenes are designated by a three-letter word, such as **abl, erb, jun, myc, ras,** and **src.**
pedunculated	Possessing a stem or stalk (peduncle); characteristic of some polypoid tumors.
pharmacokinetics	Study of the distribution and removal of drugs in the body over a period of time.
protocol	An explicit, detailed plan for treatment.
radiation	Energy carried by a stream of particles. Various forms of radiation can cause cancer.
radiocurable tumor	Cells that are eradicated by radiation therapy.
radioresistant tumor	Cells that require large doses of radiation to be destroyed.
radiosensitive tumor	A tumor in which radiation can cause death of cells.
radiosensitizers	Drugs that increase the sensitivity of tumors to x-rays.
radiotherapy	Treatment using radiation.
relapse	Return of symptoms of disease.
remission	Absence of symptoms of disease.
ribonucleic acid (RNA)	Cellular substance (located within and outside the nucleus) that, along with DNA, plays an important role in the synthesis of proteins in a cell.
sarcoma	Cancerous tumor derived from connective tissue.

serous	Pertaining to a thin, watery fluid (serum).
sessile	Having no stem; characteristic of some polypoid tumors.
solid tumor	Tumor composed of mass of cells.
staging of tumors	System of evaluating the extent of spread of tumors. An example is the TNM system (tumor, nodes, and metastasis).
steroids	Complex, naturally occurring chemicals, such as hormones, that are used as chemotherapeutic agents.
surgical procedures to treat cancer	Methods of removing cancerous tissue: cryosurgery, electrocauterization, en bloc resection, excisional biopsy, exenteration, fulguration, incisional biopsy.
ultraviolet radiation	Rays given off by the sun.
viral oncogenes	Pieces of DNA from viruses that infect a normal cell and cause it to become malignant.
virus	An infectious agent that reproduces by entering a host cell and using the host's genetic material to make copies of itself.

IX. Combining Forms, Suffixes, Prefixes, and Terminology

Write the meaning of the medical term in the space provided.

Combining Forms			
Combining Form	Meaning	Terminology	Meaning
alveol/o	small sac	alveolar _____ *Microscopic description of tumor cell arrangement (found in connective tissue tumors).*	
cac/o	bad	cachexia _____ *General ill health and malnutrition associated with chronic disease (-hexia means habit).*	
carcin/o	cancer, cancerous	carcinoma in situ _____ *Localized cancer; confined to the site of origin.*	
cauter/o	burn, heat	electrocauterization _____	

chem/o	chemical, drug	chemotherapy _____
cry/o	cold	cryosurgery _____
cyst/o	sac of fluid	cystic tumor _____
fibr/o	fibers	fibrosarcoma _____
follicul/o	small glandular sacs	follicular _____ *A microscopic description of cellular arrangement in glandular tumors.*
fung/o	fungus, mushroom	fungating tumor _____
medull/o	soft, inner part	medullary tumor _____
mut/a	genetic change	mutation _____ *-ation means process.*
mutagen/o	causing genetic change	mutagenic _____
onc/o	tumor	oncology _____
papill/o	nipple-like	papillary _____ *A microscopic description of tumor cell growth.*
pharmac/o	chemical, drug	pharmacokinetics _____ *-kinetic means pertaining to movement.*
plas/o	formation	dysplastic _____ *Microscopic description of cells that are highly abnormal but not clearly cancerous.*
ple/o	many, more	pleomorphic _____ *Microscopic description of tumors that are composed of a variety of cells.*
polyp/o	polyp	polypoid tumor _____ *-oid means resembling.*
radi/o	rays, x-rays	radiotherapy _____

sarc/o	flesh, connective tissue	osteo<u>sarc</u>oma _____
scirrh/o	hard	<u>scirrh</u>ous _____

Microscopic description of densely packed, fibrous tumor cell composition.

Suffixes

Suffix	Meaning	Terminology	Meaning
-blast	immature	retino<u>blast</u>oma _____	
		neuro<u>blast</u>oma _____	

This sarcoma of nervous system origin affects infants and children up to 10 years old, usually arising in the autonomic nervous system or adrenal medulla.

Suffix	Meaning	Terminology	Meaning
-oma	mass, tumor	adenocarcin<u>oma</u> _____	
-plasia	formation, growth	hyper<u>plasia</u> _____	
-plasm	formation, growth	neo<u>plasm</u> _____	
-therapy	treatment	biological <u>therapy</u> _____	

Prefixes

Prefix	Meaning	Terminology	Meaning
ana-	backward	<u>ana</u>plasia _____	
apo-	off, away	<u>apo</u>ptosis _____	
epi-	upon	<u>epi</u>dermoid _____	

Microscopic description of tumor cells that resemble epidermal tissue.

Prefix	Meaning	Terminology	Meaning
meta-	beyond	<u>meta</u>stasis _____	

X. Laboratory Tests

These tests measure proteins produced by tumors. Some are present in the bloodstream, whereas others are measured in the tumor itself.

acid phosphatase	Enzyme found in high concentration in the blood of patients with prostate cancer.
alpha-fetoprotein test	Detects the presence in serum of alpha-fetoprotein, which is found in patients with liver and testicular cancer.
beta-HCG test	Detects **human chorionic gonadotropin** (HCG) in the serum of patients with testicular cancer.
CA-125	Cell surface protein produced by ovarian cancer cells.
CEA test	Detects **carcinoembryonic antigen** (CEA) in the bloodstream of patients with tumors of gastrointestinal (GI) origin.
estrogen (estradiol) receptor assay	Measures the concentration of estrogen receptor sites in tumor cells of breast cancer patients. If a tumor is found to be estrogen receptor positive, a patient will likely respond to antiestrogen hormone therapy.
prostate specific antigen (PSA)	A protein produced by prostate cancer cells and found in the bloodstream.

XI. Clinical Procedures

bone marrow biopsy	A small amount of bone marrow tissue is aspirated and examined under the microscope for evidence of cancerous cells.
exfoliative cytology	Cells are scraped (exfoliated) from the region of suspected disease and examined under the microscope. The Pap test (smear), to determine carcinoma of the cervix or vagina, is an example of exfoliative cytology (Fig. 19–5).
lymphangiography	Contrast dye is injected into the lymphatic vessels of the feet, and x-rays are taken of the lymphatic system to detect enlarged lymph nodes, blockage of the lymphatic system, and the presence of tumors.
needle biopsy	A needle is inserted into the tissue in question, and a core of tissue is removed. Aspiration (suction) may be used to withdraw free cells from a fluid-filled cavity, such as in cystic areas of the breast, or from a solid lump of tumor.
peritoneoscopy	This procedure (also called **laparoscopy**) is used to inspect the abdominal (peritoneal) cavity for tumors. A laparoscope (peritoneoscope) is inserted into the peritoneal cavity through a small incision in the abdominal wall.

staging laparotomy   This is a wide surgical incision of the abdomen that allows the physician to explore the abdominal cavity to determine the extent of malignant disease.

radionuclide scans   Radioactive substances (called radionuclides) are injected intravenously, and pictures (scans) are taken of the organs in question. In liver and spleen scans, irregular distribution of radioactivity or absence of radioactivity indicates possible liver disease, whereas on bone scans, abnormal areas of concentration of radioactivity may indicate bone destruction and repair, processes that are associated with metastasis. Abnormalities in brain scans

Figure 19–5

Papanicolaou's smears of cervical cytology. *(A)* Normal cells. *(B)* Cancer cells. *(A* and *B,* From Kumar V, Cotran RS, Robbins SL: Basic Pathology, Philadelphia, 5th ed. WB Saunders, 1992, p 209.)

appear as increased accumulation of radioactivity (normal brain tissue does not take up radioactivity because of the blood-brain barrier). Some of the radioactive substances used in obtaining scans are: **gallium-67** (^{67}Ga)—whole body scan to detect head and neck tumors, Hodgkin's disease, lymphoma, lung tumors, and bone tumors; **rose bengal**—liver scan; **technetium-99** (^{99m}Tc)—liver and spleen scans; and ^{99m}**Tc polyphosphate**—bone scan.

XII. ABBREVIATIONS

bx	Biopsy	mets	Metastases
Ca	Cancer	NED	No evidence of disease
CEA	Carcinoembryonic antigen	NHL	Non-Hodgkin's lymphoma
chem	Chemotherapy	Pap smear	Papanicolaou's smear
CMF	Cytoxan, methotrexate, 5-fluorouracil (combination chemotherapy)	PR	Partial response (tumor is one-half of its original size)
CR	Complete response	prot.	Protocol
DES	Diethylstilbestrol	PSA	Prostate specific antigen
DNA	Deoxyribonucleic acid	RNA	Ribonucleic acid
ER	Estrogen receptor	TNM	Tumor, nodes, metastases
5-FU	5-fluorouracil	XRT	Radiation therapy
Ga	Gallium		

XIII. Practical Applications

This section contains an actual medical report using terms that you have studied in this and previous chapters.

The Philadelphia Chromosome

The Philadelphia chromosome is found in the malignant cells of patient with chronic myelogenous leukemia. In these cells, chromosome 22 is unusually short, as though the end had broken off. The missing genetic material is usually found attached to chromosome 9. The shortened chromosome is referred to as the Philadelphia chromosome because it was first documented by researchers in that city.

Case Report

A 52-year-old married woman presented to her physician with a painless mass in her left breast. During breast examination a 2-cm, firm, nontender mass was palpated in the upper outer quadrant located at the 2 o'clock position, 3 cm from the areola. The mass was not fixed to the skin, and there was no cutaneous erythema or edema. No axillary or supraclavicular lymphadenopathy was noted.

An excisional biopsy of the mass was performed. The pathology report described a gross specimen of fatty breast tissue. Microscopic evaluation of the nodule revealed a scirrhous carcinoma. The margins of the excision were free of tumor. Axillary dissection of lymph nodes was performed, and all 12 lymph nodes were free of tumor.

A portion of the specimen was sent for estrogen receptor assay and proved positive. The patient was informed of the diagnosis and underwent additional studies, including chest x-ray, liver chemistries, CBC, and bone scan—all of which were negative.

The patient was staged as having a $T_1N_0M_0$, stage 1 carcinoma of the left breast. She was referred to a radiation therapist for primary radiation therapy. After completion of radiotherapy, she was treated with tamoxifen. Prognosis is excellent for cure.

Questions for the Case Report

Answers are located at the end of the Answers to Exercises section, page 708.

1. Where was the breast lesion located?
   - (A) under the pigmented area of the breast
   - (B) about an inch and a half to the upper left of the nipple and pigmented area
   - (C) near the axilla and under the shoulder blade

2. Other associated findings were
   - (A) redness and swelling
   - (B) enlarged lymph nodes under the armpit
   - (C) none of the above

3. The tumor was composed of
   - (A) dense connective tissue, giving it a hard structure
   - (B) soft, glandular tissue
   - (C) cells that had extended beyond the borders of the mass

4. What procedure gave evidence that the tumor had not yet metastasized?
   - (A) estrogen receptor assay
   - (B) excisional biopsy of the mass
   - (C) removal of lymph nodes under the arm

5. What additional therapy was undertaken?
   - (A) bone scan, liver chemistries, CBC, and chest x-ray
   - (B) radiation to the breast
   - (C) radiation to the breast and hormonal treatment

6. Tamoxifen was prescribed because
   - (A) the tumor was found to be nonresponsive to estrogen
   - (B) the tumor was found to be responsive to estrogen and tamoxifen is an antiestrogen
   - (C) the tumor was a stage 1 carcinoma

XIV. Exercises

Remember to check your answers carefully with those given in Section XV, Answers to Exercises.

A. *Identify the following characteristics of malignant tumors from their definitions below. Word parts are given as clues.*

1. loss of differentiation of cells and reversion to a more primitive cell type:

    ana _____

2. extending beyond the normal tissue boundaries: in _____

3. having the ability to enter and destroy surrounding tissue: in _____

4. spreading to a secondary site: meta _____

B. *Match the following terms or abbreviations with their meanings below.*

mutation	mitosis	DNA
RNA	chemical carcinogen	virus
ultraviolet radiation	oncogene	radiation

1. replication of cells; two identical cells are produced from a parent cell _____

2. change in the genetic material of a cell _____

3. genetic material within the nucleus that controls replication and protein synthesis

    _____

4. cellular substance (ribonucleic acid) that is important in protein synthesis

    _____

5. rays given off by the sun; can be carcinogenic _____

6. energy carried by a stream of particles; can be carcinogenic _____

7. infectious agent that reproduces by entering a host cell and using the host's genetic material to make

    copies of itself _____

8. a region of genetic material found in tumor cells or in viruses that cause cancer

    _____

9. an agent (hydrocarbon, insecticide, hormone) that causes cancer _____

C. Give the meanings for the following terms.

1. solid tumor _____

2. adenoma _____

3. adenocarcinoma _____

4. osteoma _____

5. osteosarcoma _____

6. mixed-tissue tumor _____

7. neoplasm _____

8. pharmacokinetics _____

9. benign _____

10. differentiation _____

D. Name the terms that describe microscopic tumor growth. Definitions and word parts are given.

1. small nipple-like projections: pap _____

2. abnormal formation of cells: dys _____

3. localized growth of cells: carcin _____

4. densely packed; containing fibrous tissue: _____ ous

5. patterns resembling small, microscopic sacs: alv _____

6. small, gland-type sacs: foll _____

7. variety of cell types: pleo _____

8. lacking structures typical of mature cells: un _____

9. spreading evenly throughout the tissue: di _____

10. many areas of tightly packed clusters of cells: nod _____

11. resembling epithelial cells: epiderm _____

E. Match the following gross descriptions of tumors with their meanings below.

polypoid   medullary   inflammatory
ulcerating   necrotic   verrucous
cystic   fungating

1. containing dead tissue _____

2. mushrooming pattern of growth; tumor cells pile on top of each other

   _____

3. characterized by large, open, exposed surfaces _____

4. characterized by redness, swelling, and heat _____

5. growths are projections from a base; sessile and pedunculated tumors are examples

   _____

6. tumors from large, open spaces filled with fluid; serous and mucinous tumors are examples

   _____

7. tumors resemble wart-like growths _____

8. tumors are large, soft, and fleshy _____

F. Select or supply the appropriate medical term.

1. A (carcinoma/sarcoma) is a cancerous tumor composed of cells of epithelial tissue. An example of such a

   cancerous tumor is a (an) _____ .

2. A (carcinoma/sarcoma) is a cancerous tumor composed of connective tissue. An example of such a

   cancerous tumor is a (an) _____ .

3. Retinoblastoma and polyposis coli syndrome are examples of (chemical carcinogens/inherited cancers).

4. The assessment of a tumor's degree of maturity or microscopic differentiation is (grading/staging) of the
   tumor.

5. The assessment of a tumor's extent of spread within the body is known as (grading/staging).

6. In the TNM staging system, T stands for (tissue/tumor), N stands for (node/necrotic), and M stands for
   (mitotic/metastasis).

G. *Match the surgical procedure in column I with its meaning in column II. Write the letter of the meaning in the space provided.*

Column I

1. fulguration   _____

2. en bloc resection   _____

3. incisional biopsy   _____

4. excisional biopsy   _____

5. cryosurgery   _____

6. electrocauterization _____

7. exenteration   _____

Column II

A. removal of tumor and a margin of normal tissue for diagnosis and possible cure for small tumors
B. burning a lesion to destroy tumor cells
C. wide resection involving removal of tumor, its organ of origin, and surrounding tissue in the body space
D. destruction of tissue by electric sparks generated by a high-frequency current
E. removal of entire tumor and regional lymph nodes
F. freezing a lesion to kill tumor cells
G. cutting into tumor and removing a piece to establish a diagnosis

H. *Give medical terms for the following.*

1. The method of treating cancer by use of high-energy radiation waves is called

   _____ .

2. If tumor tissue requires large doses of radiation to kill cells, it is called a (an)

   _____ tumor.

3. If radiation can cause loss of tumor cells without much damage to surrounding regions, the tumor is

   called _____ .

4. A tumor that can be completely eradicated by irradiation is known as a (an)

   _____ tumor.

5. The method of giving radiation in small, repeated doses is called _____ .

6. Drugs that increase the sensitivity of tumors to x-rays are called _____ .

7. Treatment of cancerous tumors with drugs is called _____ .

8. The study of the distribution and disappearance of drugs in the body is called

   _____ .

9. The use of two or more drugs to kill tumor cells is called _____ .

10. A large electronic device that produces high-energy x-ray beams for treatment of deep-seated tumors is called a (an) _____ .

11. Alkylating agents, antimetabolites, steroids, antibiotics and plant derivatives are all types of _____ agents.

I. Give the meanings for the following medical terms.

1. modality _____

2. adjuvant therapy _____

3. protocol _____

4. remission _____

5. relapse _____

6. morbidity _____

7. biological therapy _____

8. biological response modifiers _____

9. interferon _____

10. monoclonal antibodies _____

J. Match the test or procedure with its description below.

peritoneoscopy   beta-HCG test   bone marrow biopsy
exfoliative cytology   staging laparotomy   needle biopsy
lymphangiography   estrogen receptor assay   PSA test
CEA test

1. test for the presence of a portion of human chorionic gonadotropin hormone (a marker for testicular cancer) _____

2. incision of the abdomen to determine extent of disease _____

3. contrast injected into lymph vessels and x-rays taken _____

4. visual examination of the abdominal cavity; laparoscopy _____

5. test for the presence of a hormone receptor on breast cancer cells _____

6. removal and microscopic examination of bone marrow tissue _____

7. aspiration of tissue for microscopic examination _____

8. blood test for the presence of an antigen related to prostate cancer _____

9. blood test for carcinogenic antigen (marker for GI cancer) _____

10. cells are scraped off tissue and microscopically examined _____

K. *Select the correct term to complete each sentence.*

1. Pauline was diagnosed with a meningioma, which is usually a (an) (benign, anaplastic, necrotic) tumor. The doctor told her that it was not malignant, but that it should be removed because of the pressure it was causing on the surrounding tissues.

2. Marlene underwent surgical resection of her breast mass. Dr. Smith recommended (dedifferentiated, modality, adjuvant) therapy because her tumor was large and she had one positive lymph node.

3. Unfortunately, at the time of diagnosis, the tumor had spread to distant sites because it was (pleomorphic, metastatic, mutagenic). The oncologist recommended beginning chemotherapy as soon as possible.

4. The polyp in Lisa's colon was *not* pedunculated, and Dr. Sidney described it as flat and (fungating, scirrhous, sessile).

5. Mr. Elder had difficulty urinating and had an elevated PSA test. Dr. Jones examined him and found a hard prostate gland. (Staging laparotomy, electrocauterization, biopsy) demonstrated adenocarcinoma.

XV. Answers to Exercises

A

1. anaplasia
2. infiltrative
3. invasive
4. metastasis

B

1. mitosis
2. mutation
3. DNA (deoxyribonucleic acid)
4. RNA (ribonucleic acid)
5. ultraviolet radiation
6. ionizing radiation
7. virus
8. oncogene
9. chemical carcinogen

C

1. tumor composed of a mass of cells
2. tumor of glandular tissue (benign)
3. cancerous tumor of glandular tissue (malignant)
4. tumor of bone (benign)
5. flesh (connective tissue) tumor of bone (malignant)
6. tumor composed of different types of tissue (both epithelial and connective tissues)
7. new formation (tumor)
8. study of the distribution and removal of drugs in the body over a period of time
9. noncancerous
10. specialization of cells

D

1. papillary
2. dysplastic
3. carcinoma in situ
4. scirrhous
5. alveolar
6. follicular
7. pleomorphic
8. undifferentiated
9. diffuse
10. nodular
11. epidermoid

E

1. necrotic
2. fungating
3. ulcerating
4. inflammatory
5. polypoid
6. cystic
7. verrucous
8. medullary

F

1. carcinoma; thyroid adenocarcinoma, squamous cell carcinoma
2. sarcoma; liposarcoma, chondrosarcoma, osteogenic sarcoma
3. inherited cancers
4. grading
5. staging
6. tumor; node; metastasis

G

1. D
2. E
3. G
4. A
5. F
6. B
7. C

H

1. radiation therapy
2. radioresistant
3. radiosensitive
4. radiocurable
5. fractionation
6. radiosensitizers
7. chemotherapy
8. pharmacokinetics
9. combination chemotherapy
10. linear accelerator
11. chemotherapeutic agents

I

1. method of treatment
2. assisting treatment
3. report or plan of steps taken in an experiment or disease case
4. absence of all signs of disease
5. symptoms of disease return
6. conditions of damage to normal tissue; disease
7. treatment that uses the body's own defense mechanisms to fight tumor cells
8. substances produced by normal cells that either directly block tumor growth or stimulate the immune system
9. a biological response modifier that is made by lymphocytes
10. biological response modifiers that are made by mouse cells and are able to bind to tumor cells

J

1. beta-HCG test
2. staging laparotomy
3. lymphangiography
4. peritoneoscopy
5. estrogen receptor assay
6. bone marrow biopsy
7. needle biopsy
8. PSA test
9. CEA test
10. exfoliative cytology

K

1. benign
2. adjuvant
3. metastatic
4. sessile
5. biopsy

Answers to Practical Applications Case Report

1. B
2. C
3. A
4. C
5. C
6. B

XVI. Pronunciation of Terms

To test your understanding of the terminology in this chapter, write the meaning of each term in the space provided. In addition, you may wish to cover the terms and write them by looking at your definitions. Make sure your spelling is correct. The page number after each term indicates where it is defined or used in the text so you can easily check your responses. (If you are not sure what the pronunciation symbols mean, refer to page 21.)

Term	Pronunciation	Meaning
adenocarcinoma (697)	ăd-ĕ-nŏ-kăr-sĭ-NŌ-mă	_____
adjuvant therapy (692)	ĂD-jū-vănt THĔR-ă-pē	_____
alkylating agents (692)	ĂL-kĭ-lā-tĭng Ā-jents	_____

alveolar (695)   ăl-vē-Ō-lăr or ăl-VĒ-ō-lăr   _____

anaplasia (692)   ăn-ă-PLĀ-zē-ă   _____

antibiotics (692)   ăn-tĭ-bī-ŎT-ĭks   _____

antimetabolites (692)   ăn-tĭ-mě-TĂB-ō-līts   _____

apoptosis (692)   ăp-ō-TŌ-sĭs or ā-pŏp-TŌ-sĭs   _____

benign (692)   bē-NĪN   _____

biological response modifier   bī-ō-LŎJ-ĭ-kăl rě-SPŎNS   _____
    (693)   MŎD-ĭ-fī-ěr   _____

biological therapy (693)   bī-ō-LŎJ-ĭ-kăl THĚR-ă-pē   _____

bone marrow biopsy (698)   bōn-MĂ-rō BĪ-ŏp-sē   _____

cachexia (695)   kă-KĚK-sē-ă   _____

carcinogen (693)   kăr-SĬN-ō-jěn   _____

carcinoma in situ (695)   kăr-sĭ-NŌ-ma ĭn SĪ-too   _____

cellular oncogenes (693)   SĚL-ū-lăr ŎNGK-ō-jēnz   _____

chemotherapy (693)   kē-mō-THĚR-ă-pē   _____

cryosurgery (696)   krī-ō-SŬR-jěr-ē   _____

cystic tumor (696)   SĬS-tĭk TOO-mŏr   _____

differentiation (693)   dĭf-ěr-ěn-shē-Ā-shŭn   _____

dysplastic (696)   dĭs-PLĂS-tĭk   _____

electrocauterization (695)   ē-lěk-trō-kăw-těr-ĭ-ZĀ-shŭn   _____

en bloc resection (689)   ěn blŏk rē-SĚK-shŭn   _____

encapsulated (693)   ěn-KĂP-sū-lāt-ěd   _____

epidermoid (697)   ěp-ĭ-DĚR-moyd   _____

excisional biopsy (689)   ek-SIZH-un-al BĪ-ŏp-sē   _____

exenteration (689)   ěks-ěn-tě-RĀ-shŭn   _____

exfoliative cytology (698)   ěks-FŌ-lē-ā-tĭv sī-TŎL-ō-jē   _____

fibrosarcoma (696)   fī-brō-săr-KŌ-ma   _____

follicular (696)   fō-LĬK-ū-lăr   _____

fractionation (693)   frăk-shă-NĀ-shŭn   _____

fulguration (689)	fŭl-gū-RĀ-shŭn	_____
fungating tumor (696)	fŭng-GĀ-tĭng or FŬNG-gā-tĭng TŌŌ-mŏr	_____
grading of tumors (693)	GRĀ-ding of TŌŌ-mŏrz	_____
hyperplasia (697)	hī-pĕr-PLĀ-zē-ă	_____
incisional biopsy (689)	ĭn-SĪZH-ŭn-ăl BĪ-ŏp-sē	_____
infiltrative (693)	ĬN-fĭl-trā-tĭv	_____
invasive (693)	ĭn-VĀ-sĭv	_____
lymphangiography (698)	lĭm-făn-jē-ŎG-ră-fē	_____
malignant (693)	mă-LĬG-nănt	_____
medullary tumor (696)	MĔD-ū-lăr-ē TŌŌ-mŏr	_____
metastasis (693)	mĕ-TĂS-tă-sĭs	_____
mitosis (694)	mī-TŌ-sĭs	_____
modality (694)	mō-DĂL-ĭ-tē	_____
morbidity (694)	mŏr-BĬD-ĭ-tē	_____
mucinous (694)	MŪ-sĭ-nŭs	_____
mutagenic (696)	mū-tă-JĔN-ĭk	_____
mutation (694)	mū-TĀ-shŭn	_____
necrotic tumor (687)	nĕ-KRŎT-ĭk TŌŌ-mŏr	_____
neoplasm (694)	NĒ-ō-plăzm	_____
neuroblastoma (697)	nŭ-rō-blăs-TŌ-mă	_____
nodular (688)	NŎD-ū-lăr	_____
oncogene (694)	ŎNGK-ō-jēn	_____
oncology (696)	ŏn-KŎL-ō-jē	_____
osteosarcoma (697)	ŏs-tē-ō-săr-KŌ-mă	_____
papillary (696)	PĂP-ĭ-lăr-ē	_____
pedunculated (694)	pĕ-DŬNG-kū-lāt-ĕd	_____
peritoneoscopy (698)	pĕr-ĭ-tō-nē-ŎS-kō-pē	_____
pharmacokinetics (694)	făr-mă-kō-kī-NĔT-ĭks	_____

pleomorphic (696)	plē-ō-MŎR-fĭk	_____
polypoid tumor (696)	PŎL-ĭ-poyd TOO-mŏr	_____
protocol (694)	PRŌ-tō-kŏl	_____
radiation (694)	rā-dē-Ā-shŭn	_____
radiocurable tumor (694)	rā-dē-ō-KŪR-ă-b'l TOO-mŏr	_____
radionuclide scans (699)	rā-dē-ō-NŪ-klīd skanz	_____
radioresistant tumor (694)	rā-dē-ō-rĕ-ZĬS-tănt TOO-mŏr	_____
radiosensitive tumor (694)	rā-dē-ō-SEN-sĭ-tĭv TOO-mŏr	_____
radiosensitizer (694)	rā-dē-ō-SĔN-sĭ-tī-zer	_____
radiotherapy (694)	rā-dē-ō-THĔR-ă-pē	_____
relapse (694)	rē-LĂPS	_____
remission (694)	rē-MĬSH-ŭn	_____
retinoblastoma (697)	rĕt-ĭ-nō-blăs-TŌ-mă	_____
ribonucleic acid (694)	rī-bō-nū-KLĒ-ik ĂS-ĭd	_____
sarcoma (694)	săr-KŌ-mă	_____
scirrhous (697)	SKĬR-ŭs	_____
serous (695)	SĒ-rŭs	_____
sessile (695)	SĔS-ĭl	_____
solid tumor (695)	SŎL-ĭd TOO-mŏr	_____
staging laparotomy (699)	STĀ-jing lă-pă-RŎT-ō-mē	_____
staging of tumors (695)	STĀ-jĭng of TOO-mŏrz	_____
steroids (695)	STĒ-roydz	_____
ulcerating tumor (687)	ŬL-sĕ-rā-tĭng TOO-mŏr	_____
ultraviolet radiation (695)	ŭl-tră-VĪ-ō-lĕt rā-dē-Ā-shun	_____
verrucous tumor (687)	vĕ-ROO-kŭs or VĔR-oo-kŭs TOO-mŏr	_____
viral oncogenes (695)	VĪ-răl ŎNGK-ō-jĕnz	_____
virus (695)	VĪ-rŭs	_____

XVII. Review Sheet

Write the meaning of each combining form in the space provided and test yourself. Check your answers with the information in the chapter or in the Glossary (Medical Terms—English) at the back of the book.

Combining Forms

Combining Form	Meaning	Combining Form	Meaning
aden/o		fung/o	
alveol/o		medull/o	
cac/o		mut/a	
carcin/o		mutagen/o	
cauter/o		onc/o	
chem/o		papill/o	
cry/o		pharmac/o	
cyst/o		plas/o	
fibr/o		ple/o	
follicul/o		polyp/o	

radi/o _____   scirrh/o _____

sarc/o _____

Suffixes

Suffix	Meaning	Suffix	Meaning
-ary	_____	-plasia	_____
-blast	_____	-plasm	_____
-oid	_____	-ptosis	_____
-oma	_____	-stasis	_____

Prefixes

Prefix	Meaning	Prefix	Meaning
ana-	_____	epi-	_____
apo-	_____	hyper-	_____
dys-	_____	meta-	_____

20

Radiology, Nuclear Medicine, and Radiation Therapy

This Chapter is divided into the following sections

In this Chapter you will

- Learn the physical properties of x-rays;
- Become familiar with diagnostic and therapeutic techniques used by radiologists and radiotherapists;
- Identify the x-ray views and patient positions used in x-ray examinations;
- Learn about the role of radioactivity in the diagnosis and treatment of disease; and
- Become familiar with medical terms used in the specialties of radiology, nuclear medicine, and radiation therapy.

I. Introduction

Radiology (also called **roentgenology** after its discoverer, Wilhelm Conrad Roentgen) is the medical specialty concerned with the study of x-rays. **X-rays** are invisible waves of energy that are produced by an energy source (x-ray machine, cathode ray tube) and are useful in diagnosis and treatment of disease.

Nuclear medicine is the medical specialty that studies the characteristics and uses of **radioactive substances** in the diagnosis of disease. Radioactive substances are materials that emit high-speed particles and energy-containing rays from the interior of their matter. The emitted particles and rays are called **radioactivity** and can be of three types: **alpha particles, beta particles,** and **gamma rays. Gamma rays** are similar to x-rays in that they have no mass and are used effectively as a diagnostic label to trace the path and uptake of chemical substances in the body.

Radiation therapy (radiation oncology) is the treatment of disease using either an external source of high-energy rays (photons, electrons, protons, gamma rays) or internally implanted radioactive substances. These rays and substances are effective in damaging the DNA of cancer cells and halting their growth.

The personnel involved in these medical fields are varied. A **radiologist** is a physician who specializes in the practice of diagnostic radiology. A **nuclear physician** is a radiologist who specializes in the practice of administering diagnostic nuclear medicine procedures. A **radiation oncologist (radiotherapist),** also a physician, specializes in the practice of radiotherapy (treatment of disease using radiation).

Allied health care professionals who work with physicians in the fields of radiology, nuclear medicine, and radiotherapy are called **radiologic technologists.** Radiologic technologists can be divided into three categories: **radiographers** (aid physicians in administering diagnostic x-ray procedures), **nuclear medicine technologists** (attend to patients undergoing nuclear medicine procedures and operate devices under the direction of a nuclear physician), and **radiation therapy technologists** (deliver courses of radiation therapy prescribed by a radiotherapist).

II. Radiology

A. Characteristics of X-Rays

Several characteristics of x-rays are useful to physicians in the diagnosis and treatment of disease. Some of these characteristics are

1. **Ability to cause exposure of a photographic plate.** If a photographic plate is placed in front of a beam of x-rays, the x-rays, traveling unimpeded through the air, will expose the silver coating of the plate and cause it to blacken.

2. **Ability to penetrate different substances to varying degrees.** X-rays pass through the different types of substances in the human body (air in the lungs, water in blood vessels and lymph, fat around muscles, and metal such as calcium in bones) with varying ease. Air is the least dense substance and exhibits the greatest transmission. Fat is denser, water is next, followed by metal, which is the densest and transmits least. If the x-rays are absorbed (stopped) by the denser body substance (e.g., calcium in bones), they do not reach the photographic plate held behind the patient, and white areas are left in the x-ray film (plate). Figure 20–1 is an example of an x-ray photograph.

A substance is said to be **radiolucent** if it permits passage of most of the x-rays. Lung tissue (containing air) is an example of a radiolucent substance, and it appears black on an x-ray image. **Radiopaque** substances (bones) are those that absorb most of the x-rays they are

Figure 20–1

X-ray photograph (radiograph) of the hand. (From Poznanski AK: The Hand in Radiologic Diagnosis, 2nd ed. Philadelphia, WB Saunders, 1984, p 21.)

exposed to, allowing only a small fraction of the x-rays to reach the x-ray plate. Thus, normally radiopaque, calcium-containing bone appears white on an x-ray image.

3. **Invisibility.** X-rays cannot be detected by sight, sound, or touch. Workers exposed to x-rays must wear a **film badge** to detect and record the amount of radiation to which they have been exposed. The film badge contains a special film that is exposed by x-rays. The amount of blackness on the film is an indication of the amount of x-rays or gamma rays received by the wearer.

4. **Travel in straight lines.** This property allows the formation of precise shadow images on the x-ray plate and also permits x-ray beams to be directed accurately at a tissue site during radiotherapy.

5. **Scattering of radiation.** Scattering occurs when x-rays come in contact with any material. Greater scatter occurs with dense objects and less scatter with those substances that are radiolucent. Scatter can be a serious occupational hazard to those in the vicinity of a source of x-rays, such as an x-ray machine. In addition, because scatter can blur images and expose areas of film that otherwise would be in shadow, a grid (containing thin lead strips arranged parallel to the x-ray beams) is placed in front of the film to absorb scattered radiation before it strikes the x-ray film.

6. **Ionization.** X-rays have the ability to ionize substances through which they pass. Ionization is a chemical process in which the energy of an x-ray beam causes rearrangement and disruption within a substance, so that previously neutral particles are changed to charged particles called **ions.** This strongly ionizing ability of x-rays is a double-edged sword. In x-ray therapy, the ionizing effect of x-rays can help kill cancerous cells and stop tumor growth; however, ionizing x-rays in small doses can affect normal body cells, leading to tissue damage and malignant changes. Thus, persons exposed to high doses of x-rays are at risk of developing leukemia, thyroid tumors, breast cancer, or other malignancies.

B. Diagnostic Techniques

X-Rays

X-rays are used in a variety of ways to detect pathological conditions. The most common use of the diagnostic x-ray is dental, to locate cavities (caries) in teeth. Other areas examined include the digestive, nervous, reproductive, and endocrine systems and the chest and bones. Some special diagnostic x-ray techniques are

Computed Tomography (CT, CAT). This is a revolutionary technique in radiologic diagnosis. Machines called **CT scanners** (also called **CAT scanners**) beam ionizing x-rays through a patient at multiple angles around a specific section of the body (Fig. 20–2). The absorption of the x-rays at these angles as they pass through the body is detected and relayed to a computer that is programmed with a knowledge of the absorption capacities of the different body tissues. The computer then synthesizes all the information it receives from the many different x-ray views and projects a single composite picture of a specific "slice" of the abdomen, chest, or head on a screen. The ability of CT scanners to detect abnormalities is enhanced by the use of iodine-containing contrast agents, which outline blood vessels.

The CT scanners are highly sensitive in detecting disease in bony structures and can actually provide images of internal organs that are impossible to visualize with ordinary x-ray technique. CT scans also involve the use of contrast dyes and can detect brain tumors, hematomas, spinal cord lesions, and masses in the chest, liver, kidneys, and pancreas. Figure 20–3 shows a series of CT scans through various regions of the body.

Contrast Studies. In x-ray film, the natural differences in the density of body tissues (e.g., air in lung, calcium in bone) produce contrasting shadow images on the x-ray film. However, when x-rays pass through two adjacent body parts composed of substances of the same density, for example, the digestive organs in the abdomen, their images cannot be distinguished on the film or on the screen. It is necessary, then, to inject a **contrast medium** into the structure or fluid to be visualized so that the specific part, organ, tube, or liquid can be visualized as a negative imprint on the dense contrast agent.

The following are artificial contrast materials used in diagnostic radiological studies:

Barium Sulfate. Barium sulfate is a metallic powder that is mixed in water and used for examination of the upper and lower GI (gastrointestinal) tract. A **barium swallow (upper GI series)** involves oral ingestion of barium sulfate so that the esophagus, stomach, and duodenum can be visualized. A **small bowel series (small bowel follow-through)** traces the passage of barium in a sequential manner as it passes through the small intestine. A **barium enema** opacifies the lumen (passageway) of the large intestine using an enema containing barium sulfate. Figure 20–4 shows a radiograph of the colon after a barium enema.

A double-contrast study uses both a radiopaque and a radiolucent contrast medium. For example, the walls of the stomach or intestine are coated with barium and the lumen is filled with air. The radiographs show the pattern of mucosal ridges.

Figure 20–2

Representation of a patient inside a CT scanner. *Arrows* indicate the x-ray tubes that are positioned around the patient.

Figure 20-3

CT scans through various regions of the body. The level of the scan is indicated on the figure of the body. The bar below the figure indicates the gradient of structure density as represented by black (least dense, such as air) and white (most dense, such as bone). (*Left,* From Solomon EP, Phillips GA: Understanding Human Anatomy and Physiology. Philadelphia, WB Saunders, 1987, p 21; *right,* Courtesy of Professor Jon H. Ehringer.)

Figure 20–4

Barium enema radiograph of the colon. (From Putman CE, Ravin CE: Textbook of Diagnostic Imaging. Philadelphia, WB Saunders, 1988, p 13.)

Iodine Compounds. Radiopaque fluids containing up to 50 per cent iodine are used in the following tests:

angiography	An x-ray image of blood vessels and heart chambers is obtained after injecting a water-soluble dye through a catheter (tube) into the appropriate blood vessel or heart chamber.
arteriography	An x-ray image of an artery is obtained after injecting a radiopaque substance directly into the artery. Cerebral arteries are often examined in this manner in a search for aneurysm, blood clot, or tumor.
arthrography	Dye or air, or both, is injected into a joint, and x-rays are taken of the joint.
bronchography	An x-ray image of the bronchial tubes after injecting an iodized oil suspension into the bronchi through the trachea.
cholangiography	Dye is injected intravenously and directed by the liver into the bile ducts. X-rays are taken of the gallbladder and bile ducts. This test is frequently ordered after cholecystectomy to examine the patency (size of opening) of bile ducts.
cholecystography	A radiopaque substance is given orally; the substance collects in the gallbladder, and x-rays are taken of the gallbladder and the bile ducts. A fatty meal may then be given and follow-up x-rays taken to look for stones in the gallbladder and common bile duct.
digital subtraction angiography (DSA)	An x-ray image of contrast-injected blood vessels is produced by taking two x-rays (the first without contrast) and using a computer to subtract obscuring shadows from the image. Figure 20–5 illustrates the final x-ray image produced by DSA.
hysterosalpingography	An x-ray record of the uterine tubes is obtained after injecting dye into the

Figure 20–5

Digital subtraction angiography showing bilateral renal artery stenosis *(arrows)* in a man with hypertension. The large dark vessel is the aorta. (From Hillman BJ: Imaging and Hypertension. Philadelphia, WB Saunders, 1983, p 37.)

uterus via the vagina. This procedure can determine patency of the uterine tubes.

lymphangiography   An x-ray record of lymphatic vessels and nodes is obtained after injection of dye (Ethiodol) into the lymphatic system of the feet or hands.

myelography   An x-ray of the spinal cord is made after injecting radiopaque dye (Pantopaque) into the subarachnoid space surrounding the spinal cord. This test identifies protrusion of an intervertebral disk or bone pressing on the spinal cord or nerve roots. Tumors in or on the spinal cord can also be identified.

pyelography   X-ray images are made on the renal pelvis and urinary tract after dye is injected into a vein **(intravenous pyelogram)** or after dye is injected directly into the urethra, bladder, and ureters **(retrograde pyelogram).**

venography   An x-ray image of veins is taken after introducing contrast medium intravenously.

Some individuals experience side effects to the iodine-containing contrast substances. These effects can range from mild reactions such as flushing, nausea, warmth, or tingling sensations to severe, life-threatening reactions characterized by airway spasm, hives, laryngeal edema (swelling of the larynx), vasodilation, and tachycardia. Treatment involves immediate establishment of an airway and ventilation followed by injections of epinephrine (adrenaline), corticosteroids, or antihistamines.

Fluoroscopy. This x-ray procedure uses a fluorescent screen instead of a photographic plate to derive a visual image from the x-rays that pass through the patient. The fact that ionizing radiation such as x-rays can produce **fluorescence** (rays of light energy emitted as a result of exposure to and absorption of radiation from another source) is the basis for fluoroscopy. The fluorescent screen glows when it is struck by the x-rays. Opaque tissue, such as bone, appears as a dark shadow image on the fluorescent screen.

A major advantage of fluoroscopy over normal radiography is that internal organs, such as the heart and digestive tract organs, can be observed in motion. In addition, the patient's position can be changed constantly to provide the right view at the right time so that the most useful diagnostic information can be obtained.

Interventional radiology includes therapeutic procedures that are performed by a radiologist while the patient is undergoing fluoroscopy (or ultrasound). Examples of uses of interventional radiology are for placement of drainage catheters, drainage of abscesses, occlusion of bleeding vessels, and installation of antibiotics or chemotherapy through catheters.

Image-intensifier systems for fluoroscopy can brighten fluoroscopic images and can be combined with movie cameras and videotape recorders to obtain a permanent record of either a fluoroscopic or an x-ray examination. This procedure is called **cineradiography** (cine-means motion).

Tomography. Tomography is a technique for taking a series of x-ray pictures, so that x-rays of a desired layer of the body are obtained, while at the same time structures in front of and behind that layer are blurred out. Multiple pictures, called **tomograms** or **body sections,** are taken by changing the depth of focus of the x-ray machine while the patient remains still. Tomograms are thus x-ray "slices" taken at different depths of focus through the patient. Each tomogram obliterates all extraneous material and focuses on the one small slice that is to be viewed. Calcifications and other solid lesions that are missed on conventional x-rays can be picked up with tomography.

Ultrasound

This technique employs high-frequency, inaudible sound waves that bounce off body tissues and are then recorded to give information about the anatomy of an internal organ. An instrument is placed near or on the skin, which is covered with a thin coating of mineral oil to assure good transmission of sound waves. This instrument emits sound waves in short, repetitive pulses. The ultrasound waves move with different speeds through body tissues and detect interfaces between tissues of different density. An echo reflection of the sound waves is formed as the waves hit the various body tissues and pass back to the ultrasound monitor.

These ultrasonic echoes are then recorded as a composite picture of the area of the body over which the instrument has passed. The record produced by ultrasound is called a **sonogram** or **echogram.**

Ultrasound is used as a diagnostic tool not only by radiologists but also by neurosurgeons and ophthalmologists to detect intracranial and ophthalmic lesions, by cardiologists to detect heart valve and blood vessel disorders **(echocardiography),** by gastroenterologists to locate abdominal masses outside the digestive organs, and by obstetricians and gynecologists to differentiate single and multiple pregnancies as well as to help in performing amniocentesis and in locating tumors or cysts. Fetal size and age can also be measured using ultrasound. The measurements are made from ultrasound images taken in various fetal planes (across the head, abdomen, and femur) (Fig. 20–6).

Ultrasound has several advantages in that the sound waves are nonionizing and noninjurious to tissues at the energy ranges utilized for diagnostic purposes. Since water is an excellent conductor of the ultrasonic beams, patients are requested to drink large quantities of water prior to examination so that the urinary bladder will be distended and enable better viewing of pelvic and abdominal organs. Figure 20–7 is an example of a fetal ultrasonogram.

Two ultrasound techniques, Doppler ultrasound and color flow imaging, make it possible to record blood velocity (in diagnosing vascular disease) and to image major blood vessels in patients at risk for stroke.

Ultrasound, like fluoroscopy, has also been used in interventional radiology to guide needle biopsies for the puncture of cysts and for the placement of needles for amniocentesis.

Figure 20–6

Fetal measurements taken with ultrasound imaging. *Dashed lines* indicate the image planes for measurements of the fetal head, abdomen, and femur. (From Putman CE, Ravin CE: Diagnostic Imaging. Philadelphia, WB Saunders, 1988, p 2012.)

Magnetic Imaging or Magnetic Resonance Imaging (MRI)

This technique produces sagittal, coronal (frontal), and axial (cross-sectional) images, the latter being similar to CT scanning. MRI, however, uses no x-rays and does not require a contrast medium. The technique is based on the fact that the nuclei of some atoms behave like little magnets when a larger magnetic field is applied. The nuclei spin and emit radio waves that create an image as the nuclei move back to an equilibrium position. Hydrogen

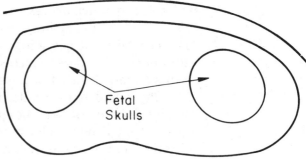

Figure 20–7

Sonogram of a pregnant uterus showing two 18 week skulls on opposite sides of the uterus. (From Leopold GR, Asher WM: Ultrasound in obstetrics and gynecology. Radiol Clin North Am 12:127, 1974.)

Figure 20–8

Magnetic resonance images. *(A)* Frontal or coronal view of the upper body. White masses in the chest are Hodgkin's disease lesions. *(B)* Transverse view of the same patient with chest mass. *(C)* Sagittal view of the head. (*C,* From Putman CE, Ravin CE: Diagnostic Imaging. Philadelphia, WB Saunders, 1988, p 5.)

nuclei, present in water and abundant in living tissue, are the nuclei used to create the image. MRI is useful in detecting edema in the brain, projecting a direct image of the spinal cord, detecting tumors in the chest and abdomen, and visualizing the cardiovascular system. Figure 20–8 shows three different MRI images (frontal, transverse, and sagittal).

Figure 20–9 reviews the radiological diagnostic techniques discussed.

Figure 20–9

Review of radiological diagnostic techniques.

C. X-Ray Positioning

In order to take the best possible view of the part of the body being radiographed, the patient, film, and x-ray tube must be positioned in the most favorable alignment possible. There are special terms used by radiologists to designate the position or direction of the x-ray beam, the patient's position, and the motion and position of the part of the body to be examined. Some of the x-ray terms describing the position of the x-ray beam are

1. **AP view** (anteroposterior). In this view, the patient is usually supine (lying on the back), and the x-ray tube is aimed from above at the anterior of the body with the beam passing from anterior to posterior. The film lies underneath the patient. The AP view may also be taken with the patient in the upright position.

2. **PA view** (posteroanterior). In this view, the patient is upright with her or his back to the x-ray machine and the film to the chest. The x-ray machine is aimed horizontally at a distance of about 6 feet from the film.

3. **Lateral view.** In this view, the x-ray beam passes from one side of the body toward the opposite side. In taking a right lateral view, the right side of the body is held closely against the x-ray film and the x-ray beam passes from the left to the right through the body.

4. **Oblique view.** In this view, the x-ray tube is positioned at an angle from the perpendicular plane. Oblique views are used to show regions that would be hidden and superimposed in routine AP and PA views.

The following terms are used to describe the position of the patient or part of the body in the x-ray examination:

abduction	Moving the part of the body away from the midline of the body or away from the body.
adduction	Moving the part of the body toward the midline of the body or toward the body.
eversion	Turning outward.
extension	Lengthening or straightening a flexed limb.
flexion	Bending a part of the body.
inversion	Turning inward.
lateral decubitus	Lying down on the side with the x-ray beam horizontally positioned; sometimes called **cross-table lateral.**
prone	Lying on the belly (face down).
recumbent	Lying down (may be prone or supine).
supine	Lying on the back (face up).

III. Nuclear Medicine

A. Radioactivity and Radionuclides

The emission of energy in the form of particles or rays coming from the interior of a substance is called **radioactivity.** A **radionuclide** (or **radioisotope**) is a substance that gives off high-energy particles or rays as it disintegrates. Radionuclides are produced in either a nuclear reactor or a charged-particle accelerator (cyclotron) or by irradiating stable substances, causing disruption and instability. **Half-life** is the time required for a radioactive substance (radionuclide) to lose half of its radioactivity by disintegration. Knowledge of a radionuclide's half-life is important in determining how long the radioactive substance will emit radioactivity when in the body. The half-life must be long enough to allow for diagnostic imaging but as short as possible to minimize patient exposure to radiation. Technetium-99m (^{99m}Tc), with a half-life of 6 hours, is an ideal radionuclide and is used most frequently in diagnostic imaging.

Radionuclides emit three types of radioactivity: **alpha particles, beta particles,** and **gamma rays.** Gamma rays, which have greater penetrating ability than alpha and beta particles, and more ionizing power, are especially useful to physicians in both the diagnosis and the treatment of disease.

B. Nuclear Medicine Tests: In Vitro and In Vivo Procedures

Nuclear medicine physicians use two types of tests in the diagnosis of disease: **in vitro** (in the test tube) procedures and **in vivo** (in the body) procedures. **In vitro** procedures involve analysis of blood and urine specimens using radioactive chemicals. For example, a **radioimmunoassay (RIA)** is an in vitro procedure that combines the use of radioactive chemicals and antibodies to detect hormones and drugs in a patient's blood. The test allows the detection of minute amounts of drug. RIA is used to monitor the amount of digitalis, a drug used to treat heart disease, in a patient's bloodstream and can detect hypothyroidism in newborn infants.

In vivo tests trace the amounts of radioactive substances within the body. They are given directly to a patient to evaluate the function of an organ or to image it. For example, in **tracer studies** a specific radionuclide is incorporated into a chemical substance and administered to a patient. The combination of the radionuclide and a drug or chemical is called a **radiopharmaceutical** (or **labeled compound**). Each radiopharmaceutical is designed to concentrate in a certain organ. The organ can then be imaged with the radiation given off by the radionuclide.

A sensitive, external detection instrument, called a **scintillation scanner,** is used to determine the distribution and localization of the radiopharmaceutical in various organs, tissues, and fluids. The amount of radiopharmaceutical at a given location is proportional to the rate at which the gamma rays are emitted. Nuclear medicine studies depict the physiological behavior (how the organ works) rather than the specific anatomy of an organ.

The procedure of making an image to follow the distribution of radioactive substance in the body is called **scanning,** and the image produced is called a **scan. Uptake** refers to the rate of absorption of the radiopharmaceutical into an organ or tissue.

Radiopharmaceuticals may be administered by many different routes to obtain a scan of a specific organ in the body. For example, in the case of a **lung scan,** the radiopharmaceutical can be given intravenously (**perfusion studies,** which rely on passage of the radioactive compound through the capillaries of the lungs) or by inhalation of xenon-133 (^{133}Xe) gas

Figure 20–10

Total-body bone scan shows darkened areas of increased radiopharmaceutical uptake in the thoracic and lumbar spine. (From James AE Jr, Squire LF: Nuclear Radiology. Philadelphia, WB Saunders, 1973, p 128.)

A

B

Figure 20–11

(A) Normal lateral brain scan. *(B)* Mass (meningioma) in the inferior frontal area of the brain. (*A* and *B,* From James AE Jr, Squire LF: Nuclear Radiology. Philadelphia, WB Saunders, 1973, pp 157, 172.)

(ventilation studies), which fills the air sacs (alveoli). The combination of these tests permits sensitive and specific diagnosis of clots in the lung (pulmonary emboli).

Other examples of diagnostic procedures that utilize radionuclides are

1. **Blood and heart scan.** Radiopharmaceutical (^{99m}Tc human serum albumin) is injected intravenously, and the blood flow is imaged as the tracer passes through the chambers of the heart and large vessels. Sequential images can be recorded on film to give a motion picture of the passage of blood through the heart. Diagnosis of various forms of heart disease is possible.

2. **Bone scan.** ^{99m}Tc is used to label phosphate substances and is intravenously injected. The phosphate compound is taken up preferentially by bone, and the skeleton can be imaged in 2 or 3 hours by use of a gamma camera. Waiting 2–3 hours allows much of the radiopharmaceutical to be excreted in urine and allows for better visualization of the skeleton. Figure 20–10 is an example of a bone scan. The scan is useful in demonstrating malignant metastases to the skeleton, which appear as areas of high uptake ("hot spots") on the scan.

3. **Brain scan.** A radiopharmaceutical (^{99m}Tc pertechnetate) is injected intravenously, and about 2 hours later images of the brain are obtained via scanning. Normal scans would show no uptake of radiopharmaceutical in the brain because of the normal functioning of the blood-brain barrier (BBB) which prevents radiopharmaceuticals from entering the brain from the blood. However, if the BBB is broken down by tumor or disease, radiopharmaceutical enters the brain and shows up on the brain scan. Brain scans are useful in detecting infarctions, abscesses, tumors, and hematomas. Figure 20–11 shows a normal and an abnormal brain scan.

4. **Gallium scan.** The radioisotope gallium-67 is injected and has an affinity for tumors and non-neoplastic lesions, such as abscesses.

5. **Liver and spleen scans.** To visualize the liver and spleen, a radiopharmaceutical (^{99m}Tc and sulfur colloid) is injected intravenously, and images are taken with a gamma camera. Areas of tumor or abscess are shown as blank spots (regions of reduced uptake). Abnormalities such as cirrhosis, abscesses, tumor, hepatomegaly, and hepatitis can be detected by liver scanning, and splenomegaly due to tumor, cyst, abscess, or rupture can be diagnosed with spleen scanning.

6. **Positron emission tomography (PET scan).** This radionuclide technique produces a cross-sectional (transverse) image of the distribution of radioactivity (through emission of positrons) in a region of the body. It is similar to the CT scan, but radioisotopes are used instead of dye and x-rays. The radionuclides are incorporated (by intravenous injection) into the tissues to be scanned, and an image is made showing where the radionuclide (such as carbon-11 [^{11}C] glucose, oxygen-15 [^{15}O] oxygen) is or is not being metabolized. For example, PET scanning has determined that schizophrenics do not metabolize glucose equally in all parts of the brain and that drug treatment can bring improvement to these regions. Thus, areas of metabolic deficiency can be pinpointed by PET, making it helpful in diagnosing and treating other neurological disorders such as stroke, epilepsy, Alzheimer's disease, and brain tumors, as well as cardiac, pulmonary, and abdominal disorders.

7. **Radioactive iodine uptake by the thyroid gland.** Radioactive iodine compound (^{131}I) is given orally by capsule (the amount of radioactive substance in the capsule is measured earlier). The amount of radioactivity taken up by the thyroid gland during the process of making thyroid hormone can be measured at 6 and 24 hours and compared with normal values. This measurement reflects the rate of hormone synthesis by the thyroid gland.

8. **Single-photon emission computed tomography (SPECT).** This technique involves an intravenous injection of radioactive tracer and the computer reconstruction of a three-dimensional image from the composite of many views. Clinical applications include

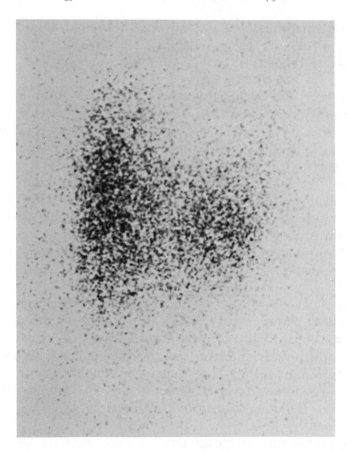

Figure 20–12

Normal thyroid scan (obtained with ^{123}I).
(From Putman CE, Ravin CE: Diagnostic
Imaging. Philadelphia, WB Saunders,
1988, p 5.)

detecting liver tumors, detecting cardiac ischemia, and evaluating bone disease of the spine.

9. **Thyroid scan.** Radionuclide is administered intravenously. The scan produced can help determine the size and shape of the thyroid gland. Hyperfunctioning thyroid nodules accumulate higher amounts of ^{131}I radioactivity and are termed "hot." Thyroid carcinoma does not concentrate radioiodine well and, therefore, is seen as a "cold" spot on the scan. Figure 20–12 shows a normal thyroid nuclear medicine image.

Figure 20–13 reviews in vitro and in vivo nuclear medicine diagnostic tests.

NUCLEAR MEDICINE TESTS

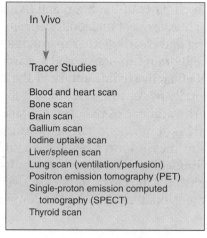

In Vitro

↓

Radioimmunoassay

In Vivo

↓

Tracer Studies

Blood and heart scan
Bone scan
Brain scan
Gallium scan
Iodine uptake scan
Liver/spleen scan
Lung scan (ventilation/perfusion)
Positron emission tomography (PET)
Single-proton emission computed
    tomography (SPECT)
Thyroid scan

Figure 20–13

Nuclear medicine tests.

IV. Radiation Therapy (Radiation Oncology)

Not only are x-rays and radionuclides helpful in detecting disease, but they can be used as therapy as well. Large doses of ionizing radiation to body tissues can be **lethal** (killing) to the cells that are **irradiated.** Radiation oncology has been particularly helpful as a method for the treatment of cancers, as discussed in Chapter 19.

The machines used for radiation oncology are different from those used for diagnosis. Therapy machines deliver rays of many times higher intensity. **Orthovoltage** machines deliver low-energy radiation, which in modern treatment centers is used in treatment of superficial skin cancers. **Megavoltage** machines generate high-energy radiation and are used to treat deeper tissues in curative radiotherapy for cancer. Two examples of such machines are the **betatron** and the **linear accelerator;** they deliver a sharply defined radiation beam to a specific area of the body while sparing overlying superficial tissue.

Radiation may be applied to a tumor from some distance **(external beam radiation)** or implanted within the tumor itself **(brachytherapy).** External beam machines (such as the linear accelerator) direct a beam of photons toward the tumor. The higher the energy of the photons, the greater the penetration of the beam. Photons can also be produced from a radioactive source (cobalt-60 [^{60}Co]); both sources of high-energy photons (linear accelerator and cobalt) are well suited for the treatment of deep-seated tumors.

Brachytherapy includes **interstitial therapy** and **intracavitary therapy.** In order to deliver interstitial therapy, a radioactive element (such as radium, gold-198 [^{198}Au], iodine-125 [^{125}I], or iridium-192 [^{192}Ir]) is surgically inserted into the tumor. This results in a very localized form of treatment, sparing normal tissues in the vicinity. The radionuclide is implanted in strands, in small sealed containers called seeds, or in removable needles. Intracavitary therapy is delivered by placing radioactive sources (radium, cesium-137 [^{137}Ce], or phosphorus-32 [^{32}P]) within a body cavity and adjacent to a tumor. This form of therapy is particularly suited for gynecological malignancies (uterus, cervix, or vagina).

Another form of radiotherapy is the administration of radioactive materials into the bloodstream. ^{131}I is used to treat hyperthyroidism and thyroid carcinoma. In hyperthyroidism, the ^{131}I, given orally, passes into the blood and accumulates in the thyroid gland, irradiating the tissue there and reducing the activity of the gland. ^{131}I is also taken up by thyroid tumors. In treating thyroid carcinoma, ^{131}I is used after partial or total thyroidectomy to inactivate any residual thyroid tissue and to treat metastases.

Radiation delivered to tissues is measured in a unit called a **gray (gy).** A gray is equal to 100 **rad** (radiation absorbed dose). Tumors and body tissues are classified as **radiosensitive** and **radioresistant,** according to the number of gray necessary to kill or injure cells. Examples of radiosensitive organs are the ovaries and testes. Radioresistant organs (such as the pituitary and adrenal glands) are less susceptible to the effects of radiation. Lymphomas are generally radiosensitive, whereas sarcomas are generally very radioresistant.

Radiotherapy, although it may be either a palliative or a curative agent, can produce undesirable side effects on normal body tissues that are incidentally irradiated. Some of these complications are reversible with time, and recovery takes place soon after the period of radiotherapy is completed. These acute reversible effects may include

1. Ulceration of mucous membranes **(mucositis);** for example, in the mouth, pharynx, vagina, bladder, or large and small intestine. **Xerostomia** (dryness of mouth) occurs after radiation to the mouth or pharynx.

2. **Nausea and vomiting** as a reaction to radiotherapy to the brain or gastrointestinal organs.

3. Bone marrow suppression **(myelosuppression),** with leukopenia and thrombocytopenia.

4. **Alopecia** (baldness).

With higher doses of radiotherapy, these complications can be associated with permanent organ damage. In addition, radiotherapy delivered in therapeutic doses may produce chronic (long-lasting) injury to any body organ that happens to be in or near the path of the radiation beam. Chronic side effects depend on the site of treatment delivery and can include pericarditis, pneumonitis, vasculitis (inflammation of blood vessels), and fibrosis of the skin and lungs.

V. Vocabulary

This list will help you review many of the new terms introduced in the text. Short definitions will reinforce your understanding of the terms. See Section XI of this chapter for help in pronouncing the more difficult terms.

betatron	Machine used in radiotherapy to deliver a dose of radiation to a patient.
brachytherapy	Radiation therapy using an implanted radioisotope radiation source (brachy means short).
cineradiography	Use of motion picture techniques to record a series of x-ray images.
cobalt-60	A radioactive substance used in radiotherapy.
computed tomography (CT)	Diagnostic x-ray procedure whereby a cross-section image of a specific body segment is produced.
contrast studies	Materials (contrast media) are injected to obtain contrast with surrounding tissue when shown on the x-ray film.
external beam radiation	Radiation applied using a distant source.
fluorescence	The emission of glowing light that results from exposure to and absorption of radiation from x-rays.
fluoroscopy	The process of using x-rays to produce a fluorescent image on a screen.
gamma rays	High-energy rays emitted by radioactive substances.
gray	Unit of absorbed radiation dose (equal to 100 rad).
half-life	Time required for a radioactive substance to lose half its radioactivity by disintegration.
interstitial therapy	Radioisotopes are surgically inserted into a tumor (-stitial means to set).
interventional radiology	Therapeutic procedures that are performed by a radiologist.
intracavitary therapy	Radioisotopes are placed within a body cavity adjacent to a tumor.
in vitro	A process, test, or procedure in which something is measured or observed outside a living organism.

in vivo	A process, test, or procedure in which something is measured or observed in a living organism.
ionization	The separation of stable substances into charged particles called ions.
irradiation	Administering radiation treatment to a patient (ir- stands for in-, meaning into).
lethal	Pertaining to that which is deadly or fatal.
linear accelerator	Machine that delivers radiation therapy.
magnetic resonance imaging	A magnetic field and radio waves are used to form sagittal, coronal, and axial images of the body.
megavoltage	High-energy radiation generated by a machine and used in curative x-ray therapy for cancer.
nuclear medicine	Medical specialty that studies the uses of radioactive substances (radionuclides) in diagnosis and treatment of disease.
orthovoltage	Low-energy radiation used in palliative radiation therapy and superficial skin cancers.
palliative	Relieving symptoms, but not curing.
positron emission tomography (PET)	Radioactive substances are given intravenously and then emit positrons, which create a cross-sectional image of the metabolism of the body, representing local concentration of the radioactive substance.
rad	Radiation absorbed dose; a unit of absorbed radiation in the body.
radiation oncology	Treatment of tumors using high-energy radiation. Also called radiotherapy or radiation therapy.
radioimmunoassay	Test that combines the use of radioactive chemicals and antibodies to detect minute quantities of substances in a patient's blood.
radioisotope	A radioactive form of a substance; radionuclide.
radiology	Medical specialty concerned with the study of x-rays and their use in diagnosis of disease; includes other forms of energy, such as ultrasound and magnetic waves.
radiolucent	Permitting the passage of most x-rays. Radiolucent structures appear black on x-ray film.
radionuclide	A radioactive chemical element that gives off energy in the form of radiation; radioisotope.
radiopaque	Obstructing the passage of x-rays. Radiopaque structures appear white on the x-ray film.

radiopharmaceutical	A radioactive drug (radionuclide plus chemical) that is administered safely for diagnostic and therapeutic purposes.
roentgenology	Study of x-rays; radiology.
scan	A general term for images of organs, parts, or transverse sections of the body produced in various ways. Most frequently used to describe images obtained from ultrasound, tracer studies, or computed tomography.
scintillation scanner	Machine used to detect radiopharmaceuticals in the body for diagnostic imaging. Scintill/o means spark.
single-photon emission computed tomography (SPECT)	A radioactive tracer substance is injected intravenously and a computer is used to create a three-dimensional image.
tagging	Attaching a radionuclide to a chemical and following its course in the body.
tomography	Diagnostic radiographic technique in which a series of pictures are taken at different depths of an organ.
tracer studies	Radionuclides are used as tags, or labels, attached to chemicals and followed as they migrate through the body.
ultrasound	Diagnostic technique that projects and retrieves high-frequency sound waves as they echo off of parts of the body.
uptake	The rate of absorption of a radionuclide into an organ or tissue.
ventilation/perfusion studies	Radiopharmaceutical is inhaled (ventilation) and injected (perfusion) and its passage through the respiratory tract is imaged.

VI. Combining Forms, Suffixes, Prefixes, and Terminology

Write the meaning of the medical term in the space provided.

Combining Forms			
Combining Form	Meaning	Terminology	Meaning
fluor/o	luminous, fluorescence	<u>fluoroscopy</u> _____ *In this term, -scopy does not refer to visual examination with an endoscope. In fluoroscopy, x-rays can be viewed directly, without*	

taking and developing x-ray photographs. Light is emitted from the fluorescent screen when it is exposed to x-rays.

| **is/o** | same | radio<u>is</u>otope _____ |

top/o means place; radioisotopes of an element have similar structures but different weights and electric charges. A radioisotope (radionuclide) is an unstable form of an element that emits radioactivity.

| **leth/o** | death | <u>leth</u>al _____ |

| **mucos/o** | mucous membrane, mucosa | <u>mucos</u>itis _____ |

This may be a side effect of radiotherapy.

| **pharmaceut/o** | drug | radio<u>pharmaceut</u>ical _____ |

In this term, radi/o stands for radioisotope (radionuclide).

| **radi/o** | x-rays | <u>radi</u>oresistant _____ |

Radioresistant tumors are not easily treated with radiotherapy.

<u>radi</u>osensitive _____

Radiosensitive tumors respond to radiotherapy and can be treated by x-rays or other radiation.

| **roentgen/o** | x-rays | <u>roentgen</u>ology _____ |

| **scintill/o** | spark | <u>scintill</u>ation scanner _____ |

| **son/o** | sound | <u>son</u>ogram _____ |

| **therapeut/o** | treatment | <u>therapeut</u>ic _____ |

| **tom/o** | to cut | <u>tom</u>ography _____ |

Several images (as if done to make slices or cuts) are made of the body to show an organ in depth.

| **vitr/o** | glass | in <u>vitr</u>o _____ |

| **viv/o** | life | in <u>viv</u>o _____ |

| **xer/o** | dry | <u>xer</u>ostomia _____ |

Radiation to the mouth and pharynx can affect the salivary glands and produce this condition.

Suffixes

Suffix	Meaning	Terminology	Meaning
-gram	record	angiogram _____	
		hysterosalpingogram _____	
		myelogram _____	
		pyelogram _____	
-graphy	process of recording	computed tomography _____	
-lucent	to shine	radiolucent _____	
		Radiolucent (indicating that x-rays pass through easily) areas on x-ray film appear dark on the exposed film.	
-opaque	obscure	radiopaque _____	
		Radiopaque (indicating that x-rays do not penetrate) areas on x-ray film appear white or light on exposed film.	
-suppression	to stop	myelosuppression _____	
		Myelosuppression may be a side effect of treatment with radiation.	
-therapy	treatment	radiotherapy _____	

Prefixes

Prefix	Meaning	Terminology	Meaning
brachy-	short, short distance	brachytherapy _____	
cine-	movement	cineradiography _____	
echo-	a repeated sound	echocardiography _____	
inter-	between	interstitial therapy _____	
		stit/o means to stand, put, or place.	
intra-	within	intracavitary therapy _____	
		cavit/o means a space.	

ultra-	beyond	ultrasonography _____

Sound waves are beyond the normal range of those that a human can hear.

VII. ABBREVIATIONS

Angio	Angiography	**KUB**	Kidneys, ureters, bladder (x-ray without contrast medium)
AP	Anteroposterior	**LAT**	Lateral
Ba	Barium	**LS Films**	Lumbosacral spine films
CAT	Computerized axial tomography	**mCi**	Millicurie (measure of radiation)
cGy	Centigray (a rad—one hundredth of a gray)	**μCi**	Microcurie (measure of radiation)
C-spine	Cervical spine films	**MRI**	Magnetic resonance imaging
CT	Computed tomography	**MUGA**	Multiple-gated acquisition scan (radioactive test to show heart function)
CXR	Chest x-ray	**PA**	Posteroanterior
Decub	Decubitus (lying down)	**PET**	Positron emission tomography
DI	Diagnostic imaging	**rad**	Radiation absorbed dose
DSA	Digital subtraction angiography	**SPECT**	Single-photon emission computed tomography; radioactive substances and a computer are used to create three-dimensional images
Fx	Fracture		
^{67}Ga	Radioactive gallium (used in whole-body and brain scans)		
Gy	Gray (unit of radiation and equal to 100 rads)	**^{99m}Tc**	Radioactive technetium (used in brain, skull, thyroid, liver, spleen, bone, and lung scans)
^{131}I	Radioactive iodine (used in thyroid uptake, liver, and kidney scans and treatment of malignant and nonmalignant conditions of the thyroid)	**UGI**	Upper gastrointestinal series
		US, U/S	Ultrasound
IVP	Intravenous pyelogram	**VQ**	Ventilation-perfusion scan of the lungs
		XRT	Radiation therapy

VIII. Practical Applications

This section contains actual medical reports using terms that you have studied in this and previous chapters.

CT Upper Abdomen Using IV Contrast

Comparison was also made with prior examination. The extensive retroperitoneal and mesenteric lymphadenopathy has shown marked reduction in size. The celiac lymph nodes are also reduced, and the outlines of the lymph nodes are in the top limits of normal at this point. In images 8 and 9 the celiac lymph nodes are no longer visible. Previously described right pleural effusion is also not present. The obstructed right kidney shows atrophy and now measures approximately 7–8 cm in size. The left kidney remains much the same as before. The adrenal glands are symmetrical with normal aorta and inferior vena cava as well as abdominal wall.

Chart Note

DX. Stage T3 N0 M0 colon carcinoma.

TX. 5-FU plus XRT.

Mr. Dean Smith returns today for general follow-up and is currently ready to begin his 5-FU and concurrent XRT in his right lower quadrant. He is without symptoms and denies any abdominal pain, diarrhea, nausea, vomiting, melena, or hematochezia. Vital signs stable, afebrile. HEENT [head, ears, eyes, nose, and throat] entirely benign. Axillary, cervical, and inguinal lymph nodes benign. Chest: lungs clear to auscultation and percussion. Abdomen: notable only for a well-healing midline abdominal scar with moderate smooth hepatomegaly.

    Laboratory. This time notable for SGOT 26 [normal: 8-20]; LDH 541 [normal 48–115]. HCT 32.2 [normal 40–54]; platelet 400,000 [normal 200,000–400,000]; WBC 10.1 [normal 4,500–11,000] with normal differential.

    Impression and Plan. Mr. Smith should begin his XRT and chemotherapy sometime early next week.

Chart Rounds: Center for Radiation Oncology

(A) Patient has metastatic carcinoma and is being treated to the costovertebral junction with 3000 palliatively.

(B) Patient is being treated for cervical esophageal carcinoma. Previously treated with a hockey field technique [RT given covering the area in the shape of a hockey stick] for breast cancer and recurrent field is only being taken to 3000 cGy.

(C) Patient is being treated for a pathological stage II-B Hodgkin's disease on the mantle [upper chest and neck]-only protocol.

(D) The patient is being treated for a parietal GBM [glioblastoma multiforme]. The plan needs to be signed. The films look fine.

Questions

    Answers are at the end of Answers to Exercises section, page 743.

1. Which patient is being treated for a brain tumor?
2. Which patient is being treated for lesions in the ribs?
3. Which patient has disease in cervical and thoracic lymph nodes?
4. Which patient is being treated for gastrointestinal cancer?

General Hospital—Nuclear Medicine Dept.—Radionuclides Available

Radionuclide	Radiopharmaceutical	Admission Route	Target Organ
^{133}Xe	xenon gas	inhaled	lungs
^{99m}Tc	albumin microspheres	IV	lungs
^{87m}Sr (strontium)	solution	IV	bone
^{99m}Tc	diphosphonate	IV	bone
^{99m}Tc	pertechnetate	IV	brain
^{99m}Tc	sulfur colloid	IV	liver/spleen
^{198}Au	colloid	IV	liver
^{199}Au	colloid	IV	spleen
^{131}I	rose bengal	IV	colon
^{99m}Tc	DTPA* or HIDA†	IV	kidney
^{197}Hg (mercury)	chlormerodrin	IV	kidney
^{131}I	iodide	oral	thyroid
^{42}K (potassium)	solution	IV	heart
^{201}Tl (thallium)	thallium chloride	IV	heart
^{99m}Tc	pyrophosphate	IV	heart
^{67}Ga (gallium)	citrate	IV	tumors and abscesses

*DTPA = diethylenetriaminepentaacetic acid
†HIDA = N-(2.6-dimethyl)iminodiacetic acid

IX. Exercises

Remember to check your answers carefully with those given in Section X, Answers to Exercises.

A. *Complete the medical term from its definition and word parts given.*

1. obstructing the passage of x-rays: radio _____

2. permitting the passage of x-rays: radio _____

3. administering radiation to a patient: irr _____

4. separation of stable substances into charge particles: _____ ization

5. deadly or fatal: _____ al

6. treatment of disease (usually cancer) by means of high-energy rays: _____

   oncology or radio _____

7. a physician who specializes in diagnostic radiology: radi _____

8. study of the uses of radioactive substances in the diagnosis of disease:

   _____ medicine

B. Match the special diagnostic technique below with its definition.

fluoroscopy   interventional radiology   cineradiography
ultrasonography   magnetic resonance imaging   contrast studies
computed tomography   tomography

1. radiopaque substances are given and x-rays taken _____

2. use of motion picture techniques to record x-ray images _____

3. series of x-rays are taken at different depths of an organ _____

4. use of echoes of high-frequency sound waves to diagnose disease _____

5. x-ray beams are focused from the body onto a screen that glows as a result of the ionizing effect of x-rays

_____

6. a magnetic field and radio waves are used to form images of the body _____

7. x-ray pictures are taken circularly around an area of the body, and a computer synthesizes the

   information into a composite cross-section picture _____

8. therapeutic procedures are performed by a radiologist under the guidance of fluoroscopy or ultrasound

_____

C. Match the diagnostic x-ray test in column I with the part of the body that is imaged in column II.

Column I   *Column II*

   1. myelography   _____   A. gallbladder
                                                B. spinal cord
   2. intravenous pyelography _____   C. uterus and fallopian tubes
                                                D. bronchial tubes
   3. arteriography   _____   E. arteries
                                                F. upper gastrointestinal tract
   4. cholecystography   _____   G. lower gastrointestinal tract
                                                H. renal pelvis of kidney
   5. lymphangiography   _____   I. bile vessels
                                                J. lymph vessels
   6. barium swallow   _____

   7. bronchography   _____

   8. cholangiography   _____

   9. barium enema   _____

  10. hysterosalpingography _____

D. Match the following x-ray views or positions in column I with their meanings in column II. Write the letter of the answer in the space provided.

Column I

1. PA   _____

2. supine   _____

3. prone   _____

4. AP   _____

5. lateral   _____

6. oblique   _____

7. lateral decubitus _____

8. adduction   _____

9. inversion   _____

10. abduction   _____

11. recumbent   _____

12. eversion   _____

13. flexion   _____

14. extension   _____

Column II

A. on the side
B. turned inward
C. movement away from the midline
D. lying on the belly
E. x-ray tube positioned on an angle
F. bending a part
G. straightening a limb
H. lying on the back
I. lying down on the side; cross-table lateral position
J. lying down; prone or supine
K. anterior to posterior view
L. turning outward
M. posterior to anterior view
N. movement toward the midline

E. Give the meanings for the following medical terms.

1. in vitro _____

2. in vivo _____

3. radiopharmaceutical _____

4. tracer studies _____

5. uptake _____

6. perfusion lung scan _____

7. ventilation lung scan _____

8. bone scan _____

9. brain scan _____

10. thyroid scan _____

F. Match the following terms with their meanings below.

palliative	lethal	orthovoltage	brachytherapy
positron emission	linear accelerator	megavoltage	radionuclide
tomography (PET)	scintillation scanner	external beam radiation	

1. Low-energy radiation used in treating superficial skin cancers is called

_____ .

2. High-energy radiation used to treat deeper tissues is called _____ .

3. Radiation therapy delivered from a shielded, distant unit is called _____ .

4. Radiation therapy using an implanted radioactive substance is called _____ .

5. A machine that delivers radiation therapy is called a (an) _____ .

6. A machine used to detect rays emitted by radioactive substances is a (an)

_____ .

7. Pertaining to that which is deadly or fatal _____ .

8. Relieving symptoms but not curative _____ .

9. A radioactive form of a substance is called a (an) _____ .

10. In this test, radioactive substances are given and metabolized by body cells; a cross-sectional image is

then produced as radioactivity (positrons) is emitted from the body _____ .

G. Give the meanings for the following terms.

1. radiosensitive _____

2. radioresistant _____

3. radioisotope _____

4. myelosuppression _____

5. interstitial therapy _____

6. echocardiography _____

7. intracavitary therapy _____

H. Give the meanings for the following terms that describe side effects produced by radiotherapy.

1. alopecia _____

2. dysphagia _____

3. hyperemesis _____

4. leukopenia _____

5. mucositis _____

6. pericarditis _____

7. xerostomia _____

8. pneumonitis _____

I. Give the meanings of the following combining forms and prefixes.

1. xer/o _____   6. viv/o _____

2. leth/o _____   7. pharmaceut/o _____

3. fluor/o _____   8. son/o _____

4. tom/o _____   9. brachy- _____

5. vitr/o _____   10. inter- _____

J. Give the meanings for the following terms and abbreviations.

1. half-life _____

2. XRT _____

3. MRI _____

4. SPECT _____

5. LAT _____

6. CXR _____

7. Decub _____

8. IVP _____

9. ^{131}I _____

10. U/S _____

11. PET _____

K. Select the correct term to complete each sentence.

1. Mr. Jones was scheduled for ultrasound-guided removal of his pleural effusion. He was sent to the (interventional radiology, radiation oncology, nuclear medicine) department for the procedure.

2. In order to better visualize Mr. Smith's colon, Dr. Wong ordered a (perfusion study, hysterosalpingography, barium enema). She hoped to determine why he was having blood in his stools.

3. After the head-on collision, Sam was brought to the emergency room in an unconscious state. The paramedics suspected head trauma, and the doctors ordered an emergency (PET scan, U/S, CT scan) of his head.

4. After her mastectomy, Lucy was referred to the department of (radiology, radiation oncology, nuclear medicine) for adjuvant treatment to her chest wall and lymph nodes.

5. In light of Sue's symptoms of fever, cough, and malaise, the doctors surmised that the consolidated, hazy (radioisotope, radiolucent, radiopaque) area on the chest x-ray represented a pneumonia.

X. Answers to Exercises

A.

1. radiopaque
2. radiolucent
3. irradiation
4. ionization
5. lethal
6. radiation oncology or radiotherapy
7. radiologist
8. nuclear medicine

B.

1. contrast studies
2. cineradiography; a type of fluoroscopy
3. tomography
4. ultrasonography
5. fluoroscopy
6. magnetic resonance imaging
7. computed tomography
8. interventional radiology

C.

1. B
2. H
3. E
4. A
5. J
6. F
7. D
8. I
9. G
10. C

D.

1. M
2. H
3. D
4. K
5. A
6. E
7. I
8. N
9. B
10. C
11. J
12. L
13. F
14. G

E.

1. Process, test, or procedure in which something is measured or observed outside a living organism.
2. Process, test, or procedure in which something is measured or observed in a living organism.
3. Radioactive drug (radionuclide plus chemical) that is given for diagnostic or therapeutic purposes.
4. Tests in which radioactive substance (radioisotopes) are used with chemicals and followed as they travel throughout the body.
5. The rate of absorption of a radionuclide into an organ or tissue.
6. A radiopharmaceutical is injected intravenously and traced within the blood vessels of the lung.
7. A radiopharmaceutical is inhaled, and its passage through the respiratory tract is imaged.
8. A radiopharmaceutical is given intravenously and taken up by bone tissue. An image as the radioactive substance is traced in the bone.
9. A radiopharmaceutical is given intravenously, and a scan (image) is made of its uptake in the brain.
10. Radioactive substance is given intravenously, and a scan (image) is made of its uptake in the thyroid gland.

F.

1. orthovoltage
2. megavoltage
3. external beam radiation
4. brachytherapy
5. linear accelerator
6. scintillation scanner
7. lethal
8. palliative
9. radionuclide
10. positron emission tomography

G.

1. tissue that is sensitive to radiation therapy
2. tissue that is resistant to the effects of radiation therapy
3. a radioactive form (radionuclide) of a substance; gives off radiation
4. bone marrow stops functioning (may be a side effect of radiation therapy)
5. radioisotopes placed in a tumor; a form of brachytherapy
6. ultrasound used to create an image of the heart
7. radioisotopes placed in a body cavity near a tumor; a form of brachytherapy

H.

1. baldness
2. difficulty swallowing
3. excessive vomiting
4. deficiency of white blood cells
5. inflammation of mucous membranes
6. inflammation of the membrane surrounding the heart
7. dry mouth
8. inflammation of the lungs

I.

1. dry
2. death
3. luminous, fluorescence
4. to cut
5. glass
6. life
7. drug
8. sound
9. short, short distance
10. between

J.

1. time that it takes a radioactive substance to lose half of its radioactivity by disintegration
2. radiation therapy
3. magnetic resonance imaging
4. single-photon emission computed tomography
5. lateral
6. chest x-ray
7. decubitus; lying down
8. intravenous pyelogram
9. radioactive iodine used in tracer studies and radiotherapy
10. ultrasound
11. positron-emission tomography (areas of metabolic activity are imaged)

K.

1. interventional radiology
2. barium enema
3. CT scan
4. radiation oncology
5. radiopaque

Answers to Practical Applications

1. D
2. A
3. C
4. B

XI. Pronunciation of Terms

To test your understanding of the terminology in this chapter, write the meaning of each term in the space provided. In addition, you may wish to cover the terms and write them by looking at your definitions. Make sure your spelling is correct. The page number after each term indicates where it is defined or used in the text so you can easily check your responses. (If you are not sure what the pronunciation symbols mean, refer to page 21.)

Term	Pronunciation	Meaning
abduction (724)	ăb-DŬK-shŭn	_____
adduction (724)	ă-DŬK-shŭn	_____
angiogram (734)	ĂN-jē-ō-grăm	_____

Term	Pronunciation	
anteroposterior (724)	ăn-tĕr-ō-pōs-TĔ-rē-ŏr	_____
arteriography (719)	ăr-tĕ-rē-ŎG-ră-fē	_____
arthrography (719)	ăr-THRŎG-ră-fē	_____
betatron (730)	BĀ-tă-trŏn	_____
brachytherapy (730)	brā-kē-THĔR-ă-pē or brăk-ē-THĔR-ă-pē	_____
cholangiography (719)	kō-lăn-jē-ŎG-ră-fē	_____
cholecystography (719)	kō-lĕ-sĭs-TŎG-ră-fē	_____
cineradiography (730)	sĭn-ē-rā-dē-ŎG-ră-fē	_____
computed tomography (730)	kŏm-PŪ-tĕd tō-MŎG-ră-fē	_____
echocardiography (734)	ĕk-ō-kăr-dē-ŎG-ră-fē	_____
eversion (724)	ē-VĔR-zhŭn	_____
extension (724)	ĕk-STĔN-shŭn	_____
external beam radiation (730)	ĕks-TĔR-năl bēm ră-dē-Ā-shŭn	_____
flexion (724)	FLĔK-shŭn	_____
fluorescence (730)	flū-RĔS-ĕns	_____
fluoroscopy (732)	flū-RŎS-kō-pē	_____
hysterosalpingogram (734)	hĭs-tĕr-ō-săl-PĬNG-gō-grăm	_____
interstitial therapy (730)	ĭn-tĕr-STĬSH-ăl THĔR-ă-pē	_____
interventional radiology (730)	ĭn-tĕr-VĔN-shŭn-ăl rā-dē-ŎL-ō-je	_____
intracavitary therapy (730)	ĭn-tră-KAV-ĭ-tār-ē THĔR-ă-pē	_____
inversion (724)	ĭn-VĔR-zhŭn	_____
in vitro (730)	in VĒ-trō	_____
in vivo (731)	in VĒ-vō	_____
ionization (731)	ī-ŏn-ĭ-ZĀ-shŭn	_____
irradiation (731)	ĭ-rā-dē-Ā-shŭn	_____
lateral decubitus (724)	LĂ-tĕr-ăl de-KŪ-bĭ-tus	_____

lethal (731)   LĒ-thăl   _____

lymphangiography (720)   limf-ăn-jē-ŎG-ră-fē   _____

magnetic resonance imaging   măg-NĔT-ik RĔZ-ō-nans   _____
(731)   IM-a-jĭng

megavoltage (731)   MĔG-ă-vōl-tăj   _____

mucositis (733)   mū-kō-SĪ-tĭs   _____

myelogram (734)   MĪ-ĕ-lō-grăm   _____

myelosuppression (734)   mī-ĕ-lō-sŭ-PRĔSH-ŭn   _____

nuclear medicine (731)   NU-klē-ar MĔD-ĭ-sĭn   _____

oblique (724)   ŏ-BLĒK   _____

orthovoltage (731)   ŎR-thō-vŏl-tăj   _____

palliative (731)   PĂL-ē-ă-tĭv   _____

positron emission   pŏs-ĭ-trŏn ē-MĬSH-ŭn   _____
tomography (731)   tō-MŎG-ră-fē

posteroanterior (724)   pōs-tĕr-ō-ăn-TĒ-rē-ŏr   _____

prone (724)   prōn   _____

pyelogram (734)   PĪ-ē-lō-grăm   _____

radioimmunoassay (731)   rā-dē-ō-ĭ-mū-nō-ĂS-ā   _____

radioisotope (731)   rā-dē-ō-Ī-sō-tōp   _____

radiolucent (731)   rā-dē-ō-LŪ-sĕnt   _____

radionuclide (731)   rā-dē-ō-NŪ-klīd   _____

radiopaque (731)   rā-dē-ō-PĀK   _____

radiopharmaceutical (732)   rā-dē-ō-făr-mă-SŪ-tĭ-kăl   _____

radiotherapy (734)   rā-dē-ō-THĔR-ă-pē   _____

recumbent (724)   rē-KŬM-bĕnt   _____

roentgenology (732)   rĕnt-gĕ-NŎL-ō-jĕ   _____

scintillation scanner (732)   sĭn-tĭ-LĀ-shŭn SKĂN-ĕr   _____

sonogram (733)   SŎN-ō-grăm   _____

supine (724)   SŪ-pīn   _____ therapeutic (733) thĕr-ă-PŪ-tik _____

tomography (732) tō-MŎG-ră-fē _____

tracer studies (732) TRĀ-sĕr STŬ-dēz _____

ultrasound (732) ŭl-tră-SOWND _____

uptake (732) ŬP-tāk _____

venogram (720) VĒ-nō-grăm _____

ventilation/perfusion studies (732) vĕn-tĭ-LĀ-shŭn/pĕr-FŪ-shŭn STŬ-dēz _____

xerostomia (733) zĕ-rō-STŌ-mē-ă _____

XII. Review Sheet

Write the meaning of each combining form in the space provided and test yourself. Check your answers with the information in the text or in the Glossary (Medical Terms—English) at the back of the book.

Combining Forms

Combining Form	Meaning	Combining Form	Meaning
fluor/o	_____	roentgen/o	_____
ion/o	_____	scintill/o	_____
is/o	_____	son/o	_____
leth/o	_____	therapeut/o	_____
mucos/o	_____	tom/o	_____
myel/o	_____	vitr/o	_____
pharmaceut/o	_____	viv/o	_____
radi/o	_____	xer/o	_____

Suffixes

Suffix	Meaning	Suffix	Meaning
-gram	_____	-opaque	_____
-graphy	_____	-suppression	_____
-lucent	_____	-therapy	_____

Prefixes

Prefix	Meaning	Prefix	Meaning
brachy-	_____	inter-	_____
cine-	_____	intra-	_____
echo-	_____	ultra-	_____

Pharmacology

This Chapter is divided into the following sections

In this Chapter you will

- Learn of the various subspecialty areas of pharmacology;
- Identify the various routes of drug administration;
- Differentiate between the different classes of drugs and their actions; and
- Define medical terms using combining forms, prefixes, and suffixes that relate to pharmacology.

I. Introduction

Drugs are chemical or biological substances used in the prevention or treatment of disease, or to alter bodily functions in a beneficial way. Drugs can come from many different sources. Some drugs are obtained from parts of **plants,** such as the roots, leaves, and fruit. Examples of such drugs are digitalis (from the foxglove plant) and antibiotics such as penicillin and streptomycin (from lower plants called molds). Drugs can also be obtained from **animals;** for example, hormones are secretions from the glands of animals. Drugs can be made as chemical substances that are **synthesized** in the laboratory. Anticancer drugs,

MEDICINAL CHEMISTRY	PHARMACODYNAMICS	PHARMACOKINETICS	MOLECULAR PHARMACOLOGY
New drug synthesis	Drug effects on the body	Drug concentration in tissues and blood is measured over a period of time	Interaction of drugs and subcellular components

	CHEMOTHERAPY	TOXICOLOGY	
	Use of drugs in treatment of disease	Study of harmful chemicals and their effects on the body	

Figure 21–1

Subspecialty areas of pharmacology.

such as methotrexate and prednisone, are examples of laboratory-synthesized drugs. Some drugs are contained in food substances; these drugs are called **vitamins.** Drugs are dispensed by a **pharmacist,** whose shop or store is called a **pharmacy.**

The field of medicine that studies drugs—their nature, origin, and effect on the body—is called **pharmacology.** Pharmacology is a broad medical specialty and contains many subdivisions of study, including **medicinal chemistry, pharmacodynamics, pharmacokinetics, molecular pharmacology, chemotherapy,** and **toxicology.**

Medicinal chemistry is the study of new drug synthesis and the relationship between chemical structure and biological effects. **Pharmacodynamics** involves the study of drug effects in the body. Scientists may also study the processes of drug **absorption** (how drugs pass into the bloodstream), **metabolism** (changes drugs undergo within the body), and **excretion** (removal of the drug from the body). The mathematical description of drug disposition (appearance and disappearance) in the body over time is called **pharmacokinetics.**

Molecular pharmacology concerns the study of the interaction of drugs and subcellular entities, such as DNA, RNA, and enzymes. These studies provide important information about the mechanism of action of the drug.

Chemotherapy is the study of drugs that destroy microorganisms, parasites, or malignant cells within the body. Chemotherapy includes treatment of infectious diseases and cancer.

Toxicology is the study of harmful chemicals and their effects on the body. Toxicological studies in animals are required by law before new drugs can be tested in humans. A toxicologist is also interested in finding proper **antidotes** to any harmful effects of drugs. Antidotes are substances given to neutralize unwanted effects of drugs.

Figure 21–1 reviews the subspecialty areas of pharmacology.

II. Drug Names, Standards, and References

Names

A drug can have three different names. The **chemical name** is the chemical formula for the drug. This name, often long and complicated, is useful for the chemist because it shows the structure of the drug.

The **generic** or **official name** is a shorter, less complicated name that is recognized as identifying the drug for legal and scientific purposes. The generic name becomes public property after 17 years of use by the original manufacturer, and any drug manufacturer may use it thereafter. There is only one generic name for each drug.

The **brand (trade or proprietary) name** is the private property of the individual drug manufacturer, and no competitor may use it. Brand names often have the superscript ® after or before the name, indicating that this is a registered trade name. Most drugs have several brand names because each manufacturer producing the drug gives it a different name. When a specific brand name is ordered on a prescription by a physician, it must be dispensed by the pharmacist; no other brand name may be substituted. It is usual practice to capitalize the first letter of a brand name.

The following lists give the chemical, generic, and brand names of the antibiotic drug ampicillin; note that the drug can have several brand names but only one generic, or official, name:

Chemical Name	Generic Name	Brand Name
derivative of 6-aminopenicillanic acid	ampicillin	Amcill capsules Omnipen Polycillin Principen

Standards

Although the U.S. **Food and Drug Administration (FDA)** has the legal responsibility for deciding whether a drug may be distributed and sold, there are definite standards for drugs set by an independent committee of physicians, pharmacologists, pharmacists, and manufacturers. This committee is called the **United States Pharmacopeia (U.S.P.).** Two important standards of the U.S.P. are that the drug must be clinically useful (useful for patients) and available in pure form (made by good manufacturing methods). If a drug has U.S.P. after its name, it has met with the standards of the Pharmacopeia.

References

Libraries and hospitals have two large reference listings of drugs. The most complete and up-to-date is the **Hospital Formulary,** which gives information about the characteristics of drugs and their clinical usage (application to patient care).

The **Physicians' Desk Reference (PDR)** is published by a private firm, and drug manufacturers pay to have their products listed. The PDR is a useful reference with several different indices to identify drugs along with precautions, warnings about side effects, and information about recommended dosage and administration for each drug.

III. Administration of Drugs

The route of administration of a drug (how it is introduced into the body) is very important in determining the rate and completeness of its absorption into the bloodstream and the speed and duration of the drug's action in the body.

The various methods of administering drugs are described here:

Oral Administration. Drugs are given by mouth and are slowly absorbed into the bloodstream through the stomach or intestinal wall. This method, although convenient for the patient, has several disadvantages. If the drug is destroyed in the digestive tract by digestive juices, or if the drug is unable to pass through the intestinal mucosa, it will be ineffective. Oral administration is also disadvantageous if time is a factor in therapy.

Sublingual Administration. Drugs are not swallowed but are placed under the tongue and allowed to dissolve in the saliva. For some agents absorption may be rapid. Nitroglycerin tablets are taken in this way to treat attacks of angina pectoris.

Rectal Administration. Suppositories (cone-shaped objects containing drugs) and aqueous solutions are inserted into the rectum. At times, drugs are given by rectum when oral administration presents difficulties, such as when the patient is nauseated and vomiting.

Parenteral Administration. This type of administration is accomplished by injection of the drug from a **syringe** (tube) through a hollow needle placed under the skin, into a muscle, into a vein, or into a body cavity. There are several types of parenteral injections:

1. Subcutaneous injection (SC). This is also called a **hypodermic injection,** and it is given just under the skin. The outer surface of the arm is a usual location for this injection.

2. Intradermal injection. This shallow injection is made into the upper layers of the skin and is used chiefly in skin testing for allergic reactions.

3. Intramuscular injection (IM). The buttock or upper arm is usually the site for this injection into muscle. When drugs are irritating to the skin or when a large volume of a long-acting drug is needed, IM injections are advisable.

4. Intravenous injection (IV). This injection is given directly into the veins. It is given when an immediate effect from the drug is desired or when the drug cannot be safely given into other tissues. Good technical skill is needed for administering this injection, because leakage of drugs into surrounding tissues may result in irritation and inflammation.

5. Intrathecal injection. This injection is made into the space underlying the membranes (meninges) that surround the spinal cord and brain. Methotrexate (a cancer chemotherapeutic drug) in injected intrathecally for treatment of leukemia.

6. Intracavitary injection. This injection is made into a body cavity, such as the peritoneal or pleural cavity. For example, nitrogen mustard is injected into the pleural cavity in people who have pleural effusions due to malignant disease. The drug causes the pleural surfaces to adhere, thus obliterating the pleural space and preventing the accumulation of fluid.

Inhalation. Vapors, or gases, are taken into the nose or mouth and are absorbed into the bloodstream through the thin walls of the air sacs in the lungs. **Aerosols** (particles of drug suspended in air) are administered by inhalation, as are many anesthetics. Examples of aerosols are pentamidine, used to treat a form of pneumonia associated with acquired immunodeficiency syndrome (AIDS), and various aerosolized medicines used to treat asthma (spasm of the lung airways).

Topical Application. Drugs are locally applied on the skin or mucous membranes of the body. **Antiseptics** (against infection) and **antipruritics** (against itching) are commonly used as ointments, creams, and lotions. **Transdermal patches** are used to deliver drugs (such as estrogen, pain medications, and nicotine) continuously through the skin.

Table 21–1 summarizes the various routes of drug administration.

Table 21–1. ROUTES OF DRUG ADMINISTRATION

Oral	Sublingual	Rectal	Parenteral	Inhalation	Topical
Tablets	Tablets	Suppositories	Injections Subcutaneous Intradermal Intramuscular Intravenous Intrathecal Intracavitary	Aerosols	Lotions Creams Ointments Transdermal patches

IV. Terminology of Drug Action

When a drug enters the body, the target substance with which the drug interacts to produce its effects is called a **receptor.** The movement of the drug across a cell membrane into the cells of the receptor is called **transport.**

The following terms describe the action and interaction of drugs in the body after they have been absorbed into the bloodstream:

Additive Action. The combination of two similar drugs is equal to the **sum** of the effects of each. For example, if drug A gives 10 per cent tumor kill as a chemotherapeutic agent and drug B gives 20 per cent tumor kill, using A and B together would give 30 per cent tumor kill.

Idiosyncrasy. This is any **unexpected effect** that may appear in the patient following administration of a drug. Idiosyncratic reactions (due to genetic deficiencies of enzymes) are produced in very few patients but may be life-threatening in those few instances. For example, in some individuals penicillin is known to cause an idiosyncratic reaction such as **anaphylaxis** (acute type of hypersensitivity, including asthma and shock).

Synergism (Potentiation). A combination of two drugs can sometimes cause an effect that is **greater** than the sum of the individual effects of each drug given alone. For example, penicillin and streptomycin, two antibiotic drugs, are given together in treatment for bacterial endocarditis because of their synergistic effect.

Tolerance. The effects of a given dose diminish as treatment goes on, and increasing amounts are needed to produce the same effect. Tolerance is a feature of addiction to drugs such as morphine and merperidine hydrochloride (Demerol).

V. Drug Toxicity

Drug toxicity is the poisonous and potentially dangerous effects of some drugs. Idiosyncrasy is an example of an unpredictable type of drug toxicity.

Other types of drug toxicity are more predictable and are based on the dosage of the drug given. Physicians are trained to be aware of the potential toxic effects of all drugs that they prescribe. **Iatrogenic** (produced by treatment) disorders can occur, however, as a result of mistakes in drug use or of individual sensitivity to a given agent.

Side effects are toxic effects that routinely result from the use of a drug. They often occur with the usual therapeutic dosage of a drug and are generally tolerable. For example, nausea, vomiting, and alopecia are common side effects of the chemotherapeutic drugs used to treat cancer.

Contraindications are factors in a patient's condition that make the use of a drug dangerous and ill advised. For example, in the presence of renal failure, it is unwise to administer a drug that is normally eliminated by the kidneys. Excess drug will accumulate in the body and cause side effects.

VI. Classes of Drugs

The following are major classes of drugs with explanations of their use in the body. The names of specific drugs are included in tables for your reference (trade or brand names are capitalized; generic names begin with a small letter).

Analgesics

An analgesic (alges/o means sensitivity to pain) is a drug that relieves pain. Mild analgesics are used for mild to moderate pain, such as caused by myalgias, headache, and toothache. More potent analgesics are **narcotics** or **opioids,** because they contain or are derived from

Table 21-2. ANALGESICS AND ANESTHETICS

Analgesics	Anesthetics
MILD	GENERAL
acetaminophen (Tylenol)	ether
aspirin	halothane (Fluothane)
NARCOTIC (opioid)	nitrous oxide
codeine	thiopental (Pentothal)
hydromorphone (Dilaudid)	LOCAL
morphine	hydrocortisone acetate (Orabase)
oxycodone (Percodan)	lidocaine (Xylocaine)
NONSTEROIDAL ANTI-INFLAMMATORY DRUG (NSAID)	
ibuprofen (Motrin, Advil)	
naproxen (Naprosyn)	

opium. They induce stupor (condition of near unconsciousness with reduced mental and physical activity). These are used only to relieve severe pain because they may produce dependence (habit formation) and tolerance. Morphine is an example of a narcotic analgesic.

Some non-narcotic analgesics reduce fever, pain, and inflammation and are used in rheumatic (joint) disorders. These agents are not steroid hormones (such as cortisone) and are known as **nonsteroidal anti-inflammatory drugs (NSAIDs).** NSAIDs act on tissues to inhibit prostaglandins (hormone-like substances that sensitize peripheral pain receptors).

Examples of analgesics are listed in Table 21-2.

Anesthetics

An anesthetic is an agent that reduces or eliminates sensation. This can affect the whole body **(general anesthetic)** or a particular region **(local anesthetic).** General anesthetics are used for surgical procedures and depress the activity of the central nervous system, producing loss of consciousness. Local anesthetics inhibit the conduction of impulses in sensory nerves in the region in which they are injected or applied.

Table 21-2 gives examples of specific anesthetics.

Antibiotics

An antibiotic is a chemical substance produced by a microorganism (bacterium, yeast, or mold) that inhibits or stops the growth of bacteria, fungi, or parasites. The use of antibiotics (penicillin was first in general use in 1945) has largely controlled many diseases such as pneumonia, rheumatic fever, and mastoiditis. Caution about the use of antibiotics is warranted because they are powerful agents. With indiscriminate use, pathogenic organisms can develop resistance to the antibiotic and thus destroy the antibiotic's disease-fighting capability.

Table 21-3 lists types of antibiotics and gives specific examples of each.

Table 21-3. ANTIBIOTICS

ANTIFUNGALS	ANTIVIRALS	PENICILLINS
amphotericin B (Fungizone)	acyclovir (Zovirax)	amoxicillin (Amoxil)
ketoconazole (Nizoral)	zidovudine or AZT (Retrovir)	ampicillin (Omnipen)
fluconazole (Diflucan)	CEPHALOSPORINS	penicillin V potassium (Pen-Vee K)
ANTIMALARIALS	cefaclor (Ceclor)	TETRACYCLINES
chloroquine (Aralen)	cephalothin (Keflin)	doxycycline
pyrimethamine (Daraprim)	cephradine (Anspor)	tetracycline
ANTITUBERCULARS	ERYTHROMYCINS AND LIKE DRUGS	SULFONAMIDES (SULFA DRUGS)
isoniazid (INH)	azithramycin	sulfasalazine (Azulfidine)
rifampin (Rifadin)	clarithromycin	sulfisoxazole (Gantrisin)
	erythromycin	

Table 21–4. ANTICOAGULANTS, ANTICONVULSANTS, ANTIDEPRESSANTS, ANTIDIABETICS, AND ANTIHISTAMINES

ANTICOAGULANTS	ANTIDEPRESSANTS	Oral drugs
dicumarol	amitriptyline (Elavil)	chlorpropamide (Diabinese)
heparin	fluoxetine (Prozac)	glipizide (Glucotrol)
sodium warfarin (Coumadin)	imipramine (Tofranil)	metformin (Glucophage)
tissue plasminogen activator (tPA)	nortriptyline (Pamelor)	tolbutamide (Orinase)
ANTICONVULSANTS	paroxetine (Paxil)	ANTIHISTAMINES
carbamazepine (Tegretol)	ANTIDIABETICS	chlorpheniramine maleate
phenobarbital	Insulins	(Chlor-Trimeton)
phenytoin (Dilantin)	Humulin	dimenhydrinate (Dramamine)
	Iletin	diphenhydramine (Benadryl)
	Lente	terfenadine (Seldane)

Anticoagulants

This type of drug prevents the clotting (coagulation) of blood. Anticoagulants are used to prevent the formation of clots or to break up clots in blood vessels in conditions such as thrombosis and embolism. They are also used to prevent coagulation in preserved blood used for transfusions. **Heparin** is a natural anticoagulant produced by liver cells and some white blood cells. Other anticoagulants are manufactured. Tissue-type plasminogen activator (tPA) dissolves clots and is used to open vessels after myocardial infarction.

Table 21–4 gives examples of anticoagulants.

Anticonvulsants

An anticonvulsant prevents or reduces the severity of convulsions in various types of epilepsy. Ideally, anticonvulsants depress abnormal spontaneous activity of the brain arising from areas of scar or tumor, without affecting normal brain function. Table 21–4 lists examples of anticonvulsants.

Antidepressants

These drugs treat symptoms of depression. They can elevate mood, increase physical activity and mental alertness, and improve appetite and sleep patterns. Many antidepressants are also mild sedatives and treat mild forms of depression associated with anxiety. One of the most commonly prescribed antidepressants is Prozac (fluoxetine). It works by allowing a neurotransmitter, serotonin, into nerve cells.

Table 21–4 gives the names of some antidepressants.

Antidiabetics

These drugs are used to treat diabetes mellitus (a condition in which the hormone insulin is either not produced by the pancreas or not effective in the body). Patients with type I (insulin-dependent) diabetes must receive daily injections of insulin. At present, most insulin is obtained from animals (pork or beef insulin). More recently, human insulin is produced by recombinant DNA research (biosynthesis), and this product is used as well.

Patients with type II (non–insulin-dependent) diabetes are given oral antidiabetic drugs (sulfonylurea agents) that stimulate the production and release of insulin by the pancreas. A newly approved drug called metformin is used as an option to sulfonylureas. It suppresses glucose production in the liver and increases tissue sensitivity to insulin without stimulating insulin secretion.

An insulin pump is a device strapped to the patient's waist that periodically delivers (via needle) the desired amount of insulin.

Table 21–4 lists antidiabetic drugs.

Antihistamines

These drugs block the action of histamine, which is normally released in the body in allergic reactions. Histamine causes allergic symptoms such as hives, bronchial asthma, hay fever, and in severe cases **anaphylactic shock** (dyspnea, hypotension, and loss of consciousness). Antihistamines cannot cure the allergic reaction, but they can relieve its symptoms. Many antihistamines have strong **antiemetic** (prevention of nausea) activity and are used to prevent motion sickness. The most common side effects of antihistamines are drowsiness, blurred vision, tremors, digestive upset, and lack of motor coordination.

Table 21–4 lists common antihistamines.

Cardiovascular Drugs

Cardiovascular drugs act on the heart or blood vessels. Those drugs that act on the heart by increasing the force and the efficiency of the heartbeat are called **cardiotonic** drugs. Cardiotonic drugs are useful in congestive heart disease. Other drugs, called **antiarrhythmics,** such as **beta-blockers** (they block the action of epinephrine at receptor sites in heart muscle and in the walls of blood vessels) and **calcium channel blockers** (they inhibit the entry of calcium into cells), correct abnormal heart rhythms. These drugs, along with other drugs, are also effective in preventing angina (chest pain due to insufficient oxygen reaching heart muscle). The drugs that prevent angina are called **antianginal** medications.

One type of drug that affects blood vessels is an **antihypertensive.** Antihypertensive **vasodilators** dilate the walls of blood vessels to lower blood pressure. **Diuretics** lower blood pressure by promoting the kidney to excrete urine, so that more fluid leaves the body. **ACE inhibitors** reduce hypertension by preventing the conversion of angiotensin I to angiotensin II, which is a powerful vasopressor (vasoconstrictor).

Vasoconstrictor drugs narrow the walls of blood vessels and thereby raise blood pressure. These drugs are used in cardiac and respiratory failure and in bronchial asthma (they dilate the bronchial tubes) and to prolong the action of local anesthetics.

Cholesterol-lowering drugs decrease the breakdown of body fats by reducing the amount of fat manufactured by the liver and increasing the excretion of bile acids (and cholesterol) in the stool. These drugs are prescribed for people with very high blood cholesterol levels who have not responded to dietary changes. Table 21–5 gives examples of the different types of cardiovascular drugs.

Table 21–5. CARDIOVASCULAR DRUGS

ANTIANGINAL	ANTIHYPERTENSIVE	CHOLESTEROL-LOWERING
beta-blockers*	beta-blockers*	cholestyramine resin (Questran)
calcium channel blockers†	calcium channel blockers†	gemfibrozil (Lopid)
nitroglycerin	diuretics‡	lovastatin (Mevacor)
ANTIARRHYTHMICS	vasodilators§	**VASOCONSTRICTOR**
beta-blockers*	**CARDIOTONIC**	norepinephrine
calcium channel blockers†	digitoxin	
procainamide (Pronestyl)	digoxin (Lanoxin)	

*Atenolol (Tenormin), metoprolol (Lopressor), nadolol (Corgard), propranolol (Inderal).
†Diltiazem (Cardizem), nifedipine (Procardia), verapamil (Isoptin).
‡Chlorothiazide (Diuril), furosemide (Lasix), hydrochlorothiazide and triamaterene (Dyazide).
§Captopril (Capoten), clonidine (Catapres).

Table 21–6. ENDOCRINE DRUGS

ANDROGEN	ANTIESTROGEN	PROGESTIN
fluoxymesterone (Halotestin)	tamoxifen (Novadex)	medroxyprogesterone (Provera)
methyltestosterone (Virilon)	GLUCOCORTICOID	megestrol (Megace)
ANTIANDROGEN	dexamethasone (Decadron)	THYROID HORMONE
flutamide	prednisone (Deltasone)	levothyroxine (Synthroid)
ESTROGEN		liothyronine (Cytomel)
estrogens (Premarin, Estradiol)		liotrix (Euthroid)

Endocrine Drugs

These drugs act in much the same manner as the naturally occurring (endogenous) hormones discussed in Chapter 19. **Androgens** are male hormones that are used for male hormone replacement or to treat endometriosis and breast cancer in women. An androgen antagonist is flutamide, which is used to treat prostate cancer. **Estrogens** are female hormones that are used for symptoms associated with menopause (estrogen replacement therapy) and to prevent postmenopausal osteoporosis. They are also used as chemotherapy for some types of cancer (for example, prostate cancer). An important antiestrogen drug is tamoxifen (Nolvadex), which is used to prevent recurrence of breast cancer and to treat metastatic breast cancer. **Progestins** are prescribed for abnormal uterine bleeding due to hormonal imbalance and, together with estrogen, in hormone replacement therapy and oral contraceptives. Levonorgestrel (Norplant) is a contraceptive drug imbedded under the skin.

Thyroid hormone is administered when there is a low output of hormone from the thyroid gland. **Glucocorticoids** (adrenal corticosteroids) are prescribed for reduction of inflammation and a wide range of other disorders including arthritis, severe skin and allergic conditions, respiratory and blood disorders, gastrointestinal ailments, and malignant conditions.

Table 21–6 gives examples of endocrine drugs.

Gastrointestinal Drugs

These drugs are often used to relieve uncomfortable and potentially dangerous symptoms, rather than as cures for specific diseases. **Antacids** neutralize the hydrochloric acid in the stomach to relieve symptoms of peptic ulcer, esophagitis, and epigastric discomfort. **Antiulcer** drugs block secretion of acid by cells in the lining of the stomach and are prescribed for patients with gastric and duodenal ulcers.

Antidiarrheal drugs relieve diarrhea and decrease the rapid movement of the walls of the colon. **Cathartics** relieve constipation and promote defecation for diagnostic and operative procedures and are used in the treatment of disorders of the gastrointestinal tract. Some cathartics increase the intestinal salt content to cause fluid to fill the intestines; others increase the bulk of the feces to promote peristalsis (movement of the intestinal wall). Another type of cathartic lubricates the intestinal tract to produce soft stools. **Laxatives** are mild cathartics, and **purgatives** are strong cathartics.

Antinauseants (antiemetics) relieve nausea and vomiting and also overcome vertigo, dizziness, motion sickness, and labyrinthitis (inflammation of the inner ear) as well.

Table 21–7 lists the various types of gastrointestinal drugs and examples of each.

Table 21-7. GASTROINTESTINAL DRUGS

ANTACID	ANTINAUSEANT (ANTIEMETIC)
aluminum and magnesium antacid (Gaviscon)	meclizine (Antivert)
magnesium antacid (milk of magnesia)	metoclopramide (Reglan)
aluminum antacid (Rolaids)	ondansetron (Zofran)
ANTIDIARRHEAL	prochlorperazine maleate (Compazine)
diphenoxylate and atropine (Lomotil)	ANTIULCER
loperamide (Imodium)	cimetidine (Tagamet)
paregoric	ranitidine (Zantac)
	CATHARTIC
	casanthranol and docusate sodium (Peri-Colace)

Respiratory Drugs

These drugs are prescribed for the treatment of emphysema, asthma, and respiratory infections, such as pneumonia and bronchitis. Bronchodilators are used to open the air passages (bronchial tubes) and can be administered by injection or aerosol (inhalers). Table 21–8 lists common bronchodilators and a steroid drug that is used as an inhaler or intranasal product to reduce inflammation in nasal passages.

Sedatives

Sedatives are drugs that relax and calm nervousness. They work by depressing the central nervous system (brain) causing reduced mental activity and weakness. **Hypnotics** are sedative drugs that produce sleep. **Barbiturates** are a type of sedative-hypnotic derived from barbituric acid. A patient can develop tolerance to barbiturates, making the drugs habit-forming. Table 21–8 lists sedatives-hypnotics and barbiturates.

Stimulants

These drugs act on the brain and are used to speed up vital processes (heart and respiration) in cases of shock and collapse. They also increase alertness and inhibit hyperactive behavior in children. High doses can produce restlessness, insomnia, and hypertension. Examples of stimulants are **amphetamines**—used to prevent narcolepsy (seizures of sleep), to suppress appetite, and to calm hyperkinetic children. **Caffeine** is also a cerebral stimulant. It is used in drugs to relieve certain types of headache by constricting cerebral blood vessels. Table 21–9 lists examples of stimulants.

Table 21-8. RESPIRATORY DRUGS AND SEDATIVES

Respiratory Drugs	Sedative-Hypnotics	Barbiturates
BRONCHODILATORS	flurazepam (Dalmane)	phenobarbital
albuterol (Proventil)	temazepam (Restoril)	secobarbital (Seconal)
aminophylline (Amoline)	triazolam (Halcion)	sodium pentobarbital (Nembutal)
epinephrine	zolpiden (Ambien)	
theophylline (Theo-Dur)		
STEROID		
beclomethasone (Beclovent, Vancenase Nasal Inhaler)		

Table 21–9. STIMULANTS AND TRANQUILIZERS

Stimulants	Tranquilizers
Caffeine dextroamphetamine sulfate (Dexedrine) methylphenidate (Ritalin)	**MINOR** alprazolam (Xanax) chlordiazepoxide (Librium) clorazepate (Tranxene) diazepam (Valium) flurazepam (Dalmane) oxazepam (Serax) **MAJOR** chlorpromazine (Thorazine) lithium thioridazine (Mellaril) trifluoperazine (Stelazine)

Tranquilizers

These drugs are useful in controlling anxiety. Minor tranquilizers (benzodiazepines) are used to control minor symptoms of anxiety. Major tranquilizers (phenothiazines) are used to control more severe disturbances of behavior. Table 21–9 lists examples of minor and major tranquilizers.

VII. Vocabulary

This list will help you review many of the new terms introduced in the text. Short definitions will reinforce your understanding of the terms. See Section XIII of this chapter for help in pronouncing the more difficult terms.

General Terms

additive action	Drug action in which the combination of two similar drugs is equal to the sum of the effects of each.
aerosol	Particles of drug suspended in air.
anaphylaxis	An exaggerated hypersensitivity reaction of the body to a drug or foreign organism.
antidote	Agent given to counteract an unwanted effect of a drug.
brand name	Commercial name for a drug; trade name.
chemical name	Chemical formula for a drug.
contraindications	Factors in the patient's condition that prevent the use of a particular drug or treatment.
Food and Drug Administration (FDA)	Governmental agency having the legal responsibility for enforcing proper drug manufacture and clinical use.
generic name	The legal noncommercial name for a drug.

iatrogenic	An effect that is produced as a result of mistakes in drug use or of individual sensitivity to a drug.
idiosyncrasy	An unexpected effect produced in a particularly sensitive individual but not seen in most patients.
inhalation	Administration of drugs in gaseous or vapor form through the nose or mouth.
medicinal chemistry	Study of new drug synthesis; relationship between chemical structure and biological effects.
molecular pharmacology	Study of interaction of drugs and subcellular entities such as DNA, RNA, and enzymes.
oral administration	Drugs are given by mouth.
parenteral administration	Drugs are given by injection into the skin, muscles, or veins (any route other than through the digestive tract).
pharmacodynamics	Study of the effects of a drug within the body.
pharmacokinetics	The calculation of drug concentration in tissues and blood over a period of time.
Physicians' Desk Reference (PDR)	Reference book that lists drug products.
receptor	Target substance with which a drug interacts in the body.
rectal administration	Drugs are inserted through the anus into the rectum.
side effect	A toxic effect that routinely results from the use of a drug.
sublingual administration	Drugs are given by placement under the tongue.
synergism	Drug action in which the combination of two drugs causes an effect that is greater than the sum of the individual effects of each drug alone; potentiation.
syringe	Instrument (tube) for introducing or withdrawing fluids from the body.
tolerance	Drug action in which larger and larger doses must be given to achieve the desired effect. The patient becomes resistant to the action of a drug as treatment progresses.
topical application	Drugs are applied locally on the skin or mucous membranes of the body; ointments, creams, and lotions are applied topically.
toxicity	Harmful effects of a drug.

toxicology	A branch of pharmacology that studies harmful chemicals and their effects on the body.
transport	Movement of a drug across a cell membrane into body cells.
United States Pharmacopeia (U.S.P.)	An authoritative list of drugs, formulas, and preparations that sets a standard for drug manufacturing and dispensing.
vitamin	Substance found in foods and essential in small quantities for growth and good health.

Classes of Drugs

ACE inhibitor	Lowers blood pressure. Angiotensin-converting enzyme inhibitors block the conversion of angiotensin I to angiotensin II (a powerful vasoconstrictor).
amphetamine	Central nervous system stimulant.
analgesic	Drug that relieves pain.
anesthetic	Drug that reduces or eliminates sensation.
antacid	Gastrointestinal drug that neutralizes acid in the stomach.
antianginal	Drug that relieves angina (chest pain due to insufficient flow of blood to the heart muscle).
antiarrhythmic	Cardiovascular drug that helps restore heart rhythm to a regular cycle.
antibiotic	Chemical substance, produced by a plant or microorganism, that has the ability to inhibit or kill foreign organisms in the body.
anticoagulant	Drug that prevents blood clotting.
anticonvulsant	Drug that prevents convulsions (abnormal brain activity).
antidepressant	Drug used to relieve symptoms of depression.
antidiabetic	Drug used to prevent diabetes mellitus.
antidiarrheal	Drug used to prevent diarrhea.
antiemetic	Agent that prevents nausea and vomiting.
antihistamine	Drug that blocks the action of histamine and helps prevent symptoms of allergy.
antihypertensive	Agent that lowers blood pressure.
antinauseant	Agent that relieves nausea and vomiting; antiemetic.
antiulcer drug	Drug that inhibits the secretion of acid by cells of the lining of the stomach.

barbituate	Sedative-hypnotic drug derived from barbituric acid.
beta-blocker	Drug that blocks the action of epinephrine at sites on receptors of heart muscle cells, the muscle lining of blood vessels, and bronchial tubes; antiarrhythmics, antianginals, and antihypertensives.
caffeine	Central nervous system stimulant.
calcium channel blocker	Drug that blocks the entrance of calcium into heart muscle and muscle lining of blood vessels; used as antiarrhythmics, antianginals, and antihypertensives.
cardiotonic	Drug that promotes the force and efficiency of the heart.
cathartic	Drug that relieves constipation.
diuretic	Drug that increases the production of urine and thus reduces the volume of fluid in the body; antihypertensive.
emetic	Drug that promotes vomiting.
glucocorticoid	Hormone from the adrenal cortex that raises blood sugar and reduces inflammation.
hypnotic	Agent that produces sleep.
laxative	Weak cathartic.
narcotic	Habit-forming drug (potent analgesic) that relieves pain by producing stupor or insensibility.
purgative	Strong cathartic.
sedative	Mildly hypnotic drug that relaxes without necessarily producing sleep.
stimulant	Agent that excites and promotes activity.
tranquilizer	Drug used to control anxiety and severe disturbances of behavior.

VIII. Combining Forms, Prefixes, and Terminology

Write the meaning of the medical term in the space provided.

Combining Forms			
Combining Form	Meaning	Terminology	Meaning
aer/o	air	aerosol _____	
		-sol means solution.	

alges/o	sensitivity to pain	analgesic _____
bronch/o	bronchial tube	bronchodilator _____

Theophylline is a smooth muscle relaxant used to treat asthma, emphysema, and chronic bronchitis.

chem/o	drug	chemotherapy _____
cras/o	mixture	idiosyncrasy _____

idi/o means individual, peculiar; syn- means together. An idiosyncrasy is an abnormal unexpected effect of a drug that is peculiar to an individual.

cutane/o	skin	subcutaneous _____
derm/o	skin	hypodermic _____
erg/o	work	synergism _____
esthes/o	feeling, sensation	anesthesia _____
hist/o	tissue	antihistamine _____

-amine indicates a nitrogen-containing compound. Histamine is a substance found in all body tissues (it causes capillary dilation and gastric acid secretion and constricts bronchial tube smooth muscle); excess of histamine is released when the body comes in contact with substances to which it is sensitive.

hypn/o	sleep	hypnotic _____
iatr/o	treatment	iatrogenic _____
lingu/o	tongue	sublingual _____
myc/o	mold, fungus	erythromycin _____
narc/o	stupor	narcotic _____
pharmac/o	drug	pharmacology _____
prurit/o	itching	antipruritic _____
pyret/o	fever	antipyretic _____
thec/o	sheath (of brain and spinal cord)	intrathecal _____

Table 21–10. VITAMINS

Vitamin	Name	Food Source
Vitamin A	Retinol; dehydroretinol	Green leafy and yellow vegetables; liver, eggs, cod liver oil
Vitamin B$_1$	Thiamine	Yeast, ham, liver, peanuts, milk
Vitamin B$_2$	Riboflavin	Milk, liver, green vegetables
Niacin	Nicotinic acid	Yeast, liver, peanuts, fish, poultry
Vitamin B$_6$	Pyridoxine	Liver, fish, yeast
Vitamin B$_{12}$	Cyanocobalamin	Milk, eggs, liver
Vitamin C	Ascorbic acid	Citrus fruits, vegetables
Vitamin D	Calciferol	Cod liver oil, milk, egg yolk
Vitamin E	α-tocopherol	Wheat germ oil, cereals, egg yolk
Vitamin K	Phytonadione; menaquinone; menadione	Alfalfa, spinach, cabbage

tox/o   poison   toxic _____

toxic/o   poison   toxicology _____

vas/o   vessel   vasodilator _____

ven/o   vein   intravenous _____

vit/o   life   vitamin _____

The first vitamins discovered were nitrogen-containing substances called amines. Table 21–10 lists vitamins, their medical names, and foods that are a major source of each.

Prefixes			
Prefix	Meaning	Terminology	Meaning
ana-	upward, excessive, again	anaphylaxis _____ *-phylaxis means protection.*	
anti-	against	antidote _____ *-dote comes from the Greek, meaning what is given.* antibiotic _____	
contra-	against, opposite	contraindication _____	
par-	other than, apart from	parenteral _____ *enter/o means intestine.*	
syn-	together, with	synergistic _____	

IX. ABBREVIATIONS

ac	before meals	**PDR**	Physicians' Desk Reference
ad lib	freely as desired	**po**	by mouth
bid	two times a day	**prn**	when requested; *pro re nata* (required)
c̄	with	**Q(q)**	every
caps	capsule	**qam**	every morning
cc	cubic centimeter	**qd**	every day
FDA	Food and Drug Administration	**qh**	every hour
gm	gram	**qhs**	at bedtime
gt, gtt	drops	**qid**	four times a day
h	hour	**qns**	quantity not sufficient
IM	intramuscular	**qod**	every other day
IV	intravenous	**qpm**	every evening
mg	milligram	**s̄**	without
NPO	nothing by mouth	**subq**	subcutaneous injection
NSAID	nonsteroidal anti-inflammatory drug	**sig.**	let it be labeled
os	mouth	**sos**	if necessary *(si opus sit)*
oz.	ounce	**tab**	tablet
pc	after meals	**tid**	three times a day

X. Practical Applications

The following are the top 20 prescription drugs dispensed in U.S. community pharmacies, new and refill prescriptions in 1993 (from American Druggist, February 1994).

Top 20 Prescription Drugs–1993

Drug (Trade Name)	Generic Name	Type
1. Premarin	estrogen	Hormone
2. Zantac	ranitidine	Antiulcer
3. Amoxil	amoxicillin	Antibiotic (penicillin-type)
4. Synthroid	levothyroxine	Hormone (thyroid)
5. Procardia	nifedipine	Calcium channel blocker
6. Lanoxin	digoxin	Cardiotonic
7. Xanax	alprazolam	Tranquilizer
8. Trimox	amoxicillin	Antibiotic (penicillin-type)
9. Vasotec	enalapril	Antihypertensive

10. Cardizem	diltiazem HCl	Calcium channel blocker
11. Ceclor	cephalosporin	Antibiotic
12. Augmentin	amoxicillin/clavulanic acid	Antibiotic
13. Proventil	albuterol	Bronchodilator
14. Naprosyn	naproxen	NSAID (analgesic)
15. Provera	medroxyprogesterone	Hormone
16. Prozac	fluoxetine HCl	Antidepressant
17. Mevacor	lovastatin	Cholesterol-lowering drug
18. Seldane	terfenadine	Antihistamine
19. Ortho-Novum 7/7/7	estrogen and progesterone	Oral contraceptive
20. Capoten	captopril	Antihypertensive (ACE inhibitor)

Prescriptions

The usual order of drug prescription is name of the drug, dosage, route of administration, time of administration. At times the physician will include a qualifying phrase to indicate why the prescription is written. Not all information is listed with every prescription. Consider the following:

1. Fluoxetine (Prozac) 20 mg po bid
2. Dimenhydrinate (Dramamine) 10 mg 2 tab q 4–6h
3. Ondansetron (Zofran) 4 mg 1 tab/caps tid prn for nausea
4. Ranitidine (Zantac) 300 mg 1 tab pc qd
5. Pseudoephedrine (Sudafed) 60 mg 1 caps qid for 15 days
6. Acetaminophen (300 mg) & codeine (30 mg) 1 tab qid prn for pain

XI. Exercises

Remember to check your answers carefully with those given in Section XII, Answers to Exercises.

A. *Match the pharmacological specialty with its description below.*

1. use of drugs in the treatment of disease _____

2. study of new drug synthesis _____

3. study of how drugs interact with subcellular parts _____

4. study of the harmful effects of drugs _____

5. study of drug effects in the body _____

6. measurement of drug concentrations in tissues and in blood over a period of time

B. Select from the following terms to complete the sentences below.

antidote   trade (brand) name   toxicologist
generic name   Food and Drug Administration   chemical name
Physicians' Desk Reference   pharmacologist   pharmacist
United States Pharmacopeia

1. A person specializing in the study of the harmful effects of drugs on the body is known as a (an)

   _____ .

2. An agent given to counteract harmful effects of a drug is a (an) _____ .

3. The governmental agency that has legal responsibility for enforcing proper drug manufacture and

   clinical use is known as the _____ .

4. The _____
   is the commercial name for a drug.

5. The _____
   is the complicated chemical formula for a drug.

6. The _____
   is the legal noncommercial name for a drug.

7. A person who dispenses drugs from a store is known as a (an) _____ .

8. A person (often a medical doctor) who specializes in the study of the actions of drugs is known as a (an)

   _____ .

9. A reference book that lists drug products is known as the _____ .

10. An authoritative list of drugs, formulas, and preparations that sets a standard for drug manufacturing

    and dispensing is known as the _____ .

C. Name the route of drug administration from its description below.

1. Drug is administered via suppository or fluid into the anus. _____

2. Drug is administered via vapor or gas into the nose or mouth. _____

3. Drug is administered under the tongue. _____

4. Drug is applied locally on skin or mucous membrane. _____

5. Drug is injected via syringe under the skin, into a vein, muscle, or body cavity.

   _____

CHAPTER 21 ■ Pharmacology **767**

6. Drug is given by mouth and absorbed through the stomach or intestinal wall.

_____

D. Give the meanings for the following terms.

1. intravenous _____

2. intrathecal _____

3. antiseptic _____

4. antipruritic _____

5. aerosol _____

6. intramuscular _____

7. subcutaneous _____

8. intracavitary _____

E. Match the routes of drug administration in column I with the medications or procedures in column II. Write the letter of the answer in the space provided.

Column I

1. intravenous _____

2. rectal _____

3. oral _____

4. topical _____

5. inhalation _____

6. intrathecal _____

7. intramuscular _____

8. intradermal _____

Column II

A. lotions, creams, ointments
B. tablets and capsules
C. skin testing for allergy
D. lumbar puncture
E. deep injection, usually in buttock
F. suppositories
G. blood transfusions
H. aerosol medications

F. The following are descriptions of drug actions. Supply the proper name that fits the description.

1. the combination of two drugs that causes an effect that is greater than the sum of the individual effects

    of each drug given alone _____

2. the combination of two drugs that is equal to the sum of the effects of each _____

3. the effects of a given drug dose become less as treatment continues, and larger and larger doses must

be given to achieve the desired effect _____

4. any unexpected effect that may appear in a patient following administration of a drug

_____

G. *Give the meanings for the following terms that describe classes of drugs.*

1. antibiotic _____

2. antidepressant _____

3. antihistamine _____

4. analgesic _____

5. anticoagulant _____

6. anesthetic _____

7. antidiabetic _____

8. sedative _____

9. stimulant _____

10. tranquilizer _____

H. *Match the term in column I with an associated term in column II. Write the letter of the answer in the space provided.*

Column I

1. antihistamine _____

2. analgesic _____

3. antidiabetic _____

4. anticoagulant _____

5. antibiotic _____

6. stimulant _____

7. sedative _____

8. tranquilizer _____

Column II

A. caffeine or amphetamines
B. penicillin or erythromycin
C. insulin
D. barbiturate
E. heparin
F. nonsteroidal anti-inflammatory drug
G. phenothiazine
H. anaphylactic shock

I. Select from the following terms to complete the definitions below that relate to cardiovascular drugs.

antiarrhythmic   antianginal   vasodilator
cardiotonic   diuretic   antihypertensive
vasoconstrictor   cholesterol-lowering drug

1. drug that prevents chest pain due to ischemia _____

2. drug that narrows blood vessels _____

3. drug that promotes excretion of urine and lowers blood pressure _____

4. drug that strengthens force and efficiency of the heartbeat _____

5. drug that reduces lipids in the blood _____

6. drug that widens blood vessels _____

7. drug that corrects abnormal heart rhythms _____

8. any drug that reduces blood pressure _____

J. Give the meanings for the following terms.

1. beta-blocker _____

2. androgen _____

3. glucocorticoid _____

4. calcium channel blocker _____

5. estrogen _____

6. antacid _____

7. cathartic _____

8. antiemetic _____

9. bronchodilator _____

10. hypnotic _____

K. *Match the type of drug in column I with the condition it treats in column II. Write the letter of the answer in the space provided.*

Column I

1. anticonvulsant   _____

2. anticoagulant   _____

3. antacid   _____

4. progestins   _____

5. antibiotic   _____

6. cardiotonic   _____

7. antihypertensive   _____

8. antihistamine   _____

9. tranquilizer   _____

10. analgesic   _____

Column II

A. abnormal uterine bleeding due to hormonal imbalance

B. severe behavior disturbances and anxiety

C. epilepsy

D. congestive heart failure

E. epigastric discomfort

F. myalgia

G. anaphylactic shock

H. thrombosis and embolism

I. bacterial pneumonia

J. high blood pressure

L. *Complete the following terms from their definitions.*

1. an agent that reduces fever: anti _____

2. an agent that reduces itching: anti _____

3. a habit-forming analgesic: _____ tic

4. two drugs cause an effect greater than the sum of each alone: syn _____

5. an antibiotic derived from a red mold: _____ mycin

6. the legal nonproprietary name of a drug: _____ name

7. factor in a patient's condition that prevents use of a particular drug:

   contra _____

8. drug that produces no sensation or feeling: an _____

M. *Give the meanings for the following abbreviations.*

1. NSAID _____

2. prn _____

3. qid _____

4. ad lib _____

5. tid _____

6. mg _____

7. c̄ _____

8. s̄ _____

9. NPO _____

10. pc _____

11. bid _____

12. qh _____

13. po _____

14. q _____

15. qod _____

N. Circle the term that best completes the meaning of the sentence.

1. After his heart attack, Bernie was supposed to take many drugs including diuretics and a(an) (progestin, laxative, anticoagulant) to prevent blood clots.

2. Estelle was always anxious and had a hard time sleeping. Dr. Max felt that a mild (antacid, anticonvulsant, tranquilizer) would help her relax and concentrate on her work.

3. During chemotherapy Helen was very nauseated. Dr. Cohen prescribed an (antihypertensive, anti-emetic, antianginal) to relieve her symptoms of queasy stomach.

4. The two antibiotics worked together and were therefore (idiosyncratic, generic, synergistic) in killing the bacteria in Susan's bloodstream.

5. The label warned that the drug might impair fine motor skills. It listed the (side effects, antidote, pharmacodynamics) to taking the sedative.

XII. Answers to Exercises

A

1. chemotherapy
2. medicinal chemistry
3. molecular pharmacology
4. toxicology
5. pharmacodynamics
6. pharmacokinetics

B

1. toxicologist
2. antidote
3. Food and Drug Administration
4. trade (brand) name
5. chemical name
6. generic name
7. pharmacist
8. pharmacologist
9. Physicians' Desk Reference
10. United States Pharmacopeia

C

1. rectal
2. inhalation
3. sublingual
4. topical
5. parenteral
6. oral

D

1. within a vein
2. within a sheath (membranes around the spinal cord or brain)
3. an agent that is against infection
4. an agent that is against itching
5. a solution of particles (drug) in air (vapor or gas)
6. within a muscle
7. under the skin
8. within a cavity

E

1. G
2. F
3. B
4. A
5. H
6. D
7. E
8. C

F

1. synergism (potentiation)
2. additive action
3. tolerance
4. idiosyncrasy

G

1. an agent that inhibits or kills germ life (microorganisms)
2. an agent that relieves the symptoms of depression
3. an agent that blocks the action of histamine and relieves allergic symptoms
4. an agent that relieves pain
5. an agent that prevents blood clotting
6. an agent that reduces or eliminates sensation
7. an agent used to prevent diabetes mellitus
8. an agent (mildly hypnotic) that relaxes and calms nervousness
9. an agent that excites and promotes activity
10. a drug used to control anxiety and severe disturbances of behavior

H

1. H
2. F
3. C
4. E
5. B
6. A
7. D
8. G

I

1. antianginal
2. vasoconstrictor
3. diuretic
4. cardiotonic
5. cholesterol-lowering drug
6. vasodilator
7. antiarrhythmic
8. antihypertensive

J

1. drug that blocks the action of epinephrine at sites of receptors of heart muscles, blood vessels, and bronchial tubes (antihypertensive, antianginal, and antiarrhythmic)
2. a drug that produces male sexual characteristics
3. a hormone from the adrenal glands that reduces inflammation and raises blood sugar
4. drug that blocks the entrance of calcium into heart muscle and blood vessel walls (antianginal, antiarrhythmic, and antihypertensive)
5. a hormone that produces female sexual characteristics
6. a drug that neutralizes acid in the stomach
7. a drug that relieves constipation
8. a drug that prevents nausea and vomiting
9. a drug that opens air passages
10. an agent that produces sleep

K

1. C
2. H
3. E
4. A
5. I
6. D
7. J
8. G
9. B
10. F

L

1. antipyretic
2. antipruritic
3. narcotic
4. synergism
5. erythromycin
6. generic
7. contraindication
8. anesthetic

M

1. nonsteroidal anti-inflammatory drug
2. when requested
3. four times a day
4. freely as desired
5. three times a day

6. milligram
7. with
8. without
9. nothing by mouth
10. after meals

11. twice a day
12. every hour
13. by mouth
14. every
15. every other day

N

1. anticoagulant
2. tranquilizer
3. antiemetic

4. synergistic
5. side effects

XIII. Pronunciation of Terms

To test your understanding of the terminology in this chapter, write the meaning of each term in the space provided. In addition, you may wish to cover the terms and write them by looking at your definitions. Make sure your spelling is correct. The page number after each term indicates where it is defined or used in the text so you can easily check your responses. (If you are not sure what the pronunciation symbols mean, refer to page 21.)

Term	Pronunciation	Meaning
additive action (758)	AD-ĭ-tĭv ĂK-shŭn	
aerosol (758)	Ā-ĕr-ō-sōl	
amphetamine (760)	ăm-FĔT-ă-mēn	
analgesic (760)	ăn-ăl-JĒ-zĭk	
anaphylaxis (758)	ăn-ă-fĭ-LĂK-sĭs	
anesthesia (762)	ăn-ĕs-THĒ-zē-ă	
anesthetic (760)	ăn-ĕs-THĔ-tĭk	
antacid (760)	ănt-ĂS-ĭd	
antianginal (760)	ăn-tĭ-ĂN-jĭ-nal	
antiarrhythmic (760)	ăn-tĭ-ă-RĬTH-mĭk	
antibiotic (760)	ăn-tĭ-bī-ŎT-ĭk	
anticoagulant (760)	ăn-tĭ-kō-ĂG-ū-lănt	
anticonvulsant (760)	ăn-tĭ-kŏn-VŬL-sănt	
antidepressant (760)	ăn-tĭ-dĕ-PRĔS-ănt	
antidiabetic (760)	ăn-tĭ-dī-ă-BĔ-tik	
antidiarrheal (760)	ăn-tĭ-dī-ă-RĒ-ăl	
antidote (758)	ĂN-tĭ-dōt	

antiemetic (760)	ăn-tĭ-ĕ-MĚ-tĭk	_____
antihistamine (760)	ăn-tĭ-HĬS-tă-mēn	_____
antihypertensive (760)	ăn-tĭ-hī-pĕr-TĔN-sĭv	_____
antinauseant (760)	ăn-tĭ-NAW-zē-ănt	_____
antipyretic (762)	ăn-tĭ-pī-RĔT-ĭk	_____
barbiturate (761)	băr-BĬT-ū-rāt	_____
beta-blocker (761)	BĀ-tă-BLŎK-ĕr	_____
bronchodilator (762)	brŏng-kō-DĪ-lā-tĕr	_____
caffeine (761)	kăf-ĒN	_____
calcium channel blocker (761)	KĂL-sē-ŭm CHĂ-năl BLŎK-ĕr	_____
cardiotonic (761)	kăr-dē-ō-TŎN-ĭk	_____
cathartic (761)	kă-THĂR-tĭk	_____
chemotherapy (762)	kē-mō-THĔR-ă-pē	_____
contraindication (758)	kŏn-tră-ĭn-dĭ-KĀ-shŭn	_____
diuretic (761)	dī-ū-RĔT-ĭk	_____
emetic (761)	ĕ-MĚT-ĭk	_____
erythromycin (762)	ĕ-rīth-rō-MĪ-sĭn	_____
generic name (758)	jĕ-NĔR-ĭk nām	_____
glucocorticoid (761)	glōō-kō-KŌR-tĭ-koyd	_____
hypnotic (761)	hĭp-NŎT-ĭk	_____
hypodermic (762)	hī-pō-DĔR-mĭk	_____
iatrogenic (759)	ī-ăt-rō-JĚN-ĭk	_____
idiosyncrasy (759)	ĭd-ē-ō-SĬN-kră-sē	_____
inhalation (759)	ĭn-hă-LĀ-shŭn	_____
intrathecal (762)	ĭn-tră-THĒ-kăl	_____
laxative (761)	LĂK-să-tĭv	_____
medicinal chemistry (759)	mĕ-DĬ-sĭ-năl KĔM-ĭs-trē	_____

molecular pharmacology (759)	mō-LĔK-ū-lăr făr-mă-KŎL-ō-jē	_____
narcotic (761)	năr-KŎT-ĭk	_____
parenteral (759)	pă-RĔN-tĕr-ăl	_____
pharmacodynamics (759)	făr-mă-kō-dī-NĂM-ĭks	_____
pharmacokinetics (759)	făr-mă-kō-kĭ-NĔT-ĭks	_____
progestin (756)	prō-GĔS-tĭn	_____
purgative (761)	PŬR-gă-tĭv	_____
sedative (761)	SĔD-ă-tĭv	_____
stimulant (761)	STĬM-ū-lănt	_____
sublingual (759)	sŭb-LĬNG-wăl	_____
synergism (759)	SĬN-ĕr-jĭzm	_____
synergistic (763)	sĭn-ĕr-JĬS-tĭk	_____
syringe (759)	sĭ-RĬNJ	_____
tolerance (759)	TŎL-ĕr-ănz	_____
toxicity (759)	tŏk-SĬS-ĭ-tē	_____
toxicology (760)	tŏk-sĭ-KŎL-ō-jē	_____
tranquilizer (761)	TRĂN-kwĭ-lī-zĕr	_____
vasoconstriction (755)	văz-ō-kŏn-STRĬK-shŭn	_____
vasodilation (755)	văz-ō-dī-LĀ-shŭn	_____
vitamin (760)	VĪ-tă-mĕn	_____

XIV. Review Sheet

Write the meaning of each word part in the space provided and test yourself. Check your answers with the information in the chapter or in the Glossary (Medical Terms—English) at the back of the book.

Combining Forms

Combining Form	Meaning	Combining Form	Meaning
aer/o	_____	lingu/o	_____
alges/o	_____	myc/o	_____
bronchi/o	_____	narc/o	_____
chem/o	_____	pharmac/o	_____
cras/o	_____	prurit/o	_____
cutane/o	_____	pyret/o	_____
derm/o	_____	thec/o	_____
enter/o	_____	tox/o	_____
erg/o	_____	toxic/o	_____
esthes/o	_____	vas/o	_____
hist/o	_____	ven/o	_____
hypn/o	_____	vit/o	_____
iatr/o	_____		

Suffixes

Suffix	Meaning	Suffix	Meaning
-amine	_____	-in	_____
-dote	_____	-phylaxis	_____
-genic	_____	-sol	_____

Prefixes

Prefix	Meaning	Prefix	Meaning
ana-	_____	par-	_____
anti-	_____	syn-	_____
contra-	_____		

Psychiatry

This Chapter is divided into the following sections

In this Chapter you will

- Differentiate among a psychiatrist, a psychologist, and other psychiatric specialists;
- Learn of tests used by clinical psychologists to evaluate a patient's mental health and intelligence;
- Define terms that describe major psychiatric disorders;
- Identify terms that describe psychiatric symptoms;
- Compare different types of therapy for psychiatric disorders; and
- Define combining forms, suffixes, prefixes, and abbreviations related to psychiatry.

I. Introduction

You will find this chapter different from others in the book. Psychiatric disorders are not readily explainable in terms of abnormalities in the structure or chemistry of an organ or tissue, as are other illnesses. In addition, the etiology of mental disorders is complex. Although a chemical basis for psychiatric disorders cannot be excluded, psychological and social factors play an important role in mental illness. Our purpose here will be to provide a simple outline and definition of major psychiatric terms. For more extensive and detailed information, you may wish to consult the **Diagnostic and Statistical Manual IV-R** (American Psychiatric Association, Washington, DC, 1994), as well as other textbooks of psychiatry.

Psychiatry (psych/o means mind, **iatr/o** means treatment) is the branch of medicine that deals with the diagnosis, treatment, and prevention of mental illness. It is a specialty of clinical medicine comparable with surgery, internal medicine, pediatrics, and obstetrics.

Psychiatrists complete the same medical training (4 years of medical school) as other physicians and receive an M.D. degree. Then they spend a varying number of years training in the methods and practice of **psychotherapy** (treatment of mental disorders). Psychiatrists can also take additional years of training to specialize in certain aspects of psychiatry. **Child psychiatrists** specialize in the treatment of children; **forensic psychiatrists** specialize in the legal aspects of psychiatry, such as determination of mental competence in criminal cases. **Psychoanalysts** complete 3–5 years of training in a special psychotherapeutic technique called **psychoanalysis** in which the patient freely relates her or his thoughts to the analyst, who does not interfere in the flow of thoughts.

A **psychologist** is a nonmedical person who is trained in methods of psychotherapy, analysis, and research and completes a master's or doctor of philosophy (Ph.D.) degree in a specific field of interest, such as **clinical** (patient-oriented) **psychology, experimental psychology,** or **social psychology** (focusing on social interaction and the ways the actions of others influence the behavior of the individual). A clinical psychologist, like a psychiatrist, can use various methods of psychotherapy to treat patients but, unlike the psychiatrist, cannot use drugs or electroconvulsive therapy without the permission of a physician.

Clinical psychologists are trained in the use of tests to evaluate various aspects of a patient's mental health and intelligence. Examples are intelligence (I.Q.) tests such as the **Wechsler Adult Intelligence Scale (WAIS)** and the **Stanford-Binet Intelligence Scale.** Projective (personality) tests are the **Rorschach technique** (inkblots, as shown in Fig. 22–1, are used to bring out associations) and the **Thematic Apperception Test (TAT),** in which pictures are used as stimuli for making up a story (Fig. 22–2). Both tests are especially revealing of personality structure. Graphomotor projection tests are the **Draw a Person Test,** in which the patient is asked to draw a body, and the **Bender-Gestalt Test,** in which the patient is asked to draw certain geometric designs. These tests are useful in detecting deficiencies in movement or coordination due to brain damage. The **Minnesota Multiphasic Personality**

Figure 22–1

Inkblots like this one are presented on ten cards in the Rorschach test. The patient describes images seen in the blot.

Figure 22–2

A sample picture from the Thematic Apperception Test. A patient is asked to tell the story that the picture illustrates. (From Gleitman H: Psychology. New York: WW Norton, 1991, p 637.)

Inventory (MMPI) contains true-false questions that reveal aspects of personality, such as sense of duty or responsibility, ability to relate to others, and dominance. This test is widely used as an objective measure of psychological disorders in adolescents and adults. A patient's responses to questions are compared with responses made by patients with diagnoses of schizophrenia, depression, and so on.

II. Psychiatric Symptoms

The following terms are often used to describe abnormalities in behavior and will help you to understand Section III, Psychiatric Disorders.

amnesia	Loss of memory.
anxiety	Varying degrees of uneasiness, apprehension, or dread often accompanied by palpitations, tightness in the chest, breathlessness and choking sensations.
apathy	Absence of emotions; lack of interest or emotional involvement.
autism	Severe lack of responsiveness to others, preoccupation with inner thoughts; withdrawal and retarded language development.
compulsion	Uncontrollable urge to perform an act repeatedly.
conversion	Anxiety becomes a bodily symptom such as blindness, deafness, or paralysis, none of which have an organic basis.
delusion	A fixed, false belief that cannot be changed by logical reasoning or evidence.
dissociation	Uncomfortable feelings are separated from their real object. In order to avoid mental distress the feelings are redirected toward a second object or behavior pattern.

dysphoria	Sadness, hopelessness; depressive mood.
euphoria	Exaggerated feeling of well-being ("high").
hallucination	False or unreal sensory perception as, for example, hearing voices when none is present; an **illusion** is a false perception of an actual sensory stimulus.
labile	Unstable; undergoing rapid emotional change.
mania	State of excessive excitability; hyperactivity and agitation.
mutism	Nonreactive state; stupor.
obsession	An involuntary, persistent idea, emotion, or urge.
paranoia	Delusions of persecution or grandeur or combinations of the two.

III. Psychiatric Disorders

Sigmund Freud's ideas of personality structure play an important role in the understanding of many types of psychiatric disorders. Freud believed that personality is made up of three major parts: the **id,** the **ego,** and the **superego.** The **id** represents the unconscious instincts and psychic energy present at birth and thereafter. From the id arises basic drives that, operating according to the pleasure principle, seek immediate gratification regardless of the reality of the situation. The id is believed to predominate in the thinking of infants and to be manifest in the uncontrolled actions of certain mentally ill patients.

The **ego** is the central coordinating branch of the personality. It is the mediator between the id and the outside world. It is the part of the personality that evaluates and assesses the reality of a situation **(reality testing)** and, if necessary, postpones the gratification of a need or drive (id) until a satisfactory object or situation arises. The ego is perceived as being "self" by the individual.

The **superego** is the internalized conscience and moral part of the personality. It encompasses the sense of discipline derived from parental authority and society. Guilt feelings, for example, arise from behavior and thoughts that do not conform to the standards of the superego.

Freud believed that certain psychological disorders occur when conflicts arise between two or more of these aspects of the personality. **Defense mechanisms,** such as denial, are the techniques people employ to ward off the anxiety produced by these conflicts. For example, a person afflicted with a serious illness may avoid confronting his or her present or future problems by denial. Thus, he or she may refuse to believe the diagnosis, may miss appointments, may neglect medication, or may ignore symptoms. Whereas all persons utilize defense mechanisms to cope with difficult problems, the use of these mechanisms may be regarded as abnormal or normal according to whether that use makes a constructive or destructive contribution to the individual's personality.

The term **psychosis** is frequently used to describe mental illness. A **psychosis** involves significant impairment of reality testing, with symptoms such as **delusions** (false beliefs), **hallucinations** (false sensory perceptions), and bizarre behavior. Schizophrenic disorders are examples of psychoses. Patients exhibit a disturbed sense of self, inappropriate affect (emotional reactions), and withdrawal from the external world.

Psychiatric disorders that will be discussed in this section are **anxiety disorders, delirium** and **dementia, dissociative disorders, eating disorders, mood disorders, personality disorders, schizophrenia, sexual** and **gender identity disorders, somatoform disorders,** and substance-related disorders.

Anxiety Disorders

These disorders are characterized by anxiety—the experience of unpleasant tension, distress, troubled feelings, and avoidance behavior. Panic attacks, marked by intense fear or discomfort and symptoms such as palpitations, sweating, trembling, dizziness, and so on, occur in the context of several anxiety disorders. Examples of anxiety disorders are **phobic disorders, obsessive-compulsive disorder,** and **post-traumatic stress disorder.**

Phobic disorders are characterized by irrational or debilitating fears associated with a specific object or situation. The patient with a phobic disorder goes to extreme lengths to avoid the object of her or his fear. The object that is feared is often symbolic of an unconscious conflict that is the cause of the phobia and thus diverts the patient's attention from the conflict, keeping it unconscious.

Agoraphobia (**agora** means marketplace) is the fear of being alone or in open, crowded, public places from which escape would be difficult or in which help might not be available. Persons with agoraphobia limit their normal activities to avoid situations that trigger their anxiety. Thus, they may feel comfortable only by remaining at home or in the company of a friend or relative. Panic attacks (periods of intense apprehension and fear) can occur in anticipation of the phobic situation.

A **social phobia** is the fear of situations in which the individual is open to public scrutiny with possible embarrassment and humiliation. Fear of speaking in public, using public lavatories, or eating in public are examples of social phobias.

Other specific phobias are **claustrophobia** (fear of closed-in places; **claustr/o** means barrier), **acrophobia** (fear of heights; **acr/o** means extremity), and **zoophobia** (fear of animals; **zo/o** means animals).

Obsessive-compulsive disorder (OCD) involves recurrent thoughts (**obsessions**) and repetitive acts (**compulsions**) that dominate the patient's behavior. The patient experiences anxiety if he or she is prevented from performing special rituals, which are used to shield against overwhelming anxiety or fear. Often the OCD consumes time and significantly interferes with the individual's social or occupational functioning. An antidepressant drug, clomipramine, has been used for the treatment of OCD with some success.

Post-traumatic stress disorder is the development of symptoms (intense fear, helplessness, insomnia, nightmares, and diminished responsiveness to the external world) following exposure to a traumatic event.

Delirium and Dementia

Delirium and **dementia** are both disorders of abnormal **cognition** (mental processes of thinking, perception, reasoning, judgment).

Delirium is acute, temporary disturbance of consciousness and mental confusion. It is characterized by rambling, irrelevant, or incoherent speech, sensory misperceptions, and disorientation to time, place, or person with memory impairment. Delirium is caused by a variety of conditions, including drug intoxication or withdrawal, seizures or head trauma, and metabolic disturbances such as hypoxia, hypoglycemia, electrolyte imbalances, or hepatic or renal failure. **Delirium tremens** is brought on by withdrawal after prolonged periods of heavy alcohol ingestion.

Dementia is a general loss of intellectual abilities involving impairment of judgment, memory, and abstract thinking as well as changes in personality. Dementia may be caused by conditions, some reversible and some progressive, involving damage to the brain. The most common cause is Alzheimer's disease, but others are cerebrovascular disease, central nervous system (CNS) infection, brain trauma, tumors, and Parkinson's and Huntington's disease.

Dissociative Disorders

Dissociative disorders are chronic or sudden disturbances of memory, identity, consciousness, or perception of the environment that are not caused by the direct effects of brain damage or drug abuse. Symptoms hide the pain and anxiety of unconscious conflicts. Examples of dissociative disorders are **dissociative identity disorder,** which is the existence within the individual of two or more distinct personalities that take hold of the individual's behavior (illustrated in literature by Dr. Jekyll and Mr. Hyde); **dissociative amnesia** (inability to remember important personal information that is too extensive to be explained by ordinary forgetfulness); and **dissociative fugue** (sudden, unexpected travel away from home or customary work locale). The fugue disorder includes the assumption of a new identity and an inability to recall one's previous identity.

Eating Disorders

Eating disorders are severe disturbances in eating behavior. Examples are **anorexia nervosa** and **bulimia nervosa.** Anorexia nervosa is a refusal to maintain a minimally normal body weight. An individual is intensely afraid of gaining weight and has a disturbance in the perception of the shape or size of his or her body. (The term anorexia, meaning lack of appetite, is a misnomer because lack of appetite is rare). The condition predominantly affects adolescent females, and its principal symptom is a conscious, relentless attempt to diet along with excessive, compulsive overactivity, such as exercise, running, or gymnastics. Most postmenarcheal females with this disorder are amenorrheic.

Bulimia nervosa (bulimia means abnormal increase in hunger) is characterized by binge eating (abnormality in the amount of food consumed). Bulimic individuals can maintain normal or nearly normal weight because after binging they engage in inappropriate activities that eliminate food from the body. Examples of such behavior are self-induced vomiting; misuse of laxatives, diuretics, or enemas; and fasting or excessive exercise.

Mood Disorders

A mood disorder is a prolonged emotion, such as depression or mania (elation) that dominates a patient's entire mental life. Examples of mood disorders are **bipolar disorders** and **depressive disorders.**

Bipolar disorders (**bi** means two; **pol/o** means extreme) are characterized by one or more **manic** episodes alternating with depressive episodes. A manic episode is a period during which the predominant mood is excessively elevated (euphoria), expansive, or irritable. Associated symptoms include inflated self-esteem, decreased need for sleep, nearly continuous flow of rapid speech with rapid changes of topic, distractability, increase in goal-directed activity, and excessive involvement in pleasurable activities that have a high potential for painful consequences. Often there is increased sociability and participation in multiple activities marked by intrusive, domineering, and demanding behavior. **Hypomania** is a term used to describe a mood resembling mania, but of lesser intensity. **Cyclothymia** (**cycl/o** means cycle, **thym/o** means mind) is a mild form of bipolar disorder in which there are numerous manic or hypomanic episodes intermixed with depressive episodes, but the episodes are not as severe or of as long duration.

Depressive disorders are marked by one or more major depressive episodes without a history of mania or hypomania. **Major depression** involves severe **dysphoria** (sadness, hopelessness, worry, discouragement). Other symptoms are appetite disturbances and changes in weight, sleep disorders such as insomnia or hypersomnia, fatigue or low energy, feelings of worthlessness, hopelessness, or excessive or inappropriate guilt, difficulty thinking or concentrating, and recurrent thoughts of death or suicide. **Dysthymia** (or dysthymic disorder) is a depressive disorder involving depressive episodes but not of the same severity and duration as in major depression. Also, there are no psychotic features (delusions, hallucinations, incoherent thinking) in dysthymia, which are sometimes found in major depression.

Physicians have noted a relationship between the onset of an episode of depressive disorder and a particular 60-day period of the year. A regular appearance of depression may occur between the beginning of October and the end of November every year. This is referred to as **seasonal affective** (mood) **disorder (SAD).** A change from depression to mania or hypomania also may occur within a 60-day period from mid-February to mid-April.

Personality Disorders

Personality traits are established patterns of thinking and ways of relating to and perceiving the environment and one's self. However, when these traits become inflexible and rigid, causing impairment of functioning, distress, and conflict with others, they constitute personality disorders. Examples of personality disorders are

antisocial	No loyalty or concern for others, and without moral standards; acts only in response to desires and impulses; cannot tolerate frustration and blames others when she or he is at fault.
histrionic	Emotional, attention-seeking, immature, and dependent; irrational outbursts and tantrums; flamboyant and theatrical; having general dissatisfaction with one's self and angry feelings about the world.
narcissistic	Grandiose sense of self-importance or uniqueness and preoccupation with fantasies of success and power. **Narcissism** is a pervasive interest in one's self with a lack of empathy for others.
paranoid	Continually suspicious and mistrustful of other people; jealous and overly concerned with hidden motives of others; quick to take offense.
schizoid	Emotionally cold and aloof; indifferent to praise or criticism or to the feelings of others; few friendships and rarely appears to experience strong emotions, such as anger or joy.

Schizophrenia

This disorder is characterized by withdrawal from reality into an inner world of disorganized thinking and conflict. There is mental deterioration from a previous level of function in areas such as work, social relations, and self-care. Some characteristic symptoms of schizophrenia are:

Delusions such as thought broadcasting (the belief that one's thoughts, as they occur, are broadcast from one's head to the external world so that others can hear them).

Hallucinations, which may involve many voices the person perceives as coming from outside her or his head.

Disorganized thinking such as loosening of associations (ideas shift from one subject to another, completely unrelated or only obliquely connected). This may result in incoherent, incomprehensible speech.

Flat affect (external expression of emotion) marked by monotonous voice, immobile face, and no signs of expression. Affect may also be inappropriate (giggling and laughing when talking about torture and illness).

Impaired interpersonal functioning and relationship to the external world such as emotional detachment and social withdrawal. **Autism** (preoccupation with self-centered, illogical ideas and fantasies that exclude the external world) is often a feature of schizophrenia.

Physicians describe several types of schizophrenia, such as **catatonic type** (characterized by catatonic stupor in which the patient is mute and does not move or react to the outside environment); **disorganized type** (disorganized speech and behavior and flat or inappropriate affect); and **paranoid type** (presence of prominent delusions of grandeur or persecution and auditory hallucinations).

Sexual and Gender Identity Disorders

Sexual disorders are divided into two types: **paraphilias** and **sexual dysfunctions.** Paraphilias (**para** means abnormal, **philia** means attraction to or love) are characterized by recurrent intense sexual urges, fantasies, or behaviors that involve unusual objects, activities, or situations. Sexual dysfunctions are disturbances in sexual desire or psychosexual changes in sexual response, such as premature ejaculation and dyspareunia that are not the result of a general medical condition.

Examples of paraphilias are

exhibitionism	Compulsive need to expose one's body, particularly the genitals, to an unsuspecting stranger.
fetishism	The use of nonliving objects (articles of clothing) as substitutes for a human sexual love object.
pedophilia	Sexual urges and fantasies involving sexual activity with a prepubescent child (age 13 or younger).
sexual masochism	Sexual gratification is gained by being humiliated, beaten, bound, or otherwise made to suffer by another person.
sexual sadism	Sexual gratification is gained by inflicting physical or psychological pain or humiliation on others.
transvestic fetishism	Cross-dressing; wearing clothing of the opposite sex. This disorder has only

been described in heterosexual males who have intense sexually arousing fantasies, urges, or behaviors involving cross-dressing.

voyeurism   Sexual excitement is achieved by observing unsuspecting people who are naked, undressing, or engaging in sexual activity.

A **gender identity disorder** is a strong and persistent cross-gender identification with the opposite sex. In children, this identification is manifested in preference for cross-dressing and cross-sex roles in make believe play, or persistent fantasies of being the other sex.

Somatoform Disorders

These are a group of disorders in which the patient's mental conflicts are expressed as physical symptoms. The physical symptoms, such as abdominal or chest pain, nausea, vomiting, diarrhea, palpitations, deafness, blindness, and paralysis, are not adequately explained by a physical or other mental disorder or by injury and are not side effects of medication, drugs, or alcohol.

Examples of somatoform (**somat/o** means body) disorders are **conversion disorder** and **hypochondriasis.**

Conversion disorder is a loss of physical functioning that suggests a physical disorder but that instead is an expression of a psychological conflict or need. The patient usually has a feared or unconscious conflict that threatens to escape from **repression** (a defense mechanism in which a person removes unacceptable ideas or impulses from consciousness), but the energies associated with this conflict are experienced as a physical symptom. The conversion symptom (examples are paralysis, blindness, seizures, paresthesias, and dyskinesia) enables the individual to avoid the conflict and get support from the surrounding environment. For example, a person with repressed anger and desire to physically harm a family member may suddenly develop paralysis of the arm (conversion symptom). Another example of conversion disorder is shell shock or combat fatigue, in which a soldier becomes paralyzed and cannot participate in battle.

Hypochondriasis is a preoccupation with bodily aches, pains, and discomforts in the absence of real illness. Appropriate physical evaluation does not support the diagnosis of any physical disorder that can account for the symptoms or the person's unwarranted interpretation of them.

Table 22–1 reviews the different types of psychiatric disorders and gives examples of each type.

Substance-related Disorders

These disorders are characterized by symptoms and behavioral changes associated with regular use of substances that affect the central nervous system. Continued or periodic use of certain drugs produces a state of dependence. **Psychological dependence** is a compulsion to continue taking a drug despite adverse consequences, and **physical dependence** is characterized by the onset of withdrawal symptoms when the drug is discontinued abruptly. A significant feature of dependence is **tolerance.** Tolerance is the declining effect of the drug, so that the dose must be increased to give the same effect.

Examples of substances that are associated with drug abuse (use of a drug for purposes other than those for which it is prescribed) and dependence are:

Table 22–1. PSYCHIATRIC DISORDERS

Disorder	Examples
Anxiety disorders	Phobic disorders
	Obsessive-compulsive disorder
	Post-traumatic stress disorder
Delirium and dementia	Delirium tremens
Dissociative disorders	Dissociative identity disorder
	Dissociative amnesia
	Dissociative fugue
Eating disorders	Anorexia nervosa
	Bulimia nervosa
Mood disorders	Bipolar disorders
	Depressive disorders
Personality disorders	Antisocial, histrionic, narcissistic, paranoid, schizoid
Schizophrenia	Catatonic, disorganized and paranoid types
Sexual and gender identity disorders	Paraphilias
	Sexual dysfunctions
	Gender identity disorders
Somatoform disorders	Conversion disorder
	Hypochondriasis
Substance-related disorders	Alcohol, amphetamines, cannabis, cocaine, hallucinogens, opioids, sedatives

Alcohol. Alcohol dependence is often associated with the use and abuse of other psychoactive drugs (cannabis, cocaine, heroin, amphetamines). Signs of alcohol dependence and intoxication include slurred speech, incoordination, unsteady gait, nystagmus (rapid, rhythmic movement of the eyeball), impairment in attention or memory, stupor or coma. It is also associated with depression, but usually the depression appears to be a consequence, not a cause, of the drinking.

Amphetamines. These central nervous system stimulants are taken orally or intravenously. Examples are **amphetamine (Benzedrine), dextroamphetamine (Dexedrine),** and **methamphetamine (Desoxyn** or speed). Appetite suppressants (diet pills) are amphetamine-like drugs. Psychological and behavioral changes associated with amphetamine dependence include anger, tension or anxiety, impaired judgment, inability to enjoy what was previously pleasurable, and social isolation. Physical symptoms include tachycardia or bradycardia, pupillary dilation, nausea, elevated or low blood pressure, and muscular weakness.

Cannabis (Marijuana). This class of drugs includes all substances with psychoactive properties derived from the cannabis plant plus chemically similar synthetic substances. Examples are marijuana, hashish, and purified delta-9-tetrahydrocannabinol (THC), the major psychoactive ingredient in these substances. Psychological and physical symptoms following the smoking of cannabis include euphoria, impaired motor coordination, anxiety, sensation of slowed time, social withdrawal and impaired judgment. Other signs of cannabis intoxication are increased appetite, dry mouth, and tachycardia.

Cocaine. Cocaine is a stimulant drug that produces euphoria as well as vasoconstriction, tachycardia, and hypertension. It comes from the leaves of the coca tree, which grows in Central and South America. The form of cocaine most commonly used in the United States is cocaine hydrochloride powder, which is inhaled through the nostrils and then absorbed into the bloodstream through mucous membranes. It can also be injected intravenously and mixed with heroin (speedball). This mixture is particularly dangerous because cocaine and heroin act synergistically in depressing respiratory function. If the cocaine is separated from its powdered salt form (with ether, ammonia, or baking soda), the resulting cocaine alkaloid is commonly called freebase. This form can be smoked and is known as crack or rock. Often,

Figure 22–3

the user of cocaine is also dependent on alcohol or sedatives, which are taken in an attempt to alleviate the unpleasant aftereffects (anxiety, depression, and fatigue) of cocaine intoxication.

Hallucinogens. These drugs produce a state of central nervous system excitement, hyperactivity, hallucinations, delusions, hypertension, and mood changes. Examples of hallucinogens are **lysergic acid diethylamide (LSD), mescaline (peyote),** and **phencyclidine (PCP).** The use of hallucinogens is generally episodic because their psychoactive effects are so potent; frequent use may lead to marked tolerance.

Opioids. This group of drugs includes **heroin** and **morphine** and synthetic drugs with morphine-like action (**codeine** and **methadone).** These compounds are prescribed as analgesics, anesthetics, or cough-suppressants. Typical symptoms of opioid intoxication are pupillary constriction, euphoria, slowness in movement, drowsiness, and slurred speech. Effects of overdose are slow and shallow breathing, convulsions, coma, and possible death. Symptoms of opioid withdrawal are watery eyes, rhinorrhea, pupillary dilation, abdominal cramps and diarrhea, and muscle and joint pain.

Sedatives, hypnotics, or anxiolytics. These drugs have a soothing, relaxing, euphoric effect and can also produce sleep (hypnotics). Sleeping pills include **barbiturates** such as phenobarbital and secobarbital. Other drugs that produce a barbiturate-like effect are **diazepam (Valium)** and **meprobamate (Miltown, Equanil).** Intoxication is characterized by slurred speech and disorientation. Effects of overdose are shallow respiration, cold and clammy skin, dilated pupils, weak and rapid pulse, coma, and possibly death.

Figure 22–3 reviews the types of psychoactive substances that lead to drug dependence and abuse.

IV. Therapeutic Terminology

Some major therapeutic techniques for psychiatric disorders are **psychotherapy, electroconvulsive therapy,** and **drug therapy.**

Psychotherapy

This is the treatment of emotional problems by psychological techniques. The following are psychotherapeutic techniques used by both psychiatrists and psychologists:

Behavior Therapy. Conditioning (changing behavior patterns and responses by training and repetition) is used to relieve anxiety and treat phobias.

Family Therapy. Treatment of an entire family to resolve and understand their conflicts and problems.

Group Therapy. A group of patients with similar problems gain insight into their own personalities through discussions and interaction, together. In **psychodrama** patients express their feelings by acting out roles along with other patient-actors on a stage. After a scene has been presented, the audience (composed of other patients) is asked to make comments and offer interpretations about what they have observed.

Hypnosis. A **trance** (state of altered consciousness) is created to increase the speed of psychotherapy or to help recovery of deeply repressed memories.

Play Therapy. Therapy in which a child, through play, uses toys to express conflicts and feelings that she or he is unable to communicate in a direct manner.

Psychoanalysis. Developed by Sigmund Freud, this long-term and intense form of psychotherapy seeks to influence behavior and resolve internal conflicts by allowing patients to bring their unconscious emotions to the surface. Through techniques such as **free association** (speaking one's thoughts one after another without censorship), **transference** (relating to the therapist as one had to a person who figured prominently in early childhood, such as a parent or sibling), and **dream interpretation,** the patient is able to bring to awareness his or her unconscious emotional conflicts and thus can overcome these problems.

Sex Therapy. This form of therapy helps individuals to overcome sexual dysfunctions such as **frigidity** (inhibited sexual response in women), **impotence** (inability of a man to achieve and/or maintain an erection), and **premature ejaculation** (release of semen before coitus can be achieved).

Electroconvulsive Therapy (ECT)

A treatment in which an electric current applied to the brain to produce convulsions (involuntary muscular contractions) and sometimes unconsciousness. It is used chiefly for serious depression and the depressive phase of bipolar (manic-depressive) disorder. With the introduction of antidepressant drug therapy, there are fewer indications for electroconvulsive therapy.

Drug Therapy

Neuroleptic drugs are those that modify psychotic symptoms. Categories of these drugs are:

Antianxiety Agents. These drugs (minor tranquilizers and sedatives) lessen anxiety. Examples are barbiturates and drugs such as diazepam (Valium) and chlordiazepoxide hydrochloride (Librium).

Antidepressants. These drugs reverse depressive symptoms and produce feelings of well-being. The basis of depression is thought to be an imbalance in the levels of neurotransmitters in the brain. An example of a commonly prescribed antidepressant is fluoxetine (Prozac). Prozac allows the passage of serotonin (a neurotransmitter) into nerve cells. It improves mood, mental alertness, physical activity, and sleep patterns. Other examples of antidepressants are:

Monoamine Oxidase (MAO) Inhibitors. These drugs suppress an enzyme (MAO) that normally degrades neurotransmitters. MAO inhibitors are not as widely prescribed as other antidepressants because serious cardiovascular complications can occur with their use.

Stimulants. Amphetamines are used to produce elevation in mood.

Tricyclic Antidepressants. These drugs contain three fused rings (tricyclic) in their chemical structure. They block the reuptake of neurotransmitters at nerve endings.

Lithium. Lithium carbonate is used in the control of the manic phase of bipolar (manic-depressive) illness.

Figure 22–4

Phenothiazines. Major tranquilizers used to treat symptoms of psychoses. They reduce anxiety, tension, and hyperactivity, control agitation and aggressiveness, and modify psychotic symptoms (delusions and hallucinations).

Figure 22–4 reviews the various types of drug therapy.

V. Vocabulary

This list will help you review many of the new terms introduced in the text. Short definitions reinforce your understanding of the terms. See Section XI of this chapter for help in pronouncing the more difficult terms.

Psychiatric Symptoms and Disorders

affect	External emotion or emotional response.
amnesia	Loss of memory.
anorexia nervosa	An eating disorder of excessive dieting and refusal to maintain a normal body weight.
anxiety disorders	Characterized by unpleasant tension, distress, and avoidance behavior; examples are phobias, obsessive-compulsive disorder and post-traumatic stress disorder.
apathy	Absence of emotions; lack of interest or emotional involvement.
autism	Severe lack of response to other people; withdrawal, inability to interact, and retarded language development.
bipolar disorder	Intermixed periods of mania and depression.
bulimia nervosa	An eating disorder of binge eating followed by vomiting and depression.
compulsion	Uncontrollable urge to perform an act repeatedly.

conversion disorder	A physical symptom, with no organic basis, that appears as a result of anxiety and conflict.
defense mechanism	Unconscious technique a person uses to resolve or conceal conflicts and anxiety.
delirium	Confusion in thinking; faulty perceptions and irrational behavior. Delirium tremens is associated with alcohol withdrawal.
delusion	Fixed, false belief that cannot be changed by logical reasoning or evidence.
dementia	Loss of intellectual abilities with impairment of memory, judgment, and reasoning as well as changes in personality.
depression	Major mood disorder with chronic sadness, loss of energy, hopelessness, worry, and discouragement.
dissociative disorder	Chronic or sudden disturbance of memory, identity, or consciousness; dissociative identity disorder, amnesia, and fugue.
ego	The central coordinating branch of the personality.
fugue	Amnesia with flight from customary surroundings.
gender identity disorder	Strong and persistent cross-gender identification with the opposite sex.
hallucination	False sensory perception.
id	The major unconscious part of the personality; energy from instinctual drives and desires.
labile	Unstable; undergoing rapid emotional change.
mania	Extreme excitement, hyperactivity, inflated self-esteem.
mood disorders	Prolonged emotion dominates a person's life; examples are bipolar and depressive disorders.
mutism	Nonreactive state; stupor.
obsessive-compulsive disorder	An anxiety disorder in which recurrent thoughts and repetitive acts dominate behavior.
paranoia	Delusions of persecution or grandeur or combinations of the two.
paraphilia	Recurrent intense sexual urge, fantasy, or behavior that involves unusual objects, activities, or situations.
personality disorders	Lifelong personality patterns marked by inflexibility and impairment of social functioning.

phobia	Irrational or disabling fear of an object or situation.
post-traumatic stress disorder	Anxiety-related symptoms appear following exposure to personal experience of a traumatic event.
psychosis	Impairment of mental capacity to recognize reality, communicate, and relate to others.
reality testing	Ability to perceive fact from fantasy; severely impaired in psychoses.
repression	Defense mechanism by which unacceptable thoughts, feelings, and impulses are pushed into the unconscious.
sexual disorders	Disorders of paraphilias and sexual dysfunctions.
schizophrenia	Withdrawal from reality into an inner world of disorganized thinking and conflict.
somatoform disorders	Having physical symptoms that cannot be explained by any actual physical disorder.
substance-related disorders	Regular use of psychoactive substances (alcohol, amphetamines, cannabis, cocaine, hallucinogens, opioids and sedatives) that affect the central nervous system.
superego	Internalized conscience and moral part of the personality.

Therapy

amphetamines	Central nervous system stimulants that may be used to treat depression.
behavior therapy	Conditioning (changing behavior patterns by training and repetition) is used to relieve anxiety and improve symptoms of illness.
electroconvulsive therapy	Electric current is used to produce convulsions in the treatment of depression.
family therapy	Treatment of an entire family to resolve and understand conflicts.
free association	A psychoanalytic technique in which the patient verbalizes, without censorship, the passing contents of his or her mind.
group therapy	A group of patients with similar problems gain insight into their personalities through discussion and interaction together.
hypnosis	Trance (state of altered consciousness) is used to increase the pace of psychotherapy.
lithium	Substance used to treat the manic stage of manic-depressive illness.

neuroleptic drug	Any drug that favorably modifies psychotic symptoms. Examples are phenothiazines.
phenothiazines	Tranquilizers used to treat psychoses.
play therapy	Treatment in which a child, through use of toys and playroom setting, expresses conflicts and feelings unable to be communicated in a direct manner.
psychoanalysis	A treatment that allows the patient to explore inner emotions and conflicts to understand and change current behavior.
psychodrama	Group therapy in which a patient expresses feelings by acting out roles with other patients.
sedatives	Drugs that lessen anxiety.
transference	Psychoanalytic process in which the patient relates to the therapist as he or she had to a prominent childhood figure.
tricyclic antidepressants	Drugs used to treat severe depression; three-ringed fused structure.

VI. Combining Forms, Suffixes, Prefixes, and Terminology

Write the meaning of the medical term in the space provided.

Combining Forms

Combining Form	Meaning	Terminology	Meaning
anxi/o	uneasy, anxious, distressed	anxiolytic _____ *This type of drug relieves anxiety.*	
aut/o	self	autism _____	
hallucin/o	hallucination, to wander in the mind	hallucinogen _____ *A hallucination is a sensory perception in the absence of any external stimuli, and an illusion is an error in perception in which sensory stimuli are present but incorrectly interpreted.*	
hypn/o	sleep	hypnosis _____ *The Greek god of sleep (Hypnos) put people to sleep by touching them with his magic wand or by fanning them with his dark wings.*	

iatr/o	treatment	psychiatrist _____	
ment/o	mind	mental _____	
neur/o	nerve	neurosis _____	

A term formerly used to describe mental disorders in which symptoms are distressing but reality testing is intact.

phil/o	attraction to, love	paraphilia _____	

para- means abnormal.

phren/o	mind	schizophrenia _____	

schiz/o means split.

psych/o	mind	psychosis _____	

Significant impairment of reality testing with symptoms such as delusions, hallucinations, and bizarre behavior.

psychotherapy _____

schiz/o	split	schizoid _____	

Used to describe a mild form of schizophrenia or a withdrawn, introverted personality.

somat/o	body	psychosomatic _____	

somatoform disorder _____

-form means resembling. Symptoms of these disorders resemble those of actual physical disease, but the origins are in the mind (psychogenic).

Suffixes

Suffix	Meaning	Terminology	Meaning
-genic	produced by	psychogenic _____	
-leptic	to seize hold of	neuroleptic drugs _____	
-mania	obsessive preoccupation	kleptomania _____	

klept/o means to steal.

pyromania _____

pyr/o means fire, heat.

Table 22–2. PHOBIAS

Phobia	Medical Term
Air	Aerophobia
Animals	Zoophobia
Bees	Apiphobia, melissophobia
Blood or bleeding	Hematophobia, hemophobia
Books	Bibliophobia
Cats	Ailurophobia
Corpses	Necrophobia
Crossing a bridge	Gephyrophobia
Darkness	Nyctophobia, scotophobia
Death	Thanatophobia
Dogs	Cynophobia
Drugs	Pharmacophobia
Eating	Phagophobia
Enclosed places	Claustrophobia
Hair	Trichophobia, trichopathophobia
Heights	Acrophobia
Insects	Entomophobia
Light	Photophobia
Marriage	Gamophobia
Men	Androphobia
Needles	Belonephobia
Sexual intercourse	Coitophobia, cypridophobia
Sleep	Hypnophobia
Snakes	Ophidiophobia
Spiders	Arachnophobia
Traveling	Hodophobia
Vomiting	Emetophobia
Women	Gynephobia
Worms	Helminthophobia
Writing	Graphophobia

-phobia	fear (irrational and often disabling)	agoraphobia _____

agora- means marketplace. Agoraphobics fear being left alone and feel anxious when away from familiar surroundings.

xenophobia _____

xen/o means stranger. Table 22-2 lists examples of other phobias.

-phoria	feeling, bearing	euphoria _____

dysphoria _____

-thymia	mind	cyclothymia _____

cycl/o means circle, recurring. Alternating periods of hypomania and depression.

dysthymia _____

Depressed mood that is not as severe as major depression.

Prefixes

Prefix	Meaning	Terminology	Meaning
a-, an-	no, not	apathy _____	
cata-	down	catatonic stupor _____	

ton/o means tension. A type of schizophrenia in which the patient has a decrease in activity and reactivity to the environment.

hypo-	deficient, less than, below	hypomania _____	
		hypochondriasis _____	

chondr/o means cartilage. The Greeks believed that the liver and spleen (under the cartilage of the ribs) were the seat of melancholy or sadness.

para-	abnormal	paranoia _____	

no- comes from the Greek word nous, *meaning mind.*

VII. ABBREVIATIONS

AD	Alzheimer's disease (dementia)	**MAO**	Monoamine oxidase
ADHD	Attention-deficit hyperactivity disorder	**M.A.**	Mental age (as determined by psychological tests)
C.A.	Chronological age	**MMPI**	Minnesota Multiphasic Personality Inventory
CNS	Central nervous system		
DSM	Diagnostic and Statistical Manual of Mental Disorders	**PCP**	Phencyclidine (hallucinogen)
		SAD	Seasonal affective disorder
DT	Delirium tremens	**TAT**	Thematic Apperception Test
ECT	Electroconvulsive therapy	**THC**	delta-9-tetrahydrocannabinol (active ingredient in marijuana)
I.Q.	Intelligence quotient. The average person is considered to have an I.Q. of between 90 and 110. Those who score below 70 are considered mentally retarded.		
		WAIS	Wechsler Adult Intelligence Scale
		WISC	Wechsler Intelligence Scale for Children
LSD	Lysergic acid diethylamide (hallucinogen)		

VIII. Practical Applications

This section contains an actual medical report using terms that you have studied in this and previous chapters.

Catatonic Schizophrenia: Case Report

A young, unmarried woman, aged 20, was admitted to a psychiatric hospital because she had become violent toward her parents, had been observed gazing into space with a rapt expression, and had been talking to invisible persons. She had been seen to strike odd poses. Her speech had become incoherent. The patient received voice messages telling her to do certain things. Then pictures began to appear on the wall, most of them ugly and sneering. These pictures had names—one was named shyness, another distress, another envy.

The patient was agitated and noisy and uncooperative in the hospital for several weeks after she arrived, and she required sedation. She was given several courses of electroconvulsive treatment, which failed to influence the schizophrenic process to any significant degree. Ten years later, when neuroleptic [antipsychotic] drugs became available, she received pharmacotherapy.

Despite therapeutic efforts, her condition throughout her many years of stay in a mental hospital has remained one of chronic catatonic stupor. She is mute and practically devoid of any spontaneity, but she responds to simple requests. She stays in the same position for many hours or sits in a chair in a curled-up position. Her facial expression is fixed and stony.

Major Depression: Case Report

Mrs. C, a 58-year-old widow, was brought to an emergency ward by her daughter, who found her at home in bed in the middle of the day. For a period of months, Mrs. C had become increasingly withdrawn and dysphoric, without any precipitating events. She had become progressively less active and even required encouragement to eat and perform her daily tasks. Her daughter and son-in-law became alarmed but did not know what to do. Mrs. C's medical history was unremarkable, but her psychiatric history revealed an episode of postpartum depression following the birth of one of her children.

On examination, the ER physician noted that Mrs. C was withdrawn and negativistic, refusing to cooperate with the examination, and even refusing to open her mouth. There were signs of acute dehydration and decline in personal hygiene and grooming.

Further questioning of Mrs. C's daughter revealed that Mrs. C had become increasingly paranoid and had delusions of sinfulness and guilt. Recently, she had shown signs of increasing mutism.

The physician recognized signs of major depression and arranged for immediate hospitalization. Mrs. C responded favorably to combined use of an antipsychotic and an antidepressant drug. An alternative treatment would have been a course of electroconvulsive therapy, which also produces favorable results.

Somatoform Disorder: Case Report

A 35-year-old man presented with a 6-year history of abdominal pain that he was convinced was cancer. For most of his life, the patient had been dominated by a tyrannical father who never gave him the love he craved. When the patient was 29, his father died of carcinoma of the colon, and soon after the patient developed abdominal pain. His complaints gradually increased as his identification with his father, as well as his unconscious hostility toward him, increased. The patient began to present to the clinic almost daily with complaints of bloody stools (the feces were found to be free of blood) and the belief that he had cancer. He felt that none of the clinic doctors listened to him, just as his father had not.

Treatment included a long-standing, trusting, positive relationship with one of the clinic physicians who allowed the patient time to talk about the illness. His hypochondriasis gradually subsided during a 12-month period of a supportive physician-patient relationship.

IX. Exercises

Remember to check your answers carefully with those given in Section X, Answers to Exercises.

A. *Give the terms for the following definitions.*

1. a physician specializing in treating mental illness: _____

2. a nonphysician trained in treatment of mental illness: _____

3. a therapist who practices psychoanalysis: _____

4. branch of psychiatry dealing with legal matters: _____ psychiatry

5. unconscious part of the personality: _____

6. conscious, coordinating part of the personality: _____

7. conscience or moral part of the personality: _____

8. the ability to perceive fact from fantasy: _____ testing

9. unconscious technique used to resolve or conceal conflicts and anxiety: _____ mechanism

10. branch of psychology dealing with patient care: _____ psychology

B. Match the following psychiatric symptoms with their meanings below.

delusion   conversion   autism
compulsion   mutism   mania
hallucination   amnesia   apathy
dissociation   anxiety   obsession

1. a nonreactive state; stupor _____

2. state of excessive excitability; agitation _____

3. loss of memory _____

4. uncontrollable urge to perform an act repeatedly _____

5. persistent idea, emotion, or urge _____

6. feelings of apprehension, uneasiness, dread _____

7. uncomfortable feelings are separated from their real object and redirected toward a second object or

behavior pattern _____

8. anxiety becomes a bodily symptom that has no organic basis _____

9. lack of responsiveness to others _____

10. absence of emotions _____

11. fixed false belief that cannot be changed by logical reasoning or evidence

_____

12. false or unreal sensory perception _____

C. Give the meanings for the following terms.

1. dysphoria _____

2. euphoria _____

3. amnesia _____

4. paranoia _____

5. psychosis _____

6. neurosis _____

7. phobia _____

8. agoraphobia _____

9. labile _____

10. affect _____

D. Select from the following terms to complete the sentences below.

anxiety disorders   dissociative disorders   substance-related disorders
mood disorders   eating disorder   delirium
sexual disorders   personality disorder   dementia
somatoform disorders

1. Mental symptoms (disturbances of memory and identity) that hide the anxiety of unconscious conflicts

   are _____ .

2. Troubled feelings, unpleasant tensions, distress, and avoidance behavior are hallmarks of

   _____ .

3. Illnesses related to regular use of drugs and alcohol are _____ .

4. Bulimia nervosa is an example of a (an) _____ .

5. Disorders involving paraphilias are _____ .

6. Illnesses marked by prolonged emotions (mania and depression) are _____ .

7. Mental disorders in which physical symptoms cannot be explained by an actual physical disorder are

   _____ .

8. A lifelong personality pattern that is inflexible and causes impairment of social functioning, distress,

   and conflict is a (an) _____ .

9. Loss of intellectual abilities with impairment of memory, judgment, and reasoning is known as a (an)

   _____ .

10. Confusion in thinking with faulty perceptions and irrational behavior is a (an)

    _____ .

E. Give the meanings for the following terms.

1. obsessive-compulsive disorder _____

2. post-traumatic stress disorder _____

3. bipolar disorder _____

4. fugue _____

5. paranoia _____

6. amphetamines _____

7. cannabis _____

8. schizophrenia _____

9. sexual sadism _____

10. hypochondriasis _____

F. *Match the general psychiatric disorder in column I with its example in column II. Write the letter of the answer in the space provided.*

Column I

1. somatoform disorder   _____

2. sexual disorder   _____

3. anxiety disorder   _____

4. mood disorder   _____

5. substance-related disorder   _____

6. schizophrenia   _____

7. dissociative disorder   _____

8. personality disorder   _____

Column II

A. conversion disorder
B. cocaine abuse
C. phobia
D. catatonia
E. pedophilia
F. fugue
G. bipolar disorder
H. narcissistic type

G. *Give the meanings for the following terms.*

1. anorexia nervosa _____

2. bulimia nervosa _____

3. repression _____

4. dementia _____

5. hypomania _____

6. hallucinogen _____

7. opioids _____

8. cocaine _____

H. *Identify the personality disorder from its description below.*

1. flamboyant, theatrical, emotionally immature _____

2. no loyalty or concern for others; does not tolerate frustration and blames others when he or she is at fault

_____

3. has fantasies of success and power and a grandiose sense of self-importance

_____

4. pervasive, unwarranted suspiciousness and mistrust of people

_____

5. emotionally cold, aloof, indifferent to praise or criticism or to the feelings of others

_____

I. *Identify the psychotherapeutic technique from its description below.*

1. patients express feelings by acting out roles with other patients _____

2. a trance is used to help the patient recover deeply repressed feelings _____

3. long-term and intense exploration of unconscious feelings using techniques such as transference and free

association _____

4. toys are used to help a child express conflicts and feelings _____

5. conditioning that changes actual behavior patterns rather than focusing on subconscious thoughts and

feelings _____

6. techniques that help patients overcome sexual dysfunctions _____

7. electric current is applied to the brain to produce convulsions and reverse major depression

_____

8. neuroleptic substances are used to relieve symptoms of psychiatric disorders

_____

J. Select from the following terms to complete the sentences below.

amphetamines   tricyclic antidepressants   kleptomania
MAO inhibitors   minor tranquilizers and   agoraphobia
phenothiazines   sedatives   dysthymia
cyclothymia   pyromania   xenophobia

1. Fear of strangers is _____.

2. Obsessive preoccupation with stealing is _____.

3. Antidepressant agents that work by blocking the action of a specific enzyme are

   _____.

4. A mood disorder marked by depressive periods that are milder than major depression is

   _____.

5. Antipsychotic tranquilizers such as Thorazine are _____.

6. Fear of being left alone in unfamiliar surroundings is _____.

7. Stimulants that are used as therapy for mood disorders or for treatment of children with attention-

   deficit hyperactivity disorder are _____.

8. A mild form of bipolar disorder in which hypomanic episodes alternate with depression is

   _____.

9. An obsessive preoccupation with fire is _____.

10. Drugs (such as Elavil or Tofranil) that are used to elevate mood and increase physical activity and mental

    alertness are called _____.

11. Anxiolytic agents used to reduce tension are _____.

K. Give the meanings for the following word parts.

1. aut/o _____

2. phren/o _____

3. hypn/o _____

4. somat/o _____

5. phil/o _____

6. iatr/o _____

7. schiz/o _____

8. -mania _____

9. -phobia _____

10. -thymia _____

11. -tropic _____

12. -genic _____

13. para- _____

14. hypo- _____

15. cata- _____

L. Circle the term that best completes the meaning of the sentence.

1. Robin fluctuated between bouts of depression and mania and was finally diagnosed as having a (xenophobic, histrionic, bipolar) disorder.

2. Although the root of Jon's problems could hardly be addressed simply with medication, his personality disorder as well as depression was treated with a new drug called (lithium, Prozac, Valium).

3. Hillary had an enormous fear of open-air markets, shopping malls, and stadiums. She was diagnosed as having (agoraphobia, xenophobia, pyromania).

4. When Sam was admitted to the hospital after his automobile accident his physicians were told of his alcoholism. They needed to know Sam's history so that they could prevent (dementia, dysthymia, delirium tremens).

5. Hanna was afraid of everyone she met. She had the (paranoid, narcissistic, schizoid) delusion that everyone was out to get her.

X. Answers to Exercises

A

1. psychiatrist	5. id	8. reality
2. psychologist	6. ego	9. defense
3. psychoanalyst	7. superego	10. clinical
4. forensic		

B

1. mutism	5. obsession	9. autism
2. mania	6. anxiety	10. apathy
3. amnesia	7. dissociation	11. delusion
4. compulsion	8. conversion	12. hallucination

C

1. sadness, hopelessness, despair
2. exaggerated feeling of well-being ("high")
3. loss of memory
4. delusions of grandeur or persecution
5. severe mental disorder in which the patient withdraws from reality into a world of disorganized thinking and feeling or

cannot function in basic ways owing to severe impairment of mood
6. emotional disorder, such as anxiety or fear, that disturbs a person's ability to function or impairs a person's physical health
7. an irrational fear of an object or a situation

8. fear of being alone or in open, public places from which escape may be difficult
9. unstable; undergoing rapid emotional change
10. a person's external emotional reactions

D

1. dissociative disorders
2. anxiety disorders
3. substance-related disorders
4. eating disorder

5. sexual disorders
6. mood disorders
7. somatoform disorders

8. personality disorder
9. dementia
10. delirium

E

1. recurrent thoughts and repetitive acts that dominate a person's behavior
2. anxiety-related symptoms appear following exposure to personal experience of a traumatic event
3. intermixed periods of mania and depression
4. amnesia with flight from customary surroundings

5. delusions of persecution or grandeur
6. CNS stimulants
7. marijuana
8. withdrawal from reality into an inner world of disorganized thinking and conflict

9. achievement of sexual gratification by inflicting physical or psychological pain
10. preoccupation with bodily aches, pains, and discomforts (in the absence of real illness)

F

1. A
2. E
3. C

4. G
5. B
6. D

7. F
8. H

G

1. eating disorder marked by excessive dieting because of emotional factors
2. eating disorder characterized by binge eating followed by vomiting and depression
3. a defense mechanism by which unacceptable thoughts, feelings, and impulses are pushed into the unconscious

4. loss of higher mental functioning, memory, judgment, and reasoning
5. mood disorder resembling mania (exaggerated excitement, hyperactivity) but of lesser intensity
6. drug that produces hallucinations (false sensory perceptions)

7. drugs that are derived from opium (morphine and heroin)
8. stimulant drug that causes euphoria and hallucinations

H

1. histrionic
2. antisocial
3. narcissistic

4. paranoid
5. schizoid

I

1. psychodrama
2. hypnosis
3. psychoanalysis

4. play therapy
5. behavioral therapy
6. sexual therapy

7. electroconvulsive therapy
8. drug therapy

J

1. xenophobia
2. kleptomania
3. MAO inhibitors
4. dysthymia

5. phenothiazines
6. agoraphobia
7. amphetamines
8. cyclothymia

9. pyromania
10. tricyclic antidepressants
11. minor tranquilizers and sedatives

K

1. self
2. mind
3. sleep
4. body
5. love, attraction to

6. treatment
7. split
8. obsessive preoccupation
9. fear
10. mind

11. to influence, turn
12. produced by
13. abnormal
14. deficient, less than, below
15. down

L

1. bipolar
2. Prozac
3. agoraphobia

4. delirium tremens
5. paranoid

XI. Pronunciation of Terms

To test your understanding of the terminology in this chapter, write the meaning of each term in the space provided. In addition, you may wish to cover the terms and write them by looking at your definitions. Make sure your spelling is correct. The page number after each term indicates where it is defined or used in the text so you can easily check your responses. (If you are not sure what the pronunciation symbols mean, refer to page 21.)

Term	Pronunciation	Meaning
affect (789)	ĂF-fĕkt	
agoraphobia (794)	ăg-ŏ-ră-FŌ-bē-ă	
amnesia (789)	ăm-NĒ-zē-ă	
amphetamines (791)	ăm-FĚT-ă-mēnz	
anorexia nervosa (789)	ăn-ō-RĔK-sē-ă nĕr-VŌ-să	
antisocial personality (783)	ăn-tē-SŌ-shăl pĕr-sŏ-NĂL-ĭ-tē	
anxiety disorders (789)	ăng-ZĪ-ĕ-tē dĭs-ŎR-derz	
anxiolytic (792)	ăng-zī-ō-LĬT-ik	
apathy (789)	ĂP-ă-thē	
autism (789)	ĂW-tĭzm	
behavior therapy (791)	bē-HĀV-yŏr THĔR-ă-pē	
bipolar disorder (789)	bī-PŌ-lăr dĭs-ŎR-dĕr	
bulimia nervosa (789)	bū-LĒ-mē-ă nĕr-VŌ-să	
cannabis (786)	KĂ-nă-bis	
catatonic stupor (795)	kăt-ă-TŎN-ĭk STŌŌ-pĕr	
claustrophobia (781)	klaws-trō-FŌ-bē-ă	
compulsion (789)	kŏm-PŬL-shŭn	
conversion disorder (790)	kŏn-VĔR-zhŭn dĭs-ŎR-dĕr	
cyclothymia (794)	sī-klō-THĪ-mē-ă	
defense mechanism (790)	dē-FĔNS mĕ-kăn-NĬ-zm	
delirium (790)	dĕ-LĬR-ē-ŭm	

delirium tremens (790)	dě-LĬR-ē-ŭm TRĔ-měnz	_____
delusion (790)	dě-LŪ-zhŭn	_____
dementia (790)	dē-MĔN-shē-ă	_____
depression (790)	dē-PRĔ-shŭn	_____
dissociative disorder (790)	dĭs-SŌ-shē-ă-tĭv dĭs-ŎR-der	_____
dysphoria (794)	dĭs-FŎR-ē-ă	_____
dysthymia (794)	dīs-THĪ-mē-ă	_____
ego (790)	Ē-gō	_____
electroconvulsive therapy (791)	ē-lěk-trō-kŏn-VŬL-sĭv THĔR-ă-pē	_____
euphoria (794)	ū-FŎR-ē-ă	_____
exhibitionism (784)	ěk-sĭ-BĬSH-ŭ-nĭzm	_____
family therapy (791)	FĂM-ĭ-lē THĔR-ă-pē	_____
fetishism (784)	FĔT-ĭsh-ĭzm	_____
free association (791)	frē ă-sō-shē-Ā-shŭn	_____
fugue (790)	fūg	_____
gender-identity disorder (790)	GĔN-děr ī-DĔN-tĭ-te dĭs-ŎR-děr	_____
group therapy (791)	grōōp THĔR-ă-pē	_____
hallucination (790)	hă-lū-sĭ-NĀ-shŭn	_____
hallucinogen (792)	hă-LŪ-sĭ-nō-jěn	_____
histrionic personality (783)	hĭs-trē-ŎN-ĭk pěr-sŏn-ĂL-ĭ-tē	_____
hypnosis (791)	hĭp-NŌ-sĭs	_____
hypochondriasis (795)	hī-pō-kŏn-DRĪ-ă-sĭs	_____
hypomania (795)	hī-pō-MĀ-nē-ă	_____
id (790)	ĭd	_____
kleptomania (793)	klěp-tō-MĀ-nē-ă	_____
labile (780)	LĀ-bĭl	_____

lithium (791)	LĬTH-ē-ŭm	_____
mania (790)	MĀ-nē-ă	_____
mental (793)	MĔN-tăl	_____
mood disorders (790)	MŌŌD dĭs-ŎR-dĕrz	_____
mutism (790)	MŪ-tĭzm	_____
narcissistic personality (783)	năr-sĭ-sĭs-tik pĕr-sĕ-NĂL-ĭ-tē	_____
neuroleptic drug (792)	nū-rō-LĔP-tik drŭg	_____
neurosis (793)	nū-RŌ-sĭs	_____
obsession (780)	ŏb-SĔSH-ŭn	_____
obsessive-compulsive disorder (790)	ŏb-SĔS-ĭv cŏm-PŬL-sĭv dĭs-ŎR-dĕr	_____
opioid (787)	Ō-pē-ŏyd	_____
paranoia (790)	păr-ă-NŎY-ă	_____
paranoid personality (783)	PĂR-ă-nŏyd pĕr-sĕ-NĂL-ĭ-tē	_____
paraphilia (790)	păr-ă-FĬL-ē-ă	_____
pedophilia (784)	pē-dō-FĬL-ē-ă	_____
personality disorders (790)	pĕr-sĕ-NĂL-ĭ-tē dĭs-ŎR-dĕrz	_____
phenothiazines (792)	fē-nō-THĪ-ă-zēnz	_____
phobia (791)	FŌ-bē-ă	_____
play therapy (792)	plā THĔR-ă-pē	_____
post-traumatic stress disorder (791)	pōst-trăw-MĂT-ĭk strĕs dĭs-ŎR-der	_____
psychiatrist (793)	sī-KĪ-ă-trĭst	_____
psychiatry (778)	sī-KĪ-ă-trē	_____
psychoanalysis (792)	sī-kō-ă-NĂL-ĭ-sĭs	_____
psychodrama (792)	sī-kō-DRĂ-mă	_____
psychogenic (793)	sī-kō-JĔN-ĭk	_____
psychologist (778)	sī-KŌL-ō-jĭst	_____

psychosis (791)   sī-KŌ-sĭs   _____

psychosomatic (793)   sī-kō-sō-MĂT-ĭk   _____

psychotherapy (793)   sī-kō-THĔR-ă-pē   _____

pyromania (793)   pī-rō-MĀ-nē-ă   _____

reality testing (791)   rē-ĂL-ĭ-tē TĔS-tĭng   _____

repression (791)   rē-PRĔ-shŭn   _____

schizoid personality (783)   SKĬZ-ŏyd or SKĬT-sŏyd   _____
                                   pĕr-sĕ-NĂL-ĭ-tē

schizophrenia (791)   skĭz-ō-FRĒ-nē-ă or   _____
                                   skĭt-sō-FRĒ-nē-ă

sedatives (792)   SĔD-ă-tĭvz   _____

sexual disorders (791)   SĔX-ū-ăl dĭs-ŎR-dĕrz   _____

sexual masochism (784)   SĔX-ū-ăl MĂS-ō-kĭzm   _____

sexual sadism (784)   SĔX-ŭ-ăl SĀ-dĭzm   _____

somatoform disorders (791)   sō-MĂT-ō-fŏrm dĭs-ŎR-dĕrz   _____

superego (791)   sū-pĕr-Ē-gō   _____

tolerance (785)   TŎL-ĕr-ănz   _____

transference (792)   trăns-FŬR-ĕns   _____

transvestic fetishism (784)   trăns-VĔS-tĭk FĔT-ĭsh-ĭzm   _____

tricyclic antidepressants   trī-SĬK-lĭk   _____
(792)   ăn-tĭ-dĕ-PRĔ-săntz

voyeurism (785)   VŎY-yĕr-ĭzm   _____

xenophobia (794)   zĕn-ō-FŌ-bē-ă   _____

Write the meaning of each word part in the space provided and test yourself. Check your answers with the information in the chapter or in the Glossary (Medical Terms—English) at the back of the book.

Combining Forms

Combining Form	Meaning	Combining Form	Meaning
anxi/o	_____	phil/o	_____
aut/o	_____	phren/o	_____
cycl/o	_____	psych/o	_____
hallucin/o	_____	pyr/o	_____
hypn/o	_____	schiz/o	_____
iatr/o	_____	somat/o	_____
klept/o	_____	ton/o	_____
ment/o	_____	xen/o	_____
neur/o	_____		

Suffixes

Suffix	Meaning	Suffix	Meaning
-form	_____	-pathy	_____
-genic	_____	-phobia	_____
-kinesia	_____	-phoria	_____
-leptic	_____	-somnia	_____
-mania	_____	-thymia	_____
-oid	_____	-tropic	_____

Prefixes

Prefix	Meaning	Prefix	Meaning
a-, an-	_____	dys-	_____
agora-	_____	hypo-	_____
cata-	_____	para-	_____

Glossary

Medical Terms—English

Combining Form, Suffix, or Prefix	Meaning
a-	no; not; without
ab-	away from
abdomin/o	abdomen
-ac	pertaining to
acanth/o	spiny; thorny
acetabul/o	acetabulum (hip socket)
acous/o	hearing
acr/o	extremities; top; extreme point
acromi/o	acromion
actin/o	light
acu/o	sharp; severe; sudden
ad-	toward
aden/o	gland
adenoid/o	adenoids
adip/o	fat
adren/o	adrenal glands
adrenal/o	adrenal glands
aer/o	air
af-	toward
agglutin/o	clumping; sticking together
-agon	to assemble, gather
agora-	marketplace
-agra	excessive pain
-al	pertaining to
alb/o	white
albin/o	white
albumin/o	albumin (protein)
alges/o	sensitivity to pain
-algesia	sensitivity to pain
-algia	pain
alveol/o	alveolus; air sac; small sac
ambly/o	dim; dull
-amine	nitrogen compound
amni/o	amnion
amyl/o	starch
an-	no; not; without
an/o	anus
ana-	up; apart; backward; excessive
andr/o	male
aneurysm/o	aneurysm

Combining Form, Suffix, or Prefix	Meaning
angi/o	vessel
anis/o	unequal
ankyl/o	crooked; bent; stiff
ante-	before; forward
anter/o	front
anthrac/o	coal
anti-	against
anxi/o	uneasy; anxious
aort/o	aorta
apheresis	removal
aphth/o	ulcer
apo-	off, away
aponeur/o	aponeurosis (type of tendon)
append/o	appendix
appendic/o	appendix
aque/o	water
-ar	pertaining to
-arche	beginning
arter/o	artery
arteri/o	artery
arteriol/o	arteriole
arthr/o	joint
-arthria	articulate (speak distinctly)
articul/o	joint
-ary	pertaining to
asbest/o	asbestos
-ase	enzyme
-asthenia	lack of strength
atel/o	incomplete
ather/o	plaque (fatty substance)
-ation	process
atri/o	atrium
audi/o	hearing
audit/o	hearing
aur/o	ear
auricul/o	ear
aut/o	self, own
auto-	self, own
axill/o	armpit
azot/o	urea; nitrogen

Combining Form, Suffix, or Prefix	Meaning
bacill/o	bacilli (bacteria)
bacteri/o	bacteria
balan/o	glans penis
bar/o	pressure; weight
bartholin/o	Bartholin's glands
bas/o	base; opposite of acid
bi-	two
bi/o	life
bil/i	bile; gall
bilirubin/o	bilirubin
-blast	embryonic; immature
blephar/o	eyelid
bol/o	cast; throw
brachi/o	arm
brachy-	short
brady-	slow
bronch/o	bronchial tube (bronchus)
bronchi/o	bronchial tube (bronchus)
bronchiol/o	bronchiole
bucc/o	cheek
bunion/o	bunion
burs/o	bursa (sac of fluid near joints)
byssin/o	cotton dust
cac/o	bad
calc/o	calcium
calci/o	calcium
calcane/o	calcaneus (heel bone)
cali/o	calyx
calic/o	calyx
capn/o	carbon dioxide
-capnia	carbon dioxide
carcin/o	cancerous
cardi/o	heart
carp/o	wrist bones
cata-	down
caud/o	tail; lower part of body
caus/o	burn; burning
cauter/o	heat; burn
cec/o	cecum
-cele	hernia
celi/o	belly; abdomen
-centesis	surgical puncture to remove fluid
cephal/o	head
cerebell/o	cerebellum
cerebr/o	brain; cerebrum
cerumin/o	cerumen
cervic/o	neck; cervix (neck of uterus)
-chalasia	relaxation

Combining Form, Suffix, or Prefix	Meaning
cheil/o	lip
chem/o	drug; chemical
-chezia	defecation; elimination of wastes
chir/o	hand
chol/e	bile; gall
cholangi/o	bile vessel
cholecyst/o	gallbladder
choledoch/o	common bile duct
cholesterol/o	cholesterol
chondr/o	cartilage
chore/o	dance
chori/o	chorion
chorion/o	chorion
choroid/o	choroid layer of eye
chrom/o	color
chron/o	time
chym/o	to pour
cib/o	meal
-cidal	pertaining to killing
cine/o	movement
cirrh/o	orange-yellow
cis/o	to cut
-clasis	to break
-clast	to break
claustr/o	enclosed space
clavicul/o	clavicle (collar bone)
-clysis	irrigation; washing
coagul/o	coagulation (clotting)
-coccus (-cocci, pl.)	berry-shaped bacterium
coccyg/o	coccyx (tailbone)
col/o	colon (large intestine)
coll/a	glue
colon/o	colon (large intestine)
colp/o	vagina
comat/o	deep sleep
con-	together, with
coni/o	dust
conjunctiv/o	conjunctiva
-constriction	narrowing
contra-	against; opposite
cor-	heart
cor/o	pupil
corne/o	cornea
coron/o	heart
corpor/o	body
cortic/o	cortex, outer region
cost/o	rib
crani/o	skull

Combining Form, Suffix, or Prefix	Meaning
cras/o	Mixture; temperament
crin/o	secrete
-crine	secrete; separate
-crit	to separate
cry/o	cold
crypt/o	hidden
culd/o	cul-de-sac
-cusis	hearing
cutane/o	skin
cyan/o	blue
cycl/o	ciliary body of eye; cycle, circle, recurring
-cyesis	pregnancy
cyst/o	urinary bladder; cyst; sac of fluid
cyt/o	cell
-cyte	cell
-cytosis	condition of cells; slight increase in numbers
dacry/o	tear; lacrimal duct; tear duct
dacryocyst/o	tear sac; lacrimal sac
dactyl/o	fingers; toes
de-	lack of; down; less; removal of
dem/o	people
dent/i	tooth
derm/o	skin
-derma	skin
dermat/o	skin
desicc/o	drying
-desis	to bind, tie together
dia-	complete; through
diaphor/o	sweat
-dilation	widening; stretching; expanding
dipl/o	double
dips/o	thirst
dist/o	far; distant
dors/o	back (of body)
dorsi-	back
-dote	what is given
-drome	to run
duct/o	to lead, carry
duoden/o	duodenum
dur/o	dura mater
-dynia	pain
dys-	bad; painful; difficult; abnormal
-eal	pertaining to
ec-	out; outside
echo-	reflected sound

Combining Form, Suffix, or Prefix	Meaning
-ectasia	stretching; dilation; expansion
-ectasis	stretching; dilation; expansion
ecto-	out; outside
-ectomy	removal; excision; resection
-edema	swelling
-elasma	flat plate
electr/o	electricity
em-	in
-ema	condition
-emesis	vomiting
-emia	blood condition
-emic	pertaining to blood condition
emmetr/o	in due measure
en-	in; within
encephal/o	brain
endo-	in; within
enter/o	intestines (usually small intestine)
eosin/o	red; rosy; dawn-colored
epi-	above; upon; on
epididym/o	epididymis
epiglott/o	epiglottis
episi/o	vulva
-er	one who
erg/o	work
erythem/o	flushed; redness
erythr/o	red
-esis	condition
eso-	inward
esophag/o	esophagus
-esthes/o	nervous sensation
esthesi/o	feeling (nervous sensation)
-esthesia	nervous sensation
estr/o	female
ethm/o	sieve
eti/o	cause
eu-	good; normal
-eurysm	widening
ex-	out; away from
exanthemat/o	rash
exo-	out; away from
extra-	outside
faci/o	face
fasci/o	fascia
femor/o	femur (thigh bone)
-ferent	to carry
fibr/o	fiber
fibros/o	fibrous connective tissue
fibul/o	fibula

Combining Form, Suffix, or Prefix	Meaning
-fication	process of making
-fida	split
flex/o	to bend
fluor/o	luminous
follicul/o	follicle; small sac
-form	resembling; in the shape of
fung/o	fungus; mushroom
furc/o	forking; branching
-fusion	to pour
galact/o	milk
ganglion/o	ganglion; collection of nerve cell bodies
gastr/o	stomach
gen/o	producing; produced by
-gen	producing; forming
-genesis	producing; forming
-genic	produced by or in
gester/o	pregnancy
gingiv/o	gum
glauc/o	gray
gli/o	glue; neuroglial tissue (supportive tissue of nervous system)
-globin	protein
-globulin	protein
glomerul/o	glomerulus
gloss/o	tongue
gluc/o	glucose; sugar
glyc/o	glucose; sugar
glycogen/o	glycogen; animal starch
glycos/o	glucose; sugar
gnos/o	knowledge
gon/o	seed
gonad/o	sex glands
goni/o	angle
-grade	to go
-gram	record
granul/o	granule(s)
-graph	instrument for recording
-graphy	process of recording
gravid/o	pregnancy
-gravida	pregnant woman
gynec/o	woman; female
hallucin/o	hallucination
hem/o	blood
hemat/o	blood
hemi-	half
hemoglobin/o	hemoglobin
hepat/o	liver
herni/o	hernia

Combining Form, Suffix, or Prefix	Meaning
-hexia	habit
hidr/o	sweat
hist/o	tissue
histi/o	tissue
home/o	sameness; unchanging; constant
hormon/o	hormone
humer/o	humerus (upper arm bone)
hydr/o	water
hyper-	above; excessive
hypn/o	sleep
hypo-	deficient; below; under
hypophys/o	pituitary gland
hyster/o	uterus; womb
-ia	condition
-iac	pertaining to
-iasis	abnormal condition
iatr/o	physician; treatment
-ic	pertaining to
-ical	pertaining to
ichthy/o	dry; scaly
idi/o	unknown; individual; distinct
ile/o	ileum
ili/o	ilium
immun/o	immune; protection; safe
in-	in; into; not
-in, -ine	a substance
-ine	pertaining to
infra-	below; inferior to; beneath
inguin/o	groin
inter-	between
intra-	within; into
iod/o	iodine
ion/o	ion; to wander
-ion	process
-ior	pertaining to
ipsi-	same
ir-	in
ir/o	iris (colored portion of eye)
irid/o	iris (colored portion of eye)
is/o	same; equal
isch/o	to hold back; back
ischi/o	ischium (part of hip bone)
-ism	process; condition
-ist	specialist
-itis	inflammation
-ium	structure; tissue
jejun/o	jejunum

Combining Form, Suffix, or Prefix	Meaning
kal/i	potassium
kary/o	nucleus
kerat/o	horny, hard; cornea
kern-	nucleus (collection of nerve cells in the brain)
ket/o	ketones; acetones
keton/o	ketones; acetones
kines/o	movement
kinesi/o	movement
-kinesia	movement
-kinesis	movement
klept/o	to steal
kyph/o	humpback
labi/o	lip
lacrim/o	tear; tear duct; lacrimal duct
lact/o	milk
lamin/o	lamina (part of vertebral arch)
lapar/o	abdominal wall; abdomen
-lapse	to slide, fall, sag
laryng/o	larynx (voice box)
later/o	side
leiomy/o	smooth (visceral) muscle
-lemma	sheath, covering
-lepsy	seizure
lept/o	thin, slender
-leptic	to seize, take hold of
leth/o	death
leuk/o	white
-lexia	word; phrase
lex/o	word; phrase
ligament/o	ligament
lingu/o	tongue
lip/o	fat; lipid
-listhesis	slipping
lith/o	stone; calculus
-lithiasis	condition of stones
-lithotomy	incision (for removal) of a stone
lob/o	lobe
log/o	study of
-logy	study of
lord/o	curve; swayback
-lucent	to shine
lumb/o	lower back; loin
lux/o	to slide
lymph/o	lymph
lymphaden/o	lymph gland
lymphangi/o	lymph vessel

Combining Form, Suffix, or Prefix	Meaning
-lysis	breakdown; separation; destruction; loosening
-lytic	to reduce, destroy
macro-	large
mal-	bad
-malacia	softening
malleol/o	malleolus
mamm/o	breast
mandibul/o	mandible (lower jaw bone)
-mania	obsessive preoccupation
mast/o	breast
mastoid/o	mastoid process
maxill/o	maxilla (upper jaw bone)
meat/o	meatus (opening)
medi/o	middle
mediastin/o	mediastinum
medull/o	medulla (inner section); middle; soft, marrow
mega-	large
-megaly	enlargement
melan/o	black
men/o	menses; menstruation
mening/o	membranes; meninges
meningi/o	membranes; meninges
ment/o	mind; chin
meso-	middle
meta-	change; beyond
metacarp/o	metacarpals (hand bones)
metatars/o	metatarsals (foot bones)
-meter	measure
metr/o	uterus; womb; measure
metri/o	uterus; womb
mi/o	smaller; less
micro-	small
-mimetic	mimic; copy
-mission	to send
mon/o	one; single
mono-	one; single
morph/o	shape; form
mort/o	death
muc/o	mucus
mucos/o	mucous membrane (mucosa)
multi-	many
mut/a	genetic change
mutagen/o	causing genetic change
my/o	muscle
myc/o	fungus
mydr/o	wide

Combining Form, Suffix, or Prefix	Meaning
myel/o	spinal cord; bone marrow
myocardi/o	myocardium (heart muscle)
myom/o	muscle tumor
myos/o	muscle
myring/o	tympanic membrane (eardrum)
myx/o	mucus
narc/o	numbness; stupor; sleep
nas/o	nose
nat/i	birth
natr/o	sodium
necr/o	death
nect/o	to bind, tie, connect
neo-	new
nephr/o	kidney
neur/o	nerve
neutr/o	neither; neutral
nid/o	nest
noct/i	night
norm/o	rule; order
nucle/o	nucleus
nulli-	none
nyct/o	night
obstetr/o	midwife
ocul/o	eye
odont/o	tooth
-oid	resembling
-ole	little; small
olecran/o	olecranon; elbow
olig/o	scanty
-oma	tumor; mass; fluid collection
om/o	shoulder
omphal/o	umbilical cord, navel
onc/o	tumor
-one	hormone
onych/o	nail
o/o	egg
oophor/o	ovary
-opaque	obscure
ophthalm/o	eye
-opia	vision
-opsia	vision
-opsy	view of
opt/o	eye; vision
optic/o	eye; vision
-or	one who
or/o	mouth
orch/o	testis
orchi/o	testis

Combining Form, Suffix, or Prefix	Meaning
orchid/o	testis
-orexia	appetite
orth/o	straight
-ose	full of, pertaining to, sugar
-osis	abnormal condition
-osmia	smell
ossicul/o	ossicle (small bone)
oste/o	bone
-ostosis	conditon of bone
ot/o	ear
-otia	ear condition
-ous	pertaining to
ov/o	egg
ovari/o	ovary
ovul/o	egg
ox/o	oxygen
-oxia	oxygen
oxy-	swift; sharp; acid
oxysm/o	sudden
pachy-	heavy; thick
palat/o	palate
palpebr/o	eyelid
pan-	all
pancreat/o	pancreas
papill/o	nipple-like; optic disk (disc)
par-	other than; abnormal
para-	near; beside; abnormal; apart from; along the side of
-para	to bear, bring forth (live births)
-parous	to bear, bring forth
parathyroid/o	parathyroid glands
-paresis	slight paralysis
-pareunia	sexual intercourse
-partum	birth; labor
patell/a	patella
patell/o	patella
path/o	disease
-pathy	disease; emotion
pector/o	chest
ped/o	child; foot
pelv/i	pelvic bone; hip
pelv/o	pelvic cavity; hip
pend/o	to hang
-penia	deficiency
-pepsia	digestion
per-	through
peri-	surrounding
perine/o	perineum
peritone/o	peritoneum
perone/o	fibula

Combining Form, Suffix, or Prefix	Meaning
-pexy	fixation; to put in place
phac/o	lens of eye
phag/o	eat; swallow
-phage	eat; swallow
-phagia	eating; swallowing
phak/o	lens of eye
phalang/o	phalanges (finger and toe)
pharmac/o	drug
pharmaceut/o	drug
pharyng/o	throat; pharynx
phas/o	speech
-phasia	speech
phe/o	dusky; dark
-pheresis	removal
phil/o	like; love; attraction to
-phil	attraction for
-philia	attraction for
phim/o	muzzle
phleb/o	vein
phob/o	fear
-phobia	fear
phon/o	voice; sound
-phonia	voice; sound
-phoresis	carrying; transmission
-phoria	to bear, carry; feeling (mental state)
-phor/o	to bear
phot/o	light
phren/o	diaphragm; mind
-phthisis	wasting away
-phylaxis	protection
phys/o	growing
physi/o	nature
-physis	to grow
phyt/o	plant
-phyte	plant
pil/o	hair
pineal/o	pineal gland
pituitar/o	pituitary gland
-plakia	plaque
plant/o	sole of the foot
plas/o	development; formation
-plasia	development; formation; growth
-plasm	formation
-plastic	pertaining to formation
-plasty	surgical repair
ple/o	more; many
-plegia	paralysis; palsy
-plegic	paralysis; palsy
pleur/o	pleura
plex/o	plexus; network (of nerves)

Combining Form, Suffix, or Prefix	Meaning
-pnea	breathing
pneum/o	lung; air
pneumon/o	lung; air
pod/o	foot
-poiesis	formation
-poietin	substance that forms
poikil/o	varied; irregular
pol/o	extreme
polio-	gray matter of brain or spinal cord
poly-	many; much
polyp/o	polyp; small growth
pont/o	pons (a part of the brain)
-porosis	lessening in density
post-	after; behind
poster/o	back (of body); behind
-prandial	meal
-praxia	action
pre-	before; in front of
presby/o	old age
primi-	first
pro-	before
proct/o	anus and rectum
pros-	before
prostat/o	prostate gland
prot/o	first
proxim/o	near
prurit/o	itching
pseudo-	false
psych/o	mind
-ptosis	droop; sag; prolapse; fall
-ptysis	spitting
pub/o	pubis (part of hip bone)
pulmon/o	lung
pupill/o	pupil
purul/o	pus-filled
py/o	pus
pyel/o	renal pelvis
pylor/o	pylorus; pyloric sphincter
pyr/o	fever; fire
pyret/o	fever
pyrex/o	fever
quadri-	four
rachi/o	spinal column; vertebrae
radi/o	x-rays; radioactivity; radius (lateral lower arm bone)
radicul/o	nerve root
re-	back; again; backward

Combining Form, Suffix, or Prefix	Meaning
rect/o	rectum
ren/o	kidney
reticul/o	network
retin/o	retina
retro-	behind; back; backward
rhabdomy/o	striated (skeletal) muscle
rheumat/o	watery flow
rhin/o	nose
roentgen/o	x-rays
-rrhage	bursting forth of blood
-rrhagia	bursting forth of blood
-rrhaphy	suture
-rrhea	flow; discharge
-rrhexis	rupture
rrhythm/o	rhythm
sacr/o	sacrum
salping/o	uterine (fallopian) tube; oviduct; auditory (eustachian) tube
-salpinx	uterine (fallopian) tube; oviduct
sarc/o	flesh (connective tissue)
scapul/o	scapula; shoulder blade
-schisis	to split
schiz/o	split
scintill/o	spark
scirrh/o	hard
scler/o	sclera (white of eye)
-sclerosis	hardening
scoli/o	crooked; bent
-scope	instrument for visual examination
-scopy	visual examination
scot/o	darkness
seb/o	sebum
sebace/o	sebum
sect/o	to cut
semi-	half
semin/i	semen; seed
seps/o	infection
sial/o	saliva
sialaden/o	salivary gland
sider/o	iron
sigmoid/o	sigmoid colon
silic/o	glass
sinus/o	sinus
-sis	state of; condition
-sol	solution
somat/o	body
-somes	bodies
somn/o	sleep
-somnia	sleep
son/o	sound

Combining Form, Suffix, or Prefix	Meaning
-spadia	to tear, cut
-spasm	sudden contraction of muscles
sperm/o	spermatozoa; sperm cells
spermat/o	spermatozoa; sperm cells
sphen/o	wedge; sphenoid bone
spher/o	globe-shaped; round
sphygm/o	pulse
-sphyxia	pulse
spin/o	spine (backbone); spinal cord
spir/o	to breathe
splen/o	spleen
spondyl/o	vertebrae (back bone)
squam/o	scale
-stalsis	contraction
staped/o	stapes (middle ear bone)
staphyl/o	clusters; uvula
-stasis	stop; control; place
-static	pertaining to stopping; controlling
steat/o	fat, lipid, sebum
-stenosis	tightening; stricture
ster/o	solid structure; steroid
stere/o	solid; three-dimensional
stern/o	sternum (breastbone)
steth/o	chest
-sthenia	strength
-stitial	to set; pertaining to standing or positioned
stomat/o	mouth
-stomy	new opening (to form a mouth)
strept/o	twisted chains
styl/o	pole or stake
sub-	under; below
submaxill/o	mandible (lower jaw bone)
-suppression	to stop
supra-	above, upper
sym-	together; with
syn-	together; with
syncop/o	to cut off, cut short
syndesm/o	ligament
synov/o	synovia; synovial membrane; sheath around a tendon
syring/o	tube
tachy-	fast
tars/o	tarsus (ankle bone)
tax/o	order; coordination
tel/o	complete
tele/o	distant
ten/o	tendon
tendin/o	tendon
terat/o	monster; malformed fetus

Combining Form, Suffix, or Prefix	**Meaning**
test/o	testis; testicle
tetra-	four
thalam/o	thalamus
thalass/o	sea
the/o	put; place
thec/o	sheath
thel/o	nipple
therapeut/o	treatment
-therapy	treatment
therm/o	heat
thorac/o	chest
-thorax	pleural cavity; chest
thromb/o	clot
thym/o	thymus gland
-thymia	mind
-thymic	pertaining to mind
thyr/o	thyroid gland; shield
thyroid/o	thyroid gland
tibi/o	tibia (shin bone)
-tic	pertaining to
-tion	process
toc/o	labor; birth
-tocia	labor; birth
-tocin	labor; birth
tom/o	to cut
-tome	instrument to cut
-tomy	process of cutting
ton/o	tension
tone/o	to stretch
tonsill/o	tonsil
top/o	place; position; location
tox/o	poison
toxic/o	poison
trache/o	trachea (windpipe)
trans-	across
-tresia	opening
tri-	three
trich/o	hair
trigon/o	trigone
-tripsy	to crush
troph/o	nourishment; development
-trophy	nourishment; development
-tropia	to turn
-tropic	turning
-tropin	stimulate; act on
tympan/o	tympanic membrane (eardrum); middle ear
-type	classification; picture
-ule	little; small
uln/o	ulna (medial lower arm bone)

Combining Form, Suffix, or Prefix	**Meaning**
ultra-	beyond; excess
-um	structure; tissue; thing
umbilic/o	navel; umbilical cord
ungu/o	nail
uni-	one
ur/o	urine; urinary tract
ureter/o	ureter
urethr/o	urethra
-uria	urination; condition of urine
urin/o	urine
-us	thing
uter/o	uterus; womb
uve/o	uvea, vascular layer of eye (iris, choroid, ciliary body)
uvul/o	uvula
vag/o	vagus nerve
vagin/o	vagina
valv/o	valve
valvul/o	valve
varic/o	varicose veins
vas/o	vessel; duct; vas deferens
vascul/o	blood vessel
ven/o	vein
venere/o	sexual intercourse
ventr/o	belly side of body
ventricul/o	ventricle (of brain or heart)
venul/o	venule; small vein
-verse	to turn
-version	to turn
vertebr/o	vertebra (back bone)
vesic/o	urinary bladder
vesicul/o	seminal vesicle
viscer/o	internal organs
vit/o	life
vitr/o	glass
viv/o	life
vol/o	to roll
vulv/o	vulva
xanth/o	yellow
xen/o	stranger
xer/o	dry
xiph/o	sword
-y	condition; process
zo/o	animal life

English—Medical Terms

Meaning	Combining Form, Prefix, or Suffix	Meaning	Combining Form, Prefix, or Suffix
abdomen	abdomin/o	arm bone, lower, lateral	radi/o
	celi/o	arm bone, lower, medial	uln/o
	lapar/o	arm bone, upper	humer/o
abdominal wall	lapar/o	armpit	axill/o
abnormal	dys-	arteriole	arteriol/o
	par-	artery	arter/o
	para-		arteri/o
abnormal condition	-iasis	articulate (speak distinctly)	-arthria
	-osis	asbestos	asbest/o
above	epi-	assemble	-agon
	hyper-	atrium	atri/o
	supra-	attraction for	-phil
acetabulum	acetabul/o		-philia
acetones	ket/o	attraction to	phil/o
	keton/o	auditory tube	salping/o
acid	oxy-	away from	ab-
acromion	acromi/o		apo-
across	trans-		ex-
action	-praxia		exo-
act on	-tropin		
adrenal glands	adren/o	back	re-
	adrenal/o		retro-
after	post-	back, lower	lumb/o
again	re-	back portion of body	dorsi-
against	anti-		dors/o
	contra-		poster/o
air	aer/o	backbone	spin/o
	pneum/o		spondyl/o
	pneumon/o		vertebr/o
air sac	alveol/o	backward	ana-
albumin	albumin/o		retro-
all	pan-	bacteria	bacteri/o
along the side of	para-	bacterium (berry-shaped)	-coccus
alveolus	alveol/o	bacilli (rod-shaped bacteria)	bacill/o
amnion	amni/o		
aneurysm	aneurysm/o	bad	cac/o
angle	goni/o		dys-
animal life	zo/o		mal-
animal starch	glycogen/o	barrier	claustr/o
ankle bone	tars/o	base (not acidic)	bas/o
anus	an/o	bear (to)	-para
anus and rectum	proct/o		-parous
anxiety	anxi/o		-phoria
apart	ana-		phor/o
apart from	para-	before	ante-
appendix	append/o		pre-
	appendic/o		pro-
appetite	-orexia		pros-
arm	brachi/o	beginning	-arche

Meaning	Combining Form, Prefix, or Suffix	Meaning	Combining Form, Prefix, or Suffix
behind	post-	breathe	spir/o
	poster/o	breathing	-pnea
	retro-	bring forth	-para
belly	celi/o		-parous
belly side of body	ventr/o	bronchial tube (bronchus)	bronch/o
below, beneath	hypo-		bronchi/o
	infra-	bronchiole	bronchiol/o
	sub-	bunion	bunion/o
bend (to)	flex/o	burn	caus/o
bent	ankyl/o		cauter/o
	scoli/o	bursa	burs/o
beside	para-	bursting forth of blood	-rrhage
between	inter-		-rrhagia
beyond	hyper-		
	meta-		
	ultra-	calcaneus	calcane/o
bile	bil/i	calcium	calc/o
	chol/e		calci/o
bile vessel	cholangi/o	calculus	lith/o
bilirubin	bilirubin/o	calyx	cali/o
bind	-desis		calic/o
	nect/o	cancerous	carcin/o
birth	nat/i	carbon dioxide	capn/o
	-partum		-capnia
	toc/o	carry	duct/o
	-tocia		-ferent
	-tocin		-phoria
births (live)	-para	carrying	-phoresis
black	melan/o	cartilage	chondr/o
blood	hem/o	cast; throw	bol/o
	hemat/o	cause	eti/o
blood condition	-emia	cecum	cec/o
	-emic	cell	cyt/o
blood vessel	vascul/o		-cyte
blue	cyan/o	cells, condition of	-cytosis
bodies	-somes	cerebellum	cerebell/o
body	corpor/o	cerebrum	cerebr/o
	somat/o	cerumen	cerumin/o
bone	oste/o	cervix	cervic/o
bone condition	-ostosis	change	meta-
bone marrow	myel/o	cheek	bucc/o
brain	encephal/o	chemical	chem/o
	cerebr/o	chest	pector/o
branching	furc/o		steth/o
break	-clasis		thorac/o
	-clast		-thorax
	-lysis	child	ped/o
breakdown		chin	ment/o
breast	mamm/o	cholesterol	cholesterol/o
	mast/o	chorion	chori/o
breastbone	stern/o		chorion/o

Meaning	Combining Form, Prefix, or Suffix	Meaning	Combining Form, Prefix, or Suffix
choroid layer	choroid/o	dance	chore/o
ciliary body	cycl/o	dark	phe/o
circle	cycl/o	darkness	scot/o
clavicle	clavicul/o	dawn-colored	eosin/o
clot	thromb/o	death	leth/o
clumping	agglutin/o		mort/o
clusters	staphyl/o		necr/o
coagulation	coagul/o	defecation	-chezia
coal dust	anthrac/o	deficiency	-penia
coccyx	coccyg/o	deficient	hypo-
cold	cry/o	destroy	-lytic
collar bone	clavicul/o	destruction	-lysis
colon	col/o	development	plas/o
	colon/o		-plasia
color	chrom/o		troph/o
common bile duct	choledoch/o		-trophy
complete	dia-	diaphragm	phren/o
	tel/o	difficult	dys-
condition	-ema	digestion	-pepsia
	-esis	dilation	-ectasia
	-ia		-ectasis
	-ism	dim	ambly/o
	-sis	discharge	-rrhea
	-y	disease	path/o
condition,	-iasis		-pathy
abnormal	-osis	distant	dist/o
connect	nect/o		tele/o
connective tissue	sarc/o	distinct	idi/o
constant	home/o	double	dipl/o
controlling	-stasis	down	cata-
contraction	-stalsis		de-
contraction of muscles,	-spasm	droop	-ptosis
sudden		drug	chem/o
coordination	tax/o		pharmac/o
copy	-mimetic		pharmaceut/o
cornea	corne/o	dry	ichthy/o
	kerat/o		xer/o
cortex	cortic/o	drying	desicc/o
cotton dust	byssin/o	duct	vas/o
crooked	ankyl/o	dull	ambly/o
	scoli/o	duodenum	duoden/o
crush (to)	-tripsy	dura mater	dur/o
curve	lord/o	dusky	phe/o
cut	cis/o	dust	coni/o
	sect/o		
	tom/o		
cut off	syncop/o	ear	aur/i
cutting, process of	-tomy		aur/o
cycle	cycl/o		auricul/o

Meaning	Combining Form, Prefix, or Suffix	Meaning	Combining Form, Prefix, or Suffix
ear (condition of)	-otia	feeling	esthesi/o
eardrum	myring/o		-phoria
	tympan/o	female	estr/o
eat	phag/o		gynec/o
	-phage	femur	femor/o
eating	-phagia	fever	pyr/o
egg cell	o/o		pyret/o
	ov/o		pyrex/o
	ovul/o	fiber	fibr/o
elbow	olecran/o	fibrous connective tissue	fibros/o
electricity	electr/o	fibula	fibul/o
elimination of wastes	-chezia		perone/o
embryonic	-blast	finger and toe bones	phalang/o
enlargement	-megaly	fingers	dactyl/o
enzyme	-ase	fire	pyr/o
epididymis	epididym/o	first	prot/o
epiglottis	epiglott/o	fixation	-pexy
equal	is/o	flat plate	-elasma
esophagus	esophag/o	flesh	sarc/o
eustachian tube	salping/o	flow	-rrhea
excess	ultra-	fluid collection	-oma
excessive	ana-	flushed	erythem/o
	hyper-	foot	pod/o
excision	-ectomy	foot bones	metatars/o
expansion	-ectasia	forking	furc/o
	-ectasis	form	morph/o
extreme	pol/o	formation	plas/o
extreme point	acr/o		-plasia
extremities	acr/o		-plasm
eye	ocul/o		-poiesis
	ophthalm/o	forming	-genesis
	opt/o	forward	ante-
	optic/o	four	quadri-
eyelid	blephar/o	front	anter/o
	palpebr/o	full of	-ose
		fungus	fung/o
			myc/o
face	faci/o		
fall	-ptosis		
fallopian tube	salping/o	gall	bil/i
	-salpinx		chol/e
false	pseudo-	gallbladder	cholecyst/o
far	dist/o	ganglion	gangli/o
fascia	fasci/o		ganglion/o
fast	tachy-	gather	-agon
fat	adip/o	genetic change	mut/a
	lip/o		mutagen/o
	steat/o	given (what is)	-dote
fear	phob/o	gland	aden/o
	-phobia	glans penis	balan/o

Meaning	Combining Form, Prefix, or Suffix	Meaning	Combining Form, Prefix, or Suffix
glass	silic/o	hip	pelv/i
	vitr/o		pelv/o
globe-shaped	spher/o	hold back	isch/o
glomerulus	glomerul/o	hormone	hormon/o
glucose	gluc/o		-one
	glyc/o	horny	kerat/o
	glycos/o	humerus	humer/o
glue	coll/a	humpback	kyph/o
	gli/o		
glycogen	glycogen/o		
go	-grade	ileum	ile/o
good	eu-	ilium	ili/o
granule(s)	granul/o	immature	-blast
gray	glauc/o	immune	immun/o
gray matter	poli/o	in, into	em-
groin	inguin/o		en-
grow	-physis		endo-
growing	phys/o		in-, intra-
growth	-plasia		ir-
gum	gingiv/o	in due measure	emmetr/o
		in front of	pre-
		incomplete	atel/o
habit	-hexia	increase in numbers (blood cells)	-cytosis
hair	pil/o		
	trich/o	individual	idi/o
half	hemi-	infection	seps/o
	semi-	inferior to	infra-
hallucination	hallucin/o	inflammation	-itis
hand	chir/o	instrument for recording	-graph
hand bones	metacarp/o	instrument for visual examination	-scope
hang (to)	pend/o		
hard	kerat/o	instrument to cut	-tome
	scirrh/o	internal organs	viscer/o
hardening	-sclerosis	intestine, large	col/o
head	cephal/o	intestine, small	enter/o
hearing	acous/o	iodine	iod/o
	audi/o	ion	ion/o
	audit/o	iris	ir/o
	-cusis		irid/o
heart	cardi/o	iron	sider/o
	cor-	irregular	poikil/o
	coron/o	irrigation	-clysis
heart muscle	myocardi/o	ischium	ischi/o
heat	cauter/o	itching	prurit/o
	therm/o		
heavy	pachy-		
heel bone	calcane/o	jaw, lower	mandibul/o
hemoglobin	hemoglobin/o		submaxill/o
hernia	-cele	jaw, upper	maxill/o
	herni/o	joint	arthr/o
hidden	crypt/o		articul/o

Meaning	Combining Form, Prefix, or Suffix	Meaning	Combining Form, Prefix, or Suffix
ketones	ket/o	make (to)	-fication
	keton/o	male	andr/o
kidney	nephr/o	malformed fetus	terat/o
	ren/o	malleolus	malleol/o
killing	-cidal	mandible	mandibul/o
knowledge	gnos/o		submaxill/o
		many	multiple/o
			ple/o
labor	-partum		poly-
	toc/o	marketplace	agora-
	-tocia	marrow	medull/o
	-tocin	mass	-oma
lack of	de-	mastoid process	mastoid/o
lack of strength	-asthenia	maxilla	maxill/o
lacrimal duct	dacry/o	meal	cib/o
	lacrim/o		-prandial
lacrimal sac	dacryocyst/o	measure	-meter
lamina	lamin/o		metr/o
large	macro-	meatus	meat/o
	mega-	mediastinum	mediastin/o
larynx	laryng/o	medulla	medull/o
lead	duct/o	membranes	mening/o
lens of eye	phac/o		meningi/o
	phak/o	meninges	mening/o
less	de-		meningi/o
	mi/o	menses	men/o
life	bi/o	menstruation	men/o
	vit/o	metacarpals	metacarp/o
	viv/o	metatarsals	metatars/o
ligament	ligament/o	middle	medi/o
	syndesm/o		medull/o
like	phil/o		meso-
lip	cheil/o	middle ear	tympan/o
	labi/o	midwife	obstetr/o
lipid	lip/o	milk	galact/o
	steat/o		lact/o
little	-ole	mimic	-mimetic
	-ule	mind	ment/o
liver	hepat/o		phren/o
lobe	lob/o		psych/o
location	top/o		-thymia
loin	lumb/o		-thymic
loosening	-lysis		
love	phil/o	mixture	cras/o
luminous	fluor/o	monster	terat/o
lung	pneum/o	more	ple/o
	pneumon/o	mouth	or/o
	pulmon/o		stomat/o
lymph	lymph/o	movement	cine/o
lymph gland	lymphaden/o		kines/o
lymph vessel	lymphangi/o		kinesi/o

Meaning	Combining Form, Prefix, or Suffix	Meaning	Combining Form, Prefix, or Suffix
	-kinesia	nucleus (collection of nerve cells in the brain)	kern-
	-kinesis		
much	poly-	numbness	narc/o
mucous membrane	mucos/o		
mucus	muc/o		
	myx/o	obscure	-opaque
muscle	my/o	obsessive preoccupation	-mania
	myos/o	off	apo-
muscle, heart	myocardi/o	old age	presby/o
muscle, smooth (visceral)	leiomy/o	olecranon	olecran/o
muscle, striated (skeletal)	rhabdomy/o	on	epi-
muscle tumor	myom/o	one	mon/o
muzzle	phim/o		mono-
myocardium	myocardi/o		uni-
		one's own	aut/o
			auto-
nail	onych/o	one who	-er
	ungu/o		-or
narrowing	-constriction	opening	-tresia
	-stenosis	opening (new)	-stomy
nature	physi/o	opposite	contra-
navel	omphal/o	optic disk (disc)	papill/o
	umbilic/o	orange-yellow	cirrh/o
near	para-	order	norm/o
	proxim/o		tax/o
neck	cervic/o	organs, internal	viscer/o
neither	neutr/o	ossicle	ossicul/o
nerve	neur/o	other than	par-
nerve root	radicul/o	out	ec-
nest	nid/o		ex-
network	reticul/o		exo-
network of nerves	plex/o	outer region	cortic/o
neutral	neutr/o	outside	ec-
night	noct/i		extra-
	nyct/o	ovary	oophor/o
nipple-like	papill/o	oviduct	salping/o
nitrogen	azot/o		-salpinx
nitrogen compound	-amine	own	idi/o
no	a-	oxygen	ox/o
	an-		-oxia
none	nulli-		
normal	eu-		
nose	nas/o	pain	-algia
	rhin/o		-dynia
not	a-	pain, excessive	-agra
	an-	pain, sensitivity to	-algesia
	in-		algesi/o
nourishment	troph/o	painful	dys-
	-trophy	palate	palat/o
nucleus	kary/o	palsy	-plegia
	nucle/o		-plegic

Meaning	Combining Form, Prefix, or Suffix	Meaning	Combining Form, Prefix, or Suffix
pancreas	pancreat/o		gravid/o
paralysis	-plegia		-gravida
	-plegic	pressure	bar/o
		process	-ation
paralysis, slight	-paresis		-ion
patella	patell/a		-ism
	patell/o		-tion
pelvic bone	pelv/i		-y
pelvic cavity	pelv/o	produced by or in	-genic
pelvis, renal	pyel/o	producing	gen/o
people	dem/o		-gen
perineum	perine/o		-genesis
peritoneum	peritone/o		-ptosis
pertaining to	-ac	prolapse	prostat/o
	-al	prostate gland	immun/o
	-ar	protection	-phylaxis
	-ary		-globin
	-eal	protein	-globulin
	-iac		pub/o
	-ic	pubis	sphygm/o
	-ical	pulse	-sphyxia
	-ine		-centesis
	-ior	puncture to remove fluid	cor/o
	-ose	pupil	core/o
	-ous		pupill/o
	-tic		py/o
phrase	-lexia	pus	purul/o
physician	iatr/o	pus-filled	the/o
pineal gland	pineal/o	put	-pexy
pituitary gland	hypophys/o	put in place	pylor/o
	pituit/o	pyloric sphincter	pylor/o
	pituitar/o	pylorus	
place	the/o		
	top/o	radioactivity	radi/o
plant	phyt/o	radius	radi/o
	-phyte	rapid	oxy-
plaque	ather/o	rash	exanthemat/o
	plakia	rays	radi/o
pleura	pleur/o	record	-gram
pleural cavity	-thorax	recording, process of	-graphy
plexus	plex/o	rectum	rect/o
poison	tox/o	recurring	cycl/o
	toxic/o	red	eosin/o
pole	styl/o		erythr/o
polyp	polyp/o	redness	erythem/o
pons	pont/o		erythemat/o
position	top/o	reduce	-lytic
potassium	kal/i	relaxation	-chalasia
pour	chym/o	removal	-apheresis
	-fusion		-ectomy
pregnancy	-cyesis		-pheresis
	gester/o		

Meaning	Combining Form, Prefix, or Suffix	Meaning	Combining Form, Prefix, or Suffix
renal pelvis	pyel/o		morph/o
resembling	-form	sharp	acu/o
	-oid		oxy-
retina	retin/o	sheath	thec/o
rib	cost/o	shield	thyr/o
roll (to)	vol/o	shin bone	tibi/o
rosy	eosin/o	shine	-lucent
round	spher/o	short	brachy-
rule	norm/o	shoulder	om/o
run	-drome	side	later/o
rupture	-rrhexis	sieve	ethm/o
		sigmoid colon	sigmoid/o
		single	mon/o
sac, small	alveol/o		mono-
	follicul/o	sinus	sinus/o
sac of fluid	cyst/o	skin	cutane/o
sacrum	sacr/o		derm/o
safe	immun/o		-derma
sag	-ptosis		dermat/o
saliva	sial/o	skull	crani/o
salivary gland	sialaden/o	sleep	hypn/o
same	ipsi-		somn/o
	is/o		-somnia
sameness	home/o	sleep (deep)	comat/o
scaly	ichthy/o	slender	lept/o
scanty	olig/o	slide (to)	-lapse
sclera	scler/o		lux/o
sea	thalass/o	slipping	-listhesis
sebum	seb/o	slow	brady-
	sebace/o	small	micro-
	steat/o		-ole
secrete	crin/o		-ule
	-crine	small intestine	enter/o
seed	gon/o	smaller	mi/o
	semin/i	smell	-osmia
seizure	-lepsy	sodium	natr/o
seize (to); take hold of	-leptic	soft	medull/o
self	aut/o	softening	-malacia
	auto-	sole (of the foot)	plant/o
semen	semin/i	solution	-sol
seminal vesicle	vesicul/o	sound	echo-
send (to)	-mission		phon/o
sensation (nervous)	-esthesia		-phonia
separate	-crine		son/o
separation	-lysis	spark	scintill/o
set (to)	-stitial	specialist	-ist
severe	acu/o	speech	phas/o
sex glands	gonad/o		-phasia
sexual intercourse	-pareunia	sperm cells (spermatozoa)	sperm/o
	venere/o		spermat/o
shape	-form	spinal column	rachi/o

Meaning	Combining Form, Prefix, or Suffix	Meaning	Combining Form, Prefix, or Suffix
spinal cord	myel/o	swayback	lord/o
	spin/o	sweat	diaphor/o
spine	spin/o		hidr/o
spiny	acanth/o	swift	oxy-
spitting	-ptysis	sword	xiph/o
spleen	splen/o	synovia	synov/o
split	-fida	synovial membrane	synov/o
	schiz/o		
split (to)	-schisis		
stake (pole)	styl/o	tail	caud/o
stapes	staped/o	tailbone	coccyg/o
starch	amyl/o	tear	dacry/o
state of	-sis		lacrim/o
steal	klept/o	tear (to cut)	-spadia
sternum	stern/o	tear duct	dacry/o
steroid	ster/o		lacrim/o
sticking together	agglutin/o	tear sac	dacryocyst/o
stiff	ankyl/o	temperament	cras/o
stimulate	-tropin	tendon	ten/o
stomach	gastr/o		tend/o
stone	lith/o		tendin/o
stop	-suppression	tension	ton/o
stopping	-stasis	testis	orch/o
	-static		orchi/o
straight	orth/o		orchid/o
stranger	xen/o		test/o
strength	-sthenia		
stretch	tone/o	thick	pachy-
stretching	-ectasia	thigh bone	femor/o
	-ectasis	thin	lept/o
stricture	-stenosis	thing	-um
structure	-ium		-us
	-um	thirst	dips/o
structure, solid	ster/o	thorny	acanth/o
study of	log/o	three	tri-
	-logy	throat	pharyng/o
stupor	narc/o	through	dia-
substance	-in	throw (to)	bol/o
	-ine	thymus gland	thym/o
substance that forms	-poietin	thyroid gland	thyr/o
sudden	acu/o		thyroid/o
	oxysm/o	tibia	tibi/o
sugar	gluc/o	tie	nect/o
	glyc/o	tie together	-desis
	glycos/o	tightening	-stenosis
	-ose	time	chron/o
surgical repair	-plasty	tissue	hist/o
surrounding	peri-		histi/o
suture	-rrhaphy		-ium
swallow	phag/o		-um
swallowing	-phagia	toes	dactyl/o

Meaning	Combining Form, Prefix, or Suffix	Meaning	Combining Form, Prefix, or Suffix
together	con-	uterine tube	salping/o
	sym-		-salpinx
	syn-	uterus	hyster/o
tongue	gloss/o		metr/o
	lingu/o		metri/o
tonsil	tonsill/o		uter/o
tooth	dent/i	uvea	uve/o
	odont/o	uvula	uvul/o
top	acr/o		staphyl/o
toward	ad-		
	af-		
trachea	trache/o	vagina	colp/o
transmission	-phoresis		vagin/o
treatment	iatr/o	vagus nerve	vag/o
	therapeut/o	valve	valv/o
	-therapy		valvul/o
trigone	trigon/o	varicose veins	varic/o
tube	syring/o	varied	poikil/o
tumor	-oma	vein	phleb/o
	onc/o		ven/o
turn	-tropia	vein, small	venul/o
	-verse	ventricle	ventricul/o
	-version	vertebra	rachi/o
turning	-tropic		spondyl/o
twisted chains	strept/o		vertebr/o
two	bi-	vessel	angi/o
tympanic membrane	myring/o		vas/o
	tympan/o	view of	-opsy
		vision	-opia
			-opsia
ulcer	aphth/o		opt/o
ulna	uln/o		optic/o
umbilical cord	omphal/o	visual examination	-scopy
	umbilic/o	voice	phon/o
unchanging	home/o		-phonia
under	hypo-	voice box	laryng/o
unequal	anis/o	vomiting	-emesis
unknown	idi/o	vulva	episi/o
up	ana-		vulv/o
upon	epi-		
urea	azot/o		
ureter	ureter/o	wander	ion/o
urethra	urethr/o	washing	-clysis
urinary bladder	cyst/o	wasting away	-phthisis
	vesic/o	water	aque/o
urinary tract	ur/o		hydr/o
urination	-uria	watery flow	rheumat/o
urine	ur/o	wedge	sphen/o
	-uria	weight	bar/o
	urin/o	white	alb/o

Meaning	Combining Form, Prefix, or Suffix	Meaning	Combining Form, Prefix, or Suffix
	albin/o	woman	gynec/o
	leuk/o	womb	hyster/o
wide	mydr/o		metr/o
widening	-dilation		metri/o
	-ectasia		uter/o
	-ectasis	word	-lexia
	-eurysm	work	erg/o
windpipe	trache/o	wrist bone	carp/o
with	con-		
	sym-		
	syn-	x-rays	radi/o
within	en-		
	endo-		
	intra-	yellow	xanth/o

Appendix I

Plurals

The rules for commonly forming plurals of medical terms are as follows:

1. For words ending in **a,** retain the **a** and add **e:**
   Examples:

Singular	Plural
vertebra	vertebrae
bursa	bursae
bulla	bullae

2. For words ending in **is,** drop the **is** and add **es:**
   Examples:

Singular	Plural
anastomosis	anastomoses
metastasis	metastases
epiphysis	epiphyses
prosthesis	prostheses

3. For words ending in **ix** and **ex,** drop the **ix** or **ex** and add **ices:**
   Examples:

Singular	Plural
apex	apices
varix	varices

4. For words ending in **on,** drop the **on** and add **a:**
   Examples:

Singular	Plural
ganglion	ganglia
spermatozoon	spermatozoa

5. For words ending in **um,** drop the **um** and add **a:**
   Examples:

Singular	Plural
bacterium	bacteria
diverticulum	diverticula
ovum	ova

6. For words ending in **us,** drop the **us** and add **i:**
   Examples:

Singular	*Plural*
calculus	calculi
bronchus	bronchi
nucleus	nuclei

   Two exceptions to this rule are viruses and sinuses.

7. Examples of other plural changes are:

Singular	*Plural*
foramen	foramina
iris	irides
femur	femora
anomaly	anomalies
biopsy	biopsies
adenoma	adenomata

Appendix II

Abbreviations

Many of these abbreviations may appear with or without periods and with either a capital or a lowercase first letter.

A2 or A$_2$	Aortic valve closure (heart sound).
AAA	Abdominal aortic aneurysm.
AAL	Anterior axillary line.
AB or ab.	Abortion.
abd	Abdomen.
ABGs	Arterial blood gases.
ABO	Three main blood types.
ac	Before meals *(ante cibum).*
ACTA	Automated computerized transverse axial scanner (machine for computed axial tomography).
ACTH	Adrenocorticotropic hormone.
AD	Right ear *(auris dextra);* Alzheimer's disease.
ADH	Antidiuretic hormone; vasopressin.
ADHD	Attention-deficit hyperactivity disorder.
ADL	Activities of daily living.
ADT	Admission, discharge, transfer.
ad lib	As desired.
AF	Atrial fibrillation.
AFB	Acid-fast bacillus (bacilli).
AFP	Alpha-fetoprotein.
AI	Aortic insufficiency.
AIDS	Acquired immunodeficiency syndrome.
AIHA	Autoimmune hemolytic anemia.
AKA	Above-knee amputation.
alb	Albumin.
alk phos (AP)	Alkaline phosphatase.
ALL	Acute lymphocytic leukemia.
ALS	Amyotrophic lateral sclerosis.
ALT	Alanine transaminase (liver and heart enzyme); formerly SGPT.
AML	Acute myelocytic (myelogenous) leukemia.
amp	Ampule.
ANA	Antinuclear antibody.
Angio	Angiography.
AP	Anteroposterior.
A&P	Auscultation and percussion; anterior and posterior.

aq.	Water *(aqua);* aqueous.
ARDS	Adult respiratory distress syndrome.
ARF	Acute renal failure.
AS	Left ear *(auris sinistra);* aortic stenosis.
ASA	Acetylsalicylic acid (aspirin).
ASD	Atrial septal defect.
ASH	Asymmetrical septal hypertrophy.
ASHD	Arteriosclerotic heart disease.
AST	Aspartate aminotransferase (liver and heart enzyme); formerly SGOT.
AU	Both ears *(auris uterque).*
Au	Gold.
ausc.	Auscultation.
AV	Arteriovenous; atrioventicular.
AVR	Aortic valve replacement.
ax	Axillary.
Ba	Barium.
bands	Banded neutrophils.
baso	Basophils.
BBB	Bundle branch block.
BC	Bone conduction.
B cells	Lymphocytes produced in the bone marrow.
BCNU	Bischloroethylnitrosourea.
BE	Barium enema.
bid	Twice a day *(bis in die).*
BKA	Below knee amputation.
BM	Bowel movement.
BMR	Basal metabolic rate.
BMT	Bone marrow transplant.
BP	Blood pressure.
BPH	Benign prostatic hypertrophy.
BRBPR	Bright red blood per rectum; hematochezia.
Bronch	Bronchoscopy.
BSO	Bilateral salpingo-oophorectomy.
BSP	Bromsulphalein (dye used in liver function test; its retention is indicative of liver damage or disease).

BT	Bleeding time.
BUN	Blood urea nitrogen.
bx	Biopsy.
C or C.	Celsius or centigrade.
c̄	With *(cum)*.
C1, C2	First, second cervical vertebra.
C_{cr}	Creatinine clearance.
CA	Chronological age; cardiac arrest.
Ca	Calcium; cancer.
CABG	Coronary artery bypass graft.
CAD	Coronary artery disease.
CAPD	Continuous ambulatory peritoneal dialysis.
caps	Capsule.
Cath	Catheter; catheterization.
CAT scan	Computed (axial) tomography.
CBC, c.b.c.	Complete blood count.
cc	Cubic centimeter (unit of volume; 1/1000 liter).
CCU	Coronary care unit.
CEA	Carcinoembryonic antigen.
cf.	Compare.
CF	Cystic fibrosis.
cGy	Centigray (one hundredth of a gray; a rad).
CHD	Coronary heart disease.
Chem	Chemotherapy.
CHF	Congestive heart failure.
chol	Cholesterol.
chr	Chronic.
μCi	Microcurie.
CIN	Cervical intraepithelial neoplasia.
CIS	Carcinoma in situ.
CK	Creatine kinase.
Cl	Chlorine.
CLD	Chronic liver disease.
CLL	Chronic lymphocytic leukemia.
cm	Centimeter (1/100 meter).
CMF	Cytoxan, methotrexate, and 5-fluorouracil.
CMG	Cystometrogram.
CML	Chronic myelogenous leukemia.
CMV	Cytomegalovirus.
CNS	Central nervous system.
Co	Cobalt.
CO_2	Carbon dioxide.
COPD	Chronic obstructive pulmonary disease.
CPA	Costophrenic angle.
CPC	Clinicopathological conference.
CPD	Cephalopelvic disproportion.
CPK	Creatine phosphokinase.
CPR	Cardiopulmonary resuscitation.
CR	Complete response.

CRF	Chronic renal failure.
CS	Cesarean section.
C&S	Culture and sensitivity.
C-section	Cesarean section.
CSF	Cerebrospinal fluid.
C-spine	Cervical spine films.
ct.	Count.
CTA	Clear to auscultation.
CTS	Carpal tunnel syndrome.
CT scan	Computed tomography.
CVA	Cerebrovascular accident; costovertebral angle.
CVP	Central venous pressure.
CVS	Cardiovascular system.
c/w	Compare with; consistent with.
CX (CXR)	Chest x-ray.
Cx	Cervix.
cysto	Cystoscopy.
D/C	Discontinue.
D&C	Dilatation (dilation) and curettage.
DD	Discharge diagnosis.
Decub.	Decubitus (lying down).
Derm.	Dermatology.
DES	Diethylstilbestrol; diffuse esophageal spasm.
DI	Diabetes insipidus; diagnostic imaging.
DIC	Disseminated intravascular coagulation.
diff.	Differential count (white blood cells).
DIG	Digoxin; digitalis.
dl	Deciliter (1/10 liter).
DLE	Discoid lupus erythematosus.
DM	Diabetes mellitus.
DNA	Deoxyribonucleic acid.
DOA	Dead on arrival.
DOB	Date of birth.
DOE	Dyspnea on exertion.
DPT	Diphtheria, pertussis, tetanus.
DRE	Digital rectal exam.
DRG	Diagnosis-related group.
DSA	Digital subtraction angiography.
DSM	Diagnostic and Statistical Manual of Mental Disorders.
DTs	Delirium tremens.
DTR	Deep tendon reflexes.
DUB	Dysfunctional uterine bleeding.
DVT	Deep venous thrombosis.
Dx	Diagnosis.
EBV	Epstein-Barr virus.
ECC	Endocervical curettage; extracorporeal circulation.
ECF	Extended-care facility.

ECG	Electrocardiogram.
ECHO	Echocardiography.
ECMO	Extracorporeal membrane oxygenation.
ECT	Electroconvulsive therapy.
EDC	Estimated date of confinement.
EEG	Electroencephalogram.
EENT	Eyes, ears, nose, and throat.
EGD	Esophagogastroduodenoscopy.
EKG	Electrocardiogram.
ELISA	Enzyme-linked immunosorbent assay (AIDS test).
EM	Electron microscope.
EMB	Endometrial biopsy.
EMG	Electromyogram.
ENT	Ear, nose, and throat.
EOM	Extraocular movement; extraocular muscle.
eos., eosins	Eosinophils.
Epo	Erythropoietin.
ER	Emergency room; estrogen receptor.
ERCP	Endoscopic retrograde cholangiopancreatography.
ERT	Estrogen replacement therapy.
ESR	Erythrocyte sedimentation rate.
ESRD	End-stage renal disease.
ESWL	Extracorporeal shock wave lithotripsy.
ETT	Exercise tolerance test.
F or F.	Fahrenheit.
FACP	Fellow, American College of Physicians.
FACS	Fellow, American College of Surgeons.
FB	Fingerbreadth; foreign body.
FBS	Fasting blood sugar.
FDA	Food and Drug Administration.
Fe	Iron.
FEF	Forced expiratory flow.
FEV	Forced expiratory volume.
FH	Family history.
FHT	Fetal heart tones.
FROM	Full range of movement/motion.
FSH	Follicle-stimulating hormone.
F/u	Follow-up.
5-FU	5-Fluorouracil.
FUO	Fever of undetermined origin.
F_x, Fx	Fracture.
µg	Microgram (one-millionth of a gram).
G	Gravida (pregnant).
g	Gram.
Ga	Gallium.
GB	Gallbladder.
GBS	Gallbladder series (x-rays).

GC	Gonorrhea.
G-CSF	Granulocyte colony stimulating factor.
GFR	Glomerular filtration rate.
GH	Growth hormone.
GI	Gastrointestinal.
gm	Gram.
Grav. 1, 2, 3	First, second, third pregnancy.
GTT	Glucose tolerance test.
gt, gtt	Drop (gutta), drops (guttae).
GU	Genitourinary.
Gy	Gray (unit of radiation and equal to 100 rads).
GYN	Gynecology.
H	Hydrogen.
h	Hour.
HCG (hCG)	Human chorionic gonadotropin.
HCl	Hydrochloric acid.
HCO_3	Bicarbonate.
Hct (HCT)	Hematocrit.
HCVD	Hypertensive cardiovascular disease.
HD	Hemodialysis.
HDL	High-density lipoprotein.
He	Helium.
HEENT	Head, eyes, ears, nose, and throat.
Hg	Mercury.
Hgb	Hemoglobin.
hGH	Human growth hormone.
H&H	Hematocrit and hemoglobin.
HIV	Human immunodeficiency virus.
HNP	Herniated nucleus pulposus.
h/o	History of.
H_2O	Water.
hpf	High-power field (microscope).
HPI	History of present illness.
hs	At bedtime (hora somni).
HSG	Hysterosalpingography.
h-s megaly	Hepatosplenomegaly.
HSV	Herpes simplex virus.
hx	History.
I	Iodine.
^{131}I	Radioactive isotope of iodine.
IBD	Inflammatory bowel disease.
ICP	Intracranial pressure.
ICSH	Interstitial cell-stimulating hormone.
ICU	Intensive care unit.
I&D	Incision and drainage.
IDDM	Insulin-dependent diabetes mellitus (Type I).
IgA, IgD, IgE, IgG, IgM	Immunoglobulins.

IHD	Ischemic heart disease.
IHSS	Idiopathic hypertrophic subaortic stenosis.
IM	Intramuscular; infectious mononucleosis.
IMV	Intermittent mandatory ventilation.
inf.	Infusion; inferior.
INH	Isoniazid (drug used to treat tuberculosis).
inj.	Injection.
IOL	Intraocular lens.
IOP	Intraocular pressure.
I.Q.	Intelligence quotient.
IUD	Intrauterine device.
IUP	Intrauterine pregnancy.
IV	Intravenous (injection).
IVP	Intravenous pyelogram.
K	Potassium.
kg	Kilogram (1000 grams).
KS	Kaposi's sarcoma.
KUB	Kidney, ureter, and bladder (abdominal x-ray).
L	Liter; left; lower.
l	Liter.
L1, L2	First, second lumbar vertebra.
LA	Left atrium.
LAD	Left anterior descending (coronary artery).
lap.	Laparotomy.
LAT; lat.	Lateral.
LB	Large bowel.
LCM	Left costal margin.
LD; LDH	Lactate dehydrogenase.
LDL	Low-density lipoprotein.
LE	Lupus erythematosus.
LES	Lower esophageal sphincter.
LFTs	Liver function tests.
LH	Luteinizing hormone.
Lin. ac.	Linear accelerator.
LLL	Left lower lobe (lung).
LLQ	Left lower quadrant (abdomen).
LMP	Last menstrual period.
LN; l.n.	Lymph node.
LOC	Loss of consciousness.
LOS	Length of stay.
LP	Lumbar puncture.
lpf	Low-power field (microscope).
LPN	Licensed practical nurse.
LS	Lumbosacral spine.
LSD	Lysergic acid diethylamide.

LSK	Liver, spleen, and kidneys.
LT	Left.
LTH	Luteotropic hormone (prolactin).
LUL	Left upper lobe (lung).
LUQ	Left upper quadrant (abdomen).
LV	Left ventricle.
L&W	Living and well.
lymphs	Lymphocytes.
lytes	Electrolytes.
MA	Mental age.
MAI	*Mycobacterium avium intracellulare.*
MAO	Monoamine oxidase.
mcg	Microgram.
MCH	Mean corpuscular hemoglobin (average amount of hemoglobin in each red blood cell).
MCHC	Mean corpuscular hemoglobin concentration (average concentration in a single red cell).
mCi	Millicurie.
μCi	Microcurie.
MCL	Midclavicular line.
MCV	Mean corpuscular volume (average volume or size of a single red cell).
mEq	Milliequivalent.
mEq/L	Milliequivalent per liter (measurement of the concentration of a solution).
mets	Metastases.
MG	Myasthenia gravis.
mg	Milligram (1/1000 gram).
mg/cc	Milligram per cubic centimeter.
mg/dl	Milligram per deciliter.
μg	Microgram (one-millionth of a gram).
MI	Myocardial infarction; mitral insufficiency.
ml	Milliliter (1/1000 liter).
mm	Millimeter (1/1000 meter; 0.039 inch).
mmHg	Millimeters of mercury.
MMPI	Minnesota Multiphasic Personality Inventory.
mμ	Millimicron (1/1000 micron; a micron is 10^{-3} mm).
mono	Monocyte.
MR	Mitral regurgitation.
MRI	Magnetic resonance imaging.
mRNA	Messenger RNA.
MS	Mitral stenosis; multiple sclerosis; morphine sulfate.
MSL	Midsternal line.
MTX	Methotrexate.
MUGA	Multiple-gated acquisition scan (of heart).

multip	Multipara; multiparous.	PCP	*Pneumocystis carinii* pneumonia; phencyclidine (hallucinogen).
MVP	Mitral valve prolapse.		
MVR	Mitral valve replacement.	PD	Peritoneal dialysis.
		PDA	Patent ductus arteriosus.
		PDR	Physicians' Desk Reference.
N	Nitrogen.	PE	Physical examination; pulmonary embolism.
Na	Sodium.		
NBS	Normal bowel or breath sounds.	peds	Pediatrics.
ND	Normal delivery; normal development.	PEEP	Positive end-expiratory pressure.
NED	No evidence of disease.	PEG	Percutaneous endoscopic gastrostomy.
neg.	Negative.	per os	By mouth.
neuro	Neurological.	PERRLA	Pupils equal, round, react to light and accommodation.
NG tube	Nasogastric tube.		
NHL	Non-Hodgkin's lymphoma.	PET	Positron emission tomography.
NIDDM	Non–insulin-dependent diabetes mellitus (Type II).	PE tube	Ventilating tube for eardrum.
		PFTs	Pulmonary function tests.
nitro	Nitroglycerin.	PH	Past history.
NPO	Nothing by mouth *(nulla per os).*	pH	Hydrogen ion concentration (alkalinity and acidity measurement).
NS	Normal saline.		
NSAID	Nonsteroidal anti-inflammatory drug.	PID	Pelvic inflammatory disease.
NSVP	Normal spontaneous vaginal delivery.	PIP	Proximal interphalangeal joint.
NTP	Normal temperature and pressure.	PKU	Phenylketonuria.
		plts.	Platelets.
		PM	Post mortem; petit mal; afternoon (post meridian).
O_2	Oxygen.		
OB/GYN	Obstetrics and gynecology.	PMN	Polymorphonuclear leukocyte.
OCPs	Oral contraceptive pills.	PMS	Premenstrual syndrome.
OD or O.D.	Right eye *(oculus dexter);* overdose.	PND	Paroxysmal nocturnal dyspnea.
o.d.	Once a day.	po	By mouth *(per os).*
17-OH	17-Hydroxycorticosteroids.	p/o	Postoperative.
OR	Operating room.	poly	Polymorphonuclear leukocyte.
ORTH; Ortho.	Orthopedics.	pos.	Positive.
OS or O.S.	Left eye *(oculus sinister).*	postop	Postoperative.
os	Opening; mouth; bone.	PPBS	Postprandial blood sugar.
OT	Occupational therapy.	PPD	Purified protein derivative (test for tuberculosis).
OU	Each eye *(oculus uterque).*		
oz.	Ounce.	preop	Preoperative.
		PR	Partial response.
		primip	Primipara.
P	Phosphorus; pulse.	PRL	Prolactin.
P2 or P_2	Pulmonary valve closure (heart sound).	prn	As required *(pro re nata).*
PA	Posteroanterior.	procto	Proctoscopy.
P&A	Percussion and auscultation.	prot.	Protocol.
PAC	Premature atrial contraction.	Pro. time	Prothrombin time (test of blood clotting).
$PaCO_2$ or pCO_2	Partial pressure of carbon dioxide.		
		PSA	Prostatic specific antigen.
palp.	Palpable; palpation.	PSP	Phenylsulfonphthalein (dye test for kidney impairment).
PaO_2 or pO_2	Partial pressure of oxygen.		
Pap smear	Papanicolaou's smear.	PT	Prothrombin time; physical therapy.
Para 1, 2, 3	Unipara, bipara, tripara (number of viable births).	pt.	Patient.
		PTA	Prior to admission.
Path	Pathology.	PTCA	Percutaneous transluminal coronary angioplasty.
PA view	Posteroanterior view (x-ray position).		
pc	After meals *(post cibum).*	PTH	Parathyroid hormone.

PTT	Partial thromboplastin time.	Sed. rate	Sedimentation rate (rate of blood sedimentation).
PU	Pregnancy urine.	segs	Segmented neutrophils; polys.
PVC	Premature ventricular contraction; pulmonary venous congestion.	SGOT	Serum glutamic-oxaloacetic transaminase (AST).
PVD	Peripheral vascular disease.	SGPT	Serum glutamic-pyruvic transaminase (ALT).
		SIADH	Syndrome of inappropriate antidiuretic hormone.
Q (q)	Each; every.	SIDS	Sudden infant death syndrome.
qam	Every morning.	sig.	Let it be labeled.
qd	Every day (quaque die).	SLE	Systemic lupus erythematosus; slit lamp examination.
qh	Every hour (quaque hora).	SMA-6	6 different serum tests.
qhs	Every night (quaque hora somni).	SMA-20	Test of 20 chemical constituents.
qid	Four times daily (quater in die).	SMAC	Sequential multiple analyzer computer.
qns	Quantity not sufficient.	SOAP	Subjective, objective, assessment, and plan.
qod	Every other day.	SOB	Shortness of breath.
qpm	Every evening.	sol.	Solution.
		sos	If necessary (si opus sit).
		S/P	Status post (refers to previous disease condition).
R, r., rt.	Right.	SPECT	Single-photon emission computed tomography.
RA	Rheumatoid arthritis; right atrium.	SpG	Specific gravity.
Ra	Radium.	SR	Sustained release; systems review.
rad	Radiation absorbed dose.	Staph.	Staphylococcus.
RAI	Radioactive iodine.	stat.	Immediately (statim).
RBC	Red blood cell (corpuscle); red blood count.	STD	Sexually transmitted disease.
RCM	Right costal margin.	STH	Somatotropin (growth hormone).
RDS	Respiratory distress syndrome.	Strep.	Streptococcus.
REM	Rapid eye movement.	Subq	Subcutaneous.
RF	Rheumatoid factor.	SVC	Superior vena cava.
Rh	Rhesus (monkey) factor in blood.	SVD	Spontaneous vaginal delivery.
RIA	Radioimmunoassay.	SVT	Supraventricular tachycardia.
RIND	Reversible ischemic neurological deficit/defect.		
RLL	Right lower lobe (lung).		
RLQ	Right lower quadrant (abdomen).	T	Temperature.
RML	Right middle lobe (lung).	T1, T2	First, second thoracic vertebra.
RNA	Ribonucleic acid.	T_3	Triiodothyronine test.
R/O	Rule out.	T_4	Thyroxine test.
ROM	Range of motion.	TA	Therapeutic abortion.
ROS	Review of systems.	T&A	Tonsillectomy and adenoidectomy.
RPR	Rapid plasma reagin (test for syphilis).	tab	Tablet.
RT	Right; radiation therapy.	TAH	Total abdominal hysterectomy.
RUL	Right upper lobe (lung).	TAT	Thematic Apperception Test
RUQ	Right upper quadrant (abdomen).	TB	Tuberculosis.
RV	Right ventricle.	Tc	Technetium.
R_x	Treatment; therapy; prescription.	T cells	Lymphocytes produced in the thymus gland.
$\bar{s}$	Without (sine).	TENS	Transcutaneous electrical nerve stimulation.
S1, S2	First, second sacral vertebra.	TFT	Thyroid function test.
SA	Sinoatrial.		
SAD	Seasonal affective disorder.		
SBE	Subacute bacterial endocarditis.		

TIA	Transient ischemic attack.
tid	Three times daily *(ter in die)*.
TLC	Total lung capacity.
TMJ	Temporomandibular joint.
TNI	Total nodal irradiation.
TNM	Tumor, nodes, and metastases.
tomos	Tomograms.
top.	Topically.
tPA	Tissue plasminogen activator.
TPN	Total parenteral nutrition.
TPR	Temperature, pulse, and respiration.
Trig	Triglycerides.
TRUS	Transrectal ultrasound.
TSH	Thyroid-stimulating hormone.
TSS	Toxic shock syndrome.
TUR, TURP	Transurethral resection of the prostate.
Tx	Treatment.
U	Unit.
UA	Urinalysis.
UC	Uterine contractions.
UGI	Upper gastrointestinal series.
umb.	Navel *(umbilicus)*.
U/O	Urinary output.
Ur.	Urine.
URI	Upper respiratory infection.
Urol.	Urology.
US, U/S	Ultrasound.

UTI	Urinary tract infection.
UV	Ultraviolet.
VA	Visual acuity.
VCUG	Voiding cystourethrogram.
VD	Venereal disease.
VF	Visual field.
vis à vis	As compared with; in relation to.
VLDL	Very low density lipoproteins.
V/Q scan	Ventilation-perfusion scan.
VS	Vital signs; versus.
VSD	Ventricular septal defect.
VT	Ventricular tachycardia.
WAIS	Wechsler Adult Intelligence Scale.
WBC, wbc	White blood cell; white blood count.
WBC/hpf	White blood cells per high-power field.
W-E	Wide excision.
WISC	Wechsler Intelligence Scale for Children.
Wt	Weight.
XRT	Radiation therapy.
y/o	Year old.

Appendix III

Normal Hematologic Reference Values and Implications of Abnormal Results

The implications of abnormal results are major ones in each category. SI units are the International System of Units.

cu mm = cubic millimeter (mm^3)
dL = deciliter (1/10 liter or 100 ml)
g = gram
L = liter
mg = milligram (1/1000 gram)
mL = milliliter

mEq = milliequivalent
mill = million
mm = millimeter (1/1000 meter)
mmol = millimole
thou = thousand
U = unit
μmole = micromole (one-millionth of a mole)

Cell Counts

	Conventional Units	SI Units	Implications	
Erythrocytes (RBC)				
Females	4.2–5.4 million/mm^3	4.2–5.4 × 10^{12}/L	High	■ Polycythemia
Males	4.6–6.2 million/mm^3	4.6–6.2 × 10^{12}/L		■ Dehydration
Children	4.5–5.1 million/mm^3	4.5–5.1 × 10^{12}/L	Low	■ Iron deficiency anemia
				■ Blood loss
Leukocytes (WBC)				
Total	4500–11,000/mm^3	4.5–11.0 × 10^9/L	High	■ Bacterial infection
				■ Leukemia
Differential	%			■ Eosinophils high in allergy
Neutrophils	54–62		Low	■ Viral infection
Lymphocytes	20–40			■ Aplastic anemia
Monocytes	3–7			■ Chemotherapy
Eosinophils	1–3			
Basophils	0–1			
Platelets	200,000–400,000/mm^3	200–400 × 10^9/L	High	■ Hemorrhage
				■ Infections
				■ Malignancy
				■ Splenectomy
			Low	■ Aplastic anemia
				■ Chemotherapy
				■ Hypersplenism

Coagulation Tests

	Conventional Units	SI Units	Implications
Bleeding Time (template method)	2.75–8.0 min	2.75–8.0 min	Prolonged ■ Aspirin ingestion ■ Low platelet count
Coagulation Time	5–15 min	5–15 min	Prolonged ■ Heparin therapy
Prothrombin Time (PT)	12–14 sec	12–14 sec	Prolonged ■ Vitamin K deficiency ■ Hepatic disease ■ Oral anticoagulation therapy

Red Blood Cell Tests

	Conventional Units	SI Units	Implications
Hematocrit (Hct) Females Males	 37–47% 40–54%	 0.37–0.47 0.40–0.54	High ■ Polycythemia ■ Dehydration Low ■ Loss of blood ■ Anemia
Hemoglobin (Hgb) Females Males	 12.0–14.0 gm/dL 14.0–16.0 gm/dL	 1.86–2.48 mmol/L 2.17–2.79 mmol/L	High ■ Polycythemia ■ Dehydration Low ■ Anemia ■ Recent hemorrhage

Serum Tests

	Conventional Units	SI Units	Implications
Alanine aminotransferase (ALT, SGPT)	5–30 U/L	5–30 U/L	High ■ Liver injury
Albumin	3.5–5.5 gm/dL	35–55 g/L	Low ■ Hepatic disease ■ Malnutrition ■ Nephritis and nephrosis
Alkaline phosphatase (ALP)	20–90 U/L	20–90 U/L	High ■ Skeletal disease ■ Acute hepatic disease ■ Biliary obstruction
Aspartate aminotransferase (AST, SGOT)	10–30 U/L	10–30 U/L	High ■ Liver injury ■ Cardiac and muscle injury
Bilirubin Total Neonates	 0.3–1.1 mg/dL 1–12 mg/dL	 5.1–19 μmol/L 17–205 μmol/L	High ■ Hemolysis ■ Neonatal hepatic immaturity ■ Cirrhosis ■ Biliary tract obstruction
Blood urea nitrogen (BUN)	8–20 mg/dL	3.0–7.1 mmol/L	High ■ Renal disease ■ Reduced renal blood flow ■ Urinary tract obstruction Low ■ Hepatic damage ■ Malnutrition

		Conventional Units	SI Units	Implications
Calcium		9.0–11.0 mg/dL	2.23–2.75 mmol/L	*High* ■ Hyperparathyroidism ■ Parathyroid tumors ■ Multiple myeloma ■ Metastatic cancer *Low* ■ Hypoparathyroidism ■ Total parathyroidectomy ■ Malabsorption
Cholesterol				
Desirable range		<200 mg/dL	<5.18 mmol/L	*High* ■ High fat diet
LDL cholesterol		60–80 mg/dL	600–1800 mg/L	■ Inherited
HDL cholesterol		30–80 mg/dL	300–800 mg/L	hypercholesterolemia *Low* ■ Starvation
Creatine	Females	30–135 U/L	30–135 U/L	*High* ■ Myocardial infarction
phosphokinase	Males	55–170 U/L	55–170 U/L	■ Muscle disease
(CPK)				
Creatinine		0.6–1.2 mg/dL	53–106 µmol/L	*High* ■ Renal disease
Glucose (fasting)		70–115 mg/dL	3.89–6.38 mmol/L	*High* ■ Diabetes mellitus *Low* ■ Hyperinsulinism ■ Fasting ■ Hypothyroidism ■ Addison's disease ■ Pituitary insufficiency
Lactate dehydrogenase (LDH)		100–190 U/L	100–190 U/L	*High* ■ Tissue necrosis ■ Myocardial infarction ■ Liver disease ■ Muscle disease
Phosphate ($-PO_4$)		3.0–4.5 mg/dL	1.0–1.5 mmol/L	*High* ■ Skeletal disease ■ Hypoparathyroidism *Low* ■ Malnutrition ■ Malabsorption ■ Hyperparathyroidism
Potassium (K)		3.5–5.0 mEq/L	3.5–5.0 mmol/L	*High* ■ Burn victims ■ Renal failure ■ Diabetic ketoacidosis *Low* ■ Cushing's syndrome ■ Loss of body fluids
Sodium		136–145 mEq/L	136–145 mmol/L	*High* ■ Inadequate water intake ■ Water loss in excess of sodium *Low* ■ Adrenal insufficiency ■ Inadequate sodium intake ■ Excessive sodium loss
Thyroxine (T_4)		4.4–9.9 µg/dL	57–128 nmol/L	*High* ■ Graves' disease *Low* ■ Hypothyroidism
Uric acid	Females	1.5–7.0 mg/dL	0.09–0.42 mmol/L	*High* ■ Gout
	Males	2.5–8.0 mg/dL	0.15–0.48 mmol/L	■ Leukemia

Index

Note: Page numbers in *italics* refer to illustrations; page numbers followed by t refer to tables.